Adult-Gerontology Acute Care Nurse Practitioner Certification Review

Dawn Carpenter, DNP, ACNP-BC, CCRN, is a practicing acute care nurse practitioner in the surgical/trauma ICU and trauma service line at Guthrie Healthcare System in Sayre, Pennsylvania. Carpenter's career has spanned over 30 years as a critical care nurse, nurse practitioner, and faculty. In addition, Carpenter is an associate professor at the University of Massachusetts Chan Medical School, Tan Chingfen Graduate School of Nursing. She continues to mentor Doctor of Nursing Practice students and is the previous coordinator of the adult-gerontology acute care nurse practitioner (AGACNP) program. She possesses a passion for educating and mentoring acute and critical care nurses and nurse practitioners as they advance their careers. Carpenter is a nationally known speaker on a variety of topics including sepsis.

Dr. Carpenter or Dawn has been actively engaged at the national level with the American Association of Critical-Care Nurses (AACN), where she routinely volunteers her time and expertise. She has been an item writer and a member of the exam development committee for the ACNPC-AG® and CCRN® exams. She has been a subject matter expert for AACN for several years, advising on exam content and revising practice exam questions. Additionally, she was a member and co-chair of the Advance Practice Institute (API) planning committee and member of the nominating committee.

Alexander Menard, DNP, AGACNP-BC, is an assistant professor at the University of Massachusetts Chan Medical School, Tan Chingfen Graduate School of Nursing, where he coordinates the AGACNP program. Alex is a practicing acute care nurse practitioner in the surgical ICU at UMass Memorial Medical Center in Worcester, Massachusetts. He has worked in critical care as a nurse and nurse practitioner for over 10 years.

He is a member of the American Association of Critical-Care Nurses (AACN) where he volunteers his time to develop new offerings for critical care nurses and nurse practitioners. He is also a member of the National Organization of Nurse Practitioner Faculties (NONPF).

Adult-Gerontology Acute Care Nurse Practitioner Certification Review

Dawn Carpenter, DNP, ACNP-BC, CCRN
Alexander Menard, DNP, AGACNP-BC

Editors

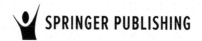 SPRINGER PUBLISHING

Springer Publishing Company, LLC
11 West 42nd Street, New York, NY 10036
www.springerpub.com

Acquisitions Editor: Jaclyn Koshofer
Compositor: diacriTech
Production Editor: Dennis Troutman

ISBN: 978-0-8261-9306-3
ebook ISBN: 978-0-8261-9307-0
DOI: 10.1891/9780826193070

23 24 25 26 27 / 5 4 3 2 1

The author and the publisher of this Work have made every effort to use sources believed to be reliable to provide information that is accurate and compatible with the standards generally accepted at the time of publication. The author and publisher shall not be liable for any special, consequential, or exemplary damages resulting, in whole or in part, from the readers' use of, or reliance on, the information contained in this book. The publisher has no responsibility for the persistence or accuracy of URLs for external or third-party Internet websites referred to in this publication and does not guarantee that any content on such websites is, or will remain, accurate or appropriate.

AGACNP-BC® is a registered service mark of the American Nurses Credentialing Center (ANCC). ACNPC-AG® is a registered service mark of the American Association of Critical-Care Nurses (AACN). Neither ANCC nor AACN sponsors or endorses this resource, nor do they have a proprietary relationship with Springer Publishing.

Library of Congress Control Number: 2023936305

Contact sales@springerpub.com to receive discount rates on bulk purchases.

Publisher's Note: **New and used products purchased from third-party sellers are not guaranteed for quality, authenticity, or access to any included digital components.**

Printed in the United States of America by Hatteras, Inc.

This book is dedicated to our current and former students, who have made us better educators and mentors. You have been the nidus to fill a gap in available resources for current and future AGACNP students. We are inspired by your commitment, dedication, and perseverance to the nursing profession.

Contents

Contributors

Martha Ofeibea Agbeli, DNP, APRN, PMHNP-BC
Assistant Professor
Tan Chingfen Graduate School of Nursing
University of Massachusetts Chan Medical School
Worcester, Massachusetts

Al-Zada "Al" Aguilar, DNP, RN, ACNP-BC, CCRN
Advanced Practice Provider
Robert Wood Johnson University Hospital—MICU
Adjunct Clinical Faculty
Rutgers University, School of Nursing AGACNP-DNP Program
New Brunswick, New Jersey

Ifeoma Asoh, PharmD
Department of Pharmacy
University of Massachusetts Memorial Medical Center
Worchester, Massachusetts

Donna Bartlett, PharmD
Associate Professor of Pharmacy Practice
Massachusetts College of Pharmacy and Health Sciences University
School of Pharmacy
Worcester, Massachusetts

Michael Bear, PharmD
Massachusetts College of Pharmacy and Health Sciences University
School of Pharmacy
Worcester, Massachusetts

Jody Beckington, DNP, APRN, ACNP-BC
Assistant Professor, Coordinator of Adult-Gerontology Acute Care Nurse Practitioner Program
University of Cincinnati College of Nursing
Cincinnati, Ohio

Paul Belliveau, PharmD
Interim Dean and Professor of Pharmacy Practice
Massachusetts College of Pharmacy and Health Sciences University
School of Pharmacy
Massachusetts

Jean Boucher, PhD, RN, ANP-BC
Professor of Nursing and Medicine, Director of DNP Program
Tan Chingfen Graduate School of Nursing
University of Massachusetts Chan Medical School
Worcester, Massachusetts

James Brinson, DNP, NP-C
Assistant Professor, DNP Department
Department of Neurology, Neurocritical Care Division
College of Nursing at Augusta University
Adult-Gerontology Acute Care Nurse Practitioner
Augusta, Georgia

Roxanne M. Buterakos, DNP, AG-ACNP-BC, PNP-BC
Associate Professor and Lead Faculty, Adult-Gerontology Acute Care Nurse Practitioner Program
University of Michigan–Flint
School of Nursing
Flint, Michigan

Katherine Carey, PharmD
Associate Professor of Pharmacy Practice
Massachusetts College of Pharmacy and Health Sciences University
School of Pharmacy
Worcester, Massachusetts

Dawn Carpenter, DNP, ACNP-BC, CCRN
Nurse Practitioner, Trauma and Surgical ICU Guthrie Healthcare System
Sayre, Pennsylvania
Associate Professor
University of Massachusetts Chan Medical School
Worcester, Massachusetts

Moneé Carter-Griffin, DNP, MAOL, APRN, ACNP-BC
Director of Education
Advanced Practice Providers, Dallas Pulmonary and Critical Care PA
Clinical Assistant Professor, University of Texas at Arlington
Arlington, Texas

Jason Cross, PharmD
Associate Professor of Pharmacy Practice
Massachusetts College of Pharmacy and Health Sciences University
School of Pharmacy
Worcester, Massachusetts

Karen Dick, PhD, GNP-BC, FAANP
Associate Professor
Tan Chingfen Graduate School of Nursing
University of Massachusetts Chan Medical School
Worcester, Massachusetts

Keri Draganic, DNP, APRN, ACNP-BC
Director, Adult-Gerontology Acute Care Nurse Practitioner Track
Clinical Assistant Professor, University of Texas at Arlington
Arlington, Texas

Henry Ellis, DNP, AGACNP
Nurse Practitioner
University of Massachusetts Memorial Medical Center, Surgical Critical Care
Assistant Professor
Tan Chingfen Graduate School of Nursing
University of Massachusetts Chan Medical School
Worcester, Massachusetts

Kerri Ellis, DNP, ACNP-BC, PMHNP-BC
University of Rhode Island, College of Nursing
Providence, Rhode Island

Margaret Emmons, PhD, ACNP-BC
University of Massachusetts Chan Medical School
Tan Chingfen Graduate School of Nursing
Worcester, Massachusetts

Kelly Esborn, FNP-C
Yale New Haven Health System, Northeast Medical Group Urgent Care
New Haven, Connecticut

Jennifer Fisher, MSN, ACNP-BC
Nurse Practitioner
Division of Neurology, Section of Neurocritical Care
Lahey Hospital and Medical Center
Burlington, Massachusetts

Jamie Gooch, APRN, ACNP-BC, DNP
Assistant Clinical Professor
University of Connecticut
Storrs, Connecticut

Shari Harding, DNP, PMHNP-BC, CPRP
Associate Professor and Coordinator of the PMHNP Track
Tan Chingfen Graduate School of Nursing
University of Massachusetts Chan Medical School
Worcester, Massachusetts

Danielle Hebert, DNP, MBA MSN, ANP-BC
Assistant Professor and Coordinator AG-PCNP Track
Tan Chingfen Graduate School of Nursing
University of Massachusetts Chan Medical School
Worcester, Massachusetts

Johnny Isenberger MSN, ACNP-BC, CCRN
Nurse Practitioner, University of Massachusetts Memorial Medical Center
Surgical Critical Care
Instructor
Tan Chingfen Graduate School of Nursing
University of Massachusetts Chan Medical School
Worcester, Massachusetts

Abir Kanaan, PharmD
Assistant Dean, Curriculum and New Programs and Professor of Pharmacy Practice
Massachusetts College of Pharmacy and Health Sciences University
School of Pharmacy
Worcester, Massachusetts

JoAnne Konick-McMahan, MSN, RN, PCCN-K
Certification Practice Specialist
American Association of Critical-Care Nurses Certification Corporation
Aliso Viejo, California

Omand Koul, PhD
Associate Professor
Tan Chingfen Graduate School of Nursing
University of Massachusetts Chan Medical School
Worcester, Massachusetts

Jennifer Lakeberg, DNP, APRN, AGACNP-BC, CPNP-AC, CPEN
Instructor
Adult-Gerontology Acute Care Nurse Practitioner Program
University of Cincinnati College of Nursing
Cincinnati, Ohio

Stefanie La Manna, PhD, MPH, APRN, FNP-C, AGACNP-BC
Associate Professor/Assistant/Associate Dean of Graduate Programs
Nova Southeastern University
Fort Lauderdale, Florida

Kimberly J. Langer, DNP, APRN, CNP, ACNP-C, FNP-BC
Winona State University
Winona, Minnesota

Gail Lis, DNP, ACNP-BC
Mercy College of Ohio
Toledo, Ohio

Donna Lynch-Smith, DNP, ACNP-BC, APRN, NE-BC, CNL
Associate Professor and AGACNP Concentration Coordinator
University of Tennessee Health Science Center College of Nursing
Memphis, Tennessee

Paula McCauley, DNP, ACNP-BC, CMC, CSC, FAANP
Research Professor
University of Connecticut School of Nursing
Storrs, Connecticut

Mary Anne McCoy, PhD., ACNS, ACNP-BC, FAANP
College of Nursing
Wayne State University
Detroit, Michigan

Beth McLear, DNP, FNP-C, ACNP-BC
Associate Professor, ACNP-BC and AGACNP Concentration Coordinator
Augusta University
Athens, Georgia

Alexander Menard, DNP, AGACNP-BC
Assistant Professor
University of Massachusetts Chan Medical School
Tan Chingfen Graduate School of Nursing
Nurse Practitioner
University of Massachusetts Memorial Medical Center
Surgical Critical Care
Worcester, Massachusetts

Christine Merman Woolf, PhD
Director, Academic Enrichment Programs
Center for Academic Achievement
Assistant Professor in the Department of Medicine
University of Massachusetts Chan Medical School
Worcester, Massachusetts

Helen Miley, PhD, RN, AGACNP-BC
CCRN Retired, Robert Wood Johnson University Hospital–MICU
Retired, Rutgers University, School of Nursing
Adjunct Instructor
Montclair State University
Montclair, New Jersey

Samar Nicolas, PharmD
Assistant Professor of Pharmacy Practice
Massachusetts College of Pharmacy and Health Sciences
School of Pharmacy
Worcester/Manchester, Massachusetts

Karen Pawelek, DNP, ACNP-BC
Yale New Haven Health System, Northeast Medical Group Urgent Care
New Haven, Connecticut

Helen Pervanas, PharmD
Professor of Pharmacy Practice
Massachusetts College of Pharmacy and Health Sciences
School of Pharmacy
Worcester, Massachusetts

Matthew Silva, PharmD
Professor of Pharmacy Practice
Massachusetts College of Pharmacy and Health Sciences University
School of Pharmacy
Worcester, Massachusetts

Elizabeth Singh, DNP, AGACNP
Nurse Practitioner Cardiovascular Medicine
Hartford Hospital
Hartford, Connecticut

Diane Thompkins, MS, RN
Interim Assistant Director, Certification Services
Governance and Accreditation
American Nurses Credentialing Center
Silver Spring, Maryland

Christina Vest, DNP, APRN, AGACNP-BC, CNRN
Assistant Professor, Adult-Gerontology Acute Care Nurse Practitioner Program
University of Cincinnati College of Nursing
Cincinnati, Ohio

Dinesh Yogaratnam, PharmD
Associate Professor of Pharmacy Practice
Massachusetts College of Pharmacy and Health Sciences University
School of Pharmacy
Worcester, Massachusetts

Reviewers

Tracy M. Brinkmeier, MSN, RN
Certification Specialist
American Association of Critical-Care Nurses Certification Corporation
Aliso Viejo, California

Kasia Dodman, ACNPC-AG, MBA
Nurse Practitioner
Hematology/Oncology BMT
University of Massachusetts Memorial Medical Center
Worcester, Massachusetts

Henry Ellis, DNP, AGACNP
Nurse Practitioner
University of Massachusetts Memorial Medical Center, Surgical Critical Care
Assistant Professor
Tan Chingfen Graduate School of Nursing
University of Massachusetts Chan Medical School
Worcester, Massachusetts

Laura J. McNamara, MSN, RN, CCNS, CCRN-K, ICE-CCP
Certification Practice Specialist
American Association of Critical-Care Nurses Certification Corporation
Aliso Viejo, California

Julie Stanik-Hutt, PhD, ACNP/GNP-BC, CCNS, FAAN
Professor (Clinical) and Director, AG-ACNP Program
University of Iowa
Iowa City, Iowa

Preface

Welcome to the first edition of *Adult-Gerontology Acute Care Nurse Practitioner Certification Review*. This book was created specifically for AGACNP students and new AGACNP graduates to prepare to successfully pass the national certification examinations. This book presents material and practice questions found on both the American Association of Critical-Care Nurses (AACN) and American Nurses Credentialing Center (ANCC) exams. The content is presented in a succinct, direct, easy-to-read and understand manner. The practice questions are written by faculty, many of whom have written questions for these certification exams.

This book can also be used to support student education during their nurse practitioner educational program. Students can use this book to enhance study habits, review for academic exams, hone test-taking skills, reinforce knowledge, and avoid test-taking errors. Faculty can use this book and practice questions throughout their curriculum by integrating them into polling technology, classroom discussion, case studies, and before and after lecture to evaluate assimilation of knowledge.

Unique to this book, a detailed overview of each certification exam is written by the certification organizations themselves. They discuss key information relevant to their respective exams. The eligibility requirements, process of how to apply for the exam, and tips for successfully passing the exam are included.

Distinctive to this book is a detailed step-by-step process outlining how to develop a study plan, create a study schedule, and use the practice questions and practice exam. This chapter is written by an education specialist, who is exceptional at coaching students to improve their study and test-taking habits. She outlines how to diagnose and avoid common test-taking errors.

This book has an outstanding review of foundational knowledge needed by AGACNPs. Review of advanced pathophysiology, pharmacology, and health assessment provide the underpinning for the rest of the content. These key chapters review fundamental history, exam findings, and select pathological states needed by AGACNPs to successfully pass the exam. Normal and pathologic geriatric changes set the stage to comprehend older adults' atypical presentations of common disease processes.

An exquisitely robust pharmacology chapter enhances new prescribers' comprehension of subtleties of cardiovascular and other drugs. Furthermore, most new AGACNPs struggle with antibiotic prescribing. The pharmacology chapter highlights application of antibiotics to facilitate learners' transition into practice.

The largest section of the book contains detailed content and practice questions that are on the exam blueprints. Practice questions have specific rationales explaining why the correct answer is correct and the distractors are incorrect. These questions will build and reinforce your knowledge base. A full-scale practice exam, which is representative in length, variety, and complexity of the board exam, is provided and can be taken in a timed format to assess your abilities under pressure.

We are eager to receive feedback and suggestions on this book. Please send any comments, suggestions, feedback, or criticisms to Dawn Carpenter at Dawn.Carpenter@umassmed.edu or Alex Menard at Alexander.Menard@umassmed.edu.

Dawn Carpenter
Alexander Menard

Acknowledgments

This book could not have been possible without our expert contributors. Your expertise will assist the next generation of AGACNPs to become our future peers and caregivers to our family, friends, and colleagues. Additionally, we appreciate the input from staff at the American Association of Critical-Care Nurses (AACN) and American Nurses Credentialing Center (ANCC) for providing content specific to their respective exams to support our test-takers.

We want to extend sincerest gratitude to all our colleagues at the University of Massachusetts Chan Medical School, Tan Chingfen Graduate School of Nursing, Guthrie Healthcare System, and UMass Memorial Medical Center for providing support and encouragement throughout this process.

Thank you to Jaclyn Koshofer and Jennifer Ehlers at Springer Publishing Company for providing the opportunity to publish this book. We appreciate the faith you have had in us and your guidance and unwavering support. You have been essential to making this project come to fruition. It has been an absolute pleasure to work with you!

Dawn: Most importantly, I am eternally grateful to my husband Andy, who has tirelessly supported my career. You have provided infinite love and patience to help make this book a reality—I love you!

Alex: I am thankful for my wife Heather and two children, Madelynn and Isabelle, who have continued to be inspiration and support.

Pass Guarantee

If you use this resource to prepare for your exam and do not pass, you may return it for a refund of your full purchase price, excluding tax, shipping, and handling. To receive a refund, return your product along with a copy of your exam score report and original receipt showing purchase of new product (not used). Product must be returned and received within 180 days of the original purchase date. Refunds will be issued within 8 weeks from acceptance and approval. One offer per person and address. This offer is valid for U.S. residents only. Void where prohibited. To initiate a refund, please contact Customer Service at csexamprep@springerpub.com.

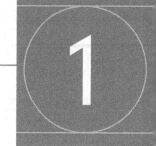

Introduction to the AGACNP Exams

Dawn Carpenter, Diane Thompkins, and JoAnne Konick-McMahan[*]

▶ INTRODUCTION

Congratulations! By purchasing this book, you've taken a crucial step toward successfully passing a national certification examination to become an AGACNP. While your AGACNP program provided a solid foundation, specific knowledge is needed to pass the exams. We recommend the use of multiple modalities to prepare for the exam, including review of this book, materials from your courses, and exam blueprint/test plans; a comprehensive certification exam review course; and review of the exam bibliography.

▶ ABOUT THIS BOOK

This book is intended for AGACNP program students/graduates to:

- prepare for quizzes and exams during the AGACNP program
- review and reinforce knowledge
- prepare for an AGACNP certification exam
- provide knowledge for practice
- identify gaps in knowledge

Faculty can use the content for:

- in-class review
- pre- and posttest assessments
- new faculty to learn how board exam questions are formatted

This book is *not* intended to do the following:

- Replace comprehensive and detailed reading, in-depth studying, or mastery of content. In other words, this book is *not* the "CliffsNotes®" to prepare for certifying exams.
- Promise or guarantee you'll pass the certification exam. Mastery of these questions will help you prepare but will not be the only material you will need to know or review to pass the exams.

▶ OVERVIEW OF CERTIFICATION EXAMS

The purpose of national certification exams is to ensure that the AGACNP meets a minimal competency level for safe entry into practice. There are two exam options for national board certification as an AGACNP. The two organizations offering an AGACNP national certification exam are the American Association of Critical-Care Nurses (AACN) Certification Corporation (AACN Cert Corp) and the American Nurses Credentialing Center (ANCC). AACN Cert Corp uses the acronym ACNPC-AG® for "acute care nurse

---

[*] The authors would like to thank Carol Hartigan for her work on Chapter 1 in *Adult-Gerontology Acute Care Nurse Practitioner Q&A Review*, which informed the creation of this chapter.

practitioner certified in adult-gerontology," whereas ANCC uses the acronym AGACNP-BC® for "adult-gerontology acute care nurse practitioner-BC." Both certifications are recognized by all 50 state boards of nursing (SBONs). Employers accept either certification exam. In this book, we use AGACNP to refer to adult-gerontology acute care nurse practitioners regardless of which certification is held, not in deference to ANCC.

Certification exams and the questions within them are written by experienced, actively practicing AGACNPs who possess diverse clinical experience; many of them are faculty members of colleges and universities. Additionally, item writers have been well educated on the process of writing items. Content for items and their answers are based on well-established standards of care.

In addition to scope and standards and competency documents, exam content is based on current surveys of AGACNPs working with acutely and critically ill patients. Exams test both medical and nursing knowledge and integrate foundational material such as advanced pathophysiology, advanced pharmacology, evidence-based practice, and advanced health assessment concepts. Both exams test the ability to:

- diagnose and treat conditions
- identify and manage complications and side effects
- recognize indications, contraindications, and complications of procedures
- effectively communicate with patients and families
- recognize and respond to medical-legal issues
- work within the scope of practice
- apply evidence-based practice concepts
- manage healthcare systems and policy challenges

Exam blueprints, also known as test plans, are readily available on the respective certification websites. We recommend that you become familiar with the exam blueprints before deciding which exam to take.

WHICH EXAM TO TAKE

This is a very personal decision that warrants thoughtful consideration. An informed decision can be made by exploring and understanding the two exams. This chapter provides an overview of the respective exams and is written by experts from each of the certifying organizations. Thoroughly explore each of the exam websites, blueprints, and styles of practice questions. The practice questions found in this book contain the type and style of questions found on both exams.

ABOUT THE CONTENT AND QUESTIONS

Content on the certifying exams is based on well-established standards of care. Exams are routinely updated every few years. As such, there is lag time, sometimes up to 2 to 3 years, between when new evidence and guidelines are published and when the content is integrated into the exams.

The exams consist of multiple-choice questions with four possible answers. All of the answer options are written to be plausible, but only one answer is correct. The questions in this book are written to be representative of the style of questions found on both exams, including content that could be on the exam. The questions are written in the same format and at the same level of difficulty and cover similar content areas.

The information in the following two sections is drawn from the respective national board certification exam organizations, the AACN Cert Corp and the ANCC. These sections highlight key information you'll need to know for their respective exams. Please note that website links can change over time. The best way to access the most current information for what you are seeking is to visit the websites.

▶ AMERICAN ASSOCIATION OF CRITICAL-CARE NURSES CERTIFICATION CORPORATION

ABOUT THE AMERICAN ASSOCIATION OF CRITICAL-CARE NURSES CERTIFICATION CORPORATION

The AACN Cert Corp drives patient health and safety through comprehensive credentialing of acute and critical-care nurses and began certifying RNs in critical care in 1975. The ACNPC-AG certification program aligns with AACN's expertise as the specialty organization that understands the practice of AGACNPs. In 1995, AACN Cert Corp joined with ANCC to offer the first AGACNP certification exam program. From 1995 through 2001, adult AGACNPs were jointly credentialed by both organizations. In 2001, AACN Cert Corp sold its share of the program to ANCC. In 2007, AACN Cert Corp relaunched its Adult ACNP program and integrated gerontology components to offer AGACNP board certification.

ACNPC-AG BOARD CERTIFICATION

The ACNPC-AG exam is nationally accredited by the National Commission for Certifying Agencies, meets the National Council of State Boards of Nursing (NCSBN) criteria for advanced practice registered nurse (APRN) certification exams, and is compliant with the Consensus Model for APRN Regulation: Licensure, Accreditation, Certification, and Education. The exam meets regulatory sufficiency for all SBONs as a proxy AGACNP licensure exam.

DETERMINING EXAM CONTENT

The first step in exam development is to determine the content. To be used for regulatory (licensure) purposes, an exam must be targeted to entry-level practice; measure only job-related knowledge, skills, and abilities; assess competence at the minimum level required for safe and effective practice; and be psychometrically sound. To ensure job relatedness, certification organizations conduct studies variously referred to as studies of practice, job analysis studies, role delineation studies, and so on, in order to learn the critical abilities required for the target practitioner to perform safely and effectively in practice. At this point in the exam development process, we often see some divergence in the focus of the educational community/professional associations and the certification/regulatory community. The role of the education/professional community is to advance the profession and to set standards for excellence in clinical practice. The role of the certification/regulatory community in conducting a job analysis is to provide for patient safety by documenting the key components of the actual practice of competent practitioners as it currently exists, not to analyze practice as we wish it would be delivered and then develop an exam based on that ideal scenario.

To develop the study of practice survey instrument, AACN Cert Corp convenes an expert panel composed of geographically and demographically representative current practitioners in the role, which may include faculty from AGACNP programs and from a variety of practice settings, including large and small facilities, rural and urban sites, and teaching and community hospitals. All exam development panels are oriented to their roles and assisted in their activities by the test service psychometrician and AACN Cert Corp staff nurses. Because AGACNPs practice in a variety of different environments, it is essential that the panel be diverse. The panel consults the current literature, as well as other resources, to determine current disease and acuity trends in constructing the survey. After a pilot test, the survey is sent to current practitioners to gather demographic information about their practice settings and conditions, as well as the types of patients they care for on a regular basis.

All of AACN Cert Corp's certification exams include the AACN Synergy Model for Patient Care (Synergy Model) as one of the major content domains, or organizing structures. The Synergy Model was developed to link nursing clinical practice with patient outcomes. The Synergy Model APRN competencies have been incorporated into the national competencies used to develop the AACN Cert Corp's ACNPC-AG exam. The purpose of the exam program is to help ensure public protection. New graduate AGACNPs are required to pass a legally defensible and psychometrically sound exam that measures the advanced practice competencies needed to perform safely and effectively as a newly licensed, entry-level AGACNP. NCSBN criteria and SBON requirements for regulatory sufficiency state that APRN exams must test both core role and population-focused competencies, as validated by the most recent job analysis survey or study of practice, and must cover the entire test plan.

The final job analysis survey consists of the AGACNP core competencies, the adult-gerontology competencies, patient care problems, and nursing interventions or procedures, as well as a series of demographic questions. The job analysis survey is sent to current practitioners, and they are asked to rate each item on its importance to and frequency in their practice. When the survey results are received, the panel members are assisted by a psychometric expert from the testing service to interpret the data. The volunteer subject matter experts (SMEs) determine, based on the responses, what content must be included on the exam and what percentage of the total exam should be devoted to each content area. Because the exam is national, a variety of subgroup analyses are conducted to be certain that the exam is not biased toward a particular region of the country or, for example, toward urban areas or toward community hospitals. All candidates must have an equal opportunity to pass the exam. The content panel's recommendations are shared with the board of directors, who approves the finalized test plan. Job analysis studies are conducted every 5 years for all AACN Cert Corp exam programs.

EXAM DEVELOPMENT PROCESS

The ACNPC-AG exam takes 3.5 hours and consists of 175 multiple-choice items, 150 of which are scored. The remaining 25 are pretest items that are indistinguishable from the scored items. In the stem, or question, only the information needed to respond is provided; no extraneous data are given. There are no "trick" questions or negative stems (e.g., "all of the following *except*"; "which of the following is *not*"). Medications may be listed with generic names (e.g., dopamine) only.

With guidance from AACN Cert Corp staff and the testing service psychometrician, multiple volunteer SMEs collaborate on creating the exam. The Item Writing Committee develops new exam items, written at the application or analysis level, that are linked to a skill and/or competency and an original reference. The Item Review Committee reviews and fine-tunes the item pool for pretesting, validating the correct answer for each item, and confirms the reference and linkage to the test plan.

The Exam Review Committee validates each item, reviews the statistical data on items administered as unscored pretest items, and evaluates the current item pool as relevant for continued use. The Score Evaluation Committee analyzes the difficulty of the items within the final item pool to determine the exam passing standard (also known as the cut score). Each exam generated from the final pool is equated based on statistical characteristics of the items and alignment with the test plan.

EXAM ELIGIBILITY

Completion of a graduate-level advanced practice education program that meets the following requirements is necessary:

- The program is through a college or university that offers a master's or higher degree in nursing with a concentration as an AGACNP and that holds accreditation through the Commission on Collegiate Nursing Education (CCNE) or the Accreditation Commission for Education in Nursing (ACEN). The program must include in-depth competencies to care for the entire adult population—young adults (including late adolescents) through older adults (including frail elderly).
- The program has demonstrated compliance with the National Task Force Criteria for Evaluation of Nurse Practitioner Programs.
- Both direct and indirect clinical supervision must be congruent with current AACN and nursing accreditation guidelines.
- The curriculum includes but is not limited to
  - biological, behavioral, medical, and nursing sciences relevant to practice as an AGACNP, including advanced pathophysiology, pharmacology, and physical assessment
  - legal, ethical, and professional responsibilities of the AGACNP
  - supervised clinical practice relevant to the specialty of acute care
- The curriculum meets the following criteria:
  - The curriculum is consistent with competencies of AGACNP practice.
  - The instructional track/major has a minimum of 500 supervised clinical hours. (This requirement may increase to 750 hours in the future.)
  - All clinical hours are focused on the direct care of acutely ill adult-gerontology patients and are completed within the United States. (International clinical experiences may be eligible in the future.)
  - The supervised clinical experience is directly related to the knowledge and all role components of the AGACNP.
  - Didactic coursework with content specific to the care of acutely ill adult-gerontology patients is required.

The program director of the education program must complete an ACNPC-AG Educational Eligibility Form that verifies completion of the required courses. You must submit originals of all graduate-level educational transcripts showing degree(s) conferred. A secure, electronic transcript may be provided by your school directly to APRNcert@aacn.org.

Current, unencumbered U.S. RN or APRN licensure is required. An unencumbered license is not currently being subjected to formal discipline by any SBON and has no provisions or conditions that limit the nurse's practice in any way. This applies to all RN or APRN licenses you currently hold. Candidates and ACNPC-AG–certified nurses must notify AACN Cert Corp within 30 days if any restriction is placed on their RN or APRN license(s). Nurses who hold an encumbered license may be eligible for conditional certification; email APRNcert@aacn.org to inquire.

APPLYING FOR THE EXAM

You may submit your exam application any time before or after graduation. At the time you apply, you will receive the following:

- access to a digital Practice Exam and Questions product with items and rationales presented in the same style as the actual exam
- consultation with a nurse specialist on exam preparation strategies (available upon request)

Have your official, final transcript showing date degree/certificate was awarded sent to AACN Cert Corp, along with official, final transcripts of any graduate-level coursework from other schools. You will receive an email confirming that your application has been received and forwarded to a certification nurse specialist for evaluation; this certification nurse specialist will be partnered with you to answer questions and provide updates. Your eligibility will be evaluated within 2 to 3 business days of required documents being received. You will receive an email notifying you that your application has been approved and providing instructions for scheduling your exam. AACN Cert Corp exams may be taken at a testing center or via live remote proctoring.

AFTER YOU TEST

Upon completion of computer-based exams, results will show on screen, and a score report with a breakdown by content area will be emailed to you within 24 to 48 hours. For purposes of evaluating educational programs, results will be reported to your program director. Within 1 week of certification, certificants, employers, SBONs, and others can verify certification status free of charge at www.aacn.org/verifycert.

ACNPC-AG certification is valid for 5 years. Renewal requirements include completion of the following: 1,000 clinical practice hours; 150 continuing education (CE) points, 25 in pharmacology; and/or retaking and passing the exam. Annual AACN membership entitles you to take advantage of free CE offerings and discounted attendance at AACN's annual National Teaching Institute/Advanced Practice Institute educational conference. To learn more, go to www.aacn.org or email APRNcert@aacn.org.

▶ AMERICAN NURSES CREDENTIALING CENTER

ABOUT THE AMERICAN NURSES CREDENTIALING CENTER

The ANCC's mission is to promote excellence in nursing and healthcare globally through credentialing programs. ANCC's internationally renowned credentialing programs board certify AGACNPs, clinical nurse specialists, and RNs in specialty areas of practice. ANCC also recognizes healthcare organizations that promote nursing excellence and quality patient outcomes while providing safe, positive work environments. ANCC accredits healthcare organizations that provide and approve continuing nursing education, interprofessional CE, residency and fellowship programs, and skills-based competency programs.

AMERICAN NURSES CREDENTIALING CENTER AGACNP BOARD CERTIFICATION

The ANCC AGACNP-BC exam is a competency-based, entry-level exam that provides a valid and reliable assessment of the entry-level clinical knowledge and skills of the AGACNP. The AGACNP-BC® exam aligns with the Consensus Model for APRN Regulation: Licensure, Accreditation, Certification, and Education (Consensus Model). The AGACNP-BC certification is accredited by the Accreditation Board for Specialty Nursing Certification.

The ANCC AGACNP-BC certification exam is accepted by the NCSBN and SBONs for licensure. The U.S. Department of Veterans Affairs, Centers for Medicare and Medicaid Services, and health insurance companies recognize ANCC AGACNP-BC certification.

The ANCC AGACNP-BC certification exam is computer based and in a multiple-choice format. The certification examination is available year-round in a Prometric testing center or via a live remote proctored session. You may apply at any time. Once you meet eligibility criteria to take the examination, you are provided a 90-day window to schedule the exam at any of the Prometric testing centers or as a live remote proctored session in the United States or internationally. Because you have two options to test, ANCC recommends you review information on their website at https://www.nursingworld.org/~4a5491/globalassets/docs/ancc/considerations-for--choosing-a-testing-option.pdf to make the best decision.

You are provided 3.5 hours to answer 150 scored and 25 pilot (unscored) multiple-choice questions. After you leave the testing center or complete your live remote proctored session, you will receive an email notification from Prometric, with a link to view your test results via the Prometric Report Validation Portal at https://scorereports.prometric.com/. To access your test results, you must enter your exam confirmation number and last name.

After successfully passing the exam, you are awarded the AGACNP-BC credential. This credential is valid for 5 years. You can continue to use this credential by maintaining your license to practice and meeting the renewal requirements of the certifying body that are in place at the time you are seeking renewal of AGACNP-BC certification.

OVERVIEW OF THE AGACNP-BC EXAM CONTENT

The AGACNP-BC certification exam includes clinical knowledge of young adults, including late adolescents, through the elderly and frail elderly. You are expected to apply knowledge from the APRN core content (advanced pharmacology, advanced health assessment, and advanced pathophysiology) as well as to demonstrate understanding of the AGACNP role and healthcare systems.

OVERVIEW OF THE AGACNP-BC EXAM DEVELOPMENT PROCESS

The AGACNP-BC® exam is developed by ANCC in cooperation with a content expert panel (CEP) composed of carefully selected AGACNP SMEs. CEPs analyze the professional skills and abilities from a Role Delineation Study (RDS), which provides evidence for the exam content outline or the exam blueprint.

Exam questions, or items, are written by AGACNP-certified SMEs who have received training by ANCC staff in writing exam questions. The items are then reviewed by the CEP with the ANCC staff and pilot tested to ensure validity and psychometric quality before being used as scored items on the actual examination. ANCC adheres to exam development standards to ensure that the items are appropriate. This includes editing and coding items, referencing items to the approved exam content outlines and reference books, and screening items for bias and stereotypes. The validity and reliability of the exam are monitored by ANCC staff. Certification exams are updated approximately every 3 to 5 years.

ELIGIBILITY FOR THE AGACNP-BC EXAM

AGACNP-BC eligibility criteria align with the Consensus Model requirements for graduate preparation for APRNs. Because eligibility criteria are regularly reviewed, consult the ANCC website for the most current version. A general overview of AGACNP-BC eligibility criteria is as follows:

- Hold a current, active RN license in a state or territory of the United States or hold the professional, legally recognized equivalent in another country.
- Hold a master's, postgraduate, or doctor of nursing practice degree from an AGACNP program accredited by the CCNE, the ACEN, or the National League for Nursing Commission for Nursing Education Accreditation. The graduate's AGACNP program must be able to demonstrate the following:
  - A minimum of 500 faculty-supervised clinical hours in the AGACNP role and population. This minimum will increase to 750 faculty-supervised hours in the future as a result of the revised National Organization of Nurse Practitioner Faculties (NONPF); National Task Force (NTF) Standards.

- Three separate, comprehensive graduate-level APRN core courses in:
  - ❏ advanced physiology/pathophysiology, including general principles that apply across the life span
  - ❏ advanced health assessment, which includes assessment of all human systems, advanced assessment techniques, concepts, and approaches
  - ❏ advanced pharmacology, which includes pharmacodynamics, pharmacokinetics, and pharmacotherapeutics of all broad categories of agents
  - ❏ content covering health promotion and/or maintenance and differential diagnosis and disease management

Note: Candidates may be authorized to sit for the examination after all coursework and faculty-supervised clinical practice hours for the degree are complete, prior to degree conferral and graduation, provided that all other eligibility requirements are met. The Validation of Education form and official/unofficial transcripts showing that coursework (and faculty-supervised clinical practice hours) is completed are required before authorization to test will be issued. ANCC will retain the candidate's exam result and will issue certification on the date that the final, degree-conferred and official transcript is received, all other eligibility requirements are met, and a passing result is on file. Contact ANCC directly at certification@ana.org for more information.

PREPARING FOR THE CERTIFICATION EXAMINATION

ANCC provides the current AGACNP-BC exam content outline, sample questions with answers, and a reference list at the ANCC website for free. ANCC also offers an AGACNP Readiness test. After completing the readiness test, you will receive diagnostic feedback for each test domain to assist you as you prepare for the AGACNP-BC exam. There is a small fee to take the test. You are not required to take the AGACNP Readiness test, and your performance on the AGACNP Readiness test is not an indicator or predictor of your actual performance on the AGACNP-BC® exam. You can obtain detailed information about the AGACNP Readiness test at https://www.nursingworld.org/certification/readiness-tests/readiness-agacnp/.

ANCC certification does not endorse any review materials, books or courses, or companies. Completing any review materials, including the AGACNP Readiness test or a review course, does not guarantee you will pass the exam.

CREATE YOUR AMERICAN NURSES CREDENTIALING CENTER ONLINE ACCOUNT

At any time, create your ANCC certification online account. You will be able to complete your application to take the exam via this account. In addition, this site offers the opportunity to store all of your professional development activities throughout the certification period. This provides an efficient means to complete the application for initial certification or recertification.

EXAM CONTENT OUTLINE

The AGACNP-BC exam content outline, also known as the exam blueprint, identifies the content areas covered on the exam. In addition, it provides the number and percentage of items (test questions) in each major category or domain.

SAMPLE QUESTIONS

For practice, there are free sample questions that are similar to those on the actual examination but do not represent the full range of content or levels of difficulty. There is no time limit associated with reviewing the sample questions, and you can review them as many times as you wish, for free.

REFERENCE LIST

For additional reading, a review of authoritative texts is recommended. While the list is not all-inclusive, it may act as a guide for preparation. Your school materials and resources are also excellent resources.

PRIMARY SOURCE VERIFICATION OF CERTIFICATION

After testing, AACN automatically sends a verification of certification to the State Board(s) of Nursing specified in your application. Verification of ACNPC-AG certification may also be requested online at www.aacn.org/verifycert.

MAINTAINING AGACNP CERTIFICATION

After you successfully pass the exam, you are awarded the AGACNP-BC credential. This credential and certification are valid for 5 years. You can maintain your certification, also known as certification renewal or recertification, and continue to use the AGACNP-BC credential by maintaining your license to practice and meeting the mandatory 75 CE hours, 25 of which must be in pharmacology and in at least one of the eight renewal categories in place at the time you renew AGACNP-BC certification. Additional information about ANCC Certification Credentials is found at www.nursingworld.org/certification/certification-policies/certification-credentials/. For any questions, you can send an email to certification@ana.org or call 1.800.284.2378.

▶ SUMMARY

The AGACNP student should undertake a review of both certification exam options before deciding which exam to take. Assess their websites and sample questions, review the exam blueprints, and then develop a study plan (see Chapter 2).

● KEY BIBLIOGRAPHY

Only key resources appear in the print edition. Access the full bibliography for this chapter on ExamPrepConnect.com.

AACN Certification Corporation. (2022). *ACNPC-AG exam handbook.* https://www.aacn.org/~/media/aacn-website/certification/get-certified/handbooks/acnpcagexamhandbook.pdf?la=en

Adult-Gerontology NP Competencies Work Group. (2016). *Adult-gerontology acute care and primary care NP competencies.* https://cdn.ymaws.com/www.nonpf.org/resource/resmgr/files/np_competencies_2.pdf

American Association of Nurse Practitioners. (2019). *Scope of practice for nurse practitioners.* https://www.aanp.org/advocacy/advocacy-resource/position-statements/scope-of-practice-for-nurse-practitioners

APRN Consensus Work Group & National Council of State Boards of Nurses APRN Advisory Committee. (2008). *Consensus model for APRN regulation: Licensure, accreditation, certification and education.* https://www.nursingworld.org/~4aa7d9/globalassets/certification/aprn_consensus_model_report_7-7-08.pdf

Bell, L., & Cain, C. (2021). *AACN Scope and standards for adult gerontology and pediatric acute care nurse practitioners 2021.* American Association of Critical-Care Nurses.

Buppert, C. (2018). *Nurse practitioner's business practice and legal guide* (6th ed.). Jones & Bartlett.

National Task Force. (2022). *Standards for quality nurse practitioner education, A report of the national task force on quality nurse practitioner education* (6th ed.). American Association of Colleges of Nursing. https://www.aacnnursing.org/Portals/42/CCNE/PDF/NTFS-NP-Final.pdf

Test-Taking Tips and Strategies

Christine Merman Woolf

▶ INTRODUCTION

Two national exams are available for AGACNP students to take (see Chapter 1). Regardless of which exam you elect to take, you will need to develop a study plan and hone your test-taking skills in preparation. This chapter reviews how to develop a detailed study plan, reviews test-taking tips, and aids in diagnosing errors on exam items deemed incorrect. This chapter is the first step in preparing to successfully pass an AGACNP certification exam.

▶ REVIEW OF EXAM BLUEPRINTS

Each national exam governing body publishes a test exam outline or blueprint. Download these from their websites and keep at your fingertips. Carefully review each exam outline/blueprint before deciding which exam to take.

STUDY MATERIALS

Once you have determined which exam you will take, use that exam's blueprint as your study guide. The test blueprint provides an outline of the content on the exam, along with the percentage of coverage of each topic. Next, assemble resources to study. Use your notes, textbooks, articles, and presentations from your AGACNP program. In addition, each certification organization has a list of references it uses to create exam items. Use these resources as you prepare for the exam. Use clinical practice guidelines that are at least 2 years old, as newer guidelines may not have yet been incorporated into the exam.

Use this book as a higher level summary of topics covered on the certification exam. Practice questions train you in how to reason through questions and apply your knowledge. Your performance on the questions throughout this book will highlight areas where you need to do additional studying.

Answering practice questions is essential to your success. Often, students want to put off reviewing practice questions. They may feel as if the questions are a precious resource that should not be used until very close to test day. Rather, it is wiser to integrate these questions into your studying, so that you know how to apply the material you are learning to questions similar to those you will see on the test. You will also learn which content needs additional review, if you need another resource to help you understand concepts better, and how to address any test-taking issues. Save some practice questions and practice exams to use within the last couple of weeks of studying, but do not hesitate to use many practice questions before that time.

▶ DEVELOP A STUDY PLAN

The first step in developing a study plan is to assess how much time you have to prepare for the exam. If you performed well and had comprehensive exams throughout your program, you may be ready to take the exam relatively soon after graduation. Try a few of the questions in each area of this book. If you perform very well on the practice questions, then consider taking the practice exam. The sooner you take the exam after completing your academic program, the better, as your knowledge will be fresh.

STUDY PLANNING

Formulate a study plan. Decide how many days and how many hours each day you can devote to studying. Be realistic and note if you need time for work, family events, appointments, and so on. Build these dates and times into your plan to avoid stress later on. Table 2.1 shows an example of the last 3 weeks of studying.

Table 2.1 Sample Study Plan

Monday	Tuesday	Wednesday	Thursday	Friday	Saturday	Sunday
22	23	24	25	26	27	28
4 hr	4 hr	0 hr	5 hr	5-hr catch-up	3 hr	6 hr
29	30	31	1	2	3	4
4 hr	4 hr	0 hr	5 hr	5 hr	3-hr practice exam	6-hr catch-up/off
5	6	7	8	9	10	11
4 hr	4 hr	0 hr	5 hr	0 hr	Exam	Celebrate!

▶ PRIORITIZE CONTENT

The exam includes both clinical content and nonclinical material. Nonclinical material focuses on role, scope of practice, health relationship, communication, patient education, ethics, patient advocacy, and so on. It is important to study both types of content.

CLINICAL CONTENT

Review the clinical content in the exam blueprints (Table 2.2). For the American Nurses Credentialing Center (ANCC) exam, clinical practice composes 45% of the exam, whereas for the American Association of Critical-Care Nurses (AACN), clinical judgment composes 80% of the exam.

Table 2.2 Clinical Content by System by Exam

ANCC	AACN
■ Head, eyes, ears, nose, and throat ■ Respiratory ■ Cardiovascular ■ Gastrointestinal ■ Genitourinary ■ Musculoskeletal ■ Neurologic ■ Psychiatric ■ Endocrine ■ Hematopoietic ■ Immune ■ Integumentary ■ Reproductive	■ Cardiovascular ■ Respiratory ■ Endocrine ■ Musculoskeletal ■ Hematology/immunology/oncology ■ Neurology ■ Gastrointestinal ■ Renal ■ Genitourinary ■ Integumentary ■ Multisystem ■ Psychosocial/behavioral/cognitive health

AACN, American Association of Critical-Care Nurses; ANCC, American Nurses Credentialing Center.

Both exams assess your knowledge in an integrated manner; thus, it is important to review content in all systems. Look at the list previously given for the exam you are taking, and note next to each list item your level of comfort with the material in that system. Rate them as:

■ 1 (very challenging—top priority)
■ 2 (somewhat challenging—middle priority)
■ 3 (feel fine with content, but still need to review)

As you rate each area, consider the following:

- How did you score on your academic exams for each of these systems?
- How much clinical experience or exposure did you get related to the systems?
- Consider how long ago you studied or clinically experienced these systems.

Read the details of the test blueprint; note specifics within each system and decide if you want to change your previously noted level of priority. For the AACN exam, you have an extra step: add the percentage of exam content next to each system. Rank priorities with content areas by their percentage on the exam. The following is an example.

PRIORITY 1 (VERY CHALLENGING—TOP PRIORITY)
- Neurology (8%)
- Hematology/immunology/oncology (6%)
- Musculoskeletal (3%)
- Psychosocial/behavioral/cognitive health (3%)

NONCLINICAL CONTENT
While physiologic organ systems compose the majority of both exams, the other, nonclinical content is essential to review. On the ANCC (2022) exam, 32% of the content tests professional role. On the AACN (2022) exam, professional caring and ethical practice account for 20% of the assessment.

Review the topics in the blueprint and determine how many hours you need to review this content. If you are unsure, complete some of the questions in this book from those sections. Determine if these topics are priority level 1, 2, or 3.

▶ CREATE A STUDY SCHEDULE

Start with the end in mind. Enter review time into the schedule for the week before the exam. These days are helpful to allow you to address unexpected challenges. During this review week, you will take the comprehensive practice exam in this book. Then, go to the first day of the calendar and add your top-priority topics into the calendar. Once you have decided how many study hours you have in each day, decide how many days you want or need to study each topic. If you feel significantly concerned about a particular topic, consider if you should stop after 3 days on the topic. Often, after 3 days, it is hard to stay as focused on one topic. For example, you may be worried about your level of knowledge of endocrinology and would like to spend weeks on endocrinology. However, after 2 or 3 days on the topic, you might be ready to focus on something else. You can always go back to a topic, if necessary. After you list your priority topics in order and for as many days/hours as you would prefer, see if you need to make any adjustments.

REORDER THE SCHEDULE
If you work through your top priorities and feel frustrated or overwhelmed, it is acceptable to reorder topics. However, do not move a high-priority topic to the end of the calendar. Reprioritize the schedule based on the percentage of coverage of the topic on the exam. Do not change your exam date unless absolutely necessary. Make the decision to change your exam date after you have engaged in some studying.

▶ WHAT TO DO DURING STUDY TIME

For each content area, plan time to

- engage in focused study on the topic of the day and actively prepare as you would for an exam during your academic program;
- complete and review practice questions on the topic of the day, note any concerns, and review material;

- complete practice questions on content previously reviewed and learn from the rationales; and
- go back and review information of concern for topics already studied but for which you got questions incorrect, and repeat practice questions if needed.

Start to study by working through your highest priorities first. By studying them, you will feel more confident. Realize that the topics at the end of your calendar should be more familiar, and thus less demanding, and should go more smoothly.

REVIEW CONTENT

Spend time actively reviewing content for part of the day. Create a system that allows you to capture essential information and is easily accessed. Tables and images may already be available in your resources; if so, mark them so they can easily be found again. Drawing can help you to recall information. Review the most essential content for the topic, without neglecting aspects that you know best. Be mindful of how you are dedicating your time to the subtopics within the topic. Spend the most time on areas of concern while still reviewing the entire topic. Identify the level of knowledge needed to become proficient with that material. Be sure to understand the entirety of the disease of concern as identified through your performance on the questions.

TAKE PRACTICE QUESTIONS

During part of each day, you will take practice questions in this book for the content area you are currently studying. Do some studying on the topic, take a break or do some other study activity, and then return to take questions on the topic you studied earlier in the day. Having time between when you completed your content review and when you take the related questions will test your recall ability.

If you feel very confident about your knowledge of a topic and only have a short time to review the material, or if it is a topic not heavily covered on the exam, then you may want to start with practice questions before studying the resources. By starting with the questions, you will know which areas need more review, and then you can use your time efficiently by focusing on specific subtopics of concern within your resources.

During part of each day, take practice questions on topics you have already studied. When you do these questions, draw from multiple topic areas. By mixing questions, you will switch your thinking from one system to another system rapidly, which will mimic the national board exam. There will be questions you do not know the answer to right away. Reason through them, reflect on what you do know, and apply it to the question.

READ THE QUESTIONS

Carefully read each question. A major mistake is to skim the question, risking misreading or omitting important information. You need to reason and process what you are reading to address the question correctly. If you miss information, the question may take longer to solve due to missing key details. Reading carefully will save you time. Reading too quickly will lead to you having to reread the stem multiple times to get the key elements, or to you reasoning through options without all of the needed information and thus being unable to determine the right answer. Both of those outcomes can lead to frustration and anxiety during the test.

Read the question, also known as the *stem*, for key words such as *assess*, *teach*, *diagnose*, or *treat*. These words direct you to what action is expected by the AGACNP in the scenario. Identify what the question is asking, and use your diagnostic reasoning skills to problem-solve. Highlight important words or phrases or write them on the paper or whiteboard provided by the testing center. Pay particular attention to details in the scenario. These details are specifically included to help you identify the correct answer.

Avoid reading into the stem; stay with the information given. The test writers provide the information needed to answer correctly. By going beyond the information presented, you lose focus on what they are telling you. Do not be distracted by information that is not presented in the question but that you are adding on your own.

EVALUATE THE ANSWERS

After reading the stem, pause for a few seconds to formulate an answer before you look at the options. Then look to see if the answer you thought of is among the possible answers or if one of them closely approximates your thoughts. You do not want to forget it by reasoning through other possibilities that were not your initial thought. After you click the one that most relates to your initial idea, then read each option carefully. These are well-written questions and options, so you need to confirm that you selected the right response. It may be that once you read all the options, you may think another one is clearly more correct. Every option deserves to be considered. Most likely your first selection is the best one.

Eliminate options that you know to be incorrect. If any part of an answer is wrong, the entire option is wrong. However, do not discount an option unless you are sure it does not apply. You must consider it, even if only for a few seconds, before eliminating it. If, as you continue to work through the options, you cannot settle on one that seems right, reconsider at least briefly the ones discounted. Maybe you discounted the correct answer.

REPHRASE THE QUESTION

Turn the question around. That is, take the distractor and turn that into a statement. For example, "Which of the following medications may increase liver enzymes?" If an answer option is vancomycin, then simply think, "Does vancomycin increase liver enzymes?" No? Then look for another answer. Avoid rewriting the question in your head as you think it "should" be worded.

USE EVIDENCE

Use knowledge of evidence-based practice (EBP) to answer the question. Avoid the tendency to apply your personal anecdotal experience to determine the correct answer. Do not think of what is done in your hospital. Consider the best evidence to make a diagnosis or treatment decision. A good way to avoid this issue is to become very familiar with the exam blueprint and the questions in this book, which are based on the exam blueprints. These resources focus on what the AACN and ANCC desire you to do in the situations presented in the questions. If you find yourself thinking of individual patients from work, remind yourself to consider what the EBP resources and textbooks have noted.

PROBLEM-SOLVE

There will be questions whose topic you are not familiar with. If the question is about a patient on asthma medication, and you think, "I do not remember asthma medication information," do not guess. Instead, relax and think about breaking down the parts and elements you do know. Reason through it.

Also, when you are unsure of an answer, think, "Why would they tell me this information? What makes it important?" Just pausing to consider those questions may prompt you to recall something from your studies. Remember, you passed your classes, studied material related to the blueprints, practiced questions, and learned from the feedback, so calm down and focus. You know something that can help you determine the correct answer.

CHANGING ANSWERS

There are only four reasons to change your answer. It is acceptable to change your answers only if the following are true:

- You misread the question or did not read the entire item and all the answer options.
- You did not consider all the information when you read the item. Did you see an option, presume it to be correct, and not fully read and consider the other options?
- You have new information to consider when you read the item again. This may happen if a question later in the exam prompts you to remember something about a disease that you had forgotten when you first read the question.
- You marked the wrong answer and discovered the error upon reviewing the exam.

REVIEW QUESTION RATIONALE/FEEDBACK

Review the rationales on questions you got both correct and incorrect to reinforce your knowledge. The rationales assume you have a foundation of knowledge. If you do not have a deep enough understanding, review additional content from the reference material and study/learn/relearn this material. Do not rush this process. If you did not know the content, go back to your study materials and reread and update your notes or cards.

When reviewing question feedback, do not just focus on the right answer. Learn why the right answer was right and the wrong answers were wrong. Study how the options relate to each other. There may be two correct answers, but one is more correct. Learn these subtle differences so when you see similar questions in the future, you can compare these options with one another.

PACING

If your pacing has been fine in classroom exams, then doing the practice questions in an untimed mode is fine initially. As the test date gets closer, though, you should do many timed practice questions. If you are someone who had pacing issues throughout your coursework, then consider doing all of your questions in timed mode, going from one question to the next without checking answers until all questions are completed. When you do the mixed review questions, do them in a timed mode as it may be more challenging.

Later, when you are taking multiple hours of questions—for example, when you take the practice exam at the end of this book—track where in the exam you get more questions incorrect (i.e., in the first third, second third, or last third of a test). If you find that you miss more questions later in the exam, it may be due to fatigue. Take longer sets of practice question sessions to condition you for the longer testing period of 3 to 4 hours.

PACING CHALLENGES

Moving on from one question can be challenging when you believe the answer will come to you if you just spend a little more time on it. The concern is that a little time can end up being 2 or more minutes spent on one question. This concern becomes a real issue when 2 or more minutes is spent on multiple questions, leading to a lack of time for other questions that you could have answered correctly. The issue needs to be addressed if you

- spend a lot of time on some questions and have to rush at the end to finish questions;
- finish other questions by completely guessing answers without reading the questions thoroughly, to make up for lost time;
- leave questions blank because you ran out of time; or
- get anxious or frustrated when spending too much time on a question, which may negatively impact future questions.

CONSEQUENCES

By spending too much time on a challenging question, you may rush and get questions incorrect that you would have otherwise answered correctly. You may end up skimming questions just to finish them and read questions too quickly, missing essential information needed to get a question right. If you run out of time before getting to all the questions, you may not see multiple questions you could have easily answered correctly.

Spending too much time on certain items can increase your anxiety, stress, and frustration level or create a negative feedback loop. Negative messages like these are counterproductive. Mark the item, move on, and tell yourself, "I can come back to it." Perhaps another question will trigger your recollection of additional information.

When you have spent about 2 minutes on a question, tell yourself it's not worth getting other questions wrong. You have a lower chance of getting that challenging question correct and a better chance of getting other questions correct. Keep moving forward.

ASSESS PRACTICE DATA

Mark questions you are unsure of during practice questions. Keep a list of these questions, and assess how many you dwelled on that you answered correctly. Then count how many items you rushed through, skipped, or completely guessed at, and assess results. Did you know the answers to all, most, or some of these questions? If so, then it was not worth spending so much time on the other questions. Not only did you potentially lose points, but you also caused yourself unnecessary stress during the exam.

REDUCE TIME ON QUESTIONS

To reduce extended time on individual questions, review the content. You spent time on these questions because you thought the answers were within your reach. Therefore, take time to learn the content so it is retrievable the next time you see a similar question. Make sure you are progressing through the exam at the pace needed, by periodically checking the clock. This system is especially helpful to those who are unaware that they are spending too much time on individual questions. Alternatively, employ regular time checks after a specific number of questions. For example, you have 1 hour to finish 50 questions. Teach yourself to check the time on every 10th item. You have 12 minutes for each set of 10 questions. Create a grid on paper:

- Item 10, want 48 minutes remaining
- Item 20, want 36 minutes remaining
- Item 30, want 24 minutes remaining
- Item 40, want 12 minutes remaining
- Item 50, want 0 minutes remaining

Do not rush through your first pass of the items just to save time to review them later, but also do not slow down just to use the time. Do not go back through the set of 10 to see if you want to change anything. Keep moving forward. It could be that other questions in the next set are more challenging and may take more time. Some may take an extra few seconds, and you can feel good knowing you had a few seconds to spare from previous sections of 10 items. However, do not think you have the time to dwell or spend over 2 minutes on challenging questions. Remember, you do not want to end up rushing at the end.

If you end up having time at the end of the test, then go back and review your marked answers. Remember during your initial pass to mark the questions on which you were spending too much time or were unsure of the answer. If you find that checking the time every 10 minutes is overwhelming, then check at item 25. At a minimum, use this system for the practice exam to see if you find it helpful.

TRACKING CHANGED ANSWERS

When you are taking practice questions, track why you changed answers. Develop a data-tracking sheet to assess these reasons. Table 2.3 can be filled out quickly while you are taking questions.

Table 2.3 Changing Answer Tracking Form

Question Number That Was Changed	Changed From (You do not need to log the one you changed to because you have that information)	Reason Changed N (new information) M (misread first time) C (considered info for first time) D (doubted self) O (other)
9	B	M
17	A	N

Identify when changing answers works for you, and change the answer only in those instances. At the end of the practice questions, analyze the data. Do you always change to incorrect? If so, stop changing answers. If changing answers negatively impacts your score, then you can write yourself a note: "Don't change answers!" Does it work for you when you logged N, M, and C, but not when you logged the reason as D (see Table 2.3)? If so, then do not change an answer when the only reason was D. Do you change some from incorrect to correct, but mostly change from correct to incorrect? If so, and if it is too hard for you to determine the reason you changed, or if you are running out of time and do not have the ability to change anyway, then consider deciding not to do a second pass at the items.

If changing answers causes a lot of stress, then you may want to decide not to mark any items or to limit which ones you mark. You should only mark those that you think you have a chance of getting correct later. If you read the item and realize you did not study that and have no idea how to answer it, then do not mark it. It might just cause you more stress to have many items marked, and that may lead you to rushing through the test. If you have a lot marked and many of them you do not have a chance of getting anyway, then you are rushing through ones you actually have a chance of getting correct just to get back to ones you have a low chance of getting correct.

▶ PRACTICE EXAM

There is a sample practice exam at the end of this book. Save this exam until you have completed studying materials, about a week before your exam date. If you plan to do multiple practice tests, then start them 2 or 3 weeks before the test date. Use the practice test in this book to evaluate overall performance. Results will determine where additional studying is required prior to taking the national examination.

Take your practice exam as a timed exam, without checking answers until you have finished all of the questions. This will mirror your exam-day experience. Be sure to take this practice exam in a quiet, distraction-free environment. Take it when you are able to focus. Before starting the questions, set your timer for 175 questions in 3.5 hours, meaning you will have 72 seconds per question.

▶ ACADEMIC ACCOMMODATIONS

Both national board certification exams are compliant with the Americans with Disabilities Act (ADA). Students who have a history of learning, mental health, or medical conditions requiring accommodations are encouraged to request reasonable accommodations during their application process. The process and format for supporting documentation differ with each certifying body. Seek the assistance of your school's disability office or academic achievement department when filling out forms or submitting your request and supporting documentation. Review the form requirements and the test administration process with your provider. This allows you to have a comprehensive discussion about your specific needs and results and ensure accurate completion of the request. Specific requirements are included on each organization's website.

Certifying bodies may request additional documentation or clarification. Thus, it is important that you do *not* schedule your exam date until you have an answer to your request for accommodations and have ensured that the testing center can facilitate your approved accommodations. Once accommodations have been approved, then you can schedule your exam date and time. Should you receive a denial letter, you should seek the assistance of your school's disability office, student ADA coordinator, and/or provider for guidance.

First and foremost, if you were granted and used accommodations during your academic career, we highly recommend you seek accommodations for your national board certification exam. We advise *against* trying to take the exam without accommodations. The risk of failing the exam without accommodations may go up exponentially. In addition, failing the exam negatively impacts your confidence level, making the second exam encounter even more intimidating.

Second, your request must match the recommendations the provider submits. Submit a copy of your request or form to the provider so they see what has been requested, or meet together and complete the forms so they are consistent.

Third, include all application paperwork/documentation, such as request and supporting letters for accommodations, in one envelope/email for ease and efficiency of processing.

Fourth, processing paperwork takes time. Submit the accommodations and application paperwork as soon as your program indicates that you are eligible to sit for the exam.

▶ SUCCEEDING ON EXAM DAY

WHAT TO EXPECT THE DAY OF THE EXAM

Be prepared for exam day. Review all the relevant information at the relevant exam website. Procedures change over time, so be certain you read the current exam policies. Do not rely on statements from peers and coworkers about these issues. You do not want to have an unexpected outcome on exam day.

These are questions you should be able to answer:

- What forms of identification do I need to bring?
- What proof is needed to show I am taking the exam on the certification exam day?
- Do I need to bring documentation showing I am to receive accommodations?
- What are the security procedures?
- How do I take breaks, and how do they impact my exam time?
- What can I bring to the exam center?

VISIT THE EXAM CENTER

Prior to taking the exam, travel to the site. This helps you plan your travel time and lessen anxiety. If you are driving, note traffic patterns, and plan your drive for around the same day of the week and time that you will take your exam. Be sure to give yourself sufficient time for any unexpected delays. Arrive early to allow time for check-in procedures.

ATTIRE

Wear comfortable clothes and shoes. Remember, you will be sitting for a few hours. Exam rooms may be cool or hot, so dress accordingly, and try to wear layers so you can remove or add clothing as needed.

ON EXAM DAY

Remember—you have the knowledge you need to succeed. You have passed many exams, so you are an experienced test taker. The questions you worked through on a regular basis are similar to the ones you will see on the exam.

Pacing on Exam Day

At times, examinees are nervous; this can throw off your usual pacing. Once you notice you are not following your practiced system, pause, take a deep breath, and try your best to relax and remind yourself that your system works.

Use the Tools Provided on Exam Day

Use the whiteboard or scratch paper you receive at the exam center to help you keep track of key words, reasoning or questions you want to review, and reasons for changing answers. You most likely used paper to perform those tasks when working with practice questions, so use the tools at the center the same way.

Manage Anxiety

Do not exaggerate the importance or significance of the exam. Avoid negative feedback, as it will increase your anxiety. If you are nervous, take 30 to 60 seconds to sit back and relax. Practice mindfulness and relaxation techniques. Focus on each item and not on your anxiety. Do not let emotions distract you. Recall what you did when you were upset during practice questions and tests, and do the same.

▶ SUMMARY

In summary, success on exam day starts with adequate preparation. Preparation begins with developing a thorough and detailed study plan. And be sure to practice lots of questions to refine the test-taking skills needed to pass enough questions to pass the exam. Be sure to practice taking timed sample questions, and perform the timed practice exam in this book. Following these steps will help ensure success on exam day.

● KEY BIBLIOGRAPHY

Only key resources appear in the print edition. Access the full bibliography for this chapter on ExamPrepConnect.com.

American Association of Critical-Care Nurses. (2022). *Certification corporation ACNPC-AG certification handbook.* https://www.aacn.org/~/media/aacn-website/certification/get-certified/handbooks/acnpcagexamhandbook.pdf?la=en

American Nurses Credentialing Center. (2022). *Adult-gerontology acute care nurse practitioner.* https://www.nursingworld.org/~4a8053/globalassets/certification/certification-specialty-pages/resources/test-content-outlines/exam-62-agacnp-tco-2020-01-13_for-web-posting.pdf

National Institutes of Health. (2012). *Asthma care quick reference: Diagnosing and managing asthma.* https://www.nhlbi.nih.gov/files/docs/guidelines/asthma_qrg.pdf

Nolting, P. D. (1997). *Winning at math.* Academic Success Press.

Thompson, D. L. (2016). Useful test-taking strategies when preparing for the WOCNCB continence examination. *Journal of Wound, Ostomy and Continence Nursing, 43*(4), 425–426. https://doi.org/10.1097/WON.0000000000000246

Part II: Foundational Knowledge
Advanced Pathophysiology Review

Omand Koul

▶ INTRODUCTION

Pathophysiology is the study of alterations in and dysfunction of various processes in the human body during an illness. In a healthy individual, the chemical and physical processes at the biochemical, cellular, and organ and system levels that occur in an integrated manner are physiological to maintain homeostasis. However, in an individual with an illness, these processes have become abnormal and are dysfunctional. Illnesses result in an altered state of cells/organs (pathology), and the alterations in the processes are pathophysiological. Hence, the study of pathophysiology leads to an understanding of the abnormalities in physiology that result in a disease/pathology and helps in designing possible interventions to restore normalcy. In this chapter, a select few of the most important pathologies are reviewed, including the inflammatory process, atherosclerosis, and renal impairment, as these are encountered by AGACNPs on a daily basis.

▶ INJURY/INFLAMMATION/DISEASE

Diseases begin with some type of injury caused by an agent that is physical, chemical, or infectious. No matter the type of injury, it is followed by inflammation. Inflammation is a protective action launched by the body in response to an injury. Inflammation that begins immediately after an injury and ends in a few days is categorized as acute. Acute inflammation lacks specificity, is a protective response, and hence is beneficial. However, inflammation has the potential to be destructive if the regulatory feedback systems that stop it become dysfunctional and a state of chronic inflammation occurs. In certain cases, organ damage occurs, which can lead to a poor outcome. Usually, the state of chronic inflammation is due to the inability to clear the agent of injury, and the processes of inflammation and injury continue together and can last for months or years.

Acute inflammation is initiated within minutes of an injury and manifests as five cardinal signs of pain (dolor), redness (rubor), edema (tumor), heat/fever (calor), and loss of function of the tissue/organ (functio laesa). These signs are a manifestation or result of the signaling events initiated by an injury. The signaling processes promote secretion of chemokines and cytokines, recruitment of immune cells such as neutrophils and macrophages, activation of complement proteins and the coagulation cascade, and induction of acute phase response by the liver, eventually leading to healing or repair.

AGENTS OF INJURY AND INFLAMMATION: INFECTIOUS AND NONINFECTIOUS

Cells and tissues are injured by infectious agents such as microbes. Infectious agents such as bacteria, viruses, and others can infect and damage cells. Microbial agents normally contain characteristic molecules that are proinflammatory by themselves and are designated as pathogen-associated molecular patterns (PAMPs). In contrast to PAMPs, cellular damage caused by noninfectious agents releases cellular contents that can induce inflammation and is defined as a damage (or danger)-associated molecular pattern (DAMP). DAMPs include molecules released by damage of cells by physical, chemical, or radiation injury. Molecules such as glucose, fatty acids, toxins, and silica can be grouped into this noninfectious category of agents of injury. In addition, microbial exotoxins and virulence factors produced by some pathogenic helminths also damage cells and release DAMPs. Thus, inflammation is categorized as of the infectious and the noninfectious/sterile type.

PATHOGEN-ASSOCIATED MOLECULAR PATTERNS AND RECOGNITION BY THE PATTERN RECOGNITION RECEPTORS: INFECTIOUS INFLAMMATION

The infecting organisms, such as bacteria, contain and carry characteristic molecules designated as PAMPs. An example of PAMPs are the bacterial endotoxins that are cell wall components of mostly gram-negative bacteria (Table 3.1). Such PAMPs are recognized by pattern recognition receptors (PRRs) that are present as soluble receptors in body fluids or are membrane-bound to macrophages or other cells of the host (Table 3.2). The crucial step of interaction between PAMPs and PRRs initiates a cascade of events that results in inflammation. Recognition of PAMPs activates the synthesis and secretion of cytokines and chemokines, leading to inflammatory response.

Table 3.1 Properties, Types, and Examples of Pathogen-Associated Molecular Patterns

Properties	Types	Examples
Not present in host Present in pathogens Relatively invariant Mutation resistant Class specific Constitutive expression	Proteins, carbohydrates, lipids, nucleic acids, glycoconjugates	Flagellin Peptidoglycan in gram-positive bacteria Lipopolysaccharide in gram-negative bacteria Double-stranded RNA, unmethylated DNA

Table 3.2 Pattern Recognition Receptors: Properties, Types, and Functions

Properties	Types	Functions
Present in host Nonclonal (expressed on all cells of a given type) Germline encoded No immunologic memory	Secreted PRRs Macrophage cell surface PRRs Toll-like receptors NOD receptors RAGE	Activate complement Induce production of cytokines, interferons Induce acute phase response

NOD, nucleotide oligomerization domain; PRRs, pattern recognition receptors; RAGE, receptors for advanced glycation end products.

SOLUBLE RECEPTORS AND SOLUBLE PATTERN RECOGNITION MOLECULES

Soluble receptors are produced by the liver during acute phase response and by immune cells. They include complement proteins, mannan-binding lectin, collectins, pentraxins, and ficolins and mostly recognize PAMPs from microbes. The recognition of PAMPs by these pattern recognition molecules activates various immune cells and the complement system. The activated complement proteins act as chemotactic factors, vasoactive compounds, and cytolytic agents, and some lead to opsonization of invading organisms and facilitate phagocytosis. In addition, certain activated complement proteins organize themselves into Membrane Attack Complexes (MAC) that are responsible for fenestration of bacteria and subsequent lysis (Tables 3.3 and 3.4).

Table 3.3 Activators of Soluble Receptors and Products of Activation

Activators of Soluble Receptors	Products of Activation/Functions
▪ Dying cells (tissue necrosis debris) ▪ Endotoxins (gram-negative bacteria) ▪ Peptidoglycan (gram-positive bacteria) ▪ Antigen–antibody complexes (infection) ▪ Clotting cascade and fibrinolysis	▪ C5a, C3a: chemotactic, vasoactive, mast cell activator ▪ C5, C6, C7: chemotactic for neutrophils ▪ C5, C9: cytolytic ▪ C4b, C2a, C3b: lead to opsonization and phagocytosis ▪ Membrane attack complex ▪ Fibrin bands

Table 3.4 Dysfunctional Activation of Complement Proteins

Too Much	Too Little

■ Increased permeability
■ Chemotaxis: too many phagocytic cells intruding at site of injury
■ Lysis of host cells: complement-mediated lysis
  ● Rheumatic disease
  ● Immune hemolytic anemia
  ● Immune thrombocytopenic purpura
  ● Age-related macular degeneration
  ● Multiple sclerosis
  ● Reperfusion injury (stroke)
	■ Autoimmune disease (systemic lupus erythematosus)
	■ Solubilizing antigen–antibody complexes: Failure of this function can lead to immune complex disorders.
	■ Recurrent infections (bacterial, viral, and fungal)

CELL SURFACE RECEPTORS ON MACROPHAGES

Cell surface receptors recognize PAMPs and activate macrophages. The activated macrophages produce and secrete proinflammatory cytokines such as interleukin (IL)-1, tumor necrosis factor (TNF)-alpha, and IL-6 that induce acute phase response in the liver (Figure 3.1).

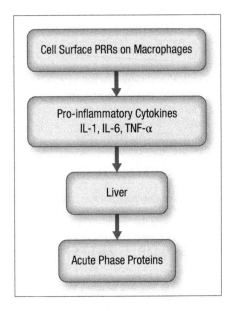

Figure 3.1 Role of macrophage PRRs. PRRs on macrophages recognize the PAMPs and initiate production of cytokines such as IL-1, IL-6, and TNF-α. These cytokines induce acute phase response in the liver and production of acute phase proteins.
IL, interleukin; PAMPs, pathogen-associated molecular patterns; PRR, pattern recognition receptor; TNF, tumor necrosis factor.

TOLL-LIKE RECEPTORS

Several different toll-like receptors (TLRs) have been identified that are present on the cell surface or intracellularly of host cells. Binding of PAMPs to TLRs promotes transcription and synthesis of various proinflammatory cytokines, chemokines, and interferons. TLRs recognize many different types of ligands that are either exogenous as PAMPs or endogenous as DAMPs. These receptors are especially important for a robust immune response, as activation of TLRs during the inflammatory process (the innate immune response) provides a bridge for cross talk between the innate and adaptive immune response of the host (Table 3.5).

Table 3.5 Toll-Like Receptors Recognize Both Exogenous and Endogenous Ligands

TLR Type	Exogenous Ligands (PAMPs)	Endogenous Ligands (DAMPs)
TLR1/TLR2	Triacyl lipopeptides	Unknown
TLR2/TLR6	Diacyl lipopeptides, LTA, PGN	HSP-60, HMGB1
TLR3	dsRNA, Poly I:C	mRNA, stathmin
TLR4	LPS, Lipid A	HMGB1, HSP 22, fibronectin, defensin, oxLDL
TLR5	Flagellin	Unknown
TLR7	ssRNA, loxoribine	Self RNA, microRNA
TLR8	ssRNA, imidazoquinoline	microRNA
TLR9	Unmethylated DNA	Self DNA
TLR11	Bacteria, profilin-like molecules	Unknown
NOD	PGN	ATP, S100, uric acid

ATP, adenosine triphosphate; dsRNA, double-stranded RNA; HMGB, high mobility group box; HSP, heat shock protein; LPS, lipopolysaccharide; LTA, lipoteichoic acid; NOD, nucleotide oligomerization domain; oxLDL, oxidized low-density lipoprotein; PGN, peptidoglycan; polyI:C, polyinosinic-polycytidylic acid; ssRNA, single-stranded RNA; TLR, toll-like receptor.
Source: Adapted from Liu, T., & Ji, R.-R. (2014). Toll-like receptors and itch. In E. Carstens & T. Akiyama, *Itch: Mechanisms and treatment* (pp. 257–270). CRC Press/Taylor & Francis Group.

ACUTE PHASE RESPONSE

Several proinflammatory cytokines released after interaction of PRRs with PAMPs, such as IL-1, TNF-α, and IL-6, activate the liver and initiate the synthesis of acute phase response proteins (Figure 3.2). These include haptoglobin, serum amyloid, fibrinogen, C-reactive protein, and acid glycoprotein. In a patient, the combined systemic proinflammatory effect of acute phase proteins and proinflammatory cytokines is the induction of neutrophilia, fever, lethargy, inappetence, capillary permeability, and weight loss. Concurrently, the acute phase response activates a feedback production of adrenal cortisol that has the potential to dampen the proinflammatory cascade and promote healing and repair.

DAMAGE-ASSOCIATED MOLECULAR PATTERNS AND PATTERN RECOGNITION RECEPTORS: STERILE/NONINFECTIOUS INFLAMMATION

When cells are damaged in an organ, the intracellular contents are released into the interstitial/extracellular compartment. These components include mitochondrial contents, mRNA, or adenosine triphosphate (ATP). These molecules, present in their non-native location, come under surveillance of the immune system as DAMPs. DAMPs are recognized by the PRRs, TLRs, and nucleotide oligomerization domain (NOD)-like receptors and initiate an inflammatory signaling response. DAMPs are released after injury to cells by a noninfectious event as well as after damage caused by an infection. Hence, even after the clearance of an infectious agent, DAMPs continue to be recognized, and inflammation signaling continues to damage organs and tissues.

An agent of completely sterile injury and inducer of noninfectious inflammation is glycated protein from glycation. The glycated proteins transform into advanced glycation end products (AGE). The AGE binds to and activates receptors for AGE (RAGE) followed by an inflammatory response leading to microvascular and macrovascular damage. In patients with diabetes, hyperglycemia accelerates the process of glycation, formation of AGE, and inflammation by activation of RAGE.

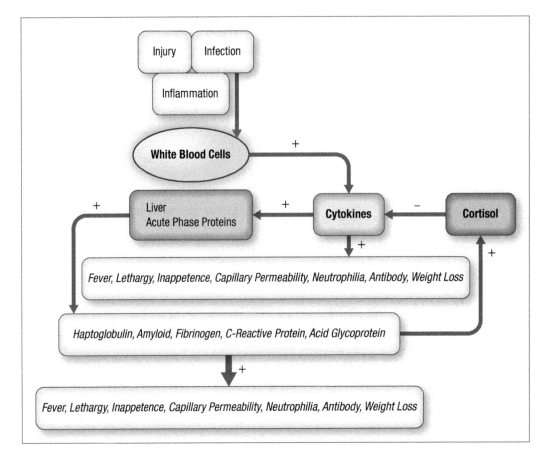

Figure 3.2 Role of cytokines in promoting inflammatory acute phase response by the liver and blunting inflammation by negative feedback by adrenal cortisol.

INFLAMMASOME AND KEY SIGNALING MOLECULES IN INFLAMMATORY RESPONSE: ROLE OF NUCLEAR FACTOR KAPPA B, CASPASES, AND PATTERN RECOGNITION RECEPTORS

Inflammasome is a multiprotein signaling complex in cells that is central to processes of inflammation. The complex includes nuclear factor kappa b, caspases, and several types of PRRs. Eventually, the activation of nuclear factor kappa b and caspases that initiate production of active proinflammatory cytokines leads to the multistep inflammatory response meant to heal and repair the damage. Here it is important to note that activation of inflammasome occurs because of PAMPs and DAMPs (Figure 3.3).

REGULATION OF INFLAMMATORY RESPONSE: FEEDBACK SYSTEMS

Acute inflammation begins within minutes of an injury with the production of proinflammatory cytokines such as IL-1. However, a little later, another set of cytokines—the anti-inflammatory cytokines—such as IL-10 begin to be produced that initiate a slowing down of the process (Figure 3.4).

One of the signaling systems that initiates this feedback is the suppressor of the cytokine signaling pathway. This pathway prevents uncontrolled production of proinflammatory cytokines and an unwanted effect of continued inflammation. This negative feedback system stops expression of cytokines such as IL-6, granulocyte colony-stimulating factor (G-CSF), and interferon gamma (IFN-γ). The feedback systems help in restoration of homeostatic balance (Figures 3.5 and 3.6; see also Figure 3.4).

However, under certain circumstances, the feedback systems fail, the inflammatory response does not shut down, and the damage continues. This could happen for several reasons—for example, due to enormity of injury with the production of large amounts of proinflammatory cytokines whose activity

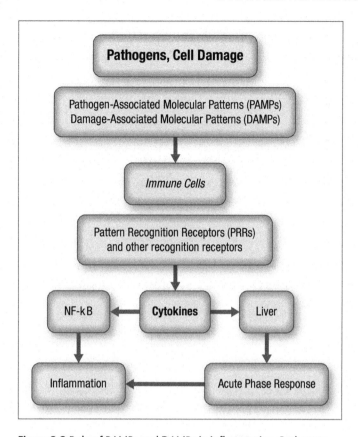

Figure 3.3 Role of PAMPs and DAMPs in inflammation. Pathogens and damaged cells release PAMPs and DAMPs. Various receptors including PRRs recognize PAMPs and DAMPs and initiate inflammatory response. The proinflammatory cytokines activate the liver and induce acute phase response, and also activate factors such as nuclear factor kappa b to initiate the inflammatory response.

cannot easily be reversed by the feedback inhibitory systems. This state of hypercytokinemia is known as the "cytokine storm." Hypercytokinemia continues to promote the effect of proinflammatory cytokines damaging vital organs, and the patient eventually progresses to systemic inflammatory response syndrome and multiorgan failure.

▶ CARDIOVASCULAR SYSTEM

ATHEROSCLEROSIS AND ACUTE CORONARY SYNDROME
Atherosclerosis is a multifactorial disorder that involves multiple genes and various lifestyle risk factors. A confluence of several risk factors along with an increase in levels of low-density lipoprotein (LDL) in plasma can precipitate acute coronary syndrome (ACS). LDL is a vehicle for delivery of fat needed by organs throughout the body. The unwanted deposition of this fat under the intimal layer of blood vessels and its oxidation and formation of foam cells and fatty plaques narrow the lumen of blood vessels (stenosis). Although stenosis and ACS can occur by a slow buildup of plaques in coronary arteries, it can also occur secondary to rupture of a fatty plaque and formation of thrombus blocking downstream blood vessel(s). The result is a condition of either myocardial ischemia because of decreased blood flow to a part of heart musculature or ischemia followed by loss of cardiomyocytes by myocardial infarction (MI) of the heart muscle.

During the early stages, dysfunction of endothelial cells of the coronary arteries also contributes to the development of ACS. Normally, endothelial cells secrete prostacyclin and nitric oxide that induce

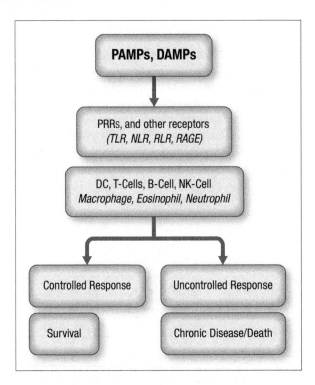

Figure 3.4 Survival or chronic disease/death. The extent of inflammatory response launched after recognition of PAMPs and DAMPs by various PRRs determine the outcomes. A controlled response with appropriately timed anti-inflammatory feedback will help with healing and repair, whereas an uncontrolled response without a timely and adequate anti-inflammatory feedback will not. DAMP, damage-associated molecular pattern; DC, dendritic cell; NK, natural killer; NLR, nucleotide-binding leucine-rich repeat; PAMP, pathogen-associated molecular pattern; PRRs, pattern recognition receptors; TLR, toll-like receptor; RAGE, receptors for advanced glycation end products; RLR, RIG-I-like receptor.

relaxation of blood vessels. The dysfunctional coronary endothelial cells, in the absence of relaxing factors, cause coronary vasospasm, bleeding, clot formation, and occlusion of the lumen.

In hypoxic cardiomyocytes (in myocardial ischemia), ionic pumps become dysfunctional across muscle membranes and alter the efficiency of cardiac muscle contraction/relaxation. Hypoxia-induced ischemia of myocardium often manifests as chest pain or angina and associated clinical symptoms. Chronic ischemia eventually leads to irreversible injury to myocytes, followed by infarction, inflammation, and necrosis. Eventually, chronic ischemia leads to impaired mechanical and electrical activity of the heart that can lead to heart attack, dysrhythmias, and heart failure (HF).

This continuum of events, beginning with signs and symptoms of myocardial ischemia and later infarction of the cardiac muscle, is ACS that can culminate in HF and dysrhythmias. However, the precursor events to ACS are mostly cumulative changes that occur in the coronary arteries over time.

Because LDL in plasma is one of the major risk factors for atherosclerosis and ACS, various methods have been developed to estimate its concentration. Current laboratory methods are based on chemical analysis of cholesterol content in LDL (LDL-C). However, this estimation ignores the fact that LDL particles vary in their physical size, and the smaller, heavier particles are more atherogenic in comparison to other sizes.

Physical techniques to analyze LDL particles (LDL-P) to determine their size and number are based on their nuclear magnetic resonance (NMR) spectra. Several researchers have compared the data obtained from these techniques to those obtained from current chemical analyses in predicting risk for ACS, and

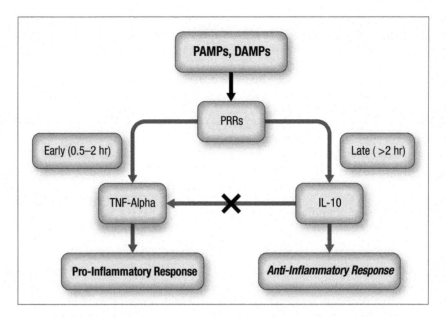

Figure 3.5 Two phases of inflammation: proinflammatory and anti-inflammatory. Recognition of PAMPs and DAMPs by the PRRs and other receptors immediately initiates an early secretion of proinflammatory cytokines and an inflammatory response. A short while later, secretion of anti-inflammatory cytokines initiates signaling to slow down/stop the inflammation and to restore homeostasis. DAMP, damage-associated molecular pattern; IL, interleukin; PAMP, pathogen-associated molecular pattern; PRR, pattern recognition receptor; TNF, tumor necrosis factor.

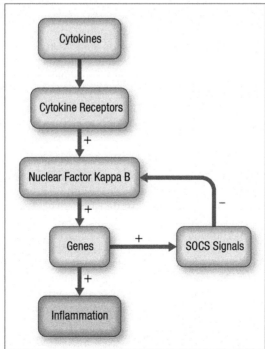

Figure 3.6 Suppressor of cytokine system (SOCS) pathway. Proinflammatory cytokines activate nuclear factor kappa B, and later the activation of another set of genes activates this pathway, shutting down the inflammatory response.

the results have not been convincing enough to recommend replacing them. However, using LDL-P data by NMR would add more individuals to the category of higher risk for cardiovascular disease. In addition to atherosclerosis, several other conditions such as infections or coronary artery vascular spasms can also impair blood flow to cardiomyocytes and precipitate myocardial ischemia.

ACS is an imbalance between oxygen supply and demand that causes myocardial ischemia and injury and, if not corrected, progresses to MI and loss of cardiac muscle function. The set of symptoms experienced by a patient reflects the state of cardiac muscle at a given time on this evolving syndrome. The classical symptoms include feeling restless or apprehensive, substernal chest pain (angina) as an aching pressure or a burning pain, and dyspnea with unusual or unexplained fatigue. The pain or discomfort can radiate to shoulders, arms, back, neck, or jaw. In addition, associated symptoms can include dyspnea, diaphoresis, lightheadedness or fainting, indigestion, and nausea or vomiting. Classic symptoms may not be experienced by women, patients with diabetes, or older adults, who instead might feel unusually fatigued. Classic symptoms might be confused with manifestations of musculoskeletal, gastrointestinal, pulmonary, or even neurologic dysfunction.

Based on symptoms of angina/dyspnea, patients may be classified to have unstable, stable, or Prinzmetal angina as manifestations of slightly different pathophysiological processes.

UNSTABLE ANGINA

Unstable angina is characterized by pain that occurs at any time during normal daily routine and is not completely relieved by vasodilators such as nitroglycerin. A major cause of unstable angina is thrombus in coronary arteries from a disrupted atherosclerotic plaque. It may be a nonocclusive thrombus that narrows the lumen, decreasing the amount of blood reaching the myocardium.

STABLE ANGINA

Stable angina occurs during exertion, and relief occurs after a little rest or with nitroglycerin. Stable angina results when demand for oxygen in myocardium exceeds supply. In this case, the major cause of the decreased supply of oxygen/blood and myocardial ischemia is coronary stenosis. Coronary stenosis is promoted by multiple factors, including endothelial cell injury due to hypertension, stress, and atherosclerosis.

PRINZMETAL ANGINA

Prinzmetal angina can occur at any time due to vasospasms and may not be related to atherosclerosis. The pain responds well to nitrates. The condition may be due to multiple factors that include dysfunction of arterial endothelial cells and smooth muscle cells and an imbalance in the tone regulated by the sympathetic and parasympathetic systems.

ELECTROCARDIOGRAM PROFILES: ACUTE CORONARY SYNDROME AND ANGINA

Patients with ACS and different types of angina are evaluated by EKG and tracked with cardio biomarkers such as troponin. In early stages of ACS with some injury of the myocardium, alterations in EKG manifest a prolongation of QT interval and/or T-wave inversion with no elevation of the biomarkers. On further progression of ACS, patients will demonstrate either an elevation of the ST segment (hence denoted as ST-ACS) or no elevation of the ST segment (hence, non-ST ACS). Patients who have non-ST ACS and those who have ST-ACS have elevated cardiac biomarkers. Patients with ACS and MI are designated as either ST-elevated MI (ST-MI) or non-ST elevated MI (NSTMI). Here, it is important to note that patients with non-ST ACS (or NSTMI) also include patients with unstable angina, because they are also negative for ST elevation. However, cardiac biomarkers are elevated in both ST-MI and NSTMI but not in unstable angina. In unstable angina, flattened T-waves, hyperacute T-wave, inverted T-waves, and ST depression may be observed (Figure 3.7). EKG tracings and biomarkers help with diagnosis and designing appropriate therapeutic approaches.

MI has been classified as types 1 and 2. As shown in Figure 3.8, Type 1 is defined in cases with an erosion or rupture of a plaque in the coronary artery with or without occlusion. Type 2 includes cases in which demand for oxygen by the cardiac cells is not adequately met because the supplying artery is affected with atherosclerosis and is partially blocked, has a vasospasm, has undergone a dissection, or has some other undefined reason.

The event of an MI is an acute episode of disbalance of oxygen demand versus supply and ends with an infarction. The condition of infarction/necrosis might begin in the subendocardium and spread

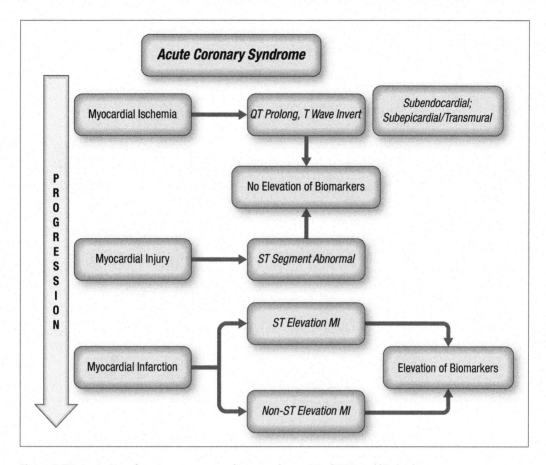

Figure 3.7 Progression of acute coronary syndrome and associated EKG and biomarkers.

up to underneath subepicardial areas. The subepicardial area has many more collateral branches of blood vessels, and hence the rate of infarction and death of cells is delayed. In an infarcted heart, cardiac function is compromised as the myocardium now has a scar, and the remodeled heart usually has segmental hypertrophy. Scar formation is due to lack of a fast, regenerative capacity of cardiac myocytes.

Therapeutic approaches address restoring blood supply to the cardiac muscle and decreasing the oxygen demand by the muscle. To remove the blockage, therapies include stents, artery bypass, or thrombolytic drugs. In most cases of ACS, a reduction of oxygen demand may be achieved by antianginal drugs and drugs to relieve vasospasms.

HEART FAILURE

HF is the condition in which pump function of the heart fails. Decreased cardiac output leads to decreased perfusion of various organs and decreased oxygenation. Patients experience shortness of breath, fatigue, and decreased capacity to exercise. HF can be a result of coronary artery disease, hypertension, diabetes, or obesity. Although genetic factors predispose some individuals to HF, several causes are modifiable, and mitigations help delay age of onset and progression. Although the pumping ability is affected in HF, the ejection fraction (EF) may be preserved (p; HFpEF), reduced (r; HFrEF), or recovered (HFrecEF). Recall that EF is dependent on diastolic filling and systolic outflow. Hence, although the EF may be intact, decreased cardiac output leads to symptoms of dyspnea and fatigue.

HF could be a systolic or a diastolic failure (HF with preserved systolic function). Systolic failure is mostly due to loss of inotropy or loss of cardiomyocytes because of infarction. In contrast, diastolic failure with preserved systolic function can be a result of loss of compliance of cardiac muscle impairing the filling ability of ventricles. In both types of failure, an increase in the end-diastolic pressure is a compensatory mechanism.

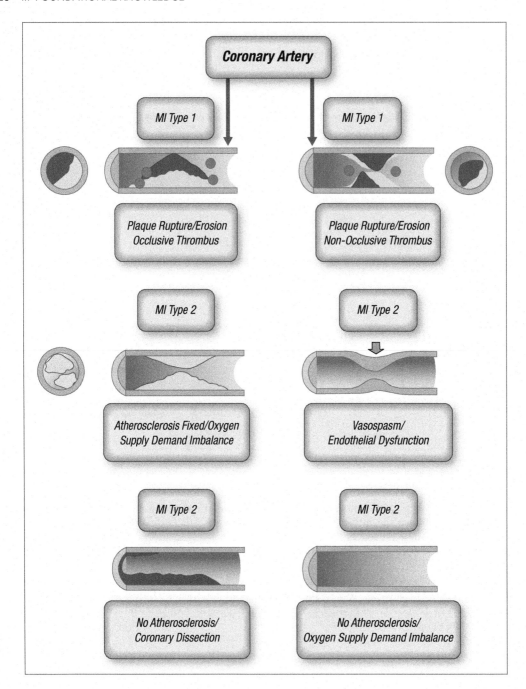

Figure 3.8 Types of acute coronary syndrome/MI.
MI, myocardial infarction.

Source: Adapted from Kristian Thygesen, Joseph S. Alpert, Allan S. Jaffe, Bernard R. Chaitman, Jeroen J. Bax, David A. Morrow, Harvey D. White, and The Executive Group on behalf of the Joint European Society of Cardiology (ESC)/American College of Cardiology (ACC)/American Heart Association (AHA)/World Heart Federation (WHF) Task Force for the Universal Definition of Myocardial Infarction. (2018). Fourth universal definition of myocardial infarction. *Journal of the American College of Cardiology, 72*(18), 2231–2264.

A patient might develop HF gradually with ongoing symptoms and progression (chronic HF). In contrast, the condition might develop suddenly (acute HF). Acute HF is a rapid-onset condition that requires hospitalized care.

CHRONIC HEART FAILURE

In patients with chronic HF, an initial decrease in cardiac output activates baroreceptors on the carotid artery, and compensatory mechanisms are initiated. These mechanisms include activation of the sympathetic system and the renin-angiotensin-aldosterone system (RAAS; Figure 3.9). Secretion of catecholamines and angiotensin II increases, and extra aldosterone and antidiuretic hormone (ADH) begin to circulate in blood. Increased norepinephrine has an inotropic effect on the heart and increases the strength of contractions to maintain the cardiac output.

Increasing the concentration of norepinephrine in plasma promotes apoptosis of cardiac cells and focal myocardial necrosis and leads to cardiac hypertrophy. When norepinephrine levels stay elevated, baroreceptor dysfunction promotes further sympathetic activity. Atrial sinus node activity is also modulated, resulting in a reduced parasympathetic effect on the rhythm. This predominance of the sympathetic and reduced vagal modulation of the sinus node is a prognostic marker with chronic HF. The stress on the heart is exacerbated by activation of the RAAS that facilitates a greater preload and afterload, and, under the influence of aldosterone, a progressively increasing retention of salt and water occurs that results in edema (Figure 3.10).

In the short term, the compensatory mechanisms are helpful but stress the cardiac muscle further because of dilation and remodeling. Eventually, the neurohumoral compensation does more harm, and decompensation begins. This precipitates the condition of acute decompensated heart failure (ADHF). Patients with ADHF, therefore, have had a history of heart disease before acute HF.

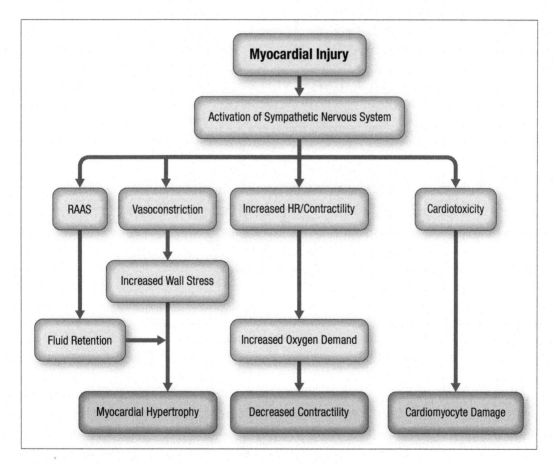

Figure 3.9 Sympathetic response after myocardial injury. Activation of sympathetic system induces compensatory mechanisms that increase venous return and increase cardiac contractility, but in the long run these mechanisms are cardiotoxic, induce cardiac hypertrophy, increase fluid retention, and add more stress to cardiac muscle. Timely, appropriate interventions designed to counter these mechanisms can improve patient outcomes.

HR, heart rate; RAAS, renin-angiotensin-aldosterone system.

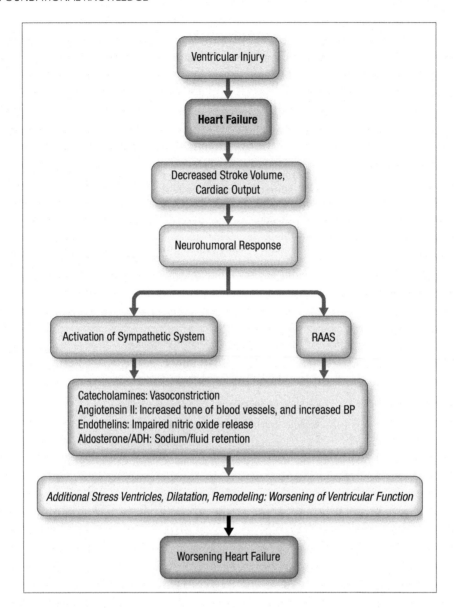

Figure 3.10 Neurohumoral response after ventricular injury and heart failure.
The decreased cardiac output activates the sympathetic system and the RAAS.
The result is increased output of catecholamines and angiotensin II that increase
vasoconstriction, and aldosterone promotes retention of sodium and water. These
events eventually worsen the heart.
ADH, antidiuretic hormone; RAAS, renin-angiotensin-aldosterone system.

In patients with chronic HF, a norepinephrine level above 5.32 nmol/L has been shown to be a prognosticator of mortality within a 2-year period. However, its precise measurement at the point of care is not practical. In contrast, more recent data indicate that sustained increase in B-type natriuretic peptide (BNP) can also be a predictor of mortality, and methods of measuring this biomarker are much less cumbersome. A decline in BNP level has been found to be associated with a better outcome.

ACUTE HEART FAILURE

A patient with acute HF has signs of congestion and fluid retention. The patient may experience exertional dyspnea, orthopnea, and dependent edema. Some of the indicators of clinical signs of congestion are pulmonary rales, peripheral bilateral edema, jugular venous distension greater than 6 cm, hepatomegaly, or hepatojugular reflux. In contrast, the presence of cold extremities or signs of oliguria or mental confusion would be taken as signs of hypoperfusion.

Because of declining cardiac output, patients have signs and symptoms that reflect the consequences of decreased perfusion. Although common presenting symptoms are dyspnea, tachycardia, and anxiety, in severe cases pallor and hypotension may also be present. Signs and symptoms are listed in Table 3.6. (See also Chapter 9.)

Table 3.6 Signs and Symptoms of Acute Heart Failure

Dyspnea on exertion
Fatigue and weakness
Reduced ability to exercise
Edema: dependent areas: legs, ankles, feet, hips
Tachycardia or irregular heartbeat
Persistent cough or wheezing with white or pink blood-tinged sputum
Nocturia
Ascites
Rapid weight gain (fluid retention)
Lack of appetite and nausea
Difficulty concentrating or decreased alertness
Sudden, severe shortness of breath and coughing up pink, frothy sputum
Angina (if heart failure caused by a myocardial infarction)

When the ventricles do not keep pace with demands of perfusion, cardiac filling pressures increase, and extracellular fluid accumulation leads to systemic congestion. The overall goal of therapy is decreasing the fluid volume overload and helping with improved ventilation.

Clinically, patients with HF could be classified as wet or dry and warm or cold, which later formed the basis of the 2016 European Society of Cardiology HF guidelines with recommended treatment approaches for each category. These guidelines provide an algorithm for assessment and designing appropriate approaches for therapy.

As indicated in Figure 3.11, in patients who show up "dry/cold" or "dry/warm," adjustment of oral therapies or inotropic agents might be needed. However, to hemodynamically stabilize patients who are in the "wet" category (with congestion) requires a more detailed workup and detailed attention to blood pressure and adjustment of pharmacological agents such as diuretics, vasodilators, or vasopressors. The 6-month mortality rate of "dry/cold" patients is 11% in comparison with "wet/cold" patients, who have a 40% mortality rate. In either case, the first action should be to correct the hypoxia concurrently with therapeutic agents that lead to vasodilation and diuresis to reduce preload and anxiety.

EFFECT OF HEART FAILURE ON NONCARDIAC ORGANS AND SYSTEMS (NEUROHUMORAL EFFECTS)

Vasculature

An increase in sympathetic activity alters the vascular tone (vasoconstriction), and one would expect an increase in peripheral resistance. Similarly, activation of the RAAS also leads to an increase in peripheral resistance as additional amounts of angiotensin II are released. Additionally, an increase in endothelin negatively affects the release of endothelium-derived relaxing factor (or nitric oxide), adding to the effect of angiotensin II. AGACNPs can teach patients about the usefulness of exercise training to improve endothelial function and mitigate the effects of endothelin. Pharmacologically, the use of angiotensin-converting enzyme inhibitors also improves endothelial function.

Skeletal Muscle Changes

The effect on skeletal muscles is a direct result of alterations in the vasculature and leads to a decreased flow of blood in the muscle and a reduction in muscle mass, muscle structure, metabolism, and function. Functionally, the patient may report fatigue, lethargy, and exercise intolerance. Sympathetic activation

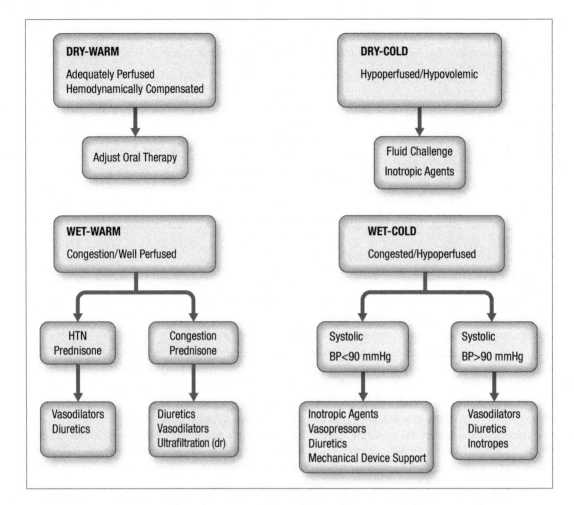

Figure 3.11 Therapeutic approaches to patients with heart failure. The patients might present in dry or wet category. Interventions are based on the algorithm so that outcomes can be improved.
BP, blood pressure; HTN, hypertension.

leads to a passive congestion in the gut manifesting as intestinal edema. Such changes in the gastrointestinal system also alter absorption of drugs given orally.

HF adversely affects cardiac output and perfusion of tissues. Noncardiac organs/tissue are impacted not only by a decrease in perfusion but also by the neurohumoral response.

▶ RESPIRATORY SYSTEM

To discuss pathophysiology of the respiratory system, recall that functional areas of gas exchange are the alveoli that contain the respiratory membrane. The respiratory membrane is a composite structure made up of three distinct membranes. The first belongs to the alveolar epithelial cell membrane, the second is of the blood capillary endothelial cell membrane, and the third is a composite acellular basement membrane between the cellular membranes. The alveolar side of the membrane is slightly moist, allowing dissolution and diffusion of gases across it, and it also lowers surface tension because of the surfactant. The important properties of this membrane that help in gas exchange are its thinness, moistness, and permeability to gases.

Inspiration of air into the lungs is regulated by the concentration of carbon dioxide in the blood that permeates across into the brain and leads to production of hydrogen ions sensed by chemosensors and activation of the inspiratory center in the medulla oblongata. Action potentials generated by the inspiratory center travel through the phrenic nerve to the diaphragm. Contraction of the diaphragm expands the thoracic cavity, and the resultant negative pressure draws air into the lungs. The relaxation phase of the diaphragm decreases intrathoracic volume and increases intrapulmonary pressure that pushes the air out: exhalation. Hence, inspiration of air into the lungs is an active process, and expiration is a passive process.

Lungs contain elastic fibers; the resulting elastance (resistance) demands a certain amount of force for expansion during inhalation, and it also helps in returning the lungs to functional lung capacity during exhalation. Therefore, compliance allows them to be compliant during inspiration and expiration. Each of the lungs is enclosed by two layers of pleural membranes. The visceral pleura is adherent to the lung surface, and the parietal pleura is adherent to the inside of the thoracic wall. Due to this arrangement, the lungs are held in a semi-stretched condition by the pull of the thoracic wall such that the lungs are partially filled with a volume of air that is greater than the residual volume—thus the term *functional lung capacity*. Since the lungs are stretched by the pull of the thoracic wall (because of adherent parietal pleura), a negative pressure is established in the pleural space that helps in the compliance and filling of the lungs with air and at the same time keeps the lungs from complete collapse after expiration.

Functional lung capacity includes the residual volume and the expiratory reserve volume. Normal automated inspiration brings in about 500 mL of new air with each breath that is added on top of the functional lung capacity. Taking a deep breath adds to the inspiratory reserve volume of air over and above the functional lung capacity and tidal volume. Thus, the total lung volume is the sum of functional lung capacity, tidal volume, and inspiratory reserve volume.

VENTILATION PERFUSION RATIO

The lungs help oxygenate the blood brought in by the pulmonary arteries. Alveolar perfusion depends on a continuous flow of blood in the capillaries that surround the alveoli brought in with every cardiac contraction. The perfusion rate of the lungs is about 4,900 mL per minute (Q) based on cardiac output of 70 mL and heart rate of 70 bpm. Each inspiration brings about 500 mL of air into the respiratory tree, about 350 mL of which end up in the alveolar area so that the net ventilation volume per minute (V) in the alveoli is about 4,200 mL (assuming 12 breaths per minute). Thus, a normal V/Q ratio is about 0.8. This ratio is altered if the lungs have a pulmonary embolus lodged in one of the pulmonary arteries, thus reducing perfusion. This can lead to an acute condition needing immediate attention. Similarly, V/Q will also change if ventilation volume is altered, as in diseases that affect the lungs.

FRACTIONAL INSPIRATION OF OXYGEN AND PARTIAL PRESSURE OF ARTERIAL OXYGEN: VALUE IN DETERMINING RATIO

Inspiration brings in air into the lungs at normal atmospheric pressure of 760 mmHg at sea level. Normal room air is composed of about 78% nitrogen (N_2), 21% oxygen (O_2), and about 0.003% carbon dioxide (CO_2), with other gases contributing a trace amount. Hence, the fraction of oxygen in the inspired air (FIO_2) is 0.21 out of a total of 1.

Total normal atmospheric pressure is due to the sum of all the partial pressures of each of the component gases proportional to their concentration. The diffusion of O_2 and CO_2 across the respiratory membrane in the lungs depends on the gradient of their partial pressures that exists in the lungs and blood. The extent of oxygenation of arterial blood can be ascertained by the partial pressure of O_2 in the arterial blood (PaO_2). The efficiency of gas exchange at the level of the lungs can be determined by calculating the ratio of PaO_2 and FIO_2 (P/F ratio; Table 3.7).

Table 3.7 Sample Calculation of PaO_2/FIO_2 (P/F ratio)[a]

Parameters	Case A (Normal)	Case B (Patient with ARDS)
FIO_2	0.21 (21% oxygen in room air)	0.5 (patient receiving 50% oxygen)
PaO_2	100 mmHg	100 mmHg
PaO_2/FIO_2	476	200

[a]The patient is receiving oxygen at a much higher partial pressure.

ARDS, acute respiratory distress syndrome; FIO_2, fraction of inspired oxygen; PaO_2, partial pressure of arterial oxygen.

ACUTE RESPIRATORY DISTRESS SYNDROME

Acute respiratory distress syndrome (ARDS) develops due to diffuse injury to alveolar walls and endothelial cells. Therefore, damage to blood vessels and respiratory membrane (and elastic fibers) compromises the lungs' ability to perform efficient gas exchange and lung compliance. Patients develop bilateral pulmonary infiltrates and progressive hypoxemia with life-threatening consequences. The defining criterion of ARDS is the ratio of PaO_2 to FIO_2. Patients have PaO_2/FIO_2 of less than 300. Auscultation provides evidence of chest rales in the absence of a cardiopulmonary condition.

The first phase of ARDS begins with diffuse alveolar damage with epithelial cell injury to Type I and Type II pneumocytes followed by necrosis. This accompanies diffuse microvascular injury and influx of inflammatory cells and proteinaceous fluid (exudative phase, 1 to 3 days). The second phase begins the process of lung repair manifested with hyperplasia of Type II pneumocytes followed by proliferation of fibroblasts (fibroproliferative phase, 3 to 7 days). Concurrently, because of injury of the alveolovascular system, removal of fluid from the alveolar space is impaired. In addition, injury to the Type II pneumocytes reduces the production of the surfactant and precipitates and exacerbates atelectasis that further impairs gas exchange. Because of proliferation of fibroblasts, fibrosis begins to set in, altering lung compliance.

The onset of the syndrome may occur within 7 days of a precipitating event. Initially, patients complain of dyspnea and show signs of hypoxemia that escalate such that within a short time, they require mechanical ventilation to relieve the symptoms of dyspnea and hypoxemia. The first phase of ARDS itself paves the way for infiltration of fluids and proteins into the alveolar space, leading to edema and proteinosis. Pulmonary edema affects gas exchange and causes hypoxemia. Since the injury may not equally affect all the lung segments, a nonuniform pattern of alveolar edema and compliance issues develop. This differential effect presents challenges in the clinic as external means of ventilation at a given pressure may not benefit the whole lung area equally; thus, the strategies of oxygenation must be adapted to the patient's condition with respect to dead spaces, partial or complete edema, or atelectasis. The ventilation strategy must be adjusted to provide an appropriate size of tidal volume and air pressure. Because patients receive mostly supportive care (in the absence of effective therapies), mortality rates are high. Surviving patients may subsequently develop pulmonary hypertension.

MAJOR PRECIPITANTS OF ACUTE RESPIRATORY DISTRESS SYNDROME

The syndrome nature of ARDS suggests the difficulty in pinpointing one cause, yet a common theme of varying degrees of alveolar/vascular damage provides clinical criteria for assessing the degree of ARDS. Several precipitants for the development of the syndrome have been identified (Table 3.8). Pneumonia of all causes and sepsis are noted precipitants of the syndrome. Since the beginning of the SARS-CoV-2 epidemic, a large number of patients with COVID-19 have developed ARDS and overwhelmed the healthcare system. In general, the presentation of ARDS in patients with COVID-19 is similar to that of classic ARDS.

Table 3.8 Common Precipitants of Acute Respiratory Distress Syndrome

Direct Lung Injury	Indirect Lung Injury
Pneumonia (bacterial, viral, fungus)	Sepsis and septic shock
Aspiration of gastric contents	Transfusion-related lung injury
Drownings	Acute pancreatitis
Toxic inhalation or thermal inhalation injuries	Severe trauma
Air or fat emboli	Burns
Lung contusion(s)	Drug overdose
Reperfusion after lung transplant or thrombectomy	Drug toxicity

ARDS is identified using the Berlin definition (Table 3.9). This definition provides tools for assessing mild, moderate, and severe ARDS and for possible use in providing therapeutic approaches in treating patients. The Berlin definition removed the requirement for wedge pressure to less than 18 and included the requirement of positive end-expiratory pressure (PEEP) or continuous positive airway pressure (CPAP) of ≥5. Since the clinical criteria use PEEP, patients who are not on mechanical ventilation assist may not be appropriately diagnosed based on the criteria.

Table 3.9 Berlin Definition of Acute Respiratory Distress Syndrome

Timing	≤1 Week of a Known Clinical Insult or New/Worsening Respiratory Status
Diagnostics (CXR, CT scan)	Bilateral opacities—not fully explained by effusions, lobar/lung collapse, or nodules
Etiology of edema	Respiratory failure not explained by cardiac failure or fluid overload Requires objective assessment (e.g., echocardiography) to exclude hydrostatic edema if no risk factors present
Classification	
Mild	PaO_2/FIO_2 200–300 mmHg with PEEP or CPAP $\geq$5 cm H_2O
Moderate	PaO_2/FIO_2 100–200 mmHg with PEEP $\geq$5 cm H_2O
Severe	PaO_2/FIO_2 $\leq$100 mmHg with PEEP $\geq$5 cm H_2O

CPAP, continuous positive airway pressure; CXR, chest x-ray; FIO_2, fraction of inspired oxygen; PaO_2, partial pressure of arterial oxygen; PEEP, positive end-expiratory pressure.

▶ RENAL SYSTEM

The *nephron* is the functional unit of kidneys. It performs three main functions in the production of urine: filtration, absorption, and secretion. The integrity of the filtration membrane is essential for filtration, and it gets damaged mostly by chronic conditions of hypertension and diabetes. In contrast, tubular function can be compromised acutely during acute kidney injury that might necessitate supportive dialysis.

GLOMERULAR FILTRATION RATE AND TUBULAR REABSORPTION

Filtration at the glomerulus depends on the integrity of the filtration membrane. The filtrate normally contains mostly water along with various compounds selectively allowed through as the filtration membrane is thin, fenestrated, and negatively charged. Therefore, proteins are usually excluded from the filtrate, and glucose and ions are allowed through.

The efficiency of filtration can be calculated from lab values of creatinine (Cr) in urine and plasma. Although Cr is typically the biomarker used for determining glomerular filtration rate (GFR), inulin may be used in select cases. The concentration of Cr in plasma increases when GFR decreases; hence, Cr concentration in plasma and GFR are inversely proportional. An important point to consider is that as GFR continues to decrease, a greater proportion of Cr is then excreted into the urine by secretion (rather than by filtration); therefore, under such conditions, any Cr-based estimation of GFR becomes less accurate. This is particularly important in older individuals.

Post filtration, the task of reabsorption is handled by different segments of the tubular portion of the nephron. Efficiency of reabsorption can be determined by estimation of fractional excretion of sodium (FE Na) in urine (in relation to that in plasma). Under normal conditions, with no confounding variables, most sodium is reabsorbed, and the FE Na is less than 1%.

ACUTE KIDNEY INJURY

Acute kidney injury (AKI) is characterized by a sharp decline in GFR. In older individuals, renal reserve is decreased, and in the presence of comorbid conditions the risk of AKI increases in the geriatric population. Some data indicate that individuals older than 60 years are at a greater risk of developing AKI (a three- to eight-fold progressive age-dependent increase).

AKI can occur because of prerenal, intrarenal, or postrenal causes (Table 3.10). In cases of prerenal etiology, the tubules remain mostly undamaged, GFR is decreased, and the FE Na is less than 1%. Alterations in functioning of the vascular system compounded by tendency to dehydration lead to prerenal issues of hypotension, hypovolemia, and decreased blood flow to the kidneys that can precipitate AKI. In contrast, in AKI due to intrarenal damage (e.g., acute tubular necrosis), the GFR may be normal, but the FE Na is usually greater than 2% (Table 3.11). In such cases, the excessive loss of sodium would decrease plasma volume and secondarily impact cardiovascular function as well. Older individuals with a hematologic profile of monoclonal gammopathy of unknown significance may develop AKI because of tubular obstruction due to excessive amounts of protein in the filtrate.

Although FE Na is useful in discriminating between the two types of AKI, these values should not be viewed in isolation. It is necessary and important to consider history, physical exam, clinical context, and medications the patient is taking along with the values of FE Na in deciding appropriate approaches to therapy.

Table 3.10 Prerenal Risk Factors for Acute Kidney Injury: Reduced Blood Flow to the Kidneys

Condition	Etiology
Hypovolemia	Hemorrhage, severe burns, GI losses
Hypotension	Cardiac: acute coronary syndrome, cardiogenic shock
Hypotension	Noncardiac: systemic vasodilation, septic shock, anesthesia, anaphylaxis
Vasoconstriction: renal	NSAIDs, contrast agents, amphotericin B
Vasodilation: afferent glomerular	ACE inhibitors, angiotensin receptor blockers

ACE, angiotensin-converting enzyme; GI, gastrointestinal; NSAID, nonsteroidal anti-inflammatory drug.

Table 3.11 Intrarenal Risk Factors for Acute Kidney Injury: Tubular Injury

Condition	Etiology
Acute tubular necrosis	Ischemia: prolonged prerenal injury Drugs: aminoglycosides, vancomycin, amphotericin B Rhabdomyolysis
Acute interstitial nephritis	Infections, penicillin, NSAIDs, PPIs, SLE
Glomerulonephritis	SLE, postinfectious glomerulonephritis
Intratubular obstruction	MGUS, tumor lysis syndrome, ethylene glycol

MGUS, monoclonal gammopathy of undetermined significance; NSAIDs, nonsteroidal anti-inflammatory drugs; PPIs, proton pump inhibitors; SLE, systemic lupus erythematosus.

PATIENT EDUCATION
CLINICAL EDUCATION

1. If possible, avoid use of nephrotoxic medications.
2. Avoid or decrease consumption of nonsteroidal anti-inflammatory drugs.
3. Follow your medication regimen for controlling blood pressure.
4. Ensure you are well hydrated and have normal urine output before any labs that involve contrast agents.

DIETARY EDUCATION TO DECREASE LIKELIHOOD OF PROGRESSION TO END-STAGE RENAL DISEASE

1. Restrict intake of excessive salt and fluid.
2. Avoid a high-potassium diet.
3. Consume adequate caloric intake to compensate for the catabolic state of AKI.
4. Monitor renal function to ensure slowdown of progression to end-stage renal disease.

▶ SUMMARY

This chapter describes some of the most important pathophysiological states the AGACNP must know in order to treat patients with these conditions. Understanding the pathophysiology helps the AGACNP grasp how to both prevent and treat the conditions. Additionally, patient education is foundational to the AGACNP role. Helping patients and families understand the pathophysiology can engage them in their care and advance them toward health and recovery.

KNOWLEDGE CHECK: CHAPTER 3

1. Myocardial ischemia manifests as:

   A. T-wave inversion
   B. ST elevation
   C. Peaked T-waves
   D. Prolonged PR interval

2. Angina caused by vasospasms is:

   A. Stable
   B. Unstable
   C. Refractory
   D. Prinzmetal

3. Which patient is likely to have the classic signs of ST-elevated MI (ST-MI)?

   A. 60-year-old man
   B. 75-year-old woman
   C. 50-year-old patient with diabetes
   D. 85-year-old patient with chronic obstructive pulmonary disease (COPD)

4. Severe acute respiratory distress syndrome (ARDS) is classified as a PaO_2/FIO_2 ratio of:

   A. >300 mmHg
   B. <200 to 300 mmHg
   C. 100 to 200 mmHg
   D. <100 mmHg

5. Prerenal acute kidney injury (AKI) has a fractional excretion of sodium (FE Na) of:

   A. Less than 1%
   B. Less than 2%
   C. Less than 10%
   D. Greater than 10%

6. An older adult male patient presents with complaints of a distended abdomen and acknowledges that he has not used the bathroom for a few days. Labs reveal blood urea nitrogen (BUN) 96 and creatinine 6.2. CT scan shows a distended bladder and hydronephrosis. The most likely cause of his renal failure is:

   A. Dehydration
   B. Sepsis
   C. Postrenal obstruction
   D. Acute tubular necrosis

(See answers next page.)

1. A) T-wave inversion

Myocardial ischemia manifests with QT prolongation and/or T-wave inversion. ST elevation is myocardial infarction. Peaked T-waves are seen with hyperkalemia. Prolonged QT, not prolonged PR interval, is noted with myocardial ischemia.

2. D) Prinzmetal

Prinzmetal angina occurs due to vasospasms and may not be related to atherosclerosis. The condition may be due to multiple factors that include dysfunction of arterial endothelial cells and smooth muscle cells and imbalance in the tone regulated by sympathetic and parasympathetic systems. Unstable angina is caused by a nonocclusive thrombus that narrows the lumen, decreasing the amount of blood reaching the myocardium. Stable angina occurs during exertion, and relief occurs after rest or with nitroglycerin. Refractory angina is frequent anginal attacks uncontrolled by maximal drug therapy that is not amenable to percutaneous coronary intervention (PCI) or coronary artery bypass grafting (CABG) and significantly limits a patient's" daily activities.

3. A) 60-year-old man

Classic symptoms of ST-MI include feeling restless or apprehensive, substernal chest pain (angina) as an aching pressure or a burning pain, and dyspnea with unusual or unexplained fatigue. Pain or discomfort can radiate to shoulders, arms, back, neck, or jaw. In addition, associated symptoms can include dyspnea, diaphoresis, lightheadedness or fainting, indigestion, and nausea or vomiting. Classic symptoms may not be experienced by women, patients with diabetes, or older adults, who instead might feel unusually fatigued or nauseous.

4. D) <100 mmHg

Mild ARDS has a PaO_2/FIO_2 of 200 to 300 mmHg with positive end-expiratory pressure (PEEP) or continuous positive airway pressure (CPAP) ≥ 5 cm H_2O; moderate ARDS has a PaO_2/FIO_2 of 100 to 200 mmHg with PEEP ≥ 5 cm H_2O; and severe ARDS has a PaO_2/FIO_2 ≤ 100 mmHg with PEEP ≥ 5 cm H_2O.

5. A) Less than 1%

In cases of prerenal etiology, the tubules remain mostly undamaged, glomerular filtration rate (GFR) is decreased, and the FE Na is less than 1%. Alterations in functioning of the vascular system are compounded by the tendency of dehydration to lead to prerenal issues of hypotension, hypovolemia, and a decreased blood flow to the kidneys that can precipitate AKI. In contrast, in AKI because of intrarenal damage (e.g., acute tubular necrosis), the GFR may be normal, but the FE Na is usually greater than 2%.

6. C) Postrenal obstruction

Postrenal issues that precipitate acute kidney injury (AKI) are mostly due to bladder outlet obstruction. A postrenal cause of AKI that is particularly important for older adults is obstruction of the urinary tract (intrinsic or extrinsic) at any level. In male patients, this could be because of prostate hypertrophy; in female patients, it could be due to a pelvic malignancy.

7. An older adult male patient presents with complaints of a distended abdomen and acknowledges that he has not used the bathroom for a few days. Labs reveal blood urea nitrogen (BUN) 96 and creatinine 6.2. CT scan shows a distended bladder and hydronephrosis. The *immediate first step* of the AGACNP is to:

   A. Prescribe a diuretic
   B. Consult nephrology
   C. Place a Foley catheter
   D. Order tamsulosin (Flomax)

8. Patient education for patients recovering from an acute kidney injury include:

   A. Stay well hydrated
   B. Stop antihypertensive agents
   C. Use nonsteroidal anti-inflammatory drugs (NSAIDs) for pain control
   D. Get needed CT angiography (CTA) as soon as possible

9. To decrease the risk of progressing stages of chronic kidney disease (CKD) to end-stage renal disease, instruct patients to:

   A. Avoid lab draws and CT scans
   B. Limit caloric intake
   C. Restrict excessive salt use
   D. Consume oranges daily

10. A patient presents with redness, pain, and edema of the calf. These signs and symptoms signify:

    A. Deep vein thrombosis (DVT)
    B. Trauma
    C. Infection
    D. Inflammation

11. A patient who had a recent myocardial infarction (MI) is cold to touch and presents with shortness of breath, mottled legs, and bibasilar rales. Vital signs are T 96°F, heart rate (HR) 120, blood pressure (BP) 80/40, Sat 90%. The AGACNP should:

    A. Adjust oral medications
    B. Administer inotropes
    C. Administer oral diuretics
    D. Use continuous renal replacement therapy (CRRT) to ultrafiltrate

12. A patient presents with crushing chest pain. EKG notes an ST-elevated myocardial infarction (ST-MI) in leads II, III, AVF. Troponins are significantly elevated. Cardiology is called, and a percutaneous coronary intervention (PCI) is performed with placement of stents. This myocardial infarction (MI) is type:

    A. I
    B. II
    C. III
    D. IV

(See answers next page.)

7. C) Place a Foley catheter

The patient needs immediate relief of his obstruction by placement of a Foley catheter. Tamsulosin may be indicated but is not the highest priority. Nephrology is not needed at this point but may be if relieving the obstruction is ineffective in correcting the patient's BUN/creatinine. There is no urgent need for dialysis at this time. Diuretics are not indicated; rather, hydration with intravenous fluid (IVF) to flush out the kidneys after being obstructed is indicated.

8. A) Stay well hydrated

Patients should be instructed to avoid use of nephrotoxic medications, including NSAIDs, and follow their medication regimen for controlling blood pressure. Patients should be encouraged to stay well hydrated and should achieve normal labs and urine output before any testing that involves contrast agents.

9. C) Restrict excessive salt use

Patients should be encouraged to restrict intake of excessive salt and fluid, avoid a high-potassium diet, consume adequate caloric intake (to compensate for the catabolic state of acute kidney injury [AKI]), and monitor renal function.

10. D) Inflammation

The five cardinal signs of inflammation are pain (dolor), redness (rubor), edema (tumor), heat/fever (calor), and loss of function of the tissue/organ (functio laesa). These signs are a manifestation of the signaling events initiated by tissue injury. The signaling processes promote secretion of chemokines and cytokines, recruitment of immune cells such as neutrophils and macrophages, activation of complement proteins and the coagulation cascade, and induction of acute phase response by the liver, eventually leading to healing or repair. DVTs, trauma, and infection commonly manifest as these and other symptoms; the underlying pathology is inflammation. The AGACNP must be able to recognize inflammation and seek additional information from the patient and from diagnostics testing to conclude a diagnosis.

11. B) Administer inotropes

The patient is in cardiogenic shock. They are cold, wet, and hypoperfused, thus requiring inotropic agents, vasopressors, and mechanical support devices. Adjustment of oral medications and use of oral diuretics and ultrafiltration can occur when the patient is warm and wet/congested.

12. A) I

Type I ST-MI is caused by atherosclerotic plaque rupture. Type II MI is caused by ischemic imbalance. Type III is an MI that results without positive biomarkers, type IV is an MI related to PCI or stent thrombosis, and type V is an MI related to coronary artery bypass grafting (CABG).

13. A patient is admitted with septic shock and requires Levophed and vasopressin. They now have elevated troponins and an acute kidney injury (AKI). Transthoracic echocardiography (TTE) shows global hypokinesis. The most likely type of myocardial infarction (MI) is:

A. I

B. II

C. III

D. IV

14. The patient most likely to develop acute respiratory distress syndrome (ARDS) is a patient with:

A. Cellulitis and urinary tract infection (UTI)

B. Fractured femur

C. Acute renal failure

D. Stroke who aspirated

15. A patient presents after a fall with traumatic hip fracture. On hospital Day 3 and postoperative Day 2, the patient has new and increasing oxygen requirements requiring intubation. A chest radiograph reveals bilateral opacities. The patient has a postoperative echo that reveals a normal functioning heart. What does this presentation most align with?

A. Myocardial infarction

B. Acute respiratory distress syndrome

C. Acute heart failure

D. Acute kidney injury

(See answers next page.)

13. B) II

Type II MI is caused by ischemic imbalance. In this case, the imbalance is caused by higher oxygen demands needed in septic shock. Type I ST-elevated MI (ST-MI) is caused by atherosclerotic plaque rupture. Type I MI can occur in sepsis/septic shock but would have TTE changes consistent with a specific vessel territory, not global hypokinesis. Type III is an MI that results without positive biomarkers, Type IV is an MI related to percutaneous coronary intervention (PCI) or stent thrombosis, and Type V is an MI related to coronary artery bypass grafting (CABG).

14. D) Stroke who aspirated

The patient who had a stroke and aspirated has a direct lung injury. Causes of ARDS include both direct and indirect lung injuries. Direct lung injuries include pneumonia, aspiration, drowning, toxic or thermal inhalation injuries, air or fat emboli, lung contusion, reperfusion after lung transplant, or thrombectomy. Indirect lung injury includes sepsis/septic shock, transfusion-related lung injury (TRALI), acute pancreatitis, severe trauma, burns, and drug overdose. While cellulitis and UTI can cause sepsis, infection outside the lung without systemic involvement does not cause ARDS. The fractured femur alone does not cause ARDS; a fat embolus would also be needed to potentially cause ARDS. Acute renal failure does not cause ARDS.

15. B) Acute respiratory distress syndrome

By the Berlin criteria, a diagnosis of acute respiratory distress syndrome can be made if the respiratory failure developed within 1 week of an insult and imaging shows bilateral infiltrates that are not otherwise explained by a cardiac origin. There is no evidence to suspect myocardial infraction, acute heart failure, or acute kidney injury.

KEY BIBLIOGRAPHY

Only key resources appear in the print edition. Access the full bibliography for this chapter on ExamPrepConnect.com.

Hall, J. E. (2022). *Guyton and Hall textbook of medical physiology (Guyton Physiology)* (13th ed.). Elsevier.

Heidenreich, P. A., Bozkurt, B., Aguilar, D., Allen, L. A., Byun, J. J., Colvin, M. M., Deswal, A., Drazner, M. H., Dunlay, S. H., Evers, L. R., Fang, J. C., Fedson, S. E., Fonarow, G. C., Hayek, S. S., Hernandez, A. F., Khazanie, P., Kittleson, M. M., Lee, C. S., Link, M. S., … Yancy, C. W. (2022, May 3). 2022 AHA/ACC/HFSA guideline for the management of heart failure: A report of the American College of Cardiology/American Heart Association Joint Committee on clinical practice guidelines. *Circulation, 145*(18), e895–e1032. https://doi.org/10.1161/CIR.0000000000001063

Helgason, D., Long, T. E., Helgadottir, S., Palsson, R., Sigurdsson, G. H., Gudbjartsson, T., Indridason, O. S., Gudmundsdottir, I. J., & Sigurdsson, M. I. (2018, October). Acute kidney injury following coronary angiography: A nationwide study of incidence, risk factors and long-term outcomes. *Journal of Nephrology, 31*(5), 721–730. https://doi.org/10.1007/s40620-018-0534-y

Klabunde, R. E. (2021). *Cardiovascular physiology concepts* [Online]. https://www.cvphysiology.com/CAD/CAD007

Meyer, N., Gattinoni, L., & Calfee, C. S. (2021). Acute respiratory distress syndrome. *Lancet, 398*, 622–637. https://doi.org/10.1016/S0140-6736(21)00439-6

Zuber, K., & Davis, J. (2018). The ABCs of chronic kidney disease. *JAAPA, 31*(10), 17–25. https://doi.org/10.1097/01.JAA.0000545065.71225.f5

Advanced Pharmacology Review

Dinesh Yogaratnam, Ifeoma Asoh, Donna Bartlett, Michael Bear, Paul Belliveau, Katherine Carey, Jason Cross, Karen Dick, Abir Kanaan, Samar Nicolas, Helen Pervanas, and Matthew Silva

4

▶ INTRODUCTION

Pharmacology is an integral part of AGACNP education and practice. This chapter reviews general pharmacology concepts and delves further into specific acute care medications and prescribing considerations. The focus of this chapter is acute care content pertaining to cardiovascular and pulmonary content. Antibiotic prescribing is reviewed in detail because it is an area where students commonly struggle. Pain, agitation, and sedation treatment options are also detailed given the current opioid crisis. This chapter is best used as an adjunct to the system- and disease-specific content throughout the book.

▶ GENERAL PHARMACOLOGY

PHARMACOKINETICS
Pharmacokinetics is broadly defined as the movement of drug through the body. This journey typically occurs in four main stages: absorption, distribution, metabolism, and elimination (ADME). Each phase of the ADME process can be altered in the setting of acute and critical illness. Furthermore, individuals may have altered ADME as a result of either the aging process or chronic illness. Understanding how changes in ADME can affect drug disposition can help providers better anticipate and prevent problems related to both drug dosing and drug interactions.

ABSORPTION
Absorption is the movement of drug from the site of administration to the systemic circulation. Medications can be administered by numerous routes, including intravenous (IV), oral, subcutaneous, per rectum, intradermal, intranasal, sublingual, and intraosseous. When a drug is administered outside the systemic circulation, its movement into the systemic circulation can be affected by several factors (Table 4.1).

Table 4.1 Factors Influencing Absorption

Factor	Description
Host factors	Regional blood flow, type of tissue, local acidity (pH), availability of transport proteins, surface area for absorption, gastrointestinal motility, and function
Characteristics of the drug	Degree of fat and water solubility, ability to dissociate in acidic or basic environments, pharmaceutical formulation (long acting versus rapid acting), dependence on first-pass metabolism
Presence of interacting substances	Food, divalent cations, or other molecules that bind to drugs and prevent absorption
Patient factors	Acute illness, shock states, or use of vasopressors

The rate of absorption is how quickly a drug moves from the site of administration to the systemic circulation. The rate of absorption can be affected by the chemical properties of the drug (see Box 4.1).

Box 4.1

For example, insulin is often administered as a subcutaneous injection. Regular insulin takes approximately 30 minutes to travel from the subcutaneous tissue to the systemic circulation.

Absorption Characteristics of Subcutaneously Administered Insulin Products

Insulin Type	Onset of Action	Peak Effect	Duration of Action
Lispro	~15 minutes	~2 hours	~6 hours
Regular	~30 minutes	~4 hours	~8 hours
NPH	~1–2 hours	~4–12 hours	~14–24 hours
Glargine	~3–4 hours	~10–12 hours	~24–30 hours

Insulin lispro is a chemically altered form of regular insulin that has a faster rate of absorption when administered subcutaneously. Insulin NPH and glargine are also chemically altered versions of regular insulin that have slower rates of absorption from subcutaneous tissue.

The extent of absorption is referred to as a drug's bioavailability, or "F." *Bioavailability* is the proportion of a drug that reaches the systemic circulation. Consider a 100-mg pill that is taken by mouth (Figure 4.1). In this example, of the original 100 mg, 70 mg is eliminated from the body (perhaps through fecal elimination) and does not reach systemic circulation. However, 30 mg of the original dose is absorbed into the systemic circulation. Thus, the bioavailability of this drug is 30 mg out of 100 mg, or F = 30%.

Drugs that are directly administered into the systemic circulation, such as through IV or intra-arterial injection, have both instantaneous rate and complete (100%) extent of absorption. This is always true.

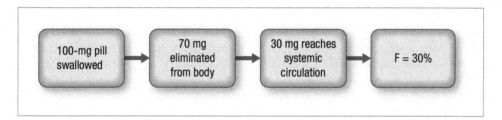

Figure 4.1 Bioavailability of a 100-mg pill. Medications that are administered orally must first pass through the liver before they reach systemic circulation. As a drug passes through the liver, a portion of the dose may be metabolized and eliminated before it has a chance to reach systemic circulation. This is known as the first-pass effect (see Box 4.2).

Box 4.2

For example, approximately 50% of orally administered metoprolol is metabolized by the liver before the drug reaches systemic circulation. By contrast, metoprolol does not undergo any first-pass effect when given IV. Thus, the effective dose of IV metoprolol is half of the oral dose. The first-pass effect explains why the following metoprolol regimens have approximately the same clinical effect at heart rate and blood pressure lowering:
- metoprolol 25 mg twice daily by mouth (50 mg/day)
- metoprolol 5 mg IV every 6 hours (20 mg/day)

Food and Drug Interactions That Affect Absorption
Food and enteral nutrition formulas may increase or decrease the absorption of some enterally administered medications, such as the following:

- Phenytoin, an antiseizure medication, has decreased absorption when administered with food.
- Ciprofloxacin, an antibiotic, has decreased absorption when administered with food.
- Rivaroxaban, an anticoagulant, has increased absorption when administered with food.

Medications that affect gastric acidity may affect the absorption of other drugs, such as the following:

- Proton pump inhibitors (PPIs) and histamine-2 receptor blockers (H2RAs) raise gastric pH.
- Atazanavir, an HIV drug, and itraconazole, an antifungal drug, have reduced absorption when gastric pH is elevated.

There are a variety of ways to minimize or avoid these interactions, such as the following:

- Use alternative medications (e.g., substitute phenytoin with an alternative like levetiracetam).
- Space out the medications (e.g., hold tube feeds 1 to 2 hours before and after the phenytoin dose).
- Use an alternative route of administration (e.g., convert from oral phenytoin to IV fosphenytoin, bypassing gastric absorption issues altogether).
- Temporarily discontinue the medication, if it is safe to do so, until absorption interactions are no longer present.

DISTRIBUTION

Distribution is the movement of drug from the systemic circulation to peripheral tissues. Volume of distribution (Vd) is a relative measure of how extensively a drug distributes from the systemic circulation to other body compartments. This is an apparent volume that relates the plasma concentration of a drug with its dose.

For a drug to move from one body compartment to another, like the systemic circulation to peripheral tissues, the drug must travel across plasma cell membranes. In general, this process is easier for fat-soluble drugs than water-soluble drugs.

The blood–brain barrier is a tight layer of capillary endothelial cells separating the central nervous system (CNS) compartment from the systemic circulation. It limits the passage of toxins, drugs, and other compounds from entering CNS through passive diffusion. It is very difficult for large and water-soluble compounds to cross this semipermeable membrane. Small and fat-soluble drug molecules tend to enter the CNS more easily.

The greater a drug's Vd, the more widely the drug distributes throughout the body. Medications with a small Vd tend to stay within the systemic circulation. Medications with a large Vd leave the systemic circulation for peripheral body compartments. This is typically quantified in liters per kilogram of body weight:

- small Vd: <0.25 L/kg, drug remains mostly in the bloodstream
- mid-range Vd: 0.25 to 0.7 L/kg, drug moderately distributes outside the bloodstream
- large Vd: >0.7 L/kg, drug distributes extensively to cells and tissues outside the bloodstream

Factors that are generally associated with larger drug distribution include:

- high degree of lipophilicity
- low degree of drug binding to plasma proteins (e.g., albumin)
- high degree of affinity for a drug's peripheral binding sites

Drugs with a high degree of lipophilicity (i.e., fat solubility) generally distribute quickly and readily outside of the systemic circulation. Patients with obesity may have larger dosing requirements for some lipophilic drugs. Drugs that are more water soluble, or hydrophilic, have a greater propensity to stay within the systemic circulation. However, in settings of acute volume overload, such as during acute heart failure (HF), acute renal failure, or aggressive volume resuscitation, drugs may display a larger volume of distribution than normal. This is because there is a larger volume of water outside of the systemic circulation.

Drugs within systemic circulation may bind to plasma proteins. These large proteins are unable to easily distribute to extravascular tissue. As a result of drug–protein binding, drug distribution is reduced; the drugs are "trapped" by proteins and remain within the bloodstream. Drugs that bind to plasma proteins are in equilibrium between a protein-bound and an unbound, or "free," state. Unbound drugs are more free to distribute to outside the systemic circulation. Albumin is the most common plasma protein to which drugs are bound. During acute and critical illness, albumin plasma concentrations may drop precipitously, resulting in an increased fraction of unbound drugs. This can result in a larger distribution of free drug that distributes to peripheral tissues.

Vd can be calculated using the following formula (see also Box 4.3):

$$Vd = (Drug\ dose)/Plasma\ concentration$$

A drug's Vd may influence its safety and efficacy for acute illness. Consider a patient with a bloodstream infection due to endocarditis. The infection is limited to the bloodstream, so an antibiotic that stays within the systemic circulation would be preferable to one that distributes widely to peripheral tissues. By contrast, for a patient with meningitis, where the infection is within the CNS, it would be preferable to use an antibiotic with a large Vd that is able to distribute across the blood–brain barrier.

Box 4.3

For example, if Drug A is administered to a patient at a dose of 1,500 mg, and the resulting plasma concentration after distribution has occurred is 50 mg/L, we can calculate the Vd of Drug A as follows:

$$Vd = 1,500\ mg \div 50\frac{mg}{L} = 30\ L$$

Of course, 30 L is not an actual physiologic volume. Rather, it represents the degree to which Drug A distributes out of the systemic circulation. We can also express Drug A's Vd relative to the patient's body weight. If the patient in this example weighed 70 kg, then the Vd of Drug A would be 30 L per 70 kg, or ~0.4 L/kg. Drug A would be classified as having a mid-range Vd.

A drug's average distribution is typically reported in the "Pharmacokinetics" section of the package insert. This information can be useful when trying to determine an optimal dose for drugs with a narrow therapeutic index and a wide interpatient variability. To do this, the Vd formula can be rearranged as follows:

$$Drug\ dose = Vd \times Plasma\ concentration$$

In this case, the plasma concentration is a desired target blood concentration (see Box 4.4).

Box 4.4

For example, phenytoin, an antiseizure medication, has an average Vd of 0.7 L/kg. In addition, the desired plasma concentration of phenytoin is between 10 and 20 mg/L for optimal safety and efficacy. For a patient weighing 70 kg, we can calculate the dose needed to achieve a plasma concentration of 15 mg/L (the middle of the desired range), as follows:

$$Drug\ dose = 0.7\ L/kg \times 70\ kg \times 15\ mg/L = 735\ mg$$

In practice, the dose could be safely rounded up to 750 mg.

METABOLISM

Metabolism (or biotransformation) is the chemical alteration of a drug to form a metabolite that is (usually) less active and more excretable than its parent compound. Not all drugs undergo metabolism; some drugs are eliminated unchanged. Metabolism most often occurs in the liver but can also occur in other organs, including small intestines, kidneys, brain, lung, and bloodstream. Reductions in liver function, whether due to acute illness, chronic disease, or advanced age, can slow the metabolism of drugs, resulting in increased and prolonged drug effects.

Phase 1 metabolism is mediated by the cytochrome P450 (CYP450) enzyme system. These enzymes facilitate chemical oxidation, reduction, and hydrolysis reactions and prepare drug substrates for further metabolic reactions. There are many different isoenzymes of the CYP450 system. Some of the more common enzymes include CYP450-1A2, CYP450-2B6, CYP450-2C9, CYP450-2C19, CYP450-2D6, CYP450-2E1, and CYP450-3A4. Not all drugs undergo phase 1 metabolism. For drugs that do undergo phase 1 metabolism, dose adjustments are typically necessary when liver dysfunction is present.

CYP450 Drug Interactions

In addition to being substrates for one or more of the CYP450 enzymes, drugs can be inducers or inhibitors of CYP450 isoenzymes. An inducer is a molecule that enhances the activity of CYP450 enzymes. When an enzyme is induced, it becomes more metabolically active, resulting in more robust metabolic clearance of drug substrates. An inhibitor is a molecule that reduces the activity of CYP450 enzymes. When an enzyme is inhibited, the metabolism of its drug substrates is reduced, resulting in slower clearance and increased drug exposure (see Box 4.5).

Box 4.5

For example, warfarin, an anticoagulant, is metabolized by CYP450-2C9. Amiodarone, an anti-arrhythmic drug, is an inhibitor of CYP450-2C9. For a patient who is on a stable dose of warfarin, the introduction of amiodarone to the patient's drug regimen could result in reduced metabolism of warfarin. This would lead to an increase in warfarin exposure with a resultant increased anticoagulant effect. Strategies to manage this drug interaction in the acute care setting could include:

- reducing the dose of warfarin and carefully monitoring the degree of anticoagulation
- transitioning to an alternative anticoagulant that is not metabolized by CYP450-2C9
- selecting an alternative anti-arrhythmic drug that does not inhibit CYP450-2C9

During *Phase 2 metabolism*, drugs are conjugated with large, polar molecules (e.g., glucuronic acid, methyl group, acetyl group, sulfate group), resulting in a compound that is more water soluble than the parent drug. The conjugated metabolite is more water soluble and more easily excreted through the urine than its unconjugated parent drug. Phase 2 metabolism is less affected by changes in liver function than phase 1 metabolism. Drugs that undergo only phase 2 metabolism often do not require dose adjustments in the setting of mild to moderate hepatic impairment.

ELIMINATION

Elimination is the removal of drug or metabolite from the body without further chemical change. *Clearance* is the volume of blood that is cleared of a specific substance (e.g., a drug) per unit time. The faster a drug's clearance, the more quickly that drug is eliminated from the body.

Many drugs are eliminated by way of passive filtration across the glomerular membrane within the kidneys. Thus, knowing a patient's glomerular filtration rate (GFR) can help estimate the ability of the kidneys to eliminate renally eliminated drugs. We can estimate a patient's GFR by determining their ability to clear creatinine. Creatinine is a breakdown product of muscle tissue; it enters the bloodstream at a steady rate, and it is eliminated from the body, unchanged, exclusively via glomerular filtration. Creatine clearance (CrCl), therefore, is used as a surrogate measurement of GFR. CrCl is the volume of blood (milliliters) that is cleared of creatinine per unit time (minutes). For the purposes of drug dosing, CrCl is typically estimated using the Cockcroft–Gault equation:

$$CrCl = \frac{(140 - \textit{Age in years})(\textit{Patient weight in kilograms})(0.85 \textit{ if female sex})}{72(Serum creatinine concentration in mg/dL)}$$

For drugs that require renal dosing adjustments for CrCl below 40 mL/min, we would choose the adjusted dose. For drugs that require renal dosing adjustments for CrCl below 30 mL/min, the decision to choose the adjusted dose should carefully consider the risks of overdosing versus underdosing.

The Cockroft–Gault formula has a few important limitations:

- It is only reliable when the patient's kidney function is stable. It will not be reliable in patients with acute worsening or improvement of renal function.
- It is not a reliable predictor of drug clearance in certain acute care situations where renal function may be temporarily enhanced (e.g., severe burns, critical illness).
- It may not reliably predict drug clearance among patients who are significantly over or under their ideal body weight.

Half-life (t1/2) is the amount of time it takes for a drug's plasma concentration to decrease by 50%. It takes approximately four to five half-lives for a drug to be considered completely removed from the body:

- After one half-life, 50% of the drug is eliminated.
- After two half-lives, 75% of the drug is eliminated.

- After three half-lives, 87.5% of the drug is eliminated.
- After four half-lives, 93.75% of the drug is eliminated.
- After five half-lives, 96.86% of the drug is eliminated.

A drug's half-life is directly proportional to its Vd and indirectly proportional to its clearance: t1/2 = 0.693 VdCl. Drugs with larger Vd and slower clearance have longer half-lives than drugs with smaller Vd and faster clearance.

STEADY STATE

Steady state is when the rate of drug entering the systemic circulation equals the rate of drug exiting the systemic circulation (rate in = rate out). This concept applies to drugs that are given on a regularly scheduled basis. Each new dose "stacks" upon the remaining previous doses. This dose stacking continues until the first dose is fully cleared from the body. Since it takes four to five half-lives to clear the first dose, it takes four to five half-lives until steady-state blood concentrations are achieved. Loading doses can help achieve therapeutic concentrations more quickly (see Box 4.6).

Box 4.6

For example:
- Lorazepam is a benzodiazepine drug used to treat alcohol withdrawal.
- Scheduled lorazepam regimens are used to treat severe cases of alcohol withdrawal.
- Lorazepam has a half-life of approximately 12 hours.
- A scheduled regimen of lorazepam would take 2 to 3 days (48–60 hours) to reach steady state.
- As blood concentrations of lorazepam slowly approach steady-state concentrations, the patient may require additional bolus doses (loading doses) to temporarily achieve therapeutic blood concentrations that effectively control withdrawal symptoms.
- The need for these as-needed loading doses should decrease as the maintenance regimen approaches its steady-state concentration.

During settings of acute or critical illness, renal function may fluctuate. As a result, renal drug elimination may also fluctuate. Estimates of renal function using clinical observations (e.g., changes in hourly urine output) or measurements (urine or serum creatinine concentrations) may help provide insight. Therapeutic drug monitoring of plasma drug concentrations (if available) and clinical endpoints for efficacy and toxicity should be diligently monitored in the setting of fluctuating renal function.

▶ PHARMACOLOGY OF ANTICOAGULATION

Many disease states and pathologies are treated or managed with anticoagulation. Therefore, the AGACNP must have an understanding of these medications. Understanding these pharmacologic properties will enable the AGACNP to make the best choice when it comes to prescribing anticoagulation. What follows is a summary of anticoagulants commonly used in clinical practice.

ANTICOAGULATION

Options for anticoagulation therapy have been expanding in recent years, providing various agents for the management of thromboembolic diseases. Choosing an anticoagulant in the inpatient setting is often informed by pharmacokinetic and pharmacodynamics considerations and formulary restrictions. Patient preference and insurance coverage are also important, especially at discharge, as it considers cost as well as route and frequency of administration, all of which can affect adherence post hospitalization.

PARENTERAL ANTICOAGULANTS

Heparins, including unfractionated heparin (UFH), low-molecular-weight heparin (LMWH) and fondaparinux, are used extensively in practice and will be the focus in this review (Table 4.2). LMWHs are derived via enzymatic or chemical depolymerization of UFH, while fondaparinux consists of the minimal antithrombin (AT)-binding region of heparin. Heparins inactivate factor Xa through an AT-dependent mechanism, but UFH also inhibits thrombin, and fondaparinux appears to exclusively target factor Xa. UFH and LMWHs do not cross the placenta and can be used in pregnancy; however, multiple dose vials may contain benzyl alcohol that crosses the placenta, potentially leading to fetal harm. If considered in pregnancy, the preservative-free preparations should be used. Fondaparinux use in pregnancy should be limited as potential concerns include its longer half-life, the possibility of underdosing as pregnancy weight increases, and the potential of crossing the placenta.

Table 4.2 Parenteral Anticoagulants

Parenteral Anticoagulant	Advantages	Limitations
UFH	▪ Rapid onset and offset of actions provide flexibility in dose titration or discontinuation when needed ▪ Easy monitoring using aPTT, anti-factor Xa activity, or ACT ▪ Lack of substantial elimination by the kidneys, allowing use in kidney disease ▪ Reversible using protamine sulfate	▪ Short half-life, typically necessitating administration via continuous infusion for therapeutic levels of anticoagulation ▪ Highly variable dose–response relationship, necessitating frequent laboratory monitoring ▪ Potential complications including HIT
LMWH	▪ Subcutaneous administration often facilitates outpatient treatment ▪ Laboratory monitoring not frequently needed ▪ Lower risk of HIT than UFH	▪ Less reversibility with protamine ▪ Requires dose adjustments in patients with renal failure (enoxaparin) ▪ When monitoring is indicated, anti-factor Xa activity testing with a rapid turnaround time may not be available
Fondaparinux	▪ Longer half-life than UFH and LMWH allowing once-daily dosing ▪ Negligible risk of HIT ▪ Laboratory monitoring not frequently needed ▪ May be used in treat HIT	▪ No approved antidote or reversal agent ▪ If monitoring is indicated, availability of fondaparinux-calibrated anti-factor Xa levels is lacking ▪ Contraindicated in renal failure

ACT, activated clotting time; aPTT, activated partial thromboplastin time; HIT, heparin-induced thrombocytopenia; LMWH, low-molecular-weight heparin; UFH, unfractionated heparin.

ORAL ANTICOAGULANTS

Available oral anticoagulants include vitamin K antagonist (warfarin), factor Xa inhibitors (apixaban, rivaroxaban, and edoxaban), and direct thrombin inhibitors (dabigatran; Table 4.3). Because edoxaban and dabigatran are not used frequently in the inpatient setting, this review focuses on warfarin, apixaban, and rivaroxaban.

Table 4.3 Oral Anticoagulants

Oral Anticoagulant	Advantages	Limitations
Warfarin	▪ Extensive clinical experience with its prescribing and monitoring ▪ Preferred agent with heparin in antiphospholipid syndrome ▪ Monitoring is widely available using INR ▪ Proven efficacy in mechanical prosthetic heart valves	▪ Pharmacokinetics is affected by vitamin K intake and production as well as induction of hepatic cytochromes ▪ Many drug interactions via hepatic cytochromes
Apixaban	▪ Lower risk of bleeding compared to warfarin ▪ Less laboratory monitoring ▪ Preferable pharmacokinetic profile ▪ Can take with or without food ▪ Used in renal failure ▪ May be used to treat HIT	▪ Not used in mechanical prosthetic heart valves ▪ Hepatically metabolized thus limiting use in severe hepatic impairment ▪ Twice-daily dosing may affect patient adherence

(continued)

Table 4.3 Oral Anticoagulants (*continued*)

Oral Anticoagulant	Advantages	Limitations
Rivaroxaban	■ Lower risk of bleeding compared to warfarin, but higher risk when compared to apixaban ■ Less laboratory monitoring ■ Preferable pharmacokinetic profile ■ Once-daily dosing may improve patient adherence ■ May be used to treat HIT	■ Not used in mechanical prosthetic heart valves ■ Hepatically metabolized thus limiting use in severe hepatic impairment ■ 15- and 20-mg dosage forms must be taken with food to improve absorption

HIT, heparin-induced thrombocytopenia; INR, international normalized ratio.

Warfarin inhibits vitamin K–dependent clotting factors and proteins C and S. Its dosing varies and is individualized based on the patient's comorbidities, concomitant medications, and international normalized ratio (INR). Factor Xa inhibitors inactivate circulating and clot-bound factor Xa. Unlike warfarin, apixaban and rivaroxaban are administered at fixed doses without monitoring. If needed, anti-Xa activity can be measured in specific circumstances (such as altered gastrointestinal [GI] anatomy, which affects drug absorption); however, the levels should be used to ensure absorption and not to inform therapeutic range. There are limited data for the use of apixaban and rivaroxaban in pregnancy, while warfarin is contraindicated in pregnancy.

TRANSITIONING BETWEEN ANTICOAGULANTS

The AGACNP will be responsible to transition patients between anticoagulants for various reasons. Knowledge of these medications is imperative (Table 4.4). Specific transitions that can occur are as follows:

■ *Heparin to warfarin*: Co-administer the two anticoagulants for a minimum of 5 days (overlapping), and discontinue the parenteral anticoagulant when the INR is therapeutic (2–3 or 2.5–3.5) for at least 24 hours.

■ *Heparin to apixaban or rivaroxaban*: The maximal anticoagulant effect of apixaban and rivaroxaban occurs 2 to 3 hours after the first dose. IV UFH can be stopped when the first dose of the apixaban or rivaroxaban is taken. When transitioning from LMWH, apixaban or rivaroxaban should be given 2 hours before the next dose of the LMWH would have been due.

■ *Apixaban/rivaroxaban to warfarin*: Discontinue apixaban/rivaroxaban and start a parenteral anticoagulant with warfarin.

■ *Warfarin to apixaban/rivaroxaban*: Discontinue warfarin and initiate apixaban when INR is less than 2; discontinue warfarin and initiate rivaroxaban when INR is less than 3.

Table 4.4 Transitioning Anticoagulants

Anticoagulant	Pharmacokinetics	Dosing (Select Indications)	Special Considerations/ Reversal Agents
Parenteral			
UFH	■ Half-life: 1–2 hours ■ Onset: IV—immediate. SUBQ ~20–30 minutes ■ Excretion: urine; nonrenal at therapeutic doses ■ Metabolism: via reticuloendothelial system	VTE prophylaxis ■ Medically ill: 5,000 units SUBQ every 8–12 hours ■ Postoperatively (hip fracture, knee or total hip arthroplasty): 5,000 units SUBQ every 8–12 hours	■ For weight-based heparin, a specific dosing nomogram may help achieve therapeutic anticoagulation while minimizing bleeding risk. ■ aPTT, anti-Xa activity, and ACT are used to monitor IV UFH depending on indication. ■ Protamine sulfate reverses the anticoagulant effects of UFH (100% neutralization).

(continued)

Table 4.4 Transitioning Anticoagulants (*continued*)

Anticoagulant	Pharmacokinetics	Dosing (Select Indications)	Special Considerations/Reversal Agents
		VTE treatment ■ 80 units/kg IV bolus followed by continuous infusion of 18 units/kg/hr ■ 5,000 units IV bolus followed by continuous infusion of 1,333 units/hr	
		ACS ■ 50–70 units/kg IV bolus followed by continuous infusion of 12 units/kg/hr *Max bolus and infusion doses may apply depending on use of fibrinolysis and reperfusion*	
		A-fib (prevention of stroke): ■ 60–80 units/kg IV bolus (max 5,000 units) followed by continuous infusion of 12–18 units/kg/hr (max 1,000 units/hr) *Used for bridging purposes in high-risk patients when oral anticoagulation is disrupted*	
Enoxaparin	■ Half-life: 4.5–7 hours ■ Onset: SUBQ 3–5 hours ■ Excretion: urine (40% as active and inactive) ■ Metabolism: hepatic via desulfation and depolymerization	VTE prophylaxis ■ Medically ill: 40 mg SUBQ every 24 hours ■ Postoperative: 40 mg SUBQ every 24 hours ■ Postoperative: 30 mg SUBQ every 12 hours ■ Trauma: 40 mg SUBQ every 12 hours	■ Duration of therapy for postoperative prophylaxis is 7–10 days. ■ When CrCl <30 mL/min, prophylaxis dose is reduced to 30 mg SUBQ daily. ■ When CrCl <30 mL/min, treatment dose is reduced to 1 m/kg SUBQ daily. ■ Protamine sulfate reverses the anticoagulant effects of LMWH (40%–60% neutralization).
		VTE treatment ■ 1 mg/kg SUBQ q12h ■ 1.5 mg/kg SUBQ once daily	
		ACS ■ NSTEMI: 1 mg/kg SUBQ q12h ■ STEMI[a]: 30-mg IV bolus followed by 1 mg/kg SUBQ q12h (max 100 mg for the first two doses only)	
Fondaparinux	■ Half-life: 17–21 hours ■ Onset: 2–3 hours ■ Excretion: urine (up to 77% as unchanged)	VTE prophylaxis ■ Medically ill: 2.5 mg SUBQ daily ■ Postoperative 2.5 mg SUBQ daily	■ Contraindicated when CrCl <30 mL/min ■ Contraindicated in VTE prophylaxis when weight <50 kg ■ No approved reversal agent
		VTE treatment Dose is weight-based: ■ <50 kg: 5 mg SUBQ daily ■ 50–100 kg: 7.5 mg SUBQ daily ■ >100 kg: 10 mg SUBQ daily	

(*continued*)

Table 4.4 Transitioning Anticoagulants (*continued*)

Anticoagulant	Pharmacokinetics	Dosing (Select Indications)	Special Considerations/ Reversal Agents
Oral			
Warfarin	▪ Half-life: 20–60 hours (depending on clotting factors) ▪ Onset: 24–72 hours; full effect may take 5–7 days ▪ Excretion: urine (92% as metabolites) ▪ Metabolism: hepatic via CYP2C9 (major), CYP3A4, CYP1A2, CYP2C8, CYP2C18, CYP2C19 (minor)	▪ Dose is chosen to maintain therapeutic INR (2–3 or 2.5–3.5) depending on indication. ▪ Starting dose is 5 mg in most patients. ● Lower doses are used in sensitive patients (1–3 mg).	▪ Not used for VTE prophylaxis in medically ill patients ▪ Drug/drug/food/disease interactions may lead to supra- or subtherapeutic INR. ▪ Vitamin K (PO or IV) reverses effects of warfarin. PCC (Kcentra) is used for major bleeding or when urgent reversal is required. Kcentra must be used with vitamin K. Fresh frozen plasma may be used but is not considered first line.

Apixaban	▪ Half-life: ~12 hours
	▪ Onset: 3–4 hours
	▪ Excretion: urine (27% as parent drug) and feces
	▪ Metabolism: hepatic via CYP3A4/5 (major), CYP1A2, CYP2C8, CYP2C9, CYP2C19 (minor)
	▪ Substrate of P-gp
		VTE prophylaxis
		▪ Postoperative: 2.5 mg every 12 hours for 12 days or 35 days, respectively
		Start 12–24 hours after surgery
		
		VTE treatment
		▪ 10 mg every 12 hours × 7 days, then 5 mg every 12 hours for 3–6 months
		
		Reducing risk of recurrent VTE
		▪ 2.5 mg every 12 hours
		
		Nonvalvular A-fib (prevention of stroke)
		▪ 5 mg every 12 hours
			▪ Andexanet alfa reverses the anticoagulant effects of apixaban. PCC (Kcentra) is also used.
			▪ No dose adjustment for renal impairment, including dialysis
			▪ No dose adjustment for mild to moderate hepatic impairment
			▪ Not recommended in severe hepatic impairment
			▪ Dose reduction is recommended for patients who are also receiving strong dual inhibitors of CYP3A4 and P-glycoprotein.
			▪ In patients with nonvalvular A-fib who meet two of the following criteria, the dose must be reduced to 2.5 mg every 12 hours:
			  ● age ≥80 years
			  ● weight ≤60 kg
			  ● SCr ≥1.5 mg/dL

(continued)

Table 4.4 Transitioning Anticoagulants (*continued*)

Anticoagulant	Pharmacokinetics	Dosing (Select Indications)	Special Considerations/ Reversal Agents
Rivaroxaban	▪ Half-life: 5–9 hours (11–13 in elderly) ▪ Onset: 2–4 hours ▪ Excretion: urine (66%; 36% as parent drug) and feces ▪ Metabolism: hepatic via CYP3A4/5 and CYP2J2 ▪ Substrate of P-gp	**VTE prophylaxis:** ▪ Medically ill[b]: 10 mg daily for 31–39 days ▪ Postoperatively[c]: 10 mg daily for 12 days or 35 days, respectively **VTE treatment** ▪ 15 mg every 12 hours × 21 days, then 20 mg daily **Reducing risk of recurrent VTE** ▪ 10 mg daily **Nonvalvular A-fib (prevention of stroke):** ▪ 20 mg daily **CAD** ▪ Reduces risk of major cardiovascular events: 2.5 mg every 12 hours + aspirin 75 mg daily **PAD** ▪ Reduces risk of major thrombotic events: 2.5 mg every 12 hours + aspirin 75 mg daily	▪ Not recommended in moderate to severe hepatic impairment ▪ Dose reduction is recommended for patients who are also receiving strong dual inhibitors of CYP3A4 and P-glycoprotein. ▪ In nonvalvular A-fib, the dose is reduced to 15 mg daily when CrCl ≤50 mL/ min. ▪ No renal dosing adjustments in CAD and PAD ▪ Avoid use when CrCl <15 mL/min in all VTE-related indications. ▪ Andexanet alfa reverses the effects of rivaroxaban. PCC (Kcentra) is also used.

Note: [a]For ≥75 years, IV bolus is not administered.
[b]Start in hospital and continue after discharge.
[c]Start 6–10 hours after surgery.
CAD, coronary artery disease; CrCl, creatine clearance; INR, international normalized ratio; IV, intravenous; LMWH, low-molecular-weight heparin; NSTEMI, non-ST elevation myocardial infarction; PAD, peripheral arterial disease; PCC, prothrombin complex concentrate; SCr, serum creatinine; STEMI, ST elevation myocardial infarction; UFH, unfractionated heparin; VTE, venous thromboembolism.

Clinical Pearls

▪ For oral factor Xa inhibitors, use the patient's actual body weight when calculating CrCl.
▪ For weight-based anticoagulants, make sure an accurate weight is documented.
▪ Check for drug interactions, and adjust doses of anticoagulants when applicable.
▪ If bleeding occurs, identify root causes and contributing factors to prevent recurrence.
▪ If discharging patients on rivaroxaban or apixaban for venous thromboembolism (VTE) treatment, the patient must have two prescriptions to cover both the initiation phase and the maintenance phase.

▶ PHARMACOLOGY OF ANTIMICROBIALS

A wide range of antimicrobial therapies is available to treat infections. Appropriate use depends on the setting, severity, infection site, organism(s) of concern, local and regional resistance, side effects, interactions, and patient-specific factors. What follows is a summary of antibiotics and antiviral and antifungal agents commonly used in clinical practice.

BETA-LACTAMS

This antibiotic class includes penicillins, cephalosporins, carbapenems, and monobactams. They disrupt bacterial cell wall synthesis by blocking key enzymes (penicillin-binding proteins [PBPs]) responsible for cell wall construction. Beta-lactams exhibit time-dependent activity; they exert the greatest antibiotic effect when their blood concentrations exceed the minimum inhibitory concentration (MIC) of the target organism. Optimized regimens are those with concentrations that exceed the MIC for at least 40% to 60% of the dosing interval. Variations in spectrum of activity between the different penicillin classes exist based on innate and acquired resistance mechanisms. Penicillins and cephalosporins may be combined with beta-lactamase (BL) inhibitors (e.g., sulbactam, tazobactam, clavulanic acid, relebactam, avibactam, vaborbactam) to overcome BL-mediated resistance.

PENICILLINS

Penicillins are bactericidal antibiotics originally derived from molds. They are effective against gram-positive and some gram-negative organisms. Semisynthetic penicillin classes have a broader microbiologic activity (Table 4.5).

Table 4.5 Penicillin-Derived Beta-Lactams: Microbiologic Activity and Common Uses

Agent (Common Route)	Microbiologic Activity	Notes/Common Uses
Natural penicillins Penicillin G (IV/IM) Penicillin VK (PO)	▪ Gram-positive coverage—*Streptococcus pyogenes, S. pneumoniae, Enterococcus* ▪ No *Staphylococcus aureus* coverage ▪ Gram-positive anaerobes	▪ Syphilis (PCN G) ▪ Pharyngitis
Aminopenicillin Ampicillin (IV/PO) Amoxicillin (IV/PO)	▪ Gram-positive coverage—*S. pyogenes, S. pneumoniae, Enterococcus* ▪ No *S. aureus* coverage ▪ Gram-positive anaerobes ▪ Some *Escherichia coli* and *Proteus mirabilis*	▪ Coverage like natural penicillins plus coverage of some *E. coli* and *Proteus mirabilis* ▪ Upper respiratory infections ▪ Community-acquired pneumonia ▪ Enterococcal infections
Aminopenicillin/BL inhibitor Ampicillin/sulbactam (IV) Amoxicillin/clavulanic acid (PO)	▪ Aminopenicillin plus MSSA, BL-positive *E. coli* and *Proteus, Haemophilus influenzae, Moraxella catarrhalis*, gram-negative anaerobic rods (*Bacteroides fragilis*)	▪ BL inhibitor adds coverage for some BL + organisms (not those producing extended-spectrum BL) ▪ Nausea/vomiting with clavulanic acid
Penicillinase resistant Nafcillin (IV) Oxacillin (IV) Dicloxacillin (PO)	▪ Gram-positive coverage: MSSA, *S. pyogenes, S. pneumoniae*	▪ Cellulitis ▪ Endocarditis ▪ Nafcillin: risk of interstitial nephritis
Extended-spectrum penicillin Piperacillin/tazobactam (IV)	▪ Aminopenicillin/BL inhibitor coverage plus *P. aeruginosa*	▪ Nosocomial pneumonia ▪ Intra-abdominal infection ▪ Severe skin and soft tissue

BL, beta-lactamase; IM, intramuscular; IV, intravenous; MSSA, methicillin-susceptible *Staphylococcus aureus*.

CEPHALOSPORINS

Cephalosporins possess similar properties to penicillins, but they are molecularly distinct from penicillins, containing different side chain components in their chemical structure. They are commonly used as first-line agents (Table 4.6). Notably, there is no enterococcal coverage as a class.

Table 4.6 Cephalosporins: Microbiologic Activity and Common Uses

Agent (Common Route)	Microbiologic Activity	Notes/Common Uses
First Generation Cefazolin (IV) Cephalexin (PO) Cefadroxil (PO)	▨ MSSA, streptococcus species ▨ *Proteus, Escherichia coli* ▨ Gram-positive anaerobes	▨ Mild skin or soft tissue infections ▨ Severe MSSA infections (cefazolin) ▨ Low CNS penetration
Second generation Cefuroxime (PO) Cefaclor (PO) Cefdinir (PO) Cefpodoxime (PO)	▨ MSSA, streptococcus species ▨ *Proteus, E. coli* ▨ *Haemophilus influenzae, Moraxella catarrhalis* ▨ Gram-positive anaerobes	▨ Sinusitis, pharyngitis, otitis media
Second generation Cefotetan (IV) Cefoxitin (IV)	▨ MSSA, streptococcus species ▨ *Proteus, E. coli* ▨ Gram-positive anaerobes ▨ Gram-negative anaerobic rods (*Bacteroides fragilis*)	▨ Surgical prophylaxis, ▨ *B. fragilis* coverage insufficient for treatment of active intra-abdominal infection
Third generation Cefotaxime (IV) Ceftriaxone (IV)	▨ Moderate-good gram-positive activity: *Streptococcus pneumoniae,* GAS ▨ Expanded gram-negative activity: Enterobacterales, respiratory bugs, *not Pseudomonas aeruginosa* ▨ Gram-positive anaerobes	▨ Community-acquired pneumonia, otitis media, upper respiratory tract infections, meningitis, UTI ▨ Ceftriaxone dosed once daily (twice daily in CNS infection)
Third generation Ceftazidime (IV)	▨ Poor gram-positive activity ▨ Expanded gram-negative activity: Enterobacterales, respiratory bugs, *P. aeruginosa*	▨ Community-acquired pneumonia, lower respiratory tract infections, meningitis, UTI, abdominal
Fourth generation Cefepime (IV)	▨ Moderate-good gram-positive activity: *S. pneumoniae,* GAS ▨ Expanded gram-negative activity: Enterobacterales, respiratory bugs, *P. aeruginosa* ▨ Gram-positive anaerobes	▨ Meningitis, febrile neutropenia, pneumonia, nosocomial infections, pyelonephritis ▨ Has the gram-positive characteristics of ceftriaxone and the gram-negative characteristics of ceftazidime
Newer Cephalosporins and Combinations with BL Inhibitors		
Fifth generation Ceftaroline (IV)	▨ Methicillin-susceptible *and* MRSA, streptococcus species ▨ *Proteus* (*not* vulgaris), *E. coli* ▨ *H. influenzae, M. catarrhalis* ▨ Gram-positive anaerobes	▨ Only cephalosporin with some MRSA coverage

(*continued*)

Table 4.6 Cephalosporins: Microbiologic Activity and Common Uses (*continued*)

Agent (Common Route)	Microbiologic Activity	Notes/Common Uses
Cephalosporin/BL inhibitor combination Ceftazidime/avibactam (IV)	▪ Ceftazidime coverage plus gram-negative organisms expressing extended-spectrum BL, *Klebsiella pneumoniae* carbapenemases, or AmpC BL	▪ Reserve for organisms expressing resistance via the described mechanisms
Cephalosporin/BL inhibitor combination Ceftolozane/ tazobactam (IV)	▪ Ceftazidime coverage plus some gram-negative organisms that may be ceftazidime-resistant and gram-negative anaerobic rods (*B. fragilis*)	▪ This combination is less susceptible to AmpC beta-lactamases
Siderophore-conjugated Cefiderocol (IV)	▪ Gram-negative coverage with little or no clinically relevant gram-positive coverage ▪ Reserve for extended-spectrum BL-producing Enterobacterales and multidrug-resistant *Pseudomonas*	▪ Unique cephalosporin that chelates free iron allowing transport through bacterial cell membrane

AmpC, ampicillin-resistance gene group C; BL, beta-lactamase; CNS, central nervous system; GAS, Group A Streptococcus; IV, intravenous; MRSA, methicillin-resistant *Staphylococcus aureus*; MSSA, methicillin-susceptible *Staphylococcus aureus*; UTI, urinary tract infection.

CARBAPENEMS

These beta-lactams have low cross-reactivity in the setting of penicillin allergy (less than 1%) and should be reserved for infections where multidrug-resistant organisms (MDROs) are suspected. Carbapenems are the antibiotic of choice for infections due to extended-spectrum beta-lactamase (ESBL)–producing organisms (Table 4.7).

Table 4.7 Carbapenem-Derived Beta-Lactams: Microbiologic Activity and Common Uses

Agent	Microbiologic Activity	Notes/Common Uses
Ertapenem (IV)	▪ Broad gram-positive and gram-negative coverage, including ESBL producers ▪ No MRSA activity ▪ No *Pseudomonas* activity	▪ UTI caused by ESBL producers ▪ Alternative when severe penicillin allergy ▪ Once-daily dosing
Meropenem (IV) Imipenem-cilastatin (IV)	▪ Broad gram-positive and gram-negative coverage, including ESBL producers and *Pseudomonas* ▪ No MRSA activity	▪ Reserved for MDROs or patients with severe penicillin allergy ▪ Decreases seizure threshold
Meropenem/vaborbactam (IV) Imipenem-cilastatin/ relebactam (IV)	▪ Expanded gram-negative coverage ▪ Covers organisms expressing *Klebsiella pneumoniae* carbapenemases and multidrug-resistant *Pseudomonas*	▪ Combinations with BL inhibitors

BL, beta-lactamase; ESBL, extended-spectrum beta-lactamase; IV, intravenous; MDRO, multidrug-resistant organism; MRSA, methicillin-resistant *Staphylococcus aureus*; UTI, urinary tract infection.

MONOBACTAMS

Monobactams are typically reserved for patients with a severe penicillin allergy. Aztreonam is the commercially available monobactam and has antipseudomonal activity but no gram-positive activity.

GENERAL BETA-LACTAM ADVERSE REACTIONS

Adverse reactions to beta-lactams include diarrhea, nausea, GI upset, rash, urticaria, *Clostridioides difficile*–associated diarrhea (more commonly associated with broad-spectrum penicillins and third-generation cephalosporins), seizure at high concentrations (notably cefepime and imipenem), bone marrow depression, and jaundice in neonates (ceftriaxone only).

BETA-LACTAM ALLERGY

Most patients with true penicillin allergies exhibit type 1 hypersensitivity. *Type 1 hypersensitivity* severity can range from rash to anaphylaxis and typically occurs 15 minutes to 2 hours after exposure. Type 2, type 3, and type 4 reactions vary in severity, may take 72 hours to weeks to manifest, and can include rash, Drug Reaction with Eosinophilia and Systemic Symptoms (DRESS), interstitial nephritis, Stevens–Johnson syndrome, and others. Cross-reactivity between penicillins and cephalosporins has been previously reported to be high as 10% but likely has a lower rate of 2% to 5%. There is a slightly increased risk of penicillins and cephalosporins having the same R1 side chain in their chemical structure (e.g., increased risk of cross-reactivity with administration of cefaclor, cephalexin, and cefadroxil in patients with ampicillin and amoxicillin allergy due to similar side chains of the drugs). Carbapenems have a low cross-reactivity (less than 1%) in patients with true penicillin allergies. Penicillin allergies should be frequently reassessed and properly documented in the patient chart. Assess and document reaction details, when the reaction occurred, how the reaction was managed, and whether similar antibiotics have been tolerated since the reaction. Penicillin skin tests followed by oral amoxicillin challenge may be appropriate to consider in certain cases.

BETA-LACTAM DRUG INTERACTIONS

There are few drug interactions with beta-lactams. One notable interaction is between carbapenems and valproic acid. Avoid this combination to prevent decreased levels of valproic acid.

GLYCOPEPTIDES (VANCOMYCIN IV/PO)

Vancomycin inhibits cell wall synthesis by binding to D-alanyl-D-alanine, resulting in efficacy against methicillin-resistant *Staphylococcus aureus* (MRSA). It has activity against gram-positive infections like those caused by staphylococci (including MRSA), streptococci, enterococci, and *C. difficile* (oral/rectal route only).

There are notable dosing and administration considerations for vancomycin. IV infusions should be administered at a maximum of 1 g/hr to avoid vancomycin infusion reactions. Vancomycin infusion reaction is a non–IgE histamine-based reaction causing rash, flushing, pruritis, and (uncommonly) hypotension; it resolves when infusion is stopped. A decreased rate of infusion of lower doses and pretreatment with hydroxyzine or diphenhydramine can allow continued therapy if reaction occurs. Serum concentration monitoring is indicated when prescribing this medication by the IV route.

Possible adverse reactions include nephrotoxicity, vancomycin infusion reaction (flushing, rash, pruritis), thrombophlebitis, thrombocytopenia, and ototoxicity.

OXAZOLIDINONES (LINEZOLID IV/PO, TEDIZOLID IV/PO)

The mechanism of action for oxazolidinones is by inhibiting protein synthesis by binding to the 50S ribosomal subunit. They have microbiologic activity against gram-positive bacteria, including MRSA and enterococcus.

Adverse effects include myelosuppression and thrombocytopenia with prolonged therapy. Significant drug–drug interactions are due to weak monoamine oxidase inhibitor (MAOI) properties. Use with caution or avoid in patients taking selective serotonin reuptake inhibitor (SSRI)/serotonin-norepinephrine reuptake inhibitor (SNRI)/MAOI therapies due to increased risk of serotonin syndrome.

CYCLIC LIPOPEPTIDE (DAPTOMYCIN IV)

The mechanism of action is by binding to the cell membrane, causing rapid depolarization of membrane potential with concentration-dependent bactericidal activity. Microbiologic activity is against gram-positives including MRSA, enterococcus, and vancomycin-resistant enterococcus.

Adverse effects include rhabdomyolysis, eosinophilic pneumonia (rare), peripheral neuropathy, chest pain, hypertension, headache, GI upset, and injection site reactions. Special consideration for prescribing includes the need for monitoring of plasma creatinine kinase and understanding that daptomycin is ineffective for pneumonia due to inactivation by pulmonary surfactant.

FLUOROQUINOLONES: CIPROFLOXACIN (IV/PO), LEVOFLOXACIN (IV/PO), OFLOXACIN (PO), MOXIFLOXACIN (IV/PO)

The mechanism of action inhibits DNA synthesis via inhibition of DNA gyrase (topoisomerase II) and topoisomerase IV. There is microbiologic activity against gram-positive organisms: penicillin-susceptible and -resistant *S. pneumoniae* (*not* ciprofloxacin); and against gram-negative organisms: Enterobacterales, *Pseudomonas aeruginosa* (ciprofloxacin, levofloxacin), *Haemophilus influenzae*, *Moraxella catarrhalis*, *Legionella pneumoniae*. (See Table 4.8 for coverage and drug choice.)

Table 4.8 Coverage and Drug Choice

Treatment	Drug
Gram-positive respiratory tract infections	Levofloxacin, ofloxacin, moxifloxacin
Gram-negative infections	Levofloxacin, ofloxacin, moxifloxacin, and ciprofloxacin (best coverage)
Urinary tract infections	Levofloxacin, ofloxacin, ciprofloxacin

Adverse effects include GI concerns (nausea, vomiting, diarrhea); *C. difficile* diarrhea (associated with infection from more virulent strain); CNS concerns (headache, dizziness, seizures, neuropsychiatric symptoms); tendinitis, tendon rupture, Achilles tendon injury; photosensitivity; QTc prolongation; peripheral neuropathy; worsening of myasthenia gravis (MG); severe decreases in blood glucose; increased risk for aortic rupture; and rash.

CLINDAMYCIN IV/PO

The mechanism of action is inhibition of protein synthesis by binding to the 50S ribosomal subunit. It has microbiologic activity against gram-positive organisms: *S. aureus*, MRSA (community-acquired only), *S. pneumoniae*; and anaerobic oral anaerobes: *Bacteroides fragilis*. Clindamycin is preferred over metronidazole for head, neck, and lung anaerobic infections; it is no longer recommended for treatment of intra-abdominal infections because of resistance from *B. fragilis* isolates.

Adverse effects include abdominal pain, *C. difficile*–associated diarrhea and colitis, diarrhea, esophagitis, nausea, and vomiting.

METRONIDAZOLE IV/PO

The mechanism of action is interaction with DNA to cause a loss of helical DNA structure and DNA degradation. There is microbiologic activity against oral anaerobes, *B. fragilis*, and *C. difficile*. Adverse effects include headache, nausea, dry mouth, and metallic taste. Metronidazole may increase concentrations of warfarin. There is also a risk of a disulfiram-like reaction with concomitant administration of alcohol-containing drug formulations.

MACROLIDES: ERYTHROMYCIN (IV/PO), CLARITHROMYCIN (PO), AZITHROMYCIN (IV/PO), FIDAXOMICIN (PO)

The mechanism of action is by inhibition of protein synthesis by binding to the 50S ribosomal subunit. Microbiologic activity for erythromycin, clarithromycin, and azithromycin includes gram-positive: *S. aureus* (not MRSA), *S. pneumoniae*; and gram-negative: *H. influenzae*, *M. catarrhalis*, *L. pneumoniae*. Fidaxomicin has microbiologic activity against *C. difficile*. Adverse effects include GI distress (nausea, vomiting, diarrhea, abdominal pain), QTc interval prolongation, and drug-induced hepatitis. Because of limited oral absorption, fidaxomicin adverse effects are limited to local GI distress. Avoid use with other agents that prolong QTc interval.

TETRACYCLINES: TETRACYCLINE (PO), DOXYCYCLINE (PO/IV)

The mechanism of action is through inhibition of protein synthesis by binding to the 30S ribosomal subunit. There is microbiologic activity against gram-positive: *S. aureus*, community-acquired MRSA (not hospital-acquired MRSA), *S. pneumoniae*; and gram-negative: *H. influenzae, M. catarrhalis, L. pneumoniae*. Adverse effects include GI intolerance, tooth discoloration in children (less of an issue with doxycycline), and photosensitivity.

TRIMETHOPRIM/SULFAMETHOXAZOLE (PO/IV)

Sulfamethoxazole and trimethoprim block sequential steps in the synthesis of folic acid, which is necessary for bacterial nucleic acid and protein formation. There is microbiologic activity against gram-positives: *S. aureus*, community-acquired MRSA, *S. pneumoniae*; and gram-negatives: *E. coli, Proteus, H. influenzae, M. catarrhalis*. Also, there is coverage of *Pneumocystis jirovecii*. Adverse effects include hypersensitivity reactions, blood dyscrasias, hyperkalemia/hyponatremia (with high-dose therapy), hypoglycemia, nausea, vomiting, and anorexia. Use caution when prescribed with drugs that can increase potassium (angiotensin-converting enzyme inhibitor [ACEI], angiotensin-receptor blocker [ARB], potassium-sparing diuretic); it may increase warfarin concentrations.

AMINOGLYCOSIDES: GENTAMICIN (IV), TOBRAMYCIN (IV), AMIKACIN (IV)

The mechanism of action is inhibition of protein synthesis by binding to the 30S ribosomal subunit. There is microbiologic activity against gram-positives: *S. aureus, Enterococcus*; and gram-negatives: rods and *Pseudomonas aeruginosa*. Adverse effects include nephrotoxicity and ototoxicity. Coadministration with other nephrotoxins may increase the risk of nephrotoxicity. Aminoglycosides are rarely used as monotherapy; they are typically combined with other antibacterial therapies for synergistic effects.

ANTIVIRALS
NEURAMINIDASE INHIBITORS: OSELTAMIVIR (PO), PERAMIVIR (IV), ZANAMIVIR INHALATION

The mechanism of action is inhibition of the influenza neuraminidase enzyme resulting in decreased viral aggregation and a reduction in the amount of virus that is released. These are effective against influenza A and B strains. Adverse effects include dose-related nausea and vomiting, confusion, delirium, and hallucination (primarily in children and adolescents). It may diminish efficacy of live/attenuated influenza vaccine if given within 2 weeks. Treatment demonstrates the best efficacy when initiated within 48 hours of symptom onset. It may be started more than 48 hours of symptoms in patients with severe disease or hospitalization. And, it can be used for treatment and exposure prophylaxis.

BALOXAVIR MARBOXIL (PO)

The mechanism of action is an endonuclease inhibitor that disrupts influenza virus replication. This is effective against influenza A and B strains. Adverse effects include nausea, diarrhea, headache, bronchitis, and nasopharyngitis. Polyvalent-cation-containing products and calcium-containing foods decrease serum concentrations of baloxavir and should be avoided. Baloxavir marboxil may diminish efficacy of live/attenuated influenza vaccine if given within 2 weeks. Treatment demonstrates best efficacy when initiated within 48 hours of symptom onset. It is given as a single dose. And, it can be used for treatment and exposure prophylaxis.

ACYCLOVIR PO/IV

The mechanism of action is inhibition of DNA synthesis and viral replication. Acyclovir has antiviral activity against herpes simplex virus, herpes zoster, and varicella zoster. Adverse effects include acute kidney injury due to renal crystal formation (risk with rapid infusion of high doses, IV administration, preexisting renal dysfunction, pediatric patients); neurotoxicity (confusion, agitation, lethargy, hallucination); thrombotic thrombocytopenic purpura (TTP); hemolytic uremic syndrome (HUS); and diarrhea, nausea, and vomiting. Renal dose adjustments are necessary. Older adults are more susceptible to CNS disturbances. Ensure patients are adequately hydrated during therapy.

VALACYCLOVIR (PO)
The mechanism of action (prodrug metabolized to acyclovir) is inhibition of DNA synthesis and viral replication. Valacyclovir has antiviral activity against herpes simplex virus and herpes zoster. Adverse effects include malaise, nausea, vomiting, increased liver function tests (LFTs), neutropenia, and elevated serum creatinine.

GANCICLOVIR (IV) AND VALGANCICLOVIR (PO)
Valganciclovir is a prodrug metabolized to ganciclovir. Ganciclovir inhibits the replication of viral DNA. There is antiviral activity against cytomegalovirus. Adverse effects include a boxed warning for myelosuppression, teratogenic and carcinogenic effects, fever, nausea, vomiting, thrombocytopenia, neutropenia, anemia, and elevated serum creatinine.

PAXLOVID
The mechanism of action is a peptidomimetic inhibitor inhibiting viral replication combined with a pharmacokinetic enhancer (ritonavir) that inhibits nirmatrelvir metabolism. This drug has antiviral activity against SARS-CoV-2. Adverse effects include hypertension, diarrhea, dysgeusia, and myalgia. There are numerous interactions due to CYP450 inhibitor properties of ritonavir.

ANTIFUNGALS
FLUCONAZOLE (PO/IV), ITRACONAZOLE (PO), KETOCONAZOLE (PO), VORICONAZOLE (PO/IV), POSACONAZOLE (PO/IV)
The mechanism of action is fungistatic activity that decreases ergosterol synthesis inhibiting cell membrane formation. There is antifungal activity against yeasts (*Candida albicans, Cryptococcus*) and dimorphic fungi; voriconazole has increased mold coverage and is the drug of choice for Aspergillosis; posaconazole has similar activity to voriconazole with added Mucormycosis and Zygomycosis activity.

Adverse effects include headache, dizziness, nausea, rash, elevated LFTs, liver toxicity, QT prolongation, hypokalemia, edema, and CNS toxicity and visual changes (voriconazole). Numerous drug interactions are due to CYP3A4, CYP2C19, and CYP2C9 inhibition; pH-dependent absorption for itraconazole and ketoconazole (decreased absorption with increased pH); and increased INR in patients on warfarin.

ECHINOCANDINS: MICONAZOLE, CASPOFUNGIN (IV)
The mechanism of action is by inhibition of the synthesis of the beta (1,3)-D-glucan component of fungal cell walls. This results in antifungal activity against yeast (multiple *Candida* species). Adverse effects include infusion reactions (rash, pruritis, facial swelling, hypotension), elevated LFTs, fever, hypokalemia, hypomagnesemia, nausea, and vomiting.

AMPHOTERICIN B (IV)
The mechanism of action is fungicidal activity to susceptible organisms via binding to ergosterol and altering membrane permeability resulting in antifungal activity against yeasts, molds, and dimorphic fungi. Adverse effects include nephrotoxicity, infusion reactions, fever, headache, hypokalemia, hypomagnesemia, and rigors. There is increased risk of nephrotoxicity when combined with other nephrotoxic agents; use with caution when combined with other agents that decrease sodium and magnesium levels

▶ PHARMACOLOGY OF THE CARDIOVASCULAR SYSTEM

Cardiovascular medications are widely prescribed and/or continued in the acute care setting. Knowledge of acute and chronic uses of these medications is a must for the AGACNP. This section reviews the pharmacology of specific cardiovascular medications.

ANGIOTENSIN-CONVERTING ENZYME INHIBITORS

ACEIs, ARBs, and direct renin inhibitors lower blood pressure (BP) by modulating various related renal mechanisms. ACEIs and ARBs are pharmacologically distinct and different, though both are effective and frequently used to manage hypertension and HF. These drugs and classes are not directly interchangeable but may be therapeutically equivalent when titrated to effect (goal BP) or when using validated dosing protocols. Each class is considered on its own, and some clinical benefits may be drug specific, apart from the class (not all drugs in the class are equal).

ACEIs lower BP and increase natriuresis by blocking ACE and limiting conversion of angiotensin I to angiotensin II. Angiotensin II interacts with angiotensin receptors to signal aldosterone secretion; in turn, aldosterone promotes renal reabsorption of sodium. ACEIs also block the breakdown of bradykinin, which is an endogenous vasodilator. The cardioprotective effects of ACEIs include the combination of bradykinin-mediated vasodilation, reduced aldosterone output, and reduced sodium reabsorption resulting in overall BP reduction. ACEI elimination is also related to renal function, so patients with renal impairment (lower GFR or CrCl) require ACEI dose reduction of 50% (Table 4.9).

Table 4.9 Examples of Angiotensin-Converting Enzyme Inhibitor

ACEI	Description
Captopril	A potent and rapid-acting sulfhydryl-based ACEI with 75% bioavailability during fasting and 50% bioavailability during a fed state. Calcium- and magnesium-based antacids should be avoided as these would limit bioavailability and interfere with BP lowering. Among ACEIs, captopril sensitivity to antacids is singular and does not result in clinical interference with other ACEIs. Captopril has a plasma peak within an hour and a half-life of elimination of 2 hours and may be used when BP lowering is needed quickly under clinical observation such as in hypertensive emergency or in hypertensive urgency.
Enalapril	A prodrug hydrolyzed by hepatic esterases into active enalaprilat which peaks in 3–4 hours; enalaprilat bioavailability is unrelated to food. Enalaprilat half-life of elimination is 11 hours, allowing oral enalapril to be administered in a single daily dose or divided over 24 hours (as done in heart failure studies). IV enalaprilat can be dosed every 6 hours and is a useful option for hypertensive emergencies in-hospital when IV access is possible.
Lisinopril	An active lysine analog of enalapril with a bioavailability also unrelated to food. Lisinopril has a plasma peak at 7 hours with a half-life of elimination of 12 hours and is suitable in a single dose over a 24-hour interval.
Benazepril	A prodrug, hydrolyzed by hepatic esterases to benazeprilat which undergoes further glucuronidation, and renal elimination of conjugates. Benazepril peaks at 1–2 hours with a half-life of elimination of 10–11 hours, allowing for once-daily dosing.
Fosinopril	A phosphorus-containing prodrug, undergoing hepatic hydrolysis and cleaved into active fosinoprilat or glucuronidated into inactive metabolites. Fosinopril peaks at 3 hours and has an elimination half-life of approximately 11.5 hours. Clearance is nonrenally dependent, with excretion into urine and bile. Patients with renal dysfunction or intravascular volume depletion will use half-dose rather than full dose.
Trandolapril	Absorption is slowed by food and has low bioavailability (approximately 10%). Once cleaved into trandolaprilat by hepatic enzymes, the active form is 70% bioavailable with 65%–94% protein binding and a half-life of elimination of 22.5 hours. Patients with mild or moderate liver disease or cirrhosis may have increased trandolaprilat concentrations, warranting caution regarding BP; as do patients with creatinine clearance lower than 30 mL/min who have twofold higher plasma trandolaprilat concentrations.
Quinapril	Is rapidly absorbed and is 60% bioavailable, then cleaved by hepatic esterases into quinaprilat with a peak plasma concentration at 1 hour, BP lowering within 2–4 hours and extensive protein binding of >97%. It has a prolonged elimination half-life of 22.5 hours due to high-affinity binding to tissue ACE, which allows for daily dosing.
Ramipril	Is slowly absorbed with a bioavailability of 50%–60% and then cleaved by hepatic esterases into ramiprilat which has a 2-hour onset. Ramiprilat extensively distributes into tissue resulting in triphasic kinetics with a distribution half-life of 2–4 hours, a plasma elimination half-life of 9–18 hours, and ramiprilat tissue dissociation half-life of more than 50 hours. Patients with a CrCl under 40 mL/min will have increased exposure and area under the curve, elevated tissue concentrations, and slower excretion of metabolites. Consider half-dose ramipril in those with stage III CKD or with acutely reduced GFR or CrCl.

(continued)

Table 4.9 Examples of Angiotensin-Converting Enzyme Inhibitor (*continued*)

ACEI	Description
Moexipril	Is hepatically cleaved and de-esterified to active moexiprilat, with a variable elimination half-life of 2–12 hours. Use half-dose moexipril in persons who are experiencing acute or chronic renal impairment, or are volume depleted.
Perindopril	Is converted to active perindoprilat by hepatic plasma esterases with biphasic kinetics. It has a variable plasma elimination half-life of 3–10 hours and slow ACE tissue dissociation of 30–120 hours.

ACE, angiotensin-converting enzyme; ACEI, angiotensin-converting enzyme inhibitors; BP, blood pressure; CKD, chronic kidney disease; CrCl, creatine clearance; GFR, glomerular filtration rate; IV, intravenous.

Other than captopril and lisinopril, most ACEIs are converted by hepatic or plasma esterases into their active form (i.e., ramiprilat). Lisinopril is active without hepatic conversion. Patients with active liver disease may not be able to convert ACEIs into the active form from the prodrug. Most ACEIs have variable plasma elimination half-lives of the active form ranging 9 to 12 hours or longer (see Table 4.9), allowing for convenient once-daily dosing (i.e., managing hypertension) or splitting the daily dose over 24 hours (i.e., guideline-directed goal doses in heart failure). Patients with acute or chronic renal impairment or volume dehydration should receive half-dose ACEI therapy and require monitoring for day-to-day ACEI tolerability, hemodynamics, and renal function (serum creatinine [SCr], serum potassium, blood urea nitrogen [BUN], GFR). Food may influence the bioavailability of the ACEI's prodrug but is not an important predictor of ACEI effects on BP.

ANGIOTENSIN-CONVERTING ENZYME INHIBITORS IN HYPERTENSION
ACE inhibition reduces systolic, diastolic, and mean 24-hour BP in persons with primary isolated systolic hypertension and in secondary hypertension. ACEIs alone are insufficient in the setting of secondary hypertension (i.e., hypertension related to primary aldosteronism.) The initial blood pressure reduction following ACEI dosing corresponds to reduction of plasma renin activity and lower angiotensin II, followed by a longer term reduction in total peripheral resistance resulting in net vasodilation in the vasculature. Renally, ACEI-mediated vasodilation increases blood flow to the afferent and efferent arterioles without increasing the GFR. Vasodilation in the large vessels reduces systolic BP, increases cardiac output, and generally does not result in exercise intolerance or postural symptoms because baroreceptor function and cardiovascular reflexes are not compromised.

Most patients with stage I hypertension respond to an ACEI and may initially reach goal BP (<130/80 mmHg); however, many patients will require additional antihypertensive therapy in addition to the ACEI. Complimentary combinations using thiazide diuretics or dihydropyridine calcium channel blockers (CCBs) may be necessary over time as BP increases, especially in persons who continue to gain weight or when lifestyle modifications are insufficient or inconsistent. ACEIs are commonly combined with beta-blockers (as well as thiazide diuretics and dihydropyridines) in persons with hypertension who have stable ischemic heart disease. Failure to lose weight (in sedentary persons with a body mass index [BMI] of 30 or more) or initiate or maintain lifestyle changes (sodium restriction, dietary modification, calorie restriction, and meeting physical activity goals) attenuates the response of ACEIs or any other pharmacotherapy intended to reduce BP.

ACEIs reduce aldosterone secretion somewhat, which is compensated for by an increase in adrenocorticotropic hormone (ACTH). Patients with stage 3 to 5 CKD or receiving supplemental potassium or on potassium-sparing diuretics may have serum hyperkalemia from potassium accumulation when also receiving an ACEI.

ANGIOTENSIN-CONVERTING ENZYME INHIBITORS IN HFPEF, HRMREF, HFREF
ACEIs are indicated in persons with left-ventricular systolic dysfunction and HF (heart failure with preserved ejection fraction [HFpEF], heart failure with mildly reduced ejection fraction [HFmrEF, 41%–49%], heart failure with reduced ejection fraction [HFrEF]). ACEIs reduce afterload and systolic wall stress and improve cardiac output, thereby improving quality of life, slowing left-ventricular disease progression, and reducing rates of hospitalization, myocardial infarction (MI), and HF-related mortality. ACEI reduction of systolic BP and improved vasodilation plus improved renal blood flow improve renal hemodynamics and natriuresis, which slows pathophysiology because of a reduction in angiotensin II and aldosterone in renal tissue. Natriuresis offloads fluid from the central compartment and reduces

right-sided venous return and simultaneously increases venodilation, which further improves venous return. ACEI vasodilation in epicardia vessels, reduction in afterload, improved return, and the reduction in aldosterone are helpful immediately after MI, and ACEIs reduce the rates of secondary cardiovascular events and cardiovascular-related hospitalization.

ANGIOTENSIN-CONVERTING ENZYME INHIBITORS IN DIABETES
Persons with type 1 and 2 diabetes and renal disease are particularly susceptible to neurovascular disease progression, and ACEIs are helpful for slowing renal disease progression related to diabetes and hypertension-related nephropathy while improving hemodynamics. ACEIs are glomerular-protective, dilating the afferent and efferent arterioles and reducing angiotensin II–mediated mesangial hypertrophy in hypertensive and diabetes nephropathy. Long-term ACEI therapy results in fewer patients with disease progression and fewer secondary cardiovascular events (MI, stroke, hospitalization related to disease progression).

ANGIOTENSIN-CONVERTING ENZYME INHIBITORS: PRESCRIBING CONSIDERATIONS
Patients who have precipitous reductions in BP after the first few ACEI doses may have plasma-renin-dependent hypertension. ACEIs may be important for management but will require monitoring for BP, postural symptoms, renal function, GFR, BUN, SCr, and serum potassium. Low- or moderate-dose ACEIs, alone or in a complementary combination (thiazides, dihydropyridine CCBs) may be very effective while being regularly monitored.

Persons with reduced renal function or with HFrEF or intravascular volume depletion may require more careful and frequent observation (postural symptoms, serum K, GFR) due to renal hemodynamics. Patients with angiotensin II and aldosterone-dependent renal artery stenosis (unilateral or bilateral) are more susceptible to renal insufficiency and hyperkalemia, including after starting an ACEI or when volume depleted or receiving nonsteroidal anti-inflammatory drugs (NSAIDs) or potassium-sparing diuretics.

ACEI vasodilation is mediated by bradykinin accumulation. Bradykinin accumulation in the oropharyngeal microvasculature and tissues of the face and neck may result in persistent, nagging cough with or without noticeable tissue swelling, redness, airway involvement, or obstruction, resulting in difficulty breathing. Cough does not require discontinuation of ACEIs but should be documented as ACEI-associated cough in the electronic health record. Up to 20% may experience ACEI cough from bradykinin accumulation; this may be managed by discontinuation and washout over three to five elimination half-lives (3–4 days) and trying (rechallenge) with another ACEI or antihypertensive. ACEI-associated skin rash may be managed by discontinuation and antihistamines.

Nonallergic angioedema from ACEIs may be minor to severe and life-threatening, requiring airway protection, hospitalization, and steroids. ACEI-mediated angioedema of the nose, lips, mouth, tongue, throat, glottis, and larynx is a medical emergency requiring airway protection and may be treated with epinephrine, steroids, and antihistamines and require overnight hospitalization for observation. Visceral angioedema may present as emesis, abdominal pain, and watery diarrhea, which may also be ACEI related and remit with discontinuation. *Note*: ACEIs are never used in pregnancy and are fetopathic due to a prominent reduction in fetal blood flow. Antacids should not be co-administered with ACEIs as antacids reduce ACEI bioavailability (Table 4.10).

Table 4.10 Angiotensin-Converting Enzyme Inhibitors: Pharmacokinetics and Dosing

Drug	Half-Life	Onset	Duration	Dosing Range	Renal Adjusted Dosing
Captopril	2–4 hours	15 minutes	Variable	6.25–50 mg TID, max 50 mg TID	½ dose every 12–18 hours
Enalapril	35 hours	1 hour	12–24 hours	5–40 mg daily, max 40 mg daily	2.5 mg daily, max 20 mg daily
Lisinopril	12 hours	1 hour	24 hours	5–40 mg daily, max 40 mg daily	2.5 mg daily
Benazepril	10–11 hours	1–2 hours	24 hours	10–40 mg daily, max 40 mg daily	5 mg daily, max 40 mg daily

(*continued*)

Table 4.10 Angiotensin-Converting Enzyme Inhibitors: Pharmacokinetics and Dosing (*continued*)

Drug	Half-Life	Onset	Duration	Dosing Range	Renal Adjusted Dosing
Fosinopril	12–14 hours	1 hour	24 hours	10–40 mg daily, max 40 mg daily	5 mg daily
Trandolapril	22.5 hours	1 hour	24 hours	0.5–8 mg daily, max 8 mg daily	0.5 mg daily
Quinapril	3 hours	1 hour	24 hours	10–80 mg daily, max 80 mg daily	2.5 mg daily
Ramipril	13–17 hours	1–2 hours	24 hours	2.5–20 mg daily, or divided BID	¼ dose daily
Moexipril	2–10 hours	1–2 hours	24 hour	3.75–7.5 mg daily, stepwise increments, max 30 mg daily or BID	3.75 mg daily, max 15 mg daily
Perindopril	3–10 hours	1–2 hours	24 hours	4–16 mg daily, max 16 mg daily	2 mg daily, max 8 mg daily

ANGIOTENSIN-RECEPTOR BLOCKERS

Angiotensin-receptor antagonists or ARBs are another means of modulating the renin-angiotensin aldosterone system (Table 4.11). ACEIs may not be tolerated by all persons, and ARBs are therapeutically similar while being pharmacologically different and working downstream by directly antagonizing the angiotensin (AT1) receptor.

Table 4.11 Examples of Angiotensin-Receptor Blockers

Drug	Description
Candesartan cilexetil	Is hydrolyzed to active candesartan in the gut during absorption by GI esterases. Candesartan onset is within 2–3 hours, with a half-life of 5–9 hours and a 24-hour duration of action allowing for once-daily dosing. Candesartan protein binding is greater than 99%; excretion is mostly in feces (67%) and less by urine (33%) with approximately 25% eliminated as unchanged drug. Mild to moderate renal dysfunction increases candesartan bioavailability and elimination half-life but was safe and tolerable in small observational evaluations.
Eprosartan	Peaks in 1–2 hours with a duration of action between 5 and 9 hours. (Eprosartan is metabolized by glucuronidation, followed by renal elimination and biliary excretion. Older age and hepatic disease increase eprosartan bioavailability requiring careful observation, individualization, and use of low doses for tolerability during blood management.)
Irbesartan	Reaches peak plasma levels within 2 hours, with an elimination half-life of 11–15 hours and dose-dependent BP lowering. (Irbesartan is partially oxidized by CYP2C9, glucuronidated to a glucuronide conjugate that is renally eliminated (20%) and hepatically excreted (80%). Clearance of irbesartan is not influenced by mild to moderate renal or hepatic dysfunction.)
Losartan	Is hepatically metabolized by CYP2C9 and CYP3A4 to 5–carboxylic acid metabolite E3174, which is 10–40 times more potent than parent drug and with fourfold greater bioavailability and a much longer terminal half-life of 5–10 hours. Plasma concentrations of losartan and E3174 are increased in mild to moderate renal insufficiency and alcohol-related liver cirrhosis. The natriuretic and uricosuric effects of losartan are helpful for BP management particularly in persons already adhering to a low-salt intake with elevated BP and elevated serum uric acid greater than 8 mg/dL.

(*continued*)

Table 4.11 Examples of Angiotensin-Receptor Blockers (*continued***)**

Drug	Description
Olmesartan medoxomil	Is hydrolyzed by GI esterases to olmesartan, reaching a plasma peak by 3 hours and with a terminal half-life of 12–18 hours. Renal and hepatic insufficiency prolong clearance but do not result in dose adjustments.
Telmisartan	Achieves a plasma peak level within 0.5–1 hour with a half-life of elimination of 24 hours. Biliary excretion of unmetabolized drug is the primary form of clearance. The typical dose for telmisartan in the treatment of hypertension and cardiovascular risk management is 40–80 mg daily. Hepatic insufficiency limits the maximum daily dose by 50%.
Valsartan	Bioavailability is best on an empty stomach, achieving a plasma peak at 2–4 hours and a half-life of elimination of 9 hours and 24-hour duration of action to permit once-daily dosing for hypertension. The dosing of valsartan is divided twice daily in heart failure and in coronary artery disease according to tolerability and BP. Clearance is 70% hepatic and influenced by hepatic insufficiency such that valsartan AUC is doubled during hepatic insufficiency, and a reduction in the valsartan dose may be reasonable based on observed BP.
Azilsartan medoxomil	Is hydrolyzed by esterases in the GI to active azilsartan. Azilsartan bioavailability is independent of food and is more effective at BP reduction compared to valsartan and olmesartan. The combination of azilsartan with chlorthalidone is safe, well-tolerated, and effective in the management of BP and a good combination option during transitions of care from hospital to home.

AUC, Area Under the Curve; BP, blood pressure; GI, gastrointestinal.

ARBs selectively and competitively antagonize or inhibit the AT1 receptor with high affinity. The physiologic effect of inhibiting the AT1 receptor with ARBs includes vasodilation, attenuated pressor response, aldosterone and catecholamine secretion, limited adrenergic neurotransmission, and a reduction in cellular hyperplasia and hypertrophy. ARBs do not result in activation of AT2 receptors, and angiotensin II may accumulate when ARBs are used, resulting in the activation of AT2 receptors that results in vasodilation.

Most ARBs have low bioavailability and high protein binding (greater than 90%), and yet concomitant dosing with antacids or acid suppression strategies does not result in clinically significant drug interactions by interfering with BP lowering. Some ARBs have unique cautions in the setting of renal or hepatic disease. Older (geriatric) patients, and those with HF, malnutrition, or mild to moderate renal or hepatic dysfunction may yet have increased bioavailability, longer half-life of elimination, and BP reductions at low or starting ARB doses.

ACEIs and ARBs were previously combined in some patients with resistant hypertension, hypertensive nephropathy, HF, and other indications. This practice is no longer indicated or appropriate owing to safety issues and an overall failure of combined ACEI and ARB therapy, a higher probability of treatment-related intolerance and other adverse events including hypotension, and a reduction in renal perfusion indicated by elevated SCr and BUN.

ARBs are oral dosage forms (Table 4.12), readily available for use in inpatient and outpatient practices, approved for the treatment of hypertension, and indicated in patients with diabetes for renal protection, as well as BP management. ARBs reduce BP and afterload that attenuate the structural remodeling of the left ventricle in persons with left-ventricular hypertrophy and HF. Similarly, ARBs are useful in patients with stable atherosclerotic cardiovascular disease following MI. ARBs are comparable to ACEIs in hypertension, post-MI management, HF, stroke prevention, and the management of hypertensive- or diabetes-related nephropathy. ARBs are complementary to thiazide diuretics and dihydropyridine CCBs when combined in the management of hypertension, post-MI management, heart failure, and stroke prevention. The benefits of ARBs for HF mortality have been inconsistent, and these are typically secondary in HF when persons do not tolerate ACEI, beta-blockers, and mineralocorticoid receptor antagonists at full doses. Valsartan, combined with sacubitril in a proprietary combination and formulation of sacubitril/valsartan tablet, is synergistic and the guideline-endorsed initial management of HF with reduced ejection fraction (EF) and reduces hospitalizations in persons with HF with reduced or preserved EF.

Table 4.12 Angiotensin-Receptor Blockers: Pharmacokinetics and Dosing

Drug	Half-Life	Onset	Duration	Dosing Range	Renal Impairment Dosing	Hepatic Impairment Dosing
Azilsartan medoxomil	11 hours	1.5–3 hours	24 hours	40 mg daily, max 80 mg daily	—	—
Candesartan cilexetil	5–9 hours	2–3 hours	24 hours	4–32 mg daily, max 32 mg daily	—	8 mg daily
Eprosartan	5–9 hours	1–2 hours	24 hours	600 mg daily, max 800 mg daily	600 mg daily	—
Irbesartan	11–15 hours	1–2 hours	24 hours	150 mg daily, max 300 mg daily	—	—
Losartan	5–10 hours	6 hours	24 hours	25–150 mg daily, max 150 mg daily	25 mg daily	—
Olmesartan medoxomil	13 hours	1–2 hours	24 hours	20–40 mg daily, max 40 mg daily	Max 20 mg daily	—
Telmisartan	24 hours	24 hours	24 hours	20–80 mg daily, max 80 mg daily	—	40 mg
Valsartan	2 hours	6 hours	24 hours	80–320 mg daily, max 320 mg daily	—	—

ANGIOTENSIN NEPRILYSIN INHIBITORS

Neprilysin is an endopeptidase that degrades endogenous vasodilating peptides including bradykinin and natriuretic peptides, thus permitting vasoconstriction, increased intravascular pressure, neurohormonal activation, and sodium retention. Sacubitril is a neprilysin inhibitor that therefore prolongs the effect of endogenous bradykinin and natriuretic peptide, promoting vasodilation, lowering vascular pressures, and attenuating neurohormonal activation and sodium retention, which slow the pathophysiologic remodeling observed in HF. Neprilysin inhibition works best when combined with the angiotensin-receptor antagonist valsartan (in proprietary combination), whereas experimental combinations with ACEIs were unsafe and not well tolerated, resulting in kidney injury and angioedema. Sacubitril/valsartan (Entresto) is now well studied and is protective in persons with HF (HF with reduced EF and HF with preserved EF), reducing the chances of HF-associated death, hospitalization, and attenuating disease progression.

The sacubitril/valsartan complex dissociates upon administration; sacubitril is moderately bioavailable (60%), highly protein bound (97%), and metabolized to active metabolite LBQ657 with an elimination half-life of 11 hours (see Table 4.11). Inhibiting neprilysin with sacubitril and valsartan results in vasodilation, reduces vascular resistance, attenuates left-ventricular and smooth muscle and vascular remodeling, and reduces HF-related disease progression. Sacubitril/valsartan is only approved in HF and is initiated at low doses, with necessary monitoring of BP, serum potassium, renal function, and tolerability at baseline and every 2 weeks until target doses are reached, and then every 1 to 3 months to ensure tolerability and renal function. Sacubitril/valsartan cannot be used in the treatment of hypertension, or in combination with other ARBs, ACEIs, or aliskiren because therapeutic duplication increases the probability of hypotension, acute kidney injury, hyperkalemia, or angioedema.

DOSING SACUBITRIL/VALSARTAN IN HFPEF

After maximizing mineralocorticoid receptor antagonists and sodium–glucose cotransporter-2 agents, use sacubitril 24 mg/valsartan 26 mg twice daily or sacubitril 49 mg/valsartan 51 mg twice daily based on starting BP. Increase the dose every 2 weeks until a -target maintenance dose of sacubitril 97 mg/valsartan 103 mg twice daily is reached.

ANTIARRHYTHMICS
BETA-BLOCKERS

Beta-blockers are used for a variety of cardiovascular diseases (acute coronary syndrome, atrial fibrillation, reduced EF HF, angina). Specific beta-1 receptor blockade causes negative inotropic and chronotropic activity, resulting in decreased workload of the heart and reduction in heart rate. Adverse effects include bradycardia, hypotension, dizziness, bronchoconstriction, depression, worsening acute decompensated HF, and withdrawal symptoms upon abrupt discontinuation.

Beta-1 Selective Beta-Blockers
Highly specific beta-1 receptor antagonism prevents catecholamine effects on cardiac myocytes. These include metoprolol tartrate, metoprolol succinate, atenolol, and bisoprolol.

Nonselective Beta-Blockers
Nonselective beta-blockers that have receptor affinity beyond beta-1 receptors are shown in Table 4.13.

Table 4.13 Nonselective Beta-Blockers

Nonselective Beta-Blocker	Receptor Activity
Carvedilol	Mixed beta-1 and alpha-1 receptor antagonist
Labetalol	Mixed beta-1 and alpha-1 receptor antagonist
Propranolol	Mixed beta-1 and beta-2 receptor antagonist
Nadolol	Mixed beta-1 and beta-2 receptor antagonist
Sotalol	Anti-arrhythmic agent with some beta-1 and beta-2 blocking activities

Clinical Pearls

- In patients with chronic HF (EF less than 40%), the only beta-blockers approved for use are carvedilol, metoprolol succinate, and bisoprolol.
- Abrupt discontinuation of beta-blockers can cause reflex tachycardia.
- Sotalol is used only in cardiac arrhythmia management.

CALCIUM CHANNEL BLOCKERS
Used for treatment of hypertension and heart rate control in a variety of cardiovascular conditions, CCBs block the influx of calcium into smooth muscle. Antagonism occurs at arterial smooth muscle or cardiac smooth muscle. Dihydropyridine CCBs have predominantly peripheral vasodilatory actions, whereas nondihydropyridine CCBs have significant sinoatrial (SA) and atrioventricular (AV) node depressant effects with lesser amounts of peripheral vasodilation. Adverse effects include hypotension, bradycardia, peripheral edema, dizziness, headache, fatigue, and worsening of acute HF.

Dihydropyridines
CCB class blocks the influx of calcium into arterial smooth muscle resulting in vasodilation. Examples are amlodipine, clevidipine, felodipine, nicardipine, and nifedipine.

Nondihydropyridines
CCB class blocks the influx of calcium into cardiac smooth muscle resulting in negative inotropic (force of contraction) and chronotropic (heart rate) activities. Examples are diltiazem and verapamil.

Clinical Pearls

- Nondihydropyridines are contraindicated in chronic HF with an EF less than 40%.
- Start nondihydropyridines at lower doses in geriatric patients due to risk of bradycardia.
- Dihydropyridines can be safely given to patients with chronic HF with an EF less than 40% who need additional treatment for angina or hypertension.

DIURETICS

Diuretics are used for treatment of hypertension and disease states involving volume overload, including HF, liver cirrhosis, and nephrotic syndrome. Agents in this class primarily inhibit the reabsorption of sodium in the renal tubules, thereby promoting sodium and water excretion. Adverse effects include electrolyte disturbances (hyponatremia, hypo-/hyperkalemia), metabolic alkalosis and acidosis, hyperuricemia, hyperglycemia, and dehydration leading to acute kidney injury. The most common diuretics seen in practice can be divided by mechanism of action and include the loop, thiazide, and potassium-sparing diuretics (Table 4.14).

Table 4.14 Diuretic Comparison

Diuretic Class	Sodium Excretion	Blood Pressure Reduction	Diuresis Efficacy (Water Loss)
Loop	30%	+	+++
Thiazide	10%	+++	++
Potassium-sparing	3%	++	+

LOOP DIURETICS

Loop diuretics block the sodium:potassium:chloride cotransporter in the ascending loop of Henle and are especially potent at promoting fluid loss. Examples of loop diuretics include furosemide, torsemide, bumetanide, and ethacrynic acid. These medications have dosing equivalents that the AGACNP must be aware of (Table 4.15).

Table 4.15 Loop Diuretic Comparison

	Furosemide	Torsemide	Bumetanide	Ethacrynic Acid
PO dose equivalents	40 mg	20 mg	1 mg	50 mg
IV:PO conversion	1:2	1:1	1:1	1:1
Bioavailability	50%	80%	80%	100%
Onset of action (IV)	5–20 minutes	1 hour (PO formulation)	2–3 minutes	30 minutes
Duration of action (IV)	2 hours	6–8 hours	2–3 hours	2 hours

IV, intravenous.

Clinical Pearls

- Assess patients for risk of hypokalemia, hyponatremia, and hypomagnesemia prior to initiation and throughout therapy. Provide potassium and magnesium supplementation as needed.
- Use with additional monitoring in patients with hypersensitivity to sulfonamide-derived antibiotics ("sulfa drugs"), including sulfamethoxazole/trimethoprim and sulfasalazine.
- Ethacrynic acid is generally reserved for use in patients who have had a hypersensitivity reaction to a sulfonamide-based loop diuretic (furosemide, bumetanide, or torsemide).
- Monitor basic metabolic panel (BMP) daily for patients on IV therapy and 1 to 2 weeks after starting oral therapy and dose changes.
- Loop diuretics can be used for fluid management in patients with chronic kidney disease, nephrotic syndrome, ascites due to liver cirrhosis, and acute or chronic HF.
- Higher doses of loop diuretics are often required for patients with decreased estimated serum GFR (eGFR; less than 30 mL/min).
- Strategies to overcome diuretic resistance in patients needing diuresis include administering both a loop and thiazide diuretic simultaneously (e.g., furosemide plus chlorthalidone or furosemide plus metolazone) and using a bolus plus continuous IV infusion of furosemide.
- Ototoxicity, including permanent deafness, has rarely been associated with loop diuretics; risk factors for development of this toxicity include using high IV doses and co-administering with nephrotoxic medications.

THIAZIDE AND THIAZIDE-LIKE DIURETICS

Thiazide and thiazide-like diuretics block the sodium:chloride cotransporter in distal tubule; they are less potent than loop diuretics, primarily used for treatment of hypertension and mild edema, and contraindicated in liver failure, severe and anuric renal failure, and gout. Examples include hydrochlorothiazide, chlorthalidone, chlorothiazide, and metolazone.

Clinical Pearls

■ Thiazide and thiazide-like diuretics are associated with hyperglycemia; monitor in patients with prediabetes and diabetes mellitus.
■ Thiazide and thiazide-like diuretics are associated with hyperuricemia; avoid use in patients with gout, and discontinue if hyperuricemia occurs.
■ Adverse effects include orthostatic hypotension, hypokalemia, hyponatremia, hypomagnesemia, increased serum calcium, and lipid changes.

POTASSIUM-SPARING DIURETICS

Potassium-sparing diuretics block sodium channels in late distal tubule and collecting duct and are the least potent at sodium excretion. They are contraindicated in hyperkalemia or severe renal failure. Examples include spironolactone and eplerenone.

MISCELLANEOUS DIURETICS

Carbonic anhydrase inhibitors (e.g., acetazolamide) block sodium and bicarbonate reabsorption in the collecting duct. This medication is used in glaucoma, diuretic resistance, acute altitude sickness, metabolic alkalosis, and idiopathic intracranial hypertension.

Osmotic diuretics (e.g., mannitol) cause diuresis independent of sodium and potassium. They are used to decrease intracranial pressure in cerebral edema.

Vasopressin receptor antagonists (e.g., tolvaptan) cause diuresis by antidiuretic hormone-mediated reabsorption in the collecting duct. They are used for treatment of chronic hyponatremia and to slow progression of kidney function decline in adults with autosomal dominant polycystic kidney disease.

VASOACTIVE AGENTS

All AGACNPs must be able to manage patients in shock. Treatment of shock, including cardiogenic, distributive, or obstructive shock, may require vasoactive support. Vasoactive agents include vasopressors, vasodilators, and inotropic agents. Additionally, vasodilators may be required for hypertensive emergencies. This section provides a review of these agents.

INOTROPES

Inotropes are prescribed for acute and chronic HF who are in cardiogenic shock (Table 4.16).

Table 4.16 Inotropes

	Dopamine	Dobutamine	Milrinone
MOA	DA and beta-1 agonist (higher doses alpha-agonist)	Beta-1 agonist	PDE-3 inhibitor
Dose	5–15 mcg/kg/min	2.5–20 mcg/kg/min	0.125–0.75 mcg/kg/min
Half-life elimination	2 minutes	2 minutes	2–3 hours
Efficacy monitoring	Increased CO and HR		
Safety monitoring	Arrhythmias Extravasation CI in sulfite allergy	Arrhythmias CI in sulfite allergy	Hypotension, Arrhythmias, SCr/BUN—requires renal dosage, adjustment, AST/ALT d/t some hepatic metabolism

ALT, alanine aminotransferase; AST, aspartate aminotransferase; BUN, blood urea nitrogen; CI, contraindicated; CO, cardiac output; DA, dopamine agonist; d/t, due to; HR, heart rate; MOA, mechanism of action; PDE, phosphodiesterase inhibitor; SCr, serum creatinine.

VASOPRESSORS

Vasopressors are commonly used in septic, neurogenic, cardiogenic, and anaphylactic shock as well as other vasodilatory states such as epidural infusion or other hypotensive states such as adrenal insufficiency (Table 4.17).

Table 4.17 Vasopressors

Drug and Doses	Mechanism of Action	Main Effects	Common Uses
Norepinephrine (Levophed) 0.5–30 mcg/min or 0.01–0.04 mcg/kg/min	α++++, β-1++	Vasoconstriction Inotropy	Main use: Septic shock; First line for most shock
Vasopressin (Pitressin) 0.01–0.06 units/min	Vasopressin +++	Vasoconstriction	Second-line septic shock
Epinephrine 0.01–0.05 mcg/kg/min Greater than 0.05 mcg/kg/min	β-1+++, β-2++ α+++, β-1++, β-2++	Vasoconstriction Inotropy Chronotropy	Anaphylaxis, asthma, cardiac arrest, third-line septic shock
Phenylephrine (Neosynephrine) 2–300 mcg/min or 0.1–1 mcg/kg/min	α++++	Vasoconstriction	Hypotension from peripheral dilation due to epidural
Dopamine 0.5–5 mcg/kg/min 5–10 mcg/kg/min 10–20 mcg/kg/min	β-1+, DA ++++ α+, β-1++, DA +++ α+++, β-1+++, DA+	Vasoconstriction Inotropy Chronotropy	Spinal cord injury

Note: The increased number of pluses equate to more activity.

INTRAVENOUS VASODILATORS

IV vasodilators are used for adjuvant therapy in patients with acute decompensated HF. Vasodilators used for this purpose include nitroglycerine and sodium nitroprusside. These medications may be used to provide relief of dyspnea in patients without symptomatic hypotension. Additionally, IV vasodilators may be administered for treatment of hypertensive crisis, defined by systolic BP greater than 180 mmHg or diastolic BP greater than 120 mmHg.

Hypertensive crises are further categorized as hypertensive emergency or urgency. Hypertensive emergency is defined by new or worsening end-organ damage, and hypertensive urgency relates severe elevation of BP without new or worsening end-organ damage. Management of hypertensive emergency involves close monitoring and IV administration of antihypertensive medications, requiring ICU admission. The preferred treatment options for hypertensive emergency depend on the end-organ damage present (Table 4.18). Ideal medications to treat hypertensive emergency are those associated with predictable BP response.

Table 4.18 Treatment Options for Hypertensive Emergency

End-Organ Damage	Treatment Options
Acute renal failure	Clevidipine Nicardipine Fenoldopam
Encephalopathy, ischemic, or hemorrhagic stroke **Avoid aggressively lowering BP**	Clevidipine Nicardipine Fenoldopam Labetalol
Acute coronary syndromes	Esmolol Nitroglycerin Labetalol
Acute aortic dissection	Esmolol ± nicardipine or clevidipine Labetalol
Acute HF and pulmonary edema	Clevidipine Nitroglycerin Nitroprusside

(continued)

Table 4.18 Treatment Options for Hypertensive Emergency (*continued*)

End-Organ Damage	Treatment Options
Preeclampsia/eclampsia	Labetalol Oral nifedipine Hydralazine
Sympathetic crisis (e.g., pheochromocytoma, postcarotid endarterectomy)	Clevidipine Nicardipine Phentolamine

BP, blood pressure; HF, heart failure.

A summary of IV vasodilators used for hypertensive emergency and dyspnea relief during acute decompensated HF is found in Table 4.19. Appropriate selection of agents involves balancing pharmacokinetic characteristics and risk of adverse effects with patient-specific characteristics. Important patient-specific characteristics to take into consideration include patient age, pregnancy status, volume status, presence of end-organ damage, and comorbidities. Patients older than 65 years should typically be started on the lower end of the dosing range. Both renal and hepatic function are important factors for dosing.

Table 4.19 Intravenous Vasodilators

Name/ Mechanism	Dosing	Pharmacokinetics (IV Dosing)	Monitoring Contraindications	Clinical Considerations
Clevidipine Third-generation dihydro-pyridine CCB	Initial dose: 1–2 mg/hr; doubled every 90 seconds until blood pressure reaches target, then adjusted every 5–10 minutes Maximum dose: 32 mg/hr	Onset: 2–4 minutes Duration: 5–15 minutes	Monitoring: triglycerides (with prolonged administration) Contraindications: patients allergic to soy, eggs, or egg products; patients with defective lipid metabolism	Dilates arterioles and reduces afterload without affecting cardiac-filling pressures or causing reflex tachycardia Unique esterase metabolism terminates action independent of renal/hepatic function
Nicardipine Dihydropyridine calcium channel blocker	Initial dose: 5 mg/hr; increase by 2.5 mg/hr every 5 minutes until therapeutic effect reached Maximum dose: 15 mg/hr	Onset: 5–15 minutes Duration: 4–6 hours	Monitoring: reflex tachycardia, headache, flushing, nausea, dizziness Contraindications: advanced aortic stenosis	May offer benefit in cerebrovascular disease due to crossing blood–brain barrier and relaxes cerebrovascular smooth muscle Does not change intracranial volume or ICP
Fenoldopam Dopamine D1-like receptor agonist; arteriolar vasodilator, natriuretic and diuretic effects	Initial dose: 0.1–0.3 mcg/kg/min; titrate dose by 0.05–0.1 mcg/kg/min every 15 minutes until therapeutic effect reached Max dose: 1.6 mcg/kg/min; do not use for longer than 48 hours	Onset: less than 5 minutes Duration: 30 minutes	Monitoring: flushing, headache, reflex tachycardia, increased intraocular pressure, dizziness Contraindications: allergy to sulfites, glaucoma, patients at risk of increased ICP	

(continued)

Table 4.19 Intravenous Vasodilators (*continued*)

Name/ Mechanism	Dosing	Pharmacokinetics (IV Dosing)	Monitoring Contraindications	Clinical Considerations
Esmolol Beta-1 blocker	Initial dose: 0.5–1.0 mg/kg over 1 minute bolus, followed by 50 mcg/kg/ min infusion; may repeat bolus dose and increase infusion rate by 50 mcg/ kg/min Maximum dose: 300 mcg/kg/min	Onset: 1 minute Duration: 10–20 minutes	Monitoring: anemia (may prolong esmolol's effect), bradycardia, hypotension, potassium (for hyperkalemia) Contraindications: concurrent beta-blocker therapy, bradycardia, second- or third-degree heart block, decompensated HF, pulmonary hypertension	Used for perioperative hypertension Safe in patients with myocardial ischemia/ infarction May exacerbate symptoms in patients with HF Although considered safe for patients with reactive airway disease, monitor patients with asthma/ COPD for worsening symptoms
Labetalol Beta and alpha-1 blocker	Initial dose: 0.3–1 mg/kg (no more than 20 mg) IV slow injection bolus; may give additional boluses of 20–80 mg every 10 minutes or start IV infusion of 0.5–2 mg/min (or 0.4–1 mg/kg/ hr) until target blood pressure reached Maximum cumulative dose: 300 mg	Onset: 2–5 minutes Duration: 2–4 minutes (single bolus) 2–4 hours (repeated bolus doses and IV infusions)	Monitoring: postural hypotension, dizziness, paresthesia, fatigue, nausea, bronchospasm, heart block Contraindications: reactive or obstructive airway disease, asthma, cardiogenic shock, increased risk of hypotension, HF, second- or third-degree heart block, severe bradycardia	Little effect on cerebral circulation and therefore not associated with increased ICP
Enalaprilat ACEI	Initial dose: 1.25 mg IV over 5 minutes every 6 hours, can increase to 5 mg every 6 hours; if patient is taking diuretic, decrease initial dose to 0.625 mg and can repeat dose in 1 hour; may give extra doses of 1.25 mg every 6 hours as needed	Onset: 15–30 minutes (peak effects may not be seen until 4 hours after administration) Duration: 12–24 hours	Monitoring: SCr/ BUN (acute kidney injury), headache, dizziness, nausea, hyperkalemia Contraindications: pregnancy, acute myocardial ischemia, bilateral renal artery stenosis, angioedema	Slow onset of action and unpredictable blood pressure response Requires renal dosage adjustment

(*continued*)

Table 4.19 Intravenous Vasodilators (*continued*)

Name/ Mechanism	Dosing	Pharmacokinetics (IV Dosing)	Monitoring Contraindications	Clinical Considerations

Hydralazine
 	
Peripheral
  arterial
  vasodilator
	Initial dose: 10–20
	  mg IV bolus
	  every 4–6 hours
	
	Maximum dose:
	  40 mg
		Onset: 10–30
		  minutes
		
		Duration: 2–4
		  hours, active
		  metabolites
		  may have
		  prolonged
		  effect
			Monitoring: heart rate
			  (tachycardia)
			
			Contraindications:
			  CAD
				Has prolonged and
				  unpredictable effects
				
				Use cautiously in
				  patients with
				  impaired renal
				  function

Sodium
  nitroprusside
 	
Arteriolar and
  venous
  vasodilator
  via nitric oxide
  donation
	Initial dose: 0.3–0.5
	  mcg/kg/min;
	  increase by 0.5
	  mcg/kg/min
	  until therapeutic
	  effect reached
	
	Maximum dose:
	  10 mcg/kg/min
	  (avoid doses
	  greater than 2
	  mcg/kg/min)
		Onset:
		  immediate
		
		Duration: 2–3
		  minutes
			Monitoring:
			  intra-arterial
			  blood pressure,
			  tachyphylaxis, if
			  available, serum
			  thiocyanate level
			  (discontinue if
			  greater than 12
			  mg/dL); metabolic
			  acidosis; red urine
			  and erythema
			
			Contraindications:
			  hypertensive
			  emergency in the
			  setting of AMI;
			  advanced aortic
			  stenosis
				May decrease cerebral
				  blood flow and
				  increase ICP; use with
				  caution in patients
				  with neurologic injury
				  or encephalopathy
				
				Can cause unpredictable
				  shifts in BP in patients
				  with hypovolemia or
				  diastolic dysfunction
				
				Avoid use in renal
				  and hepatic failure
				  and ischemic or
				  hemorrhagic stroke

Nitroglycerin
 	
Primarily a
  venous dilator
  (minimal
  arteriolar
  dilator)
	Initial dose: 5 mcg/
	  min, increase by
	  5 mcg/min every
	  3–5 minutes
	  until therapeutic
	  effect or 20
	  mcg/min
	  reached; if no
	  response at 20
	  mcg/min, may
	  increase by 10
	  mcg/min every
	  3–5 minutes
	
	Maximum dose:
	  200 mcg/min
		Onset:
		  2–5 minutes
		
		Duration:
		  1–3 minutes
			Monitoring:
			  headache, tachycardia,
			  vomiting, flushing,
			  methemoglobinemia
			  and tolerance with
			  prolonged use,
			  hypotension
			
			Contraindications:
			  volume depletion,
			  patients who have
			  taken a PDE (e.g.,
			  sildenafil, tadalafil,
			  vardenafil) within the
			  past 48 hours
				Administer low-dose
				  nitroglycerin along
				  with other IV
				  antihypertensive
				  therapy, may be
				  beneficial in patients
				  with hypertensive
				  emergencies
				  associated with ACS
				  or acute pulmonary
				  edema
				
				Tachyphylaxis develops
				  within 24–48 hours
				  of continuous
				  administration

Phentolamine
 	
Competitive
  antagonist
  of peripheral
  alpha
  receptors
	5–15 mg IV bolus;
	  continuous
	  infusion of 1 mg/
	  hr, titrate to BP
	  response, may
	  be used after
	  bolus (maximum
	  infusion rate 40
	  mg/hr)
		Onset:
		  1–2 minutes
		
		Duration:
		  10–30 minutes
			Monitoring:
			  tachycardia, flushing,
			  headache
			
			Contraindications:
			  coronary artery
			  disease, myocardial
			  infarction, angina
				Primarily used to
				  treat hypertensive
				  emergencies
				  associated with
				  pheochromocytoma,
				  cocaine toxicity,
				  amphetamine
				  overdose, or clonidine
				  withdrawal

ACEI, angiotensin-converting enzyme inhibitor; ACS, acute coronary syndromes; AMI, acute myocardial infarction; BP, blood pressure; BUN, blood urea nitrogen; CCB, calcium channel blocker; COPD, chronic obstructive pulmonary disease; HF, heart failure; ICP, intracranial pressure; IV, intravenous; PDE, phosphodiesterase inhibitor; SCr, serum creatinine.

STATINS AND OTHER MEDICATIONS FOR DYSLIPIDEMIA

Dyslipidemia is a medical condition characterized by elevated serum total cholesterol, low-density lipoprotein cholesterol (LDL-C), non-high-density lipoprotein cholesterol (non-HDL-C), triglycerides, and/or low high-density lipoprotein cholesterol (HDL-C). In addition to therapeutic lifestyle modifications, treatment of dyslipidemia frequently involves pharmacotherapy. Classes of medications to treat dyslipidemia include statins, ezetimibe, PCSK9 inhibitors, fibrates, niacin, omega-3 fatty acids, ATP citrate lyase inhibitors, and bile acid-binding resins. Statins are the most frequently used pharmacologic therapy in practice (Table 4.20).

General principles of cholesterol management are based on patient characteristics. These include:

- clinical atherosclerotic cardiovascular disease (ASCVD): high-intensity statin
- LDL-C ≥190 mg/dL: high-intensity statin
- diabetes, age 40 to 75 years, LDL 70 to 189 mg/dL: moderate-intensity statin
  - multiple ASCVD risk factors: high-intensity statin
- no diabetes, age 40 to 75 years, LDL 70 to 189 mg/dL
  - 10-year ASCVD risk ≥0%: high-intensity statin
  - 10-year ASCVD risk 7.5% to 19.8% with risk-enhancing features: moderate-intensity statin

Table 4.20 Medications to Treat Dyslipidemia

Medication Class and Name	Mechanism and Primary Cholesterol Target	Monitoring and Contraindications	Clinical Considerations
Statins: Atorvastatin (Lipitor) Fluvastatin (Lescol) Lovastatin (Mevacor) Pitavastatin (Livalo) Pravastatin (Pravachol) Rosuvastatin (Crestor) Simvastatin (Zocor)	MOA: competitively inhibits HMG-CoA reductase, the rate-limiting step of endogenous cholesterol production Primary target: LDL-C reduction (18%–55%)	Monitoring: Myalgias Arthralgias Myopathy Rhabdomyolysis Cognitive impairment Increased blood glucose and A_{1c} Increased risk of cataracts Elevations in AST/ALT Contraindications: Active liver disease Pregnancy (Cat X) Breastfeeding Strong CYP 3A4 inhibitors with simvastatin and lovastatin	Lovastatin, pitavastatin, and rosuvastatin require renal dosage adjustment. For simvastatin, do not use doses greater than 40 mg daily. Fluvastatin, lovastatin, pravastatin, and simvastatin have short half-lives and should be administered in the evening. Atorvastatin, rosuvastatin, and pitavastatin can be administered at any time of day.
Cholesterol absorption inhibitor Ezetimibe (Zetia)	MOA: inhibits intestinal and biliary cholesterol absorption Primary target: LDL-C reduce 13%–20%	Monitoring: generally well-tolerated, GI upset Contraindications: liver impairment, AKI	Preferred agent to add on to patients needing further LDL reduction despite being on maximally tolerated statin therapy

(continued)

Table 4.20 Medications to Treat Dyslipidemia (*continued*)

Medication Class and Name	Mechanism and Primary Cholesterol Target	Monitoring and Contraindications	Clinical Considerations
PCSK9 inhibitors: Alirocumab (Praluent) Evolocumab (Repatha)	MOA: humanized monoclonal antibodies that bind to PCSK9 Primary target: LDL-C reduction 43%–64%	Monitoring: injection site reaction, hypersensitivity reactions, flu-like symptoms, myalgia Contraindications: prior serious hypersensitivity reaction	Primarily used in patients with familial hypercholesterolemia Administered via subcutaneous injection
Bile acid sequestrants: Cholestyramine Colesevelam Colestipol	MOA: bind bile acids in the gut, thus increasing conversion of cholesterol to bile acids Primary target: LDL-C reduction (15%–30%)	Monitoring: constipation, hypertriglyceridemia, other GI adverse effects like flatulence, nausea, vomiting, abdominal pain Contraindications: complete biliary obstruction, bowel obstruction, serum TG >500 mg/dL or previous hypertriglyceridemia-induced pancreatitis	Primarily used for patients who cannot tolerate statins Bind absorption of other medications, so administer at least 1 hour before or 4 hours after other medications
Niacin (Niaspan)	MOA: inhibits lipolysis, causing decreased free fatty acids in the plasma and decreased hepatic esterification of TG Primary target: TG reduction (20%–50%)	Monitoring: flushing and pruritus, glucose use associated with worsening glycemic control and new-onset diabetes, hyperuricemia; discontinue if acute gout occurs Contraindications: active liver disease or unexplained elevations in transaminases, active peptic ulcer	Increases HDL-C and decreases LDL-C but has not been shown to improve cardiovascular outcomes
Fibrates: Fenofibrate Gemfibrozil	MOA: increases lipoprotein lipase activity, thus breaking down triglycerides Primary target: TG reduction (20%–50%)	Monitoring: GI adverse effects, mild increase in SCr, transient increase in transaminases, increased risk of gallstones Contraindications: CrCl < 30 mL/min, preexisting gallbladder disease	Primarily used in patients with triglycerides >500 mg/dL to reduce risk of pancreatitis May cause modest increases in LDL-C and HDL-C Gemfibrozil should not be used concomitantly with statins

AKI, acute kidney injury; ALT, alanine aminotransferase; AST, aspartate aminotransferase; CrCl, creatine clearance; GI, gastrointestinal; HDL-C, high-density lipoprotein cholesterol; HMG-CoA, hydroxymethylglutaryl-coenzyme A; LDL-C, low-density lipoprotein cholesterol; MOA, mechanism of action; PCSK, proprotein convertase subtilisin/kexin; SCr, serum creatinine; TG, triglycerides.

STATINS

Statins primarily reduce LDL-C through inhibition of HMG-CoA reductase, the enzyme that catalyzes the rate-limiting step in cholesterol synthesis (Table 4.21). Adverse effects include statin-associated muscle symptoms (SAMS) and increased risk of prediabetes and diabetes mellitus. Monitoring for statins includes baseline fasting lipid profile, AST and ALT if hepatic toxicity suspected (e.g., jaundice, dark urine, severe abdominal pain), and creatinine phosphokinase (CPK) if myopathy occurs.

Table 4.21 Statin Intensity Based on Percentage of LDL-C Lowering

High Intensity	Moderate Intensity	Low Intensity
Decrease LDL ≥ 50%	Decrease LDL 30%–49%	Decrease LDL Less than 30%
Atorvastatin 40–80 mg daily Rosuvastatin 20–40 mg daily	Atorvastatin 10–20 mg daily Rosuvastatin 5–10 mg daily Simvastatin 20–40 mg QHS Pravastatin 40–80 mg daily Lovastatin 40 mg QHS Fluvastatin 80 mg QHS Pitavastatin 2–4 mg daily	Simvastatin 10 mg QHS Pravastatin 10–20 mg daily Lovastatin 20 mg QHS Fluvastatin 20–40 mg QHS Pitavastatin 1 mg daily

LDL, low-density lipoprotein.

SAMS are the most frequently reported adverse effect of statins (5%–20% of patients). SAMS are primarily reported as subjective myalgia without other findings. Risk factors for development of SAMS include increasing age, female sex, low BMI, and comorbidities like kidney disease and hypothyroidism. Discontinue/reduce dose of any interacting medications.

Medications That Interact with Statins

- *Gemfibrozil:* Do not use this with any statin.
- *Strong CYP 3A4 inhibitors:* Do not use itraconazole, ketoconazole, posaconazole, voriconazole, erythromycin, clarithromycin, or HIV protease inhibitors with simvastatin and lovastatin.
- *Strong CYP 3A4 inhibitors:* Lower doses of simvastatin and lovastatin are required with verapamil, diltiazem, dronedarone, amiodarone, amlodipine, lomitapide, and ranolazine.

Clinical Pearls

- Do not initiate patients on simvastatin doses greater than 40 mg daily.
- In patients 75 years of age and older:
  - Initiate or continue therapy, if appropriate, in patients with LDL-C 70 to 189 mg/dL if the statin is well-tolerated.
  - Statin therapy may be discontinued in patients with physical or cognitive decline, complicated comorbidities, frailty, or limited life expectancy.

▶ PHARMACOLOGY OF PAIN, AGITATION, SEDATION, AND DELIRIUM

PAIN

Pain can be defined as an unpleasant sensory and emotional experience associated with actual or potential tissue damage. Pain categorization may be based on its duration (acute or chronic) or underlying cause (somatic, visceral, or neuropathic).

Consider the following when developing a pain regimen:

- underlying cause (e.g., somatic, visceral, neuropathic)
- intensity
- duration (acute or chronic)
- available routes of administration
- patient age
- presence of organ (hepatic or renal) dysfunction
- allergy profile or history of intolerance
- opioid-naïve status; avoid long-acting agents in opioid-naïve patients
- potential for drug–drug interactions (e.g., concurrent use of CNS depressants such as opioids and benzodiazepines)
- comorbidities (e.g., pulmonary disease, obstructive sleep apnea)

Pharmacologic interventions for pain management can be broadly classified into opioids and nonopioids.

OPIOIDS

Opioids (Table 4.22) produce analgesia through the activation of the mu receptor and undergo hepatic metabolism with subsequent renal elimination. Common adverse effects of opioids include CNS depression, constipation, cognitive impairment, hallucinations, hyperalgesia, miosis, nausea, urinary retention, pruritus, and respiratory depression.

Table 4.22 Commonly Used Opioids

Opioid	Onset (minutes)	Common Initial IV Dosing Regimens	Special Considerations
Morphine	IV: 5–10 PO: ~30	2–4 mg IV q2h 2–10 mg/hr IV infusion	▪ Histamine release (bronchospasm, vasodilation) ▪ Active metabolites may accumulate in renal dysfunction
Fentanyl	IV: less than 1	25–100 mcg IV q1h 25–100 mcg/hr IV infusion	▪ Lipophilic ▪ No allergic cross-reactivity with other opioids given structural differences compared to morphine ▪ Increased duration of action with prolonged infusions (context sensitive half-life) ▪ Potential to develop serotonin syndrome when used concomitantly with serotonergic agents
Hydrocodone	PO: ~30	2.5–10 mg PO q4–6h	▪ Preparations available in combination with nonopioid agents
Hydromorphone	IV: 5–10 PO: 15–30	0.5–2 mg IV q2h 0.5–3 mg/hr IV infusion	
Meperidine[a]	IV: 2–3	50–100 mg IV q3–4h	▪ Limited use as an analgesic ▪ Short duration of action (2–3 hr) ▪ Neurotoxic metabolite that accumulates in renal failure ▪ Significant drug interactions
Methadone	IV: 10–20 PO: 30–60	Variable	▪ NMDA antagonist ▪ Elimination half-life (15–60 hr) makes it suitable for the management of opioid dependency ▪ May prolong QTc ▪ Variable pharmacokinetics

(continued)

Table 4.22 Commonly Used Opioids (*continued*)

Opioid	Onset (minutes)	Common Initial IV Dosing Regimens	Special Considerations
Oxycodone	PO: 10–15	5–10 mg PO q4–6h	
Remifentanil[b]	IV: 1–3	0.025–0.2 mcg/kg/min infusion	■ Organ-independent elimination via plasma esterases ■ Rapid clearance within 5–10 minutes following discontinuation of infusion ■ High acquisition cost
Tramadol	PO: 60	25–50 mg PO q6h	■ Renal dose adjustment required

Note:
[a]Immediate preparations only.
[b]No enteral preparations available.
IV, intravenous; NMDA, *N*-methyl-D-aspartate.

Allergy and Intolerance

Type 1 hypersensitivity (true anaphylactic) reactions to opioids are rare. Anticipated adverse reactions are often misinterpreted as IgE-mediated responses resulting in the potential avoidance of potentially beneficial opioids (Table 4.23). Opioid-induced histamine release via mast cell degranulation resulting in pseudoallergic symptoms such as pruritus, hypotension, and flushing is a common example.

Table 4.23 Adverse Drug Reactions to Opioids

IgE Mediated	Intolerance
Rash, hives, or severe itching	Gastrointestinal upset
Angioedema	Anxiety
Respiratory compromise (e.g., wheezing, shortness of breath)	Sedation
Significant hypotension	Hallucination

Although cross-reactivity rates between opioid classes are reportedly low, a reasonable approach would be to switch to a synthetic opioid if true hypersensitivity to natural and semisynthetic opioids is demonstrated or suspected (Table 4.24).

Table 4.24 Classification of Opioids

Natural	Semisynthetic	Synthetic
Codeine	Hydrocodone	Buprenorphine
Morphine	Hydromorphone	Fentanyl
	Oxycodone	Methadone
		Tramadol

Adaptations

Chronic or prolonged use of opioids could lead to physiological and/or psychological adaptations driven in part by neurobiological changes. Opioid use disorder (OUD) refers to an aberrant pattern of opioid use comprising tolerance, dependence, and addiction with the last representing the most severe form of the disorder (Table 4.25). OUD is characterized by:

■ drug-seeking behaviors (e.g., obtaining multiple prescriptions from different clinicians)
■ intense cravings or urges
■ continued use of opioids when medically unnecessary
■ continued use despite harm and social and professional consequences

Pharmacological management of OUD involves the use of long-acting opioids that reduce cravings and withdrawal symptoms while producing less euphoria. Commonly used agents such as buprenorphine and methadone are given under medical supervision (Table 4.26).

Table 4.25 Neuroadaptations to Opioids

Tolerance	Dependence
Same amount of opioid results in a decreased therapeutic effect necessitating an increased dose to maintain the same effect	Identified when abrupt cessation or a rapid dose reduction of the opioid triggers a state of withdrawal
Withdrawal Symptoms	
Autonomic: tachypnea, hyperreflexia, tachycardia, sweating, hypertension, hyperthermia Neurologic: craving, anxiety, agitation, shaking, insomnia Gastrointestinal: abdominal cramps, diarrhea Musculoskeletal: piloerection or goosebumps, muscle pain Ophthalmic: pupil dilation, photophobia, lacrimation, or tearing Nasal: sneezing, rhinorrhea	

Table 4.26 Common Agents Used in the Management of OUD

Medication	Mechanism of Action	Notes
Buprenorphine	Partial mu receptor agonist	Initiated when mild symptoms of withdrawal present
Methadone	Opioid agonist	
Naltrexone	Opioid antagonist	Should not be initiated unless patient is motivated and has been opioid free for 7–10 days

Opioid-Induced Constipation

Constipation occurs because of opioid action on the GI mu receptors. Patients should initially receive an adequate intake of water, dietary fiber, stool softeners, and bulk laxatives but may eventually require peripherally acting mu receptor antagonists (PAMORAs). In general, PAMORAs do not cross the blood–brain barrier and therefore do not induce withdrawal (Table 4.27).

Table 4.27 Common Agents Used in the Management of Opioid-Induced Constipation

Laxatives	
Stool softeners (e.g., docusate)	■ First line ■ Stool softeners are best used to prevent OIC but have no effect if constipation is already present
Stimulants (e.g., bisacodyl, senna)	
Osmotic agents (e.g., polyethylene glycol)	
PAMORAs	
Naloxone	■ Must be given via the oral or enteral route of administration
Nalexogol	■ Pegylated formulation of naloxone that further limits crossing the blood–brain barrier ■ Oral only
Alvimopan	■ Usually reserved for the prevention and management of postoperative ileus ■ Oral only
Methylnaltrexone	■ Available orally and parenterally
Calcium Channel Activator	
Lubiprostone	■ Activation of calcium channel results in an increase of intestinal fluid ■ Oral only

OIC, opioid-induced constipation; PAMORAs, peripherally acting mu receptor antagonists.

Opioid Intoxication or Overdose

Risk factors include coadministration with other CNS depressants (e.g., benzodiazepines). Signs include depressed mental status, decreased respiratory rate, decreased tidal volume, decreased bowel sounds, and miotic pupils. Naloxone, an opioid antagonist, is the mainstay therapy for opioid overdose and may be administered intranasally, subcutaneously, IV, or intramuscularly.

Equianalgesic Dose Conversions

Opioid rotation may mitigate the tolerance that develops with chronic use. It may also be necessary in other clinical scenarios such as loss of an existing route of administration, development of renal or hepatic failure, or experience of untoward effects. Therefore, it is vital for the AGACNP to grasp the concept of equianalgesic as the conversion provides doses at which different opioids supply roughly the same amount of analgesia (Table 4.28).

Table 4.28 Equianalgesic Dosing Table

Opioid	Parenteral	PO
Morphine	10	30
Fentanyl	0.1	—
Hydrocodone	—	30
Hydromorphone	1.5	7.5
Methadone	10	20
Oxycodone	—	20–30
Tramadol	—	300

NONOPIOIDS

Multimodal Analgesia

The use of a multimodal approach to acute pain management is vital in the development of comprehensive therapy plans. Multimodal analgesia refers to a strategy that employs a variety of analgesic medications including nonopioid analgesics (Table 4.29) with different mechanisms of action, in addition to nonpharmacologic interventions to produce synergism and more effective pain relief compared with single-modality interventions.

Table 4.29 Commonly Used Nonopioid Analgesics

Medication	Mechanism of Action	Special Considerations
Acetaminophen	Unknown; possible activation of descending serotonergic inhibition pathways	May cause hepatotoxicity at doses >4 g/day Consider lower dose with advanced age, low body weights, malnutrition Avoid if heavy alcohol use suspected or determined
NSAIDs: Nonselective (COX-1 and COX-2): aspirin, ibuprofen, ketorolac, meloxicam, diclofenac, naproxen Selective (COX-2 only): celecoxib	Inhibit COX enzyme resulting in decreased formation of prostaglandin precursors Improved GI tolerability with selective inhibition of COX-2	May cause renal impairment, bleeding disorders COX-2 selective associated with increased risk of cardiovascular disease (MI, HF, stroke)

(continued)

Table 4.29 Commonly Used Nonopioid Analgesics (*continued*)

Medication	Mechanism of Action	Special Considerations
Gabapentinoids: gabapentin, pregabalin	Bind to the alpha-2-delta-1 subunit of voltage-gated calcium channels	Scope: neuropathic or perioperative pain management May cause sedation or drowsiness Renal dose adjustment required
Local anesthetics: lidocaine, bupivacaine, ropivacaine	Block peripheral and central voltage-dependent sodium channels resulting in inhibition of impulse initiation and transmission	Scope: neuropathic or perioperative pain management Local anesthetic systemic toxicity (perioral numbness, metallic taste, tachycardia, hypertension, visual changes, and seizures)
Anticonvulsants: carbamazepine oxcarbazepine	Block voltage-sensitive sodium channels	Scope: neuropathic pain Blood dyscrasias (aplastic anemia, agranulocytosis), toxic epidermal necrolysis, Stevens–Johnson syndrome; genetic testing for HLA-B*1502 allele required prior to initiation in certain populations, hepatotoxicity, hyponatremia, Carbamazepine is a strong inducer of CYP450[a] enzymes
Antidepressants: amitriptyline duloxetine venlafaxine	Serotonin and norepinephrine reuptake inhibition	Scope: neuropathic pain Anticholinergic effects (urinary retention, constipation, drowsiness), nausea Abrupt discontinuation may result in withdrawal symptoms (headache, nervousness, insomnia)

Note: [a]CYP450 enzymes play a key role in the metabolism of a wide variety of medications.
COX, cyclooxygenase; GI, gastrointestinal; MI, myocardial infarction; NSAIDs, nonsteroidal anti-inflammatory drugs.

Ketamine

Ketamine's primary mechanism of action is noncompetitive antagonism at the *N*-methyl-D-aspartate (NMDA) receptor. It also acts directly on the cortex and limbic system to produce a dissociative or cataleptic-like state. Ketamine is used as an anesthetic and has also been studied in the management of pain, sedation in critically ill patients, rapid sequence intubation, status asthmaticus, depression, and status epilepticus. Dosing is dependent on indication (Table 4.30).

Table 4.30 Common Ketamine Dosing Regimens

Dosing	Advantages	Adverse Effects
Pain: IV bolus: 0.2–0.5 mg/kg IV infusion: 0.3 mg/kg/hr	Minimal impact on the cardiopulmonary drive through preservation of the pharyngeal and laryngeal reflexes	Hypertension, tachycardia. Caution in patients with AMI, decompensated HF, ischemic CVD
Sedation: 0.5–2 mg/kg/hr	No impact on GI tract; NSAIDs that may cause GIB or opioids that may cause OIC	Increased secretion
Rapid sequence intubation: 1–2 mg/kg		Dysphoria, emergence phenomenon, confusion, nightmares, hallucinations; use caution with acute psychosis

AMI, acute myocardial infarction; CVD, cardiovascular disease; GI, gastrointestinal; GIB, gastrointestinal bleeding; HF, heart failure; NSAIDs, nonsteroidal anti-inflammatory drugs; OIC, opioid-induced constipation.

AGITATION/DELIRIUM

Agitation is often driven by underlying medical or psychological illnesses and may be acute or chronic in nature. Factors to consider during agent selection for the management of the acutely agitated patient include underlying cause of agitation, drug intoxication, alcohol withdrawal or intoxication, pain, delirium, available routes of administration, adverse effects, allergies, presence of organ (liver/ kidney) dysfunction, and patient age. Medication classes frequently used to elicit a sedative response include general anesthetics, benzodiazepines, barbiturates, alpha-2 agonists, antipsychotics, and anticonvulsants.

BENZODIAZEPINES

Benzodiazepines exert their anxiolytic, hypnotic, and anticonvulsant effects by binding to a benzodiazepine-specific site on the gamma aminobutyric acid (GABA) receptor that is different from the GABA binding site. Therefore, the CNS effects of benzodiazepines are dependent on the amount of available GABA. They are known to produce anterograde amnesia.

Long-term use of benzodiazepines may result in physical dependence, tolerance, or addiction. Physical dependence is present when abrupt cessation or a rapid dose reduction triggers a state of withdrawal. Acute withdrawal is more likely seen with abrupt discontinuation of benzodiazepines with short half-lives compared with agents with longer half-lives (Table 4.31). Signs of benzodiazepine withdrawal include anxiety, panic attacks, tremor, diaphoresis, poor concentration, sleep disturbance, insomnia, seizures, headaches, palpitations, psychosis, and perceptual disturbances.

Table 4.31 Commonly Used Benzodiazepines

Benzodiazepines	Common Initial Doses[a]	Half-Life	Comments
Alprazolam	PO: 0.25–0.5 mg	Short–intermediate	Oral formulations only
Lorazepam	IV bolus: 1–2 mg IV infusion: 0.5–5 mg/hr Onset (IV): 15–20 minutes	Short–intermediate	Useful to manage alcohol withdrawal IV administration preferred in the management of status epilepticus Propylene glycol toxicity limits use of continuous infusions
Midazolam	IV bolus: 0.5–2 mg IV infusion: 1–5 mg/hr Onset (IV): 1–5 minutes	Short, increases in renal dysfunction and/or with infusions more than 48 hours	No oral formulation available IM, IN, and buccal administration preferred for status epilepticus Requires renal dose adjustments
Clonazepam	PO: 0.25–1 mg	Long	Oral formulations only Consider in seizure management
Chlordiazepoxide	PO: 25–100 mg	Long	Only available orally Consider in alcohol withdrawal management
Diazepam	IV bolus: 5–10 mg Onset (IV): 1–5 minutes	Long	Long acting, more useful in alcohol withdrawal Rectal preparation is used in the management of status epilepticus

Note: [a]Dosing regimens are indication based.
IM, intramuscular; IN, intranasal; IV, intravenous.

Benzodiazepine Overdose

Benzodiazepine overdose is a significant toxicity. Signs of overdose include CNS depression, slurred speech, ataxia, and altered mental status.

Benzodiazepine Reversal

Flumazenil is a competitive antagonist of the benzodiazepine (BZD) receptor. Administration can precipitate withdrawal seizures. Therefore, the risks of flumazenil administration often outweigh the benefits.

■ Dose: 0.2 mg IV over 30 seconds, which may be repeated at 1-minute intervals. Usual cumulative maximum dose is 3 mg. Onset is 1 to 2 minutes. Duration is 0.7 to 1.3 hours.

BARBITURATES

Barbiturates bind to the GABA receptor at a site distinct from the benzodiazepine receptor, thereby enhancing the opening of the GABA receptor in the presence of GABA. In addition, barbiturates can directly activate GABA receptors at high concentrations, resulting in a more profound CNS depression compared with benzodiazepines. Barbiturates like benzodiazepines are metabolized hepatically and excreted by the kidneys. Barbiturates are used in the treatment and management of alcohol withdrawal, seizures, status epilepticus, induction of coma in severe brain injury, and sedation of patients requiring mechanical ventilation.

Sedation

The association of BZDs with the development of delirium in critically ill patients laid the foundation for BZD-sparing sedation strategies known as analgesia-based sedation or analgesia-first sedation. Alpha-2 agonists may have pain-sparing properties and are used as adjuncts in pain management, but propofol lacks any analgesic properties (Table 4.32).

Table 4.32 Commonly Used Nonbenzodiazepine Hypnotics

Medication Class	Onset (min)	Common Initial Regimens	Special Considerations
General Anesthetics			
Propofol	IV: 30 seconds	IV: 5–50 mcg/kg/min	Hypotension, bradycardia Urine discoloration Hypertriglyceridemia Propofol infusion syndrome
Alpha-2 agonists			
Clonidine	PO: ~1 hours TD: 2–3 days	PO: 0.1–0.2 q8h TD: 0.1–0.2 q72h	Hypotension, bradycardia
Dexmedetomidine	IV: 15–30 minutes	IV: 0.2–1.5 mcg/kg/hr	Hypotension, bradycardia

IV, intravenous; TD, transdermal.

ANTIPSYCHOTICS

Antipsychotics exert their mechanism of action via blockade of the dopamine D2 receptors. Second-generation antipsychotics have a lower propensity to cause movement disorders (extrapyramidal symptoms and tardive dyskinesia). This is because of their higher affinity for serotonin 5HT2A receptors, which may explain the lower incidence of extrapyramidal symptoms (Table 4.33). Indications for antipsychotics include acute psychosis and schizophrenia.

Table 4.33 Commonly Used Antipsychotics

Antipsychotics	Usual Starting Dose	Notes
First Generation or Typical		
Haloperidol	IV, IM: 2–5 mg PO: 0.5–5 mg Long-acting injectable is not used for acute agitation	Sedation QT prolongation Extrapyramidal symptoms Tardive dyskinesia

(continued)

Table 4.33 Commonly Used Antipsychotics (*continued*)

Antipsychotics	Usual Starting Dose	Notes
Second Generation or Atypical		
Aripiprazole	PO: 10–15 mg	
Olanzapine	IV, IM, PO: 5–10 mg	
Risperidone	PO: 1–2 mg	Long-acting preparation is not used for acute agitation
Quetiapine	PO:25–50 mg	
Ziprasidone	IM: 10 mg PO: 20–40 mg	Higher propensity for QTc prolongation

IM, intramuscular; IV, intravenous.

NEUROMUSCULAR BLOCKERS

Neuromuscular blocking agents (NMBAs) exert their action at the nicotinic acetylcholine receptor resulting in paralysis of the skeletal muscle. They may be classified as depolarizing or nondepolarizing based on their mechanism of action. Nondepolarizing agents can be further subdivided by chemical structure into aminosteroidal or benzylisoquinoline compounds (Table 4.34). Train of four monitoring with assessment of pertinent clinical parameters (e.g., ventilator compliance) should be used to guide therapy as well as the depth of paralysis. Indication for use includes rapid sequence intubation, management of life-threatening hypoxemia, shivering management in therapeutic hypothermia, and management of severe traumatic brain injury. AGACNPs must also be aware of reversal agents for neuromuscular blocking agents (Table 4.35).

Table 4.34 Commonly Used Neuromuscular Blocking Agents

Medication	Pharmacokinetics	Dosing Considerations	Special Considerations
Depolarizing: initial depolarization at the neuromuscular junction characterized by transient fasciculations followed by subsequent flaccid paralysis			
Succinylcholine	Duration: Ultra short Good option for rapid sequence intubation	No Rapidly hydrolyzed by plasma pseudocholinesterase to inactive metabolites RSI: 0.6–1.5 mg/kg	May cause life-threatening hyperkalemia, malignant hyperthermia, or myalgias Increased dose may be required in myasthenia gravis Avoid in pseudocholinesterase deficiency
Nondepolarizing: competitive antagonists by blocking the binding of acetylcholine at the receptor, thereby preventing the generation of an action potential			
Aminosteroidal Compounds			
Mivacurium	Short	No Plasma pseudocholinesterase	Histamine release Low potency requiring high doses for clinical use
Atracurium	Intermediate	No (Hoffman elimination, plasma esterases) RSI: 0.5–0.6 mg/kg Bolus: 0.1 mg/kg Infusion: 10–20 mcg/kg/min	May cause histamine release
Benzylisoquinoline Compounds			
Rocuronium	Intermediate	Hepatic RSI: 1.2 mg/kg Bolus: 0.1 mg/kg Infusion: 5–12 mcg/kg/min	Fast onset compared to other nondepolarizing NMBAs

(*continued*)

Table 4.34 Commonly Used Neuromuscular Blocking Agents (*continued*)

Medication	Pharmacokinetics	Dosing Considerations	Special Considerations
Vecuronium	Intermediate	Hepatic, renal RSI: 0.1–02 mg/kg Bolus: 0.1 mg/kg Infusion: 1–2 mcg/kg/min	Slower onset compared to succinylcholine, rocuronium
Pancuronium	Long	Renal, hepatic RSI: 0.08–0.12 Bolus: 0.02 mg/kg Infusion: not recommended	Postoperative residual neuromuscular weakness Tachycardia

NMBAs, neuromuscular blocking agents; RSI, rapid sequence intubation.

Table 4.35 Agents Used to Reverse Neuromuscular Blocking Agents

Reversal Agent	Pharmacokinetic Considerations	Notes
Neostigmine	Restores transmission at the neuromuscular junction through anticholinesterase activity Usual dose: 0.02–0.07 mg/kg IV Onset: 2–4 hours Half-life: ~65 minutes	May cause bradycardia, bronchospasm, and increased GI motility Requires simultaneous administration with anticholinergic agents (glycopyrrolate or atropine) to combat effects May not completely reverse blockade in patients with pseudocholinesterase deficiency
Sugammadex	Inactivates aminosteroidal NMBAs Usual dose: 2–4 mg/kg Onset: less than 3 minutes Half-life: ~2 hours	Higher affinity for rocuronium followed by vecuronium Will not reverse cisatracurium or atracurium

GI, gastrointestinal; IV, intravenous; NMBAs, neuromuscular blocking agents.

Special Considerations with Neuromuscular Blocking Agents

MG is an autoimmune disorder characterized by an immunologic attachment of the acetylcholine receptors resulting in skeletal muscle weakness. Treatment with anticholinesterase agents such as pyridostigmine is common. Caution should therefore be exercised and a risk–benefit assessment performed prior to the decision to use NMBAs in these patients. Succinylcholine should be avoided as these patients are considered resistant to depolarizing NMBAs because of the decreased number of acetylcholine receptors. Rocuronium or vecuronium are preferred given their intermediate-acting nature. Sugammadex, not neostigmine, should be used to reverse NMBAs in patients with MG.

Pseudocholinesterase deficiency: Succinylcholine is metabolized by pseudocholinesterase enzyme. Pseudocholinesterase deficiency refers to a defect in the pseudocholinesterase enzyme. Surveillance testing is unusual. Diagnosis often occurs when prolonged paralysis with succinylcholine is experienced

Prolonged muscle weakness: A modest risk of ICU-acquired weakness has been described with NMBA use. The odds are amplified in patients with sepsis or septic shock and the concomitant use of glucocorticoids.

▶ PHARMACOLOGY OF THE RESPIRATORY SYSTEM

Pharmacologic treatment for asthma and chronic obstructive pulmonary disease (COPD) is an important element in quality of life of older adults. The following section provides highlights for these specific health conditions.

Asthma is a chronic medical condition characterized by airflow obstruction, bronchial hyperresponsiveness, and inflammation leading to symptoms. The treatment of asthma involves the use of quick-relief or rescue medications for acute symptoms and maintenance or long-term medications to control persistent asthma. *COPD* is also an inflammation disorder that additionally can produce sputum that interferes with lung function. Smoking cessation is paramount in reducing progression of the disease state. Treatment options for both asthma and COPD are discussed next. Table 4.36 depicts maintenance/long-term control medications, and Table 4.37 depicts quick-relief/rescue medications.

Table 4.36 Maintenance/Long-Term Control Medications

Medication Class	Medications	MOA and Use	Special Considerations
ICS	Beclomethasone dipropionate, budesonide, flunisolide, fluticasone, propionate, mometasone furoate, triamcinolone, acetonide, ciclesonide	MOA: reduces inflammation, inhibits cytokine production Use: asthma and COPD (more commonly used in asthma at an earlier stage; later stage in COPD)	Gargle after inhaler use to avoid candidiasis SMART with a single inhaler of an ICS plus LABA can be used with moderate to severe persistent asthma.
LABA Inhaled agents	Formoterol, salmeterol, olodaterol, arformoterol, indacaterol	MOA: relaxes smooth muscle Use: asthma and COPD	LABA can be added to regimen of ICS if asthma is uncontrolled. Can be first line for COPD
LAMA Inhaled agents	Tiotropium, glycopyrronium, umeclidinium, aclidinium	MOA: reduces airway obstruction by inhibiting acetylcholine at muscarinic receptors causing bronchodilation Use: Asthma and COPD (typically used as first-line or second-line therapy in COPD; later use in asthma)	Used as first line for COPD Can be additive to other anticholinergic burden medications; evaluate for dry mouth, difficulty swallowing
Leukotriene modifiers Oral agents	Montelukast, zafirlukast	MOA: inhibits cysteinyl leukotriene receptor that correlates with airway edema and smooth muscle contraction Use: asthma	For asthma treatment, take in the evening as leukotrienes are increased at night.
5-Lipoxygenase Inhibitor Oral agent	Zileuton	MOA: inhibits production of leukotriene Use: asthma	
Methylxanthines Oral/IV agents	Theophylline	MOA: relaxes smooth muscle, decreases T-lymphocytes, increases contraction of diaphragm and clearance of mucous Use: asthma	Not preferred but can be used as an alternative agent Monitor serum theophylline levels
Mast cell stabilizer Inhalation via nebulizer	Cromolyn sodium	MOA: blocks early and late reaction to allergens; prevents mast cell release of histamine and leukotrienes Use: asthma	Not recommended for routine use for asthma, lower efficacy May be used for exercise or allergen-induced prevention but not first-line therapy

(continued)

Table 4.36 Maintenance/Long-Term Control Medications (*continued*)

Medication Class	Medications	MOA and Use	Special Considerations
Immunomodulators Subcutaneous injection agents	Omalizumab, mepolizumab, dupilumab, reslizumab, benralizumab	MOA: inhibits IgE binding to high-affinity IgE receptor on mast cells and basophils Use: asthma	May consider as add-on therapy for severe asthma or peripheral blood eosinophils Monitor for anaphylaxis when initiating therapy

ICS, inhaled corticosteroid; LABA: long-acting beta-agonist; LAMA, long-acting muscarinic agonist; MOA, mechanism of action; SABA, short-acting beta-agonist; SMART, single maintenance and reliever therapy.

Table 4.37 Rescue or Quick Relief Medications

Medication Class	Medications	MOA and Use	Special Considerations
SABA	Albuterol, levalbuterol, pirbuterol	MOA: relaxes bronchial muscle on beta-2 receptors Use: asthma and COPD	■ For severe exacerbations can be combined with inhaled SAMA and nebulizer treatments ■ Onset of action 5–8 minutes; duration 4–6 hours; half-life 4–5 hours ■ Used for quick rescue relief, prior to exertion or exercise ■ Best to wait a minute between inhalations
SAMA	Ipratropium bromide	MOA: causes bronchodilation by blocking acetylcholine in bronchial smooth muscle Use: asthma and COPD	Can add to anticholinergic burden; not recommended if LAMA is already employed
Oral/IV corticosteroids	Prednisone, methylprednisolone, prednisolone	MOA: anti-inflammatory Use: asthma and COPD	Oral: take earlier in the day to reduce insomnia

COPD, chronic obstructive pulmonary disease; IV, intravenous; LAMA, long-acting muscarinic antagonists; MOA, mechanism of action; SABA, short-acting beta-antagonists; SAMA, short-acting muscarinic antagonists.

CHRONIC OBSTRUCTIVE PULMONARY DISEASE

Classification of COPD using the GOLD criteria using the block levels (A-B-C-D), symptoms ratings using the Modified Medical Research Council (mMRC) Dyspnea Scale, and/or COPD Assessment Test (CAT) Score questionnaires, along with the number of exacerbations resulting in hospitalizations, is used to determine treatment.

PHOSPHODIESTERASE-4 ENZYME INHIBITOR

Roflumilast can also be used as a treatment option for refractory COPD. Roflumilast is an elective inhibition of phosphodiesterase-4 (PDE4) leading to an accumulation of cyclic AMP (cAMP) within inflammatory and structural cells important in the pathogenesis of COPD. Anti-inflammatory effects include suppression of cytokine release and inhibition of lung infiltration by neutrophils and other leukocytes. Pulmonary remodeling and mucociliary malfunction are also attenuated. This medication reduces the risk of COPD exacerbations in patients with severe COPD associated with chronic bronchitis and history of exacerbations. It is reserved for Category D treatment where high CAT and mMRC scores and hospitalizations are determined. Adverse effects include dizziness, nausea, diarrhea, headache, back pain, flu-like symptoms, insomnia, anorexia, irritability, and severe anxiety.

Clinical Pearls

- Use nebulized bronchodilators; maximize short-acting use for relief.
- If using long-acting muscarinic agonist (LAMA; better to use short-acting beta-agonist [SABA] for rescue), avoid short-acting muscarinic agonist (SAMA).
- Maximize long-acting inhalers to reduce exacerbations.
- Think of anticholinergic burden with other medications: consider side effects of dry mouth, dry throat, and difficulty swallowing as potentially medication related.
- Use corticosteroids such as methylprednisolone IV 40 to 60 mg daily for 5 to 14 days; convert to oral prednisone when able.
- Employ antibiotics only when appropriate.

ASTHMA

Teach proper inhaler technique with use of a spacer, and reassess technique at every visit/encounter to ensure proper mechanics. Stress the importance of adhering to medications. Encourage peak flow monitoring. Assess control of asthma symptoms and step-up treatment if needed followed by reassessments in 2 to 6 weeks. Use step-down therapy if asthma is controlled for 3 consecutive months. For inpatient management of asthma exacerbations, use inhaled SABA. Prescribers can use a metered dose inhaler or nebulizer treatment. Combination inhaled corticosteroids and long-acting beta-agonists (LABA) can be used for intermittent symptom relief or acute exacerbations.

▶ MEDICATION SAFETY IN THE ACUTE CARE SETTING

In 2000, *To Err Is Human* was published, highlighting patient harm caused by medical errors. The report asserted that errors are caused by system failures and established a national agenda designed to improve patient safety. *Adverse drug events* (ADEs), which include medication errors, result in more than a million ED visits annually. An ADE is defined as *harm* that patients experience from the use of a medication and includes medication errors and adverse drug reactions (ADRs). ADRs are commonly known as side effects (Table 4.38).

Table 4.38 Types of Adverse Drug Events

Type	Definition	Example
ADR	Harm or undesirable reaction that patient experiences despite proper drug prescribing and administration. ADRs include side effects and allergic reactions and are not preventable.	Patient experiences nausea (side effect) with an appropriate regimen of combined oral contraceptives.
Medication error	Harm or undesirable reaction that the patient experiences when the medication is used in error. Medication errors are preventable.	Patient experiences hypoglycemia after too much insulin is administered.

ADR, adverse drug reaction.

The National Coordinating Council for Medication Error Reporting and Prevention (NCCMERP) index classifies medication errors from Category A through I based on the severity of outcomes. Institutions may use the NCCMERP index to categorize the level of harm resulting from ADEs, where Category A is a near miss, and Category I is an error that results in patient's death. A near miss is defined as an event or situation that did not reach the patient due to chance or intervention and therefore did not cause harm.

Institutions often have high-alert medications (HAMs) on formulary (Table 4.39). HAMs are not associated with higher risk of errors; however, they tend to cause more harm when used in error. The Institute for Safe Medication Practices (ISMP) maintains a current list of HAMs with recommendations that inform safe practices.

Table 4.39 High-Alert Medications

Example	What Happens if Used in Error?
Insulin	■ Insulin overdose may lead to severe hypoglycemia, life-threatening seizures, and coma. ■ Insulin under-dose may lead to complications of severe hyperglycemia such as ketoacidosis.

Medication errors may occur at any step of the medication use process, including prescribing, processing, dispensing, administration, and monitoring. These errors are usually the result of multiple failures (Tables 4.40 and 4.41). The Swiss Cheese Model was designed to illustrate how medication errors occur. Each slice of the Swiss Cheese Model represents a barrier that prevents medication errors from happening. The holes in the Swiss cheese represent latent failures (inherent weaknesses) and active failures in the system; when lined up, a medication error ensues.

Table 4.40 Failures Involved in Medication Errors

Type and Definition	Example of Failure	Comment
Latent Failure: System failure, such as design, organization, or equipment, that is usually hidden until an error happens. System failures contribute to errors that may or may not cause harm. *Active Failure:* Human failure that is apparent and is the act that leads to the error.	Provider is ordering insulin using CPOE. IM, SUBQ, and IV ROA are options to select for insulin administration. The provider selects IM. The patient receives insulin IM and experiences a hypoglycemic event.	All holes in the Swiss Cheese lined up, perfectly leading to a hypoglycemic event. *Latent failure (i.e., system failure):* The availability of IM route of administration for insulin in CPOE *Active failure:* Selecting wrong ROA

CPOE, computerized provider order entry; IM, intramuscular; IV, intravenous; ROA, route of administration.

Table 4.41 Examples of Medication Errors

Cause of Error		Example
Illegible Handwriting		Writing prescription for famotidine but handwriting looks like furosemide
Missing Information	Comorbid conditions	Prescribing a NSAID to a patient with CHF
	Concomitant drugs	Prescribing sacubitril/valsartan to a patient taking an ACEI
	Available test results	Prescribing a potassium-sparing diuretic when serum creatinine increased by 0.3 mg/dL in 48 hours indicating AKI
	Drug allergies	Prescribing penicillin to a patient with documented severe penicillin allergy
Incorrect Drug		Prescribing potassium when the intended medication is vitamin K
Incorrect Dose		Prescribing enoxaparin without adjusting the dose for decreased renal function
Unclear/Complex Instructions		Prescribing regular insulin with complex sliding scale instructions
LASA Confusion		Prescribing hydralazine when intended medication was hydroxyzine
Drug Omission		Failure to prescribe an antiemetic medication for a patient experiencing nausea
Prescription Transmission Failure		Using electronic prescribing and failure of prescription to reach the pharmacy
Failure to Monitor Efficacy		Prescribing acetaminophen and failure to assess patient pain level
Failure to Monitor Adverse Effects		Prescribing lisinopril and failure to assess for development of cough
Misinterpret Laboratory Monitoring Parameters		Prescribing warfarin and misinterpreting the patient's INR

(continued)

Table 4.41 Examples of Medication Errors (*continued*)

Cause of Error	Example
Incorrect Timing of Monitoring	Repeating HbA$_{1c}$ level in 1 month instead of 3 months
Incorrect Timing of Serum Monitoring	Initiating lithium and checking lithium serum level before lithium reaches steady state
Cause of Error	Example
Lack of Communication with PCP	Discharging patient on a new medication and failing to communicate with PCP
Lack of Communication with Community Pharmacy	Initiating a new prescription for sertraline and failing to communicate with community pharmacy to discontinue citalopram prescription on file
Lack of Patient Counseling	Discharging patient with 1-week supply of medication and failing to counsel the patient to follow-up with their PCP to renew the prescription

ACEI, angiotensin-converting enzyme inhibitor; AKI, acute kidney injury; CHF, chronic heart failure; HbA$_{1c}$, glycated hemoglobin; INR, international normalized ratio; LASA, look-alike or sound-alike; NSAID, nonsteroidal anti-inflammatory drug; PCP, primary care physician; ROA, route of administration.

AGACNPs play a crucial role in medication safety. Follow strategies to prevent medication errors:

- Promote a just culture within your organization. A just culture is nonpunitive.
- Report medication errors and near misses to identify and implement corrective action plans.
- Be a patient safety champion! Participate in retrospective safety evaluations and event detection.
- Avoid using error-prone abbreviations, symbols, and dose designations. Review the ISMP List of Error-Prone Abbreviations.
- Use order sets to standardize prescribing practices and decrease reliance on memory.
- Encourage the implementation of Tall Man Lettering for look-alike sound-alike (LASA) medications.
- Obtain and document accurate patient height, weight, and allergies.
- Perform medication reconciliation at each patient encounter and at transitions of care.
- Maintain communications with interdisciplinary team caring for the patient.
- Subscribe to safety newsletters, such as the National Alert Network (NAN).
- Question unexpected drug reactions and suspect medication errors.

▶ PRESCRIBING CONSIDERATIONS FOR OLDER ADULTS

Caring for older adults across all healthcare settings is challenging for many reasons. It is known that patient presentation is complex, disease presentation is often atypical, and comorbid diseases are the norm. Older adults consume disproportionately more prescription and over-the-counter (OTC) medications than younger adults, increasing the risk of ADEs. Benzodiazepines, antihistamines, and NSAIDs are the most frequently identified drug classes associated with potentially inappropriate prescriptions. Multiple medications, or polypharmacy, is common given the number of coexisting chronic medical conditions; patients might have multiple specialists, all prescribing just for one condition. Polypharmacy can be rational (a three-drug regimen for HF) or irrational, where prescribers fail to take into consideration the pharmacodynamic and pharmacokinetic implications of patients taking so many medications. In addition, patient-specific factors, including cognitive and sensory impairments, limited health literacy, depression, financial constraints, and functional impairments, all may affect adherence to these types of complex regimens. Medication management in older adults calls for a more comprehensive and systematic approach to maximize patient safety. Here are several practical considerations for the AGACNP to guide prescribing decisions at different phases of care delivery.

ADMISSION

ADEs lead to millions of patients being admitted to the acute care setting each year. Always consider that the patient's complaint/condition may be due to drug–drug, drug–disease, or drug–food interactions; to side effects from a new medication being started; or to issues with drug adherence, such as abruptly stopping a medication (e.g., diuretics) or taking medications incorrectly (e.g., inhalers, insulin, anticoagulants). It is important to consider multiple sources of information when first establishing a patient's list of medications. While some patients may be able to provide a detailed list, this may not always be the case, and additional information may be needed. Family, friends, or private caregivers can be sources of information. It is perfectly appropriate to contact the patient's primary care provider and/ or pharmacy to confirm dosages, start/stop dates, or changes in dosing.

Inquiring about use of OTC preparations is also important, as even products with diphenhydramine (Benadryl) can lead to dizziness, blurred vision, urinary retention, constipation, confusion, and falls. It is also useful to match the medication list with the patient's known medical problems to identify gaps or redundancies. When making rational drug choices for older patients, always calculate renal dosing and consider the patient's body composition and nutritional state, specifically when considering drugs that are albumin bound or are highly lipophilic, which may require dosing adjustments. Physiologic changes, including changes in the blood–brain barrier, brain atrophy, neuronal loss, inflammation, and other pathologic changes may lead to sensitivity to opioids, benzodiazepines, and hypnotics, and these drugs should be used with great caution or not at all, especially as they may contribute to or worsen delirium. Use the Beers list (https://www.americangeriatrics.org/media-center/news/updated-202 2-ags-beers-criteriar-potentially-inappropriate-medication-use-older) or Screening Tool of Older Persons' Prescriptions (STOPP; https://psnet.ahrq.gov/issue/stoppstart-criteria-potentially-inap propriate-medications-potential-prescribing-omissions) as a guide for drug selection, and follow the mantra of "Start low, go slow." Prescribing decisions should always consider the individual's goals of care, risk of benefit versus harm, quality of life, and life expectancy. For example, decisions to start/ continue anticoagulation in a patient with new atrial fibrillation need to be individualized based on shared decision-making after discussion of absolute and relative risks of both stroke (CHA$_2$DS$_2$VASc score) and bleeding (HAS-BLED, ORBIT, or ATRIA scores), as well as patient values and preferences. A conversation with the patient's primary care physician (PCP) may be needed.

DISCHARGE

Medication safety for older adults becomes even more important at the time of discharge because miscommunication can lead to medication discrepancies and errors. Careful documentation needs to include medications stopped and started (especially those around the day of discharge), and dosing changes need to be highlighted. When preparing a discharge summary, always consider, what are the key points a healthcare provider would need to know about this patient if they were seeing the patient post discharge? AGACNPs should have a low threshold for referring patients to Visiting Nurses Association (VNAs) who can assess, monitor, and evaluate patients' understanding of their medication regimens and assist patients with medication management systems if needed, including prepacking medication services or obtaining blister packs through pharmacies.

▶ SUMMARY

AGACNPs regularly prescribe medications; thus, a solid foundation of pharmacology knowledge will ensure safer and more effective care. Be sure to adhere to safe medication prescribing practices. When a concern or question arises regarding a medication, reach out to a pharmacist to collaborate in making treatment and dosing decisions.

KNOWLEDGE CHECK: CHAPTER 4

1. The dose of ceftriaxone to treat urinary tract infections is 1 g intravenous (IV) once daily. However, to treat meningitis effectively, the dose of ceftriaxone needs to be increased to 2 g IV twice daily. Which pharmacokinetic parameter best explains the need for this increased dosing?

   A. Ceftriaxone experiences extensive first-pass effect when treating meningitis.
   B. Ceftriaxone has lower distribution into central nervous system (CNS) tissue than kidney/bladder tissue.
   C. Ceftriaxone has increased bioavailability when treating urinary tract infections.
   D. Ceftriaxone is eliminated more rapidly when treating meningitis.

2. A patient was prescribed aspirin for secondary prevention of stroke. After the first dose, they experienced anaphylaxis. Further investigation revealed that the patient's allergy profile listed aspirin. The prescriber and pharmacist both bypassed allergy alerts. Which of the following terms *best* describes this event?

   A. Near miss
   B. Adverse drug reaction
   C. Medication error
   D. Side effect

3. Intravenous (IV) unfractionated heparin (UFH) was given to a patient. Two hours later, an activated partial thromboplastin time (aPTT) level was drawn. The nurse adjusts the infusion rate to address a subtherapeutic aPTT level. Which of the following *best* describes the cause of this error?

   A. Incorrect timing of aPTT monitoring
   B. Failure to monitor efficacy
   C. Failure to monitor adverse effects
   D. Incorrect timing of UFH administration

4. Which of the following is considered an active failure?

   A. An infusion pump without alerts when exceeding administration rates
   B. Look-alike medications stored in the same bin
   C. Barcode malfunctions while scanning medications
   D. Administering a medication to the wrong patient

5. Which one of the following statements is correct?

   A. An adverse drug event (ADE) is always associated with a medication error.
   B. A near miss results in patient harm.
   C. Medication errors are preventable.
   D. Side effects are a result of medication errors.

6. Which of the following anticoagulant regimens is most appropriate for venous thromboembolism (VTE) prophylaxis in a medically ill patient who has creatine clearance (CrCl) of 28 mL/min?

   A. Unfractionated heparin (UFH) 5,000 units subcutaneous (SUBQ) every 24 hours
   B. Enoxaparin 30 mg SUBQ every 24 hours
   C. Fondaparinux 2.5 mg SUBQ every 24 hours
   D. Apixaban 2.5 mg PO every 12 hours

(See answers next page.)

1. **B) Ceftriaxone has lower distribution into central nervous system (CNS) tissue than kidney/bladder tissue.**

The blood–brain barrier limits the ability of drugs to distribute to the CNS. To overcome this barrier, medications must be given at higher doses to achieve adequate concentrations within this compartment. A ceftriaxone dose of 1 g once daily would result in suboptimal antibiotic concentrations to fight bacterial meningitis.

2. **C) Medication error**

The patient experienced an adverse drug event after aspirin was administered. Further investigation revealed that the patient had a known allergy to aspirin, and that was documented in their chart. Therefore, this event is a medication error. Near miss would be if this error was caught before reaching the patient. This error would be classified as an adverse drug reaction if allergy to aspirin was not documented in the patient's profile (i.e., unknown to healthcare providers). Adverse drug reaction and side effect are interchangeable terms.

3. **A) Incorrect timing of aPTT monitoring**

Based on pharmacodynamic properties, aPTT requires monitoring every 6 hours. The patient's aPTT was checked at the incorrect time (2 hours after administration). This error is not failure to monitor efficacy since aPTT was monitored. This error does not describe an adverse effect to UFH or an incorrect timing of UFH administration. Incorrect timing of aPTT monitoring best describes this error.

4. **D) Administering a medication to the wrong patient**

Active failure is a human failure that is apparent and is the act that leads to the error. An infusion pump without alerts, storage issues, and barcode malfunctioning are examples of latent failures (i.e., system failures). Administering a medication to the wrong patient is considered an active failure.

5. **C) Medication errors are preventable.**

Medication errors are preventable with the implementation of safe practices. An ADE may occur due to a side effect or a medication error. A near miss does not result in patient harm because the error is caught before reaching the patient. Side effects are not medication errors because they are inherent risks associated with proper use of the medication.

6. **B) Enoxaparin 30 mg SUBQ every 24 hours**

The patient is medically ill requiring VTE prophylaxis. Apixaban does not have a U.S. Food and Drug Administration–approved indication in this population. UFH SUBQ is an option, but the dose should be 5,000 units every 8 or 12 hours (not 24 hours). Fondaparinux is contraindicated when CrCl is <30 mL/min. Enoxaparin is renally dosed at 30 mg SUBQ every 24 hours.

7. The medical team would like to initiate rivaroxaban for a patient to treat venous thromboembolism (VTE). Which of the following is most appropriate to recommend?

   A. 15 mg PO every 12 hours for 21 days
   B. 20 mg PO every 24 hours for 7 days
   C. 10 mg PO every 12 hours for 7 days
   D. 5 mg PO every 24 hours for 21 days

8. Which of the following anticoagulants is monitored by international normalized ratio (INR)?

   A. Unfractionated heparin (UFH)
   B. Enoxaparin
   C. Warfarin
   D. Rivaroxaban

9. Which of the following anticoagulants is approved to reduce the risk of major cardiovascular events when given with aspirin?

   A. Warfarin
   B. Rivaroxaban
   C. Apixaban
   D. Fondaparinux

10. An 82-year-old man requires anticoagulation for prevention of stroke due to atrial fibrillation. He weighs 58 kg, and his creatine clearance (CrCl) is 45 mL/min. Which of the following is the most appropriate recommendation?

    A. Rivaroxaban 20 mg PO every 24 hours
    B. Apixaban 5 mg PO every 12 hours
    C. Rivaroxaban 10 mg PO every 24 hours
    D. Apixaban 2.5 mg PO every 12 hours

11. Beta-lactam efficacy is optimized by which of the following pharmacokinetic/pharmacodynamic parameters?

    A. Time above minimum inhibitory concentration (MIC)
    B. Concentration above MIC
    C. AUC relative to MIC
    D. Trough level

12. Which of the following classes of antifungals is associated with multiple drug–drug interactions?

    A. Echinocandins
    B. Amphotericin B
    C. Polyenes
    D. Azoles

13. A 75-year-old man presents to the clinic with a diagnosis of community-acquired pneumonia. He has a past medical history of diabetes, atrial fibrillation, hypertension, chronic kidney disease (CKD) stage 3, and penicillin allergy described as rash, and he previously tolerated Keflex. Which one of the following antibiotics is most appropriate to treat this patient's pneumonia in an outpatient setting?

    A. Ceftriaxone (Rocephin)
    B. Cefpodoxime (Vantin)
    C. Amoxicillin/clavulanic acid (Augmentin)
    D. Meropenem (Merrem)

(See answers next page.)

7. A) 15 mg PO every 12 hours for 21 days

Rivaroxaban is started at 15 mg PO every 12 hours for 21 days, followed by 20 mg PO daily. The 7-day duration is for apixaban (starts at 10 mg PO every 12 hours for 7 days, followed by 5 mg PO every 12 hours). Rivaroxaban is not dosed at 5 mg PO every 24 hours.

8. C) Warfarin

Warfarin is monitored using INR. UFH is monitored using activated partial thromboplastin time (aPTT), anti-Xa activity, or activated clotting time (ACT) depending on indication. Enoxaparin and rivaroxaban are monitored using anti-Xa activity.

9. B) Rivaroxaban

Rivaroxaban is the anticoagulant approved to reduce the risk of major cardiovascular events when given with aspirin. Apixaban does not have this indication, nor do warfarin or fondaparinux.

10. D) Apixaban 2.5 mg PO every 12 hours

Since the patient's CrCl is <50 mL/min, the dose of rivaroxaban should be 15 mg PO every 24 hours, not 20 mg. The 10-mg dose of rivaroxaban is not used for prevention of stroke due to atrial fibrillation but is used for venous thromboembolism (VTE) prophylaxis and to prevent VTE recurrence. Apixaban 5 mg PO every 12 hours is often used unless the patient meets two of the following criteria: age ≥80 years, weight ≤60 kg, and serum creatinine (SCr) ≥1.5 mg/dL. The patient is 82 years old (≥80 years), and his weight is 58 kg (≤ 60 kg); two criteria are met to reduce the apixaban dose to 2.5 mg PO every 12 hours.

11. A) Time above minimum inhibitory concentration (MIC)

The pharmacokinetic/pharmacodynamic parameter that best predicts beta-lactam efficacy is time above the MIC. The goal is to achieve levels above the MIC for 40% to 60% of the dosing interval to optimize the bactericidal effect of the antibiotic. Concentration and AUC are associated with other classes of antibiotics. Trough monitors vancomycin and gentamycin dosing.

12. D) Azoles

Azole antifungals have numerous drug–drug interactions due to their inhibition of cytocrome pathways (CYP) enzymes responsible for the metabolism of many drugs. Concomitant medications should be reviewed for potential interactions and adjusted, monitored, or avoided as needed.

13. B) Cefpodoxime (Vantin)

For a patient with mild penicillin allergy, cephalosporins are an appropriate class to consider. Cefpodoxime is an oral cephalosporin that can be used to treat community acquired pneumonia (CAP). Ceftriaxone is appropriate but only available in intravenous (IV) formulations. Amoxicillin/clavulanic acid is an appropriate therapy for CAP but should be avoided due to his allergy without further information or penicillin skin testing. Meropenem is only available IV and is not appropriate for CAP due to its broad antimicrobial activity.

14. What is true of all fluoroquinolones? Fluoroquinolones possess good:

    A. *Streptococcus pneumoniae* activity
    B. *Pseudomonas aeruginosa* activity
    C. *Bacteroides fragilis* activity
    D. *Enterobacterales* activity

15. Which of the following statements is true of clindamycin?

    A. Clindamycin possesses good hospital-acquired methicillin-resistant *Staphylococcus aureus* (MRSA) activity.
    B. Clindamycin is a drug of first choice for anaerobic coverage of active intra-abdominal infections.
    C. Clindamycin has been associated with development of *Clostridioides difficile*–associated diarrhea and colitis.
    D. Clindamycin is an inhibitor of CYP3A4 enzymes.

16. Which of the following antibiotics possesses activity against *Pseudomonas aeruginosa*?

    A. Ampicillin/sulbactam
    B. Ertapenem
    C. Ceftriaxone
    D. Meropenem

17. For which one of the following pathogens is there a difference in the coverage provided by azithromycin and doxycycline?

    A. Community-acquired methicillin-resistant *Staphylococcus aureus* (MRSA)
    B. *Streptococcus pneumoniae*
    C. *Escherichia coli*
    D. *Mycoplasma pneumoniae*

18. Which of the following antibiotics is *correctly* paired with a known side effect that is typically attributed to that antibiotic?

    A. Vancomycin: gastrointestinal intolerance (nausea/vomiting/diarrhea)
    B. Clindamycin: *Clostridioides difficile* diarrhea
    C. Erythromycin: nephrotoxicity
    D. Aminoglycosides: infusion reactions (flushing, rash, pruritis)

19. Which virus is treated with ganciclovir?

    A. Influenza A
    B. Herpes simplex
    C. Herpes zoster
    D. Cytomegalovirus

20. The AGACNP should follow which mantra when prescribing opioids for the older adult trauma patient:

    A. "Never give opioids to older adults."
    B. "Start low, go slow."
    C. "Higher doses equal better pain control."
    D. "Opioids go before nonopioids."

(See answers next page.)

14. D) *Enterobacterales* activity
All the fluoroquinolones possess activity against *Enterobacterales*. Most fluoroquinolones possess good activity against penicillin-susceptible and penicillin-resistant *S. pneumoniae*. However, ciprofloxacin does not cover these organisms. Some fluoroquinolones possess good activity against *P. aeruginosa*, but this is limited to ciprofloxacin and levofloxacin. Moxifloxacin is the only fluoroquinolone with *B. fragilis* activity.

15. C) Clindamycin has been associated with development of *Clostridioides difficile*–associated diarrhea and colitis.
Clindamycin has good gram-positive activity that includes community-acquired MRSA, but not hospital-acquired MRSA. Although it has activity against *Bacteroides fragilis* and had been frequently used for anaerobic coverage in active intra-abdominal infection in the past, *B. fragilis* resistance has increased and precludes current use for this indication. Clindamycin does not inhibit CYP3A4 enzymes.

16. D) Meropenem
Meropenem has activity against *P. aeruginosa*. Ampicillin/sulbactam possesses activity against some gram-negative pathogens, including some that are ampicillin-resistant due to beta-lactamase (BL) production. However, the BL inhibitor does not allow the product to have *P. aeruginosa* activity. Ertapenem is a carbapenem antibiotic with a broad spectrum of activity. Unlike the other carbapenems, it does not have activity against *P. aeruginosa*. Ceftriaxone has broad gram-negative activity, but this does not include *P. aeruginosa*.

17. A) Community-acquired methicillin-resistant *Staphylococcus aureus* (MRSA)
Doxycycline is a treatment option for community-acquired MRSA, but azithromycin has poor activity against this organism. Azithromycin and doxycycline possess activity against *S. pneumoniae* and *M. pneumoniae*. Neither have notable activity against *E. coli*.

18. B) Clindamycin: *Clostridioides difficile* diarrhea
Clindamycin is one of the antibiotics frequently implicated as being associated with *C. difficile* diarrhea. Vancomycin is not typically associated with gastrointestinal side effects. Erythromycin is not typically associated with nephrotoxicity. Vancomycin is associated with the described infusion-related side effects, but these are not typical problems observed with aminoglycosides.

19. D) Cytomegalovirus
Cytomegalovirus can be treated with ganciclovir or valganciclovir. Influenza A can be treated with oseltamivir, peramivir, zanamivir, or baloxavir. Herpes simplex and herpes zoster can be treated with acyclovir or valacyclovir.

20. B) "Start low, go slow."
Given the known physiologic changes in older adults, it is better to "start low, go slow" when introducing opioids for pain control in the older adult population. Never giving opioids to older adults is not reasonable, as some older adult patients will require opioids being added to their pain regimen, particularly in the setting of acute pain. Higher doses do not equate to better pain control; a stepwise process for increasing opioid dosing must be implemented for all patients to avoid negative side effects. Opioids should not be the initial choice of pain control given the side effect profile; nonopioid pain management should be employed first.

KEY BIBLIOGRAPHY

Only key resources appear in the print edition. Access the full bibliography for this chapter on ExamPrepConnect.com.

Dixon, D. L., Riche, D. M., & Kelly, M. S. (2021). Dyslipidemia. In J. T. DiPiro, G. C. Yee, L. L. Posey Michael, S. T. Haines, T. D. Nolin, & V. L. Ellingrod (Eds.), *DiPiro: Pharmacotherapy a pathophysiologic approach* (12th ed.). McGraw Hill.

Heidenreich, P. A., Bozkurt, B., Aguilar, D., Allen, L. A., Byun, J. J., Colvin, M. M., Deswal, A., Drazner, M. H., Dunlay, S. M., Evers, L. R., Fang, J. C., Fedson, S. E., Fonarow, G. C., Hayek, S. S., Hernandez, A. F., Khazanie, P., Kittleson, M. M., Lee, C. S., Link, M. S. … Yancy, C. W. (2022). 2022 AHA/ACC/HFSA guideline for the management of heart failure: A report of the American College of Cardiology/American Heart Association Joint Committee on clinical practice guidelines. *Circulation, 145*(18), e895–e1032. https://doi.org/10.1161/CIR.0000000000001063

National Heart, Lung, and Blood Institute. (2021, February 4). *Asthma management guidelines: Focused updates 2020*. https://www.nhlbi.nih.gov/health-topics/asthma-management-guidelines-2020-updates

Rhoney, D., & Peacock, W. F. (2009). Intravenous therapy for hypertensive emergencies, part 1. *American Journal of Health-System Pharmacy, 66*(15), 1343–1352. https://doi.org/10.2146/ajhp080348.p1

Advanced Health Assessment Review

Henry Ellis, Alexander Menard, and Dawn Carpenter

▶ INTRODUCTION

Health assessment is a conversation in which the patient provides a chief complaint (the reason for seeking care). The AGACNP elicits pertinent positives and negatives to work toward determining the diagnosis. Two main types of interviews exist: comprehensive and focused/problem oriented.

▶ HISTORY TAKING

History taking starts with a chief complaint. From there, the AGACNP will develop a list of differential diagnoses. Information gathered during the encounter narrows this list. As additional data, including physical exam and diagnostic testing results, are gathered, the primary diagnosis comes to the top of the list.

HISTORY OF PRESENTING ILLNESS
The history of presenting illness (HPI) establishes the chief complaint using the patient's own words. Investigate the chief complaint thoroughly. For multiple complaints, the AGACNP must decide if the symptoms are related or are separate problems. An effective HPI will be complete and clear and will chronologically recap the events leading to the patient presentation. Use a system to capture this data (Table 5.1).

Table 5.1 Methods to Interview Presenting Symptoms

OLDCAART	Seven Cardinal Features
■ Onset	■ Quality
■ Location	■ Location
■ Duration	■ Chronology
■ Character	■ Setting and onset
■ Aggravating and alleviating factors	■ Severity
■ Associated symptoms	■ Modifying factors
■ Radiation	■ Associated symptoms
■ Timing	

PAST MEDICAL HISTORY
Asking about other medical problems and surgeries helps to build the context of the current symptoms. Determine whether the current symptoms are a new problem, an acute exacerbation of a chronic condition, or a complication from a previous procedure:

- Start with open-ended questions: "What medical problems do you have?" (Be sure to use layperson's terms.) Then ask specifics for each diagnosis: When was the diagnosis made? Why and how was it made? How is it being managed/treated? Recent flares/exacerbations?
- Ask about specific diagnoses that are on your list of differential diagnoses.
- Include past and or recent hospitalizations, including date and duration.
- Ask about health maintenance, such as vaccinations and routine screenings.

PAST SURGICAL HISTORY

Start by asking the patient, "Have you had any surgeries or procedures?" Then ask about specific surgeries or procedures that inform the differential diagnosis list. Ask specifics for each surgery or procedure: When was the surgery or procedure done? What was the indication for the surgery or procedure? Were there complications? If yes, what were they, and how were they managed?

ALLERGIES

Ask all patients about their allergies, including their reaction and when and how it was treated. A thorough allergy history must include allergies to medications, foods, contrast dye, shellfish, and latex, as well as environmental allergies.

MEDICATIONS

A complete medication history is required for all patients and includes:

- medications: dose, frequency, route, indication, last dose, and compliance
- adherence: When asking about adherence to medications, ask, "How often do you miss a dose?" This question normalizes missing doses and allows for more accurate data.
- over-the-counter medications
- herbal and/or nutritional supplements
- other medications not prescribed, including borrowed medications (narcotics, anxiolytics)

SOCIAL HISTORY

This is a time to gather information regarding a patient's social supports and structure. A nonjudgmental and professional approach is best (Table 5.2).

Table 5.2 Social History Components and Details

Social History	Details Needed
Occupation	Exposures, injuries
Household composition	Individual, multigenerational, etc.
Military service	If yes, exposures, injuries, residual effects or deficits, PTSD
Use of nicotine	Cigarettes, cigars, electronic delivery devices, etc. Ever used? How much? How long? Interested/ready to quit?
Caffeine	Soda, coffee, tea, energy drinks, or other modes of consumption
Alcohol consumption	What kind? How much? How often? Ever have DTs or withdraw? CAGE questionnaire can provide insight.
Illicit drug use	Type of product (cannabis products or stimulants like cocaine, methamphetamines, etc.), method of use (oral intake, inhalant, injection, etc.), frequency, withdrawal
Health-related behaviors (behaviors that change risk profiles)	Amount of daily activity, exercise, stress, diet/nutrition
Sexual history	Sexual behaviors to determine risk for pregnancy and sexually transmitted infections; number of partners (male, female, or both); oral, vaginal, or rectal penetration
Violence and safety	Use of vehicle restraints; helmet use for bicycle, motorcycle, or motorized vehicles; safe storage of guns, domestic, or elder mistreatment concerns

CAGE, cut down, annoyed, guilty, eyeopener; DT, delirium tremens; PTSD, posttraumatic stress disorder.

FAMILY HISTORY

Family history (FH) can be very helpful when working through the list of differentials. Many disease states are familial and/or can be linked to similar habits that are shared among families. FH should minimally include the patient's biological parents, siblings, and children. Are they alive? If not, how/why did they pass? What medical diagnoses do/did they have? Ask for specific diagnoses that address the differential diagnoses.

REVIEW OF SYSTEMS

The review of systems (ROS) is a time for focused system-based questioning that was not elicited during the previous parts of the encounter. The goal is to further identify organ dysfunction by gathering pertinent positives and negatives. ROS is distinctly different from the HPI and elicits symptoms, not medical diagnoses. Examples of ROS questions are shown in Table 5.3.

Table 5.3 Examples of Review of System Questions by System

System	Questions	
General	▪ Feeling generally well? ▪ Fatigue? ▪ Fever? Chills? ▪ Sweats?	▪ Difficulty sleeping? ▪ Change in appetite? ▪ Weight gain or loss? If so, was it intentional?
Head, eyes, ears, neck, throat	▪ Vision difficulties? Double or blurry vision? ▪ Masses or growths? ▪ Change in voice/hoarseness? ▪ Dental problems/concerns?	▪ Hearing loss? ▪ Tinnitus? ▪ Rhinorrhea? Epistaxis? ▪ Neck pain? ▪ Otalgia? Otorrhea?
Neurological	▪ Change in mentation? ▪ Weakness? ▪ Numbness? Tingling?	▪ Dizziness? ▪ Headache? ▪ Balance issues?
Pulmonary	▪ Shortness of breath? At rest? With exertion? Lying flat? ▪ Cough? Productive? ▪ Wheezing?	▪ Hemoptysis? ▪ Recent or recurrent upper respiratory infection? ▪ Snoring or periods of apnea?
Cardiovascular	▪ Chest pain or pressure? ▪ Orthopnea? ▪ Shortness of breath? At rest? With exertion or stress? ▪ Palpitations? ▪ Syncope?	▪ Calf/leg pain with ambulation? ▪ Wounds or ulcers of the lower extremities? Slow to heal? ▪ Discoloration of the lower extremities? ▪ Leg swelling?
Gastrointestinal	▪ Heartburn? ▪ Abdominal pain? ▪ Difficulty swallowing? ▪ Nausea and/or vomiting? ▪ Abdominal distention?	▪ Hematemesis? Hematochezia? ▪ Constipation or diarrhea? ▪ Change in bowel habits? ▪ Last normal bowel movement? ▪ Incontinence?
Genitourinary	▪ Polyuria? Dysuria? ▪ Incontinence? ▪ Urgency? Frequency? ▪ Incomplete emptying? Dribbling? ▪ Pelvic pain? ▪ Testicular pain, swelling, mass?	▪ Penile discharge? ▪ Last menstrual period? ▪ Possibly pregnant? ▪ Menorrhagia? ▪ Postmenopausal bleeding? ▪ Dysmenorrhea? ▪ Vaginal discharge?
Hematology/oncology	▪ Fever? Chilling? Night sweats? ▪ Weight loss? ▪ Abnormal bruising?	▪ New or expanding lumps, bumps, or masses? ▪ Hypercoagulability?
Endocrine	▪ Polyuria? ▪ Polydipsia/polyphagia?	▪ Weight loss? Weight gain? ▪ Fatigue?
Infectious	▪ Fever? Chills?	▪ Night sweats?
Musculoskeletal	▪ Joint pain or swelling? ▪ Muscle aches?	▪ Pain in buttocks or legs while walking?
Integumentary	▪ New rashes or moles? ▪ Pruritus?	▪ Alopecia? ▪ Open wounds?
Psychiatric	▪ Sad or depressed?	▪ Anxiety?

▶ PHYSICAL EXAMINATION

The first step in any physical examination of a patient is the general survey. This is an important aspect of the exam because it is when the severity of illness is commonly determined. Is the patient "sick or not sick"? To answer this question, the AGACNP should immediately seek the following information:

- What is the patient's level of consciousness?
- Does the patient appear to be in any kind of distress:
  - struggling to breathe (sitting upright, tripod positioning, nasal flaring, muscle retractions, pursed-lip breathing)
  - uncontrolled pain
  - crying or unpleasant facial expressions
  - bleeding, pallor
- Is the patient's appearance consistent with acute or chronic illness?
- Review the patient's vital signs for abnormalities (fever, tachycardia or bradycardia, tachypnea, hyper- or hypotension, low oxygen saturation, etc.).

If the patient is in any form of distress, treat immediately. Further assessment should focus on identifying the causative factor and treating it before completing additional comprehensive assessments. Other things to consider when completing this portion of the exam include height, weight, and body mass index. There are additional visual cues to evaluate, such as patient attire, posture, and general grooming.

SKIN

- Assess for surgical scars and link to the past surgical history.
- Use ABCDE acronym for lesions consistent with skin cancer:
  - *Asymmetry*: both sides of lesion do not match
  - *Border*: irregular
  - *Color*: uneven, shades of different color
  - *Diameter*: less than 6 mm or one quarter inch
  - *Evolving*: lesion is changing in size, shape, or color

Table 5.4 discusses the primary lesions that may be seen during a physical exam.

Table 5.4 Primary Lesions

Name	Description	Examples
Macule	Flat, nonpalpable, different color than surrounding skin	Freckle
Papule	Slightly elevated (less than 1 cm), well-marked, solid lesion	Acne, warts
Vesicle	Less than 1 cm clear, fluid-filled lesion	Eczema
Bulla	Greater than 1 cm clear, fluid-filled lesion	Bullous pemphigoid
Pustule	Vesicle containing pus	Folliculitis, acne
Plaque	Elevated, flat-topped, firm, rough, superficial papule with a diameter greater than 2 cm with variable borders (well defined or ill defined)	Psoriasis
Wheal	Smooth, slightly elevated, variable diameter, and usually has surrounding erythema	Urticaria
Nodule	Small, firm lesion with greater than 1 cm elevation	Cysts, lipomas

HEAD, EYES, EARS, NOSE, THROAT

- *Head*: traumatic versus atraumatic: note any lacerations, abrasions, contusions, ecchymosis
- *Hair*: distribution, color, quantity, loss of hair (e.g., patterned baldness)

■ *Eyes*
  ● color (pupil and sclera), symmetry of gaze, conjunctiva (pale, edematous)
  ● **p**upils **e**qual **r**ound **r**eactive to **l**ight and **a**ccommodation (PERRLA)
  ● funduscopic examination using an ophthalmoscope (Table 5.5)

Table 5.5 Funduscopic Exam

Funduscopic Examination	Findings
Red reflex	Normal exam will be the orange glow in the pupil when light is shined into the pupil. (Absence of the red reflex could indicate the presence of an opaque lens, present in patients with cataracts.)
Arteries	Appear light red and smaller (veins dark red and larger)
Optic disc	Yellowing, orange structure in the shape of a cup. Swelling of the optic disc could indicate the present of papilledema, which would indicate increased intracranial pressure. Other causes could include glaucoma and retinal occlusion.
Macula	Darkened yellowish area surrounding the fovea near the retina

■ *Ears*
  ● Inspect the outer anatomy for deformity, bleeding, discharge, or impacted cerumen or foreign objects visible without otoscope
  ● hearing test
    ❏ *Weber*: testing for unilateral conductive and sensorineural hearing loss
    ❏ *Rinne*: sound transmission for air and bone conduction
    ❏ *Whisper test*: hearing test
  ● otoscopic examination
    ❏ Identify any bleeding, scarring, cerumen, or foreign objects.
    ❏ Tympanic membrane (pearly gray if normal): Look for any bulging, fluid accumulation, perforation, or bleeding.
    ❏ cone of light location (5 o'clock in right ear, 7 o'clock in left ear)
■ *Nose*
  ● *Inspect* for symmetry (any signs of deviation or deformity); nostrils to observe mucosa within the inferior and middle turbinates; note any trauma, bleeding, and so forth.
  ● *Palpate* the nose for any present of tenderness, deformity, or injury and to assess airway patency. Palpate the frontal and maxillary sinuses to elicit any pain. The presence of pain could indicate an underlying process and needs to be inquired about further.
■ *Mouth/Throat*
  ● *Inspect*
    ❏ lips for color, moisture, cracks, lesions, lacerations
    ❏ teeth and gums for any caries, loss, bleeding, abscesses
    ❏ tongue for any lesions, bleeding, cracking, dryness
    ❏ soft and hard palates
    ❏ tonsils and uvula for exudate, deviation
  ● *Palpate*: assess tongue for any lesions or painful/tender areas
■ *Neck*
  ● trachea: observe for any presence of deviation
  ● thyroid gland
    ❏ *inspection*: presence of goiter or obvious thyroid enlargement
    ❏ *palpation*
      ○ can be examined with either an anterior or a posterior approach; ensure patient swallows to feel the gland rise
      ○ assessed for any nodules or enlargement that could indicate presence of Graves' disease or malignancy
      ○ assessed for any tenderness with light palpation

◼ *Lymph nodes (Table 5.6)*
  ● Palpate and assess for any increased size, consistency, mobility, or tenderness.
  ● Investigate firm, immovable, and/or tender lymph nodes to evaluate for inflammation due to infectious process or tumors within the region that the lymph node drains.

Table 5.6 Head and Neck Lymph Nodes to Routinely Assess

1. Preauricular	**6.** Anterior cervical
2. Postauricular	**7.** Deep cervical
3. Occipital	**8.** Supraclavicular
4. Tonsillar	**9.** Submandibular
5. Posterior cervical	**10.** Submental

LUNGS

◼ *Inspection*
  ● position of patient
    ❏ Upright versus tripod; is the head of bed greater than 30 degrees for all ventilated patients? Tripod positioning would indicate dyspnea. This is a position most often adopted by a patient with chronic obstructive pulmonary disease (COPD) when having trouble breathing.
    ❏ Ability to speak in full sentences (Inability to speak in full sentences indicates impending respiratory distress/failure.)
  ● assess respirations
    ❏ *Quantity*: number per minute
    ❏ *Depth*: Is the patient breathing sufficiently deep to prevent hypercarbia? Or are they breathing too deeply? Check the tidal volume on noninvasive ventilation and on the ventilators.
    ❏ *Quality*: use of accessory muscles; pursed-lip breathing; chest rise and fall for equal rise bilaterally; nasal flaring
    ❏ *Pattern*: Eupneic, Kussmaul, Cheyne-Stokes, ataxic, and so on
◼ *Palpation:* Tactile fremitus is a vibratory sensation felt bilaterally throughout the bronchopulmonary tree as the patient is speaking. (Asymmetric tactile fremitus could indicate unilateral pleural effusion, pneumothorax, or malignancy because these would decrease the transmission of vibrations.)
◼ *Auscultation*
  ● Follow a stepwise ladder approach using the diaphragm of stethoscope.
  ● Instruct the patient to deeply inhale with mouth open and exhale with each step.
  ● See Table 5.7 for types of breath sounds and indications.
  ● See Table 5.8 for special maneuvers.

Table 5.7 Types of Breath Sounds and Their Indications

Type	Findings	Indicates
Vesicular	Normal breath sounds	Normal
Wheezes	High-pitched, continuous sounds	Asthma, COPD
Rhonchi	Low-pitched, continuous musical sounds within the large and medium airways	Bronchitis, pneumonia
Crackles (Rales)	Faint popping sounds caused by air passing through accumulated fluid within small and medium airways	CHF, infection
Stridor	Loud, high-pitched sound on inspiration produced by upper respiratory tract	Upper airway obstruction from edema or foreign body

CHF, congestive heart failure; COPD, chronic obstructive pulmonary disease.

Table 5.8 Lung Exam Special Maneuvers

Maneuver	Explanation
Whispered pectoriloquy	Auscultation while having the patient whisper a word/phrase such as "99." Normal finding would be that the words are not heard or are faintly heard. If words are clearly and distinctly heard, this would increase suspicion for underlying consolidation.
Egophony	Auscultation while having patient repeatedly say "Ee." Normal finding would be you only hear "Ee." If you hear "Aa," this would increase suspicion for underlying consolidation or effusion.
Bronchophony	While auscultating, ask the patient to say "99" repeatedly. Normally, the words will be muffled. The presence of louder or clearer words can indicate the presence of consolidation heard in pneumonia.

CARDIOVASCULAR

Assess the cardiovascular system in the following correct order: inspection, palpation, auscultation.

- *Inspection*
  - Inspect the entire anterior chest looking for location of apical impulse (not always seen) and anatomical landmarks (e.g., aortic area, pulmonic area).
  - Inspect the feet, legs, and hips for dependent edema (Table 5.9) and anasarca.
  - Inspect for increased jugular venous pressure.

Table 5.9 Grading of Edema

Grading	Definition
0+	No pitting edema
1+	Mild pitting edema, +2 mm of depression that disappears rapidly
2+	Moderate pitting edema, +4 mm of depression that disappears in ~10–15 seconds
3+	Moderately severe edema, +6 mm of depression that disappears in over 1 minute
4+	Severe pitting edema, 8 mm of depression that can last minutes

- *Palpation*
  - Palpate the second right intercostal space, the second left intercostal space, along the sternal border, and at the apex:
    - ❑ *Heaves or lifts*: Use palm flat against chest of patient. If present, there will be sustained impulses that rhythmically raise the hand off the patient. (Most often this could indicate the presence of an enlarged right or left ventricle.)
    - ❑ *Thrills*: Use the ball of the hand firmly against the patient's chest looking for a vibratory sensation. This sensation would be caused by underlying turbulent blood flow, raising the suspicion for a murmur.
  - point of maxillary impulse (PMI):
    - ❑ Start by palpating the fifth intercostal space at the midclavicular line.
    - ❑ Will only be palpable in the supine position approximately 25% of the time. If it is not palpable, have the patient roll into the left lateral decubitus position.
    - ❑ A lateral shift of the PMI can be seen in cardiomyopathy, heart failure, and ischemic heart disease.
  - peripheral pulses (Table 5.10):
    - ❑ carotid, radial, brachial, femoral, popliteal, dorsalis pedis, posterior tibial
    - ❑ If unable to palpate pulses, exam should include Doppler assessment of pulses.
  - Palpate the liver to elicit a hepatojugular reflex, which is indicative of liver congestion associated with heart failure.
  - Palpate the feet, lower extremities, and dependent areas of the hips for edema and determine whether it is pitting edema and how high up the leg the edema goes.

Table 5.10 Grading of Peripheral Pulses

Grade	Description
0	Not palpable
1+	Weak, but able to palpate, thready
2+	Normal
3+	Increased pulse, requires moderate amount of pressure to suppress
4+	Bounding, cannot suppress

- ■ *Auscultation*: Use both the diaphragm and bell.
  - ● *Diaphragm*: better with high-pitched sounds such as S1 and S2. Pay attention to quality of heart sounds. Muffled heart sounds could indicate the presence of tamponade, suggesting medical emergency for a pericardiocentesis.
  - ● *Bell*: better with low-pitched sounds such as S3 and S4. Extra heart sounds such as S3, S4 could indicate the presence of ventricular dysfunction, possibly indicating the development of heart failure.
  - ● Listen in the five locations (mnemonic: APE To Man):
    - ❑ *Aortic area*: right sternal border, second intercostal space
    - ❑ *Pulmonic area*: left sternal border, second intercostal space
    - ❑ *Erb point*: left sternal border, second intercostal space
    - ❑ *Tricuspid area*: left sternal border, fourth intercostal space
    - ❑ *Mitral area (or apex)*: fifth left intercostal space, midclavicular line
  - ● Special maneuvers: To assess for mitral stenosis, have patient in left lateral decubitus position. Place bell of stethoscope lightly on apical impulse. To assess for aortic regurgitation, have patient sit up, lean forward, and exhale completely. Following exhalation, ask patient to stop breathing briefly. Place the diaphragm of the stethoscope against the left sternal border and apex. Listen for soft diastolic decrescendo murmur.

ABDOMEN

Assess the abdomen in the following correct order: inspection, auscultation, percussion, palpation.

- ■ *Inspection*
  - ● shape, size, contour, scars, hernias
  - ● umbilicus: Bulging could indicate presence of a ventral hernia.
  - ● pulsations: Aortic pulsation is normal to see and is seen in epigastric area.
- ■ *Auscultation*
  - ● must be done prior to palpation and percussion to avoid altering bowel sounds
  - ● presence of bowel sounds (normo-/hypo-/hyperactive)
- ■ *Percussion* is used to assess the size of the presence of air in the stomach and bowels, liver span, and dullness of fluid (Table 5.11). Tenderness to percussion indicates peritonitis.
- ■ *Palpation* of the abdomen is needed to assess for abdominal tenderness, the presence of crepitus of the abdominal wall, and possible abdominal masses (Table 5.12).
  - ● *Begin with light palpation*: Gently palpate all four quadrants with one hand, paying attention to any abdominal tenderness or guarding. Watch the patient's face for signs of discomfort.
  - ● *Advance to deep palpation*: With both hands on top of each other, use the palmar surfaces of fingers to deeply palpate abdominal structures such as the liver, spleen, kidneys, and abdominal masses.

Table 5.11 Descriptions of Abdominal Percussive Sounds

Sounds	Description
Tympany	Normal; loud and hollow
Dullness	Short, high-pitched sounds heard over organs
Hyperresonance	Louder than tympany, heard over air-filled or distended intestines
Flat	Short abrupt sound; heard when no air is present (e.g., in muscle, mass, bone)

Table 5.12 Abdominal Special Maneuvers

Name of Maneuver	Description
Rovsing	Press down firmly in left lower quadrant and abruptly release pressure. Positive Rovsing is present if patient has pain in right lower quadrant when pressure is released. A positive Rovsing sign is characteristic of appendicitis.
Psoas	With patient supine, have them flex right hip against your resistance. Positive psoas is present if patient has right lower quadrant pain. A positive psoas sign is characteristic of appendicitis.
Obturator	With patient's right hip flexed, passively internally rotate the hip. Positive obturator is present if patient has pain in right lower quadrant. A positive obturator sign is characteristic of appendicitis.
Murphy	With patient supine, place fingers just under right costal margin, press slightly upward toward the right upper shoulder. Ask patient to take deep breath. A sharp, increased pain with inspiration is a positive Murphy. This is caused by the diaphragm causing the gallbladder to descend on to the examiner's fingers, thus compressing the gallbladder. The pain indicates inflammation/irritation of the gallbladder.

- Findings consistent with peritonitis
  - ❏ *Rebound tenderness*: tenderness in an area, expressed by the patient when the examiner is pressing down and suddenly releases hand
  - ❏ *Guarding*: voluntary contraction of the abdominal wall, usually accompanied by pain-expressing facial expression
  - ❏ *Rigidity*: involuntary contraction of abdominal wall that is consistent throughout abdominal exam
- Perform a digital rectal exam (DRE).

MUSCULOSKELETAL
- *Inspection*
  - Gait when ambulating: Observe for limp, hip and shoulder alignment with each other laterally, assessing for scoliosis or kyphosis.
  - muscle bulk and symmetry
- *Palpation:* during passive range of motion of all joints and active range motion against gravity and resistance; grade the strength of each extremity (Table 5.13)

Table 5.13 Grading Strength

Grade	Description
0	No response or paralysis
1	Contraction felt with palpation
2	Contraction with gravity eliminated
3	Contraction against gravity
4	Contraction against gravity and moderate resistance
5	Contraction against gravity and full resistance

GENITALIA
- *Female*
  - *External exam*: Inspect the labia minora, clitoris, urethral meatus, and vaginal opening. Look for any skin lesions, signs of infection, bleeding, or prolapse.
  - *Internal exam*: Inspect the cervix. Palpate the ovaries, and complete a bimanual exam.
- *Male*
  - *Inspection*: Inspect the penis and scrotum for any skin lesions, bleeding, or signs of infection.
  - *Palpation*: Palpate the scrotum, assessing each teste for any tenderness, signs of infection, lesions, or bleeding.

NERVOUS SYSTEM

■ *Mental status*
  ● Glasgow Coma Scale (GCS) used in patients with traumatic brain injuries (GCS score ≤ 8: intubate)
  ● National Institutes of Health Stroke Scale (NIHSS) scoring: 0 = no stroke; 1 to 4 = minor stroke; 5 to 15 = moderate stroke; 16 to 20 = moderate to severe stroke; 21 to 42 = severe stroke
■ *Cranial nerves exam (Table 5.14).* AGACNPs must know the number and name, function, and how to test each cranial nerve. Mnemonics help with learning this information.

Table 5.14 Cranial Nerve Function and Sensory Mnemonics

Cranial Nerve	Name	Mnemonic	Function	Motor or Sensory	Mnemonic
I	Olfactory	On	Smell	Sensory	Some
II	Optic	Old	Sight	Sensory	Say
III	Oculomotor	Olympus	Eye movement	Motor	Marry
IV	Trochlear	Towering	Eye movement	Motor	Money
V	Trigeminal	Tops	Facial sensation and movement	Both	But
VI	Abducens	A	Eye movement	Motor	My
VII	Facial	Fin	Face: expression and sensory	Both	Brother
VIII	Acoustic (vestibulocochlear)	And	Hearing and balance	Sensory	Says
IX	Glossopharyngeal	German	Tongue and throat	Both	Bad
X	Vagus	Viewed	Parasympathetic	Both	Business
XI	Spinal accessory	Some	Head, neck, shoulder movement, and swallow	Motor	Marries
XII	Hypoglossal	Hops	Speech, chewing, and swallowing	Motor	Money

■ *Sensation testing:* Test with both sharp and dull instruments: Test both sides of face with patient's eyes closed. Abnormal identification of sensation could indicate possible trigeminal neuralgia. Test both arms and legs as well. Abnormal findings could indicate presence of neuropathy.
■ *Proprioception:* The ability to sense passive movement and position of the body. With the patient's eyes closed, displace their great toe in three different directions, asking them to identify the direction each time.
■ *Graphesthesia:* With patient's eyes closed, draw a number/letter in their hand and ask them to identify it.
■ *Stereognosis:* With patient's eyes closed, place a three-dimensional object into their hand and ask them to identify it.
■ *Motor testing:* Observe body position during exam. Observe for involuntary movements such as tremors, tics, chorea, or fasciculations. Assess muscle bulk: Atrophy would indicate the presence of peripheral nervous disorders such as diabetic neuropathy. Assess muscle tone: the slight tension when a muscle is relaxed.
■ Cerebellar function should be tested. Impaired function of the cerebellum could indicate trauma, strokes, or masses within the cerebellum.
■ See Tables 5.15 and 5.16.

Table 5.15 Testing of Cerebellar Function

Test	Results
Finger to nose	■ With patient's arms out to side, ask them to rapidly alternate index fingers to tip of their nose. First with eyes open, then closed. ■ As a second part, ask them to alternate between the tip of their nose and the tip of your index finger, as you slowly move through the six visual fields.

(continued)

Table 5.15 Testing of Cerebellar Function (*continued*)

Test	Results
Pronator drift	Have the patient hold both arms in front of them, palms up, and close eyes. Pay close attention to any drift of either arm or any turning over of either arm, which would indicate the presence of pronator drift.
Heel to shin	Ask the patient to carefully run the heel of one foot down the shin of the opposite leg.
Romberg	While standing immediately next to the patient, have patient stand straight up and close eyes for approximately 15–30 seconds. Monitor for any swaying or imbalance.

Table 5.16 Grading Muscle Tone

Grade	Description
0	No response
1	Very slight response
2	Brisk response, normal
3	Very brisk response
4	Repeating reflex, clonus

PSYCHIATRIC

- **Patient appearance**
  - *Posture and behavior*: Is the patient sitting quietly, or are they pacing? Look for tense posture, restlessness, or fidgeting that would be associated with increased anxiety. Watch for slumped posture and slow movements that would be seen in depression.
  - *Grooming and hygiene*: Is the patient dressed appropriately for weather? Does the grooming compare with peers of their own age? These may deteriorate in patients with diagnosed mental illness such as depression, schizophrenia, or dementia.
  - *Speech*: Slower speech may be seen in depressed patients, whereas accelerated speech may be seen in individuals experiencing mania. Fluency may have interruptions caused by hesitancy and word-finding difficulties. This would be considered aphasia and can be seen in patients with a history of a stroke.
  - *Mood*: Ask the patient to describe their mood. There is a wide spectrum of moods, including sadness, contentment, joy, anger, anxiety, and worry. If symptoms of depression are elicited, identify suicide risk and its severity by asking if they have a plan for suicide and what that plan entails.
  - *Thought content*: Allow the patient to elaborate on things they have said rather than asking them questions. Elicit abnormalities such as phobias (persistent irrational fears, delusions) and false personal beliefs that will not change despite evidence indicating that they are incorrect. These can be seen in patients experiencing psychotic disorders.
- **Perception abnormalities**
  - *Illusions*: misinterpretation of real external stimuli. This could be mistaking wind for voices. This can be seen in patients experiencing grief reactions, delirium, PTSD, and schizophrenia.
  - *Hallucinations*: experiences that seem real but lack real external stimulation. These can be visual, auditory, tactile, olfactory, taste, or pain. They may occur in patients with delirium, dementia, PTSD, schizophrenia, and alcoholism.

▶ ASSESSMENT AND PLAN

The assessment and plan section of the history and physical (H&P) and daily progress notes identify the primary problem for admission, all secondary problems, and the associated plan for each problem. The plan includes additional diagnostic testing, monitoring, reassessment, and all treatments.

The assessment section is the synthesis of subjective and objective data to clearly state the primary problem and reason for admission or discuss differential diagnoses to guide the treatment plan.

Explanations of positive and negative signs and symptoms should be included. The narrative should discuss the clinical reasoning to conclude this diagnosis. When the diagnosis is not definitive, use terminology such as *presumed* or *suspected*. As additional data are obtained, subsequent documentation will be updated to reflect this data and confirm the primary diagnosis.

PRIMARY DIAGNOSIS

A primary or admitting diagnosis is usually identified during the initial workup. The AGACNP will want to "trust but verify" this diagnosis. Be sure to fully interview the patient, perform a complete assessment, and analyze the diagnostic data to confirm the correct diagnosis. Be sure to come to your own conclusion. Three primary ways exist to organize and document the patient's primary and secondary medical problems and outline the plan of care for each:

1. Problem based: lists out the problems in order of highest to lowest priority
2. System based: by physiologic systems (neurologic, pulmonary, cardiovascular, etc.)
3. Problem based within each physiologic system (combines 1 and 2)

The latter two are commonly used in ICUs where the patients are more complex. System-based problem lists are helpful to ensure comprehensiveness. This approach encourages the AGACNP to actively review clinical data from each system and problem.

The general outline of the assessment and plan for each problem is as follows:

1. State the problem and include current status (e.g., stable, improving, worsening, resolved).
2. Indicate chronicity (acute, subacute, chronic, acute on chronic).
3. List etiology (if unknown, use probable, suspected, presumed, likely).
4. State usual health status for each problem (e.g., baseline creatinine 1.1).
5. State current clinical indicators and/or supporting data (e.g., exam, vent settings, lab values). For example: AKI on CKD stage II: improving, baseline creatinine 1.1, creatinine now 1.8 down from 2.2.
6. List any additional workup being done or considered.
7. List current treatments or interventions, including monitoring and interventions.
8. Treatment plans should follow clinical practice guidelines (CPGs). Any deviations from CPGs should be explained in a narrative. For example: Patient with STEMI is bradycardic with HR 40s, thus patient was not started on a beta blocker.
9. List any consultations and their recommendations (e.g., consider nephrology consult if creatinine worsens tomorrow).

SECONDARY PROBLEMS

Documenting all secondary problems is key to demonstrating the medical complexity of the patient and provides holistic care for the patient. The AGACNP must critically appraise all information to identify secondary problems, including:

▨ Review the chart for all other active preexisting medical conditions.
▨ Assess the vital signs looking for abnormalities, including variations from normal as well as variations from the patient's baseline.
▨ Review laboratory data looking for abnormalities (e.g., hypokalemia, hypernatremia).
▨ Personally review/read all diagnostic testing results (e.g., x-ray, CT, EKG, echocardiogram) and then review the specialist's formal reads.
▨ Assess the patient's medication list. Each medication needs a diagnosis; clarify reasons with the patient because medications can have two or more indications. Do not assume you know why a patient is taking a medication.
▨ Documentation should use medical terminology. A clinical diagnosis must be listed in the problem list. In other words, just stating the lab value is not sufficient.

Secondary diagnoses help build the case mix index (CMI), which describes the acuity and complexity of the patient. The CMI determines the patient's risk of mortality while hospitalized. The CMI influences the observed-to-expected (O/E) mortality ratio. The more complex a patient is, the higher the likelihood of death. This ratio is important in publicly reportable data. O/E less than 1.0 has good patient outcomes;

O/E greater than 1.0 has not-so-good patient outcomes. The greater the ratio over 1, the worse the hospital outcomes are. Throughout the hospitalization, keep all problems in the problem list, even those that are resolved, because these problems will need to be in the discharge summary.

COMMON MISTAKES

- Do *not* use the term *postoperative* because it implies a reportable complication (e.g., ileus, bleeding, atelectasis, infection, wound).
- Complications should be clearly stated when appropriate, and always review with an attending physician before documenting.

BEST PRACTICES

The assessment and plan should address specific criteria to ensure that the patient's needs and best practices are being followed.

- spontaneous awakening trial (SAT)
- spontaneous breathing trial (SBT): If the patient fails, document why, and if not extubating the patient, state why (e.g., too many secretions, insufficient mental status).
- deep vein thrombosis (DVT) prophylaxis
- foley catheter: Specifically, state plans to keep (with rationale) or remove.
- invasive lines (central venous catheter [CVC], Aline, etc.): Include date inserted, and specifically state plans to keep (with rationale) or remove.
- daily review of antibiotics and plans to de-escalate
- current nutrition plan
- volume status: Note if patient is hypovolemic, euvolemic, hypervolemic; state if intravascular or third spaced.
- ventilator-associated pneumonia prevention: head of bed at greater than 30 degrees, plus mouth care
- bowel regimen
- glycemic control
- code status: whether patient has/had capacity, who was spoken to, date and time
- disposition: Is the patient ICU, step-down unit (SDU), or floor level of care, and is there an expected discharge plan such as long-term acute care hospital (LTACH), rehab, or home with/without services?

AGACNP notes should also include billing language. Highlight the criteria that necessitate admission or ongoing hospitalization. If a patient requires life-, limb-, or organ-saving measures, then state that the patient requires critical care. Document which organs are failing and how much time was required to provide the critical care services.

▶ SUMMARY

Health assessment is a crucial aspect of the AGACNP's role. The ability to gather information in a standardized manner will prevent missed opportunities and mistakes. Understanding normal findings during a physical exam is required to then be able to identify abnormal findings that may represent pathology. The skilled AGACNP will then synthesize the findings from all components of the health assessment to determine a plan of action best suited for the patient and scenario. Without consistent practice, the mastery of the health assessment will be difficult to attain.

KNOWLEDGE CHECK: CHAPTER 5

1. Pupillary constriction to light source assesses which cranial nerve (CN)?

   A. II
   B. III
   C. IV
   D. VI

2. A college-aged student presents with a fever of 102°F and neck pain. The patient is unable to flex the chin to the chest. This finding is known as:

   A. Kehr sign
   B. Kernig sign
   C. Nuchal rigidity
   D. Brudzinski sign

3. A patient presents with a high-pitched, whistling, musical sound with inhalation. The AGACNP recognizes this as:

   A. Rales
   B. Stridor
   C. Wheezing
   D. Bronchophony

4. A patient presents after being found on the ground. The patient cannot follow any commands to open eyes or squeeze hands. The patient does not speak or make any vocal sounds; however, pupils are 2 mm and reactive. The patient is not arousable to voice or noxious stimuli. Upon deep sternal rub, they curl their bilateral arms up to their chest and extend their legs and feet but do not reach for the examiner. What is this patient's Glasgow Coma Scale (GCS) score?

   A. 3
   B. 4
   C. 5
   D. 6

5. A patient presents with a severe traumatic brain injury. On hospital day 3, the patient's intracranial pressures are 18 to 20. What would the AGACNP expect to find on funduscopic exam?

   A. Arteriovenous nicking
   B. Papilledema
   C. Vitreous floaters
   D. Cotton wool spots

6. A patient presents with fatigue, fever, leukocytosis, increased sputum production, and infiltrate in the right lower lobe (RLL). Expected physical exam findings in the RLL include:

   A. Rales, stridor
   B. Crepitus, dullness
   C. Wheezing, tympany
   D. Fremitus, egophony

(See answers next page.)

1. A) II

CN II, the optic nerve, controls pupillary response. CN III (oculomotor), CN IV (trochlear), and CN VI (abducens) control eye movements.

2. C) Nuchal rigidity

The term *nuchal rigidity* refers to a stiff neck, specifically to the inability to flex the neck. Kernig sign is pain or resistance associated with passive extension of the knees when the knees are flexed at the hip. Brudzinski sign results in reflexive flexion of the knees and hips when the neck is passively flexed. Nuchal rigidity, Kernig sign, and Brudzinski sign are all signs of meningeal irritation, commonly seen in meningitis. Kehr sign is pain occurring in the left shoulder due to irritation of the diaphragm by blood leaking from a ruptured spleen.

3. B) Stridor

A high-pitched whistling or musical sound on inspiration is stridor, which represents airway obstruction and is an airway emergency. Causes include foreign body, edema, abscess, or tumors. Rales, also known as crackles, are intermittent, nonmusical, brief sounds representing abnormalities of the lung parenchyma, as in heart failure or pneumonia. Wheezing is a high-pitched, shrill sound heard on expiration that arises in narrowed airways. Bronchophony is the muffling of the words "99" spoken by the patient when the AGACNP is auscultating the lungs. This is consistent with consolidation of the lung tissue.

4. B) 4

The GCS measures verbal, motor, and eye-opening responses. The minimum score per category is 1 with an overall minimum score of 3. Verbal range is 1 to 5, motor range is 1 to 6, and eye opening is 1 to 4. This patient earned one point for not opening eyes to pain, one point for not verbalizing, and two points for decorticate posturing, for a total score of 4.

5. B) Papilledema

Papilledema is seen with increased intracranial pressure. Arteriovenous nicking is seen in hypertensive retinopathy. Cotton wool spots are signs of several disease processes, including diabetes mellitus and systemic hypertension. Vitreous floaters are dark specks noted between the lens and the fundus.

6. D) Fremitus, egophony

Fremitus, egophony, bronchophony, whispered pectoriloquy, and dullness are all signs of consolidation noted in pneumonia. Patients with pneumonia may have crackles or rhonchi due to the secretions. Crepitus is air in the subcutaneous tissues, typically having escaped from the lung. Wheezing is typically noted in constricted airways from chronic obstructive pulmonary disease or asthma, and rales are usually noted with heart failure exacerbations.

7. A patient who has rib fractures and was intubated an hour ago suddenly develops tachycardia and hypotension. The AGACNP suspects that this patient has a tension pneumothorax. What exam findings would the AGACNP expect to find on the affected side?

    A. Dullness
    B. Tympany
    C. Resonance
    D. Hyperresonance

8. An exam finding in a patient in left-sided heart failure would be:

    A. Pedal edema
    B. Shortness of breath
    C. Hepatojugular reflux
    D. Jugular venous distention

9. The AGACNP is assessing a new patient who has not seen a provider for 20 years. They hear an S4. The AGACNP should assess the patient for:

    A. Heart failure
    B. Hypertension
    C. ST-elevated myocardial infarction
    D. Pulmonary embolus

10. A patient presents with abdominal pain progressing over the last 48 hours. The AGACNP palpates the abdomen, noting that the patient's pain is worse when the AGACNP removes their hand. This is known as:

    A. Psoas sign
    B. Murphy sign
    C. Rovsing sign
    D. Rebound tenderness

11. A patient presents in a comatose state. Emergency medical services (EMS) report that the patient's blood sugar is 630. EMS administered naloxone (Narcan) without improvement in the patient's mental state. The AGACNP notes that the patient is breathing deeply at 35 breaths/min. These respirations are known as:

    A. Biot
    B. Ataxic
    C. Kussmaul
    D. Cheyne-Stokes

12. The AGACNP is caring for a patient with septic shock secondary to methicillin-resistant *Staphylococcus aureus* bacteremia. The patient is critically ill and now suffering from disseminated intravascular coagulations. The AGACNP notices pinpoint nonblanching spots that measure less than 2 mm in size, which affect the skin and mucous membranes. What are these spots called?

    A. Petechiae
    B. Macules
    C. Plaques
    D. Herpes zoster

(See answers next page.)

7. D) Hyperresonance

Patients with tension pneumothorax would have hyperresonance due to increased air outside the lung. Dullness represents fluid or consolidation. Resonance is an expected finding in healthy lungs. Tympany is an abdominal finding associated with increased air presence, normally found in the stomach in the left upper quadrant.

8. B) Shortness of breath

Fluid from the left side of the heart backs up into the lungs, whereas fluid from the right side of the heart backs up the venous return to the heart, resulting in liver congestion, jugular venous distention, and pedal edema.

9. B) Hypertension

An S4 is indicative of ventricular hypertrophy, causing stiffness and increased resistance; therefore, assessing the patient for hypertension is important to identify the cause of the S4.

10. D) Rebound tenderness

Rebound tenderness occurs when pressure from palpation causes worsening pain. Rebound tenderness results from peritoneal irritation. Rovsing sign is the deep palpation of the left lower quadrant and then the quick withdrawal of the hand. Murphy sign is deeply palpating the right upper quadrant and asking the patient to take a deep breath to cause the gallbladder to descend onto the fingers of the examiner, leading to irritation and compression that result in pain. To elicit the psoas sign, the examiner asks the supine patient to raise a knee against the examiner's hand, which applies resistance.

11. C) Kussmaul

Kussmaul respirations are regular, deep breaths to correct for metabolic acidosis. Cheyne-Stokes respirations are groupings of crescendo–decrescendo breaths with periods of apnea, commonly seen in patients with sleep apnea. Biot respirations are groupings of equal breaths interspersed with periods of apnea. Ataxic respirations are erratic in both rate and depth of breathing.

12. A) Petechiae

Petechiae are pinpoint nonblanching spots that measure less than 2 mm in size. They affect the skin and mucous membranes. Petechiae is not a diagnosis but a symptom of an underlying disease. Macules are flat, nonpalpable, and a different color than surrounding skin. Plaques are elevated, flat-topped, firm, rough, superficial papules with a diameter greater than 2 cm with variable borders (well defined or ill defined). Herpes zoster is a painful blistering rash that follows a dermatome.

13. A patient presents with tachycardia to the 140s, blood pressure of 180/86 mmHg, and thyroid-stimulating hormone of less than 0.5 mU/L. The AGACNP should examine the patient for:

    A. Facial edema
    B. Thinning hair
    C. Exophthalmos
    D. Weight increase

14. A patient presents with small bony growths that have appeared on the joint closest to the distal portion of the fingers. The AGACNP is concerned about:

    A. Rheumatoid arthritis
    B. Endocarditis
    C. Osteoarthritis
    D. Marfan syndrome

15. The AGACNP is caring for a trauma patient who was involved in a motorcycle crash that resulted in right femur and tibia fractures, as well as a grade 2 splenic laceration. The patient is now complaining of extreme pain and paresthesias in the right lower extremity. The AGACNP also notes that the right lower extremity is pale. The AGACNP is most concerned for:

    A. Compartment syndrome
    B. Splenic rupture
    C. Abdominal bleeding
    D. Missed injury to the right lower extremity

(*See answers next page.*)

13. C) Exophthalmos

Signs and symptoms of hyperthyroidism include exophthalmos. Facial edema, thinning hair, and weight increase are signs of hypothyroidism.

14. C) Osteoarthritis

Heberden nodes are characteristic of osteoarthritis of the hands. Endocarditis does not present with Heberden nodes but rather with Osler nodes. Marfan syndrome does not have Heberden nodes as the classic presentation. Rheumatoid arthritis presents with swan-neck fingers or boutonniere deformity of the thumb.

15. A) Compartment syndrome

The mechanism of injury (trauma) to the lower extremity and the presence of three of the 6 Ps (pain, pallor, paresthesia, pulselessness, poikilothermia, paralysis) make compartment syndrome the most plausible diagnosis for this patient.

KEY BIBLIOGRAPHY

Only key resources appear in the print edition. Access the full bibliography for this chapter on ExamPrepConnect.com.

Bickley, L. S. (2021). *Bates' guide to physical examination and history taking* (13th ed.). Wolters-Kluwer.

Carpenter, D. (2022). *Fast facts for the adult-gerontology acute care nurse practitioner*. Springer Publishing Company.

Huppert, L. A., & Dyster, T. G. (2021). Practical skills for learners. In L. A. Huppert & T. G. Dyster (Eds.), *Huppert's notes: Pathophysiology and clinical pearls for internal medicine*. McGraw-Hill.

Ingram, S. (2017). Taking a comprehensive health history: Learning through practice and reflection. *British Journal of Nursing, 26*(18), 1033–1037. https://doi.org/10.12968/bjon.2017.26.18.1033

Jameson, J. L., Kasper, D. L., Fauci, A. S., Hauser, S. L., Longo, D. L., & Loscalzo, J. (2018). *Harrison's principles of internal medicine* (20th ed.). McGraw-Hill Education.

Health Promotion, Disease Prevention, and Factors Influencing Health

Beth McLear and Stefanie La Manna

▶ INTRODUCTION

Health is considered a fundamental human right. The World Health Organization (WHO) defines it as a "state of complete physical, mental, and social well-being and not merely the absence of disease or infirmity." Health promotion, disease prevention, and understanding factors influencing health are complex. Understanding and delivering patient-centered care with health promotion and disease prevention are foundational components of advanced practice nursing. There are multiple influences on the health of an individual and a community. These include genetics; income; education level; social, economic, and physical environment; unique characteristics and behaviors; and access to healthcare. Healthy People 2030 provides a framework for data-driven national objectives to improve health and well-being over the next decade. Leading health indicators (LHIs) are key to creating these objectives. LHIs are a subset of Healthy People 2030 objectives that address essential factors that impact significant causes of death and disease in the United States. They guide organizations, communities, and states across the nation to focus their resources and efforts on improving the health and well-being of people.

Healthy People 2030 also emphasizes the impact of social determinants of health on individuals and society. The five domains of social determinants of health are economic stability, education access and quality, healthcare access and quality, neighborhood and built environment, and social and community context. Health promotion enables people to gain more control over, and improve, their health.

▶ HEALTH PROMOTION

Health promotion's primary purpose is to positively impact the health behavior of individuals and communities and the living and working conditions that affect their health. *Prevention* is an essential component of health promotion and has four levels:

1. *Primary prevention:* The goals of primary prevention are to remove or reduce disease risk factors (e.g., immunization, quitting or not starting smoking).
2. *Secondary prevention:* Secondary prevention promotes early detection of disease or precursor states (e.g., routine cervical Pap screening to detect carcinoma or dysplasia of the cervix).
3. *Tertiary prevention:* Measures included in tertiary prevention aim to limit the impact of established disease (e.g., partial mastectomy and radiation therapy to remove and control localized breast cancer).
4. *Quaternary prevention:* This is prevention of overmedicalization. AGACNPs should scrutinize whether diagnostic testing is needed and whether interventions will enhance quality of life. AGACNPs should address code and intubation status and revisit initial decisions with changes in patient conditions.

By focusing on prevention, health promotion reduces healthcare costs (both financial and human) for individuals, employers, families, insurance companies, medical facilities, and communities.

The United States Preventive Services Task Force (USPSTF), created in 1984, is a volunteer panel of national experts in prevention and evidence-based medicine. USPSTF makes evidence recommendations about clinical preventive services such as screenings, counseling services, and preventive medications. These recommendations guide health promotion and disease prevention practices in the United States.

▶ PREVENTION OF INFECTIOUS DISEASES

The risk of transmission of pathogens and infections in healthcare facilities is significant. Pathogens can be transmitted from other patients, hospital personnel, and the hospital environment. The risk is variable and depends on the patient's immune status, local prevalence of pathogens, and infection practices in combination with antimicrobial stewardship. *Standard precautions* need to be followed even when the presence of infectious agents is not apparent or they are thought to be minimal.

Standard precautions include the following:

■ Practice hand hygiene before and after patient care even if gloves are worn. Hand hygiene is the single most important measure to reduce transmission of microorganisms from one person to another. Either soap and water or alcohol-based disinfection can be used. Handwashing with soap and water should be used in association with the care of patients with known or suspected norovirus or *Clostridioides difficile* infection since alcohol does not kill *C. difficile* spores or norovirus.
■ Use gloves, gowns, and eye protection in situations where blood and body secretions are apparent.
■ Use respiratory hygiene, including masks that cover the nose and mouth and prompt disposal of used tissues.
■ Prohibit artificial nails because periungual colonization with a variety of pathogens is increased when fingernails are long and artificial nails are worn. Healthcare professionals should have clean, cut fingernails when caring for patients.
■ Isolation precautions are used to interrupt the risk of transmission of pathogens. Three isolation categories reflect the major types of pathogen transmission in nosocomial settings: contact, droplet, and airborne spread.

Contact precautions are used for patients who have multidrug-resistant organisms (MDROs) such as extended-spectrum beta-lactamase (ESBL). Patients who are on contact precautions should be in a private room. Healthcare workers should perform hand hygiene and wear gloves upon entry to the patient's room. Gowns should be worn even if direct contact with the patient or infectious material does not occur. Upon exit from the patient's hospital room, gowns and gloves should be removed, and hand hygiene should be performed immediately. Medical equipment should be dedicated to a single patient's use to avoid the transfer of pathogens via fomites.

Droplet precautions are used for patients who have an infectious disease that can be spread via coughing, sneezing, or talking. Droplets are particles of respiratory secretions that are ≥5 microns in size. Droplets remain in the air for limited but succinct periods of time. The transmission occurs when within 3 to 6 feet of the source. Healthcare workers who are caring for patients on droplet precautions should wear a surgical mask when they are within 6 ft of the patient.

Patients on *airborne precautions* should be placed in a private room with negative pressure that has a minimum of 6 to 12 air changes per hour. Doors to isolation rooms must remain closed, and all individuals who enter the room must wear a respirator with a filtering capacity of 95% and a tight seal over the nose and mouth. Airborne droplet nuclei are particles of respiratory secretions ≤5 microns. Droplet nuclei can remain suspended in the air for extended periods of time. Airborne precautions are warranted for the care of all patients with suspected or confirmed tuberculosis, measles, varicella, and smallpox. Airborne and contact precautions are also necessary for patients with severe acute respiratory syndrome (SARS) and COVID-19 who are undergoing aerosol-generating procedures. More is to be learned about the COVID-19 infection, and until more is known, airborne and contact precautions are advised.

The goal of infection control is to prevent and reduce nosocomial infections. This can be accomplished by following standard, contact, and airborne precautions when deemed necessary. Following standards will protect the patient and healthcare worker from pathogens that surround the environment.

▶ PREVENTION OF CANCER

Screening and prevention can reduce mortality from many cancers. Screening detects abnormalities before they are clinically noticeable. Detecting abnormalities early allows for intervention before cancer develops or at an early stage when treatment is most effective. Prevention strategies focus on modifying environmental and lifestyle risk factors that promote cancer.

General lifestyle factors have been associated with malignancies, including lung, colorectal, prostate, and breast cancer. Multiple risk factors have been identified, such as tobacco use, high body mass index (BMI), poor diet, and physical inactivity. The Global Burden of Disease study estimates that in 2019, 50.6% of worldwide cancer deaths in males and 36.3% of those in females were attributable to behavioral, environmental, occupational, or metabolic risk factors. Smoking was the leading risk factor for all adults, while other important risk factors included alcohol use, high BMI, and unsafe sex.

Lifestyle recommendations include the following:

- avoid tobacco
- engage in physical activity
- maintain a healthy weight
- eat a diet rich in fruits, vegetables, and whole grains and low in saturated/trans fats, red meat, and processed meat
- limit alcohol intake
- protect against sexually transmitted infections such as human papillomavirus (HPV) by getting vaccinated
- protect against the sun, and avoid tanning beds
- obtain regular screening for breast, cervical, colorectal, and lung cancer

An estimated 13% of all new cancers worldwide are due to infections. Viruses may increase cancer risk through cellular transformation, disruption of cell cycle control, increased cell turnover rates, and immune suppression. Infectious agents and cancer are growing concerns. HPV, hepatitis C virus (HCV), human T-lymphotropic virus type 1 (HTLV-1), HIV, hepatitis B virus (HBV), Epstein–Barr virus (EBV), and *Helicobacter pylori* have been linked to human cancers. Exposure prevention, preexposure prophylaxis (PrEP), screening, vaccination, and early treatment can help prevent infection-associated cancers.

Tobacco use is the most preventable cause of cancer. The health benefits of quitting smoking can be seen at all ages. Alcohol intake increases the risk of colon, breast, esophageal, and oropharyngeal cancer. Decreased physical activity and high BMI can increase cancer risk. Excessive exposure to solar radiation or artificial ultraviolet radiation can cause skin cancer. Air pollution and radon gas in enclosed environments can cause lung cancer. Arsenic in drinking water can cause bladder cancers.

Many cancers are preventable. Basic lifestyle changes can make a positive impact on the prevention of cancers. Lifestyle recommendations as mentioned earlier can play a pivotal role in maintaining the health and well-being of individuals.

▶ PREVENTION OF OSTEOPOROSIS

Osteoporosis is common among women and older patients and is distinguished by low bone mass, microarchitectural disruption, and skeletal fragility. Osteoporosis is the most common bone disease in humans and represents a major public health problem. Osteoporosis has been characterized as a silent disease because fractures occur late in the disease process. Screening to allow early diagnosis is the key to prevention. A clinical diagnosis of osteoporosis may be made in the presence of fragility fracture, including the spine, hip, wrist, humerus, rib, and pelvis, without measurement of bone mineral density (BMD). In the absence of a fragility fracture, BMD assessment by dual-energy x-ray absorptiometry (DXA) is the gold standard to diagnose osteoporosis, according to WHO classification.

Other factors that can decrease BMD are cigarette smoking and excess alcohol intake. Certain medications such as glucocorticoids and anticonvulsants should be minimized in dose and duration because they can decrease BMD. Prevention is important. When BMD is measured by DXA, it will decrease fracture risk, and the goal is to maintain bone strength and prevent fractures. Physical activity has beneficial effects on bone accumulation; however, excessive exercise can be harmful to skeletal health when it is accompanied by poor nutrition and reduced body fat.

All older adults need to be screened to identify their level of risk for development of osteoporosis by using the fracture risk assessment tool (FRAX) to determine the 10-year likelihood of fracture. The overall goal is to prevent fractures. Basic treatment and prevention include diet, exercise, and fall prevention strategies. Adequate intake of calcium and vitamin D is essential to decrease bone loss and bone turnover (Table 6.1). The USPSTF recommends screening women older than 65 years and women younger than 65 years who have a 10-year fracture risk equal to that of a woman 65 years old. The USPSTF indicates that there are insufficient data to make recommendations for screening men. Education is recommended for people with osteoporosis. AGACNPs play an integral role by recommending patient groups, senior exercise classes, and dietary consulting. With education and a multidisciplinary approach, osteoporosis can be successfully prevented. Medications can also be used to prevent and treat osteoporosis (Table 6.2).

Table 6.1 Calcium and Vitamin D Recommendations by Age

Age Groups	Calcium RDA (mg/day)	Vitamin D RDA (IU/day)
14 to 18 years old	1,300	600
19 to 30 years old	1,000	600
31 to 50 years old	1,000	600
51 to 70 years old, male	1,000	600
51 to 70 years old, female	1,200	600
Older than 70 years old	1,200	800
14 to 18 years old, pregnant/lactating	1,300	600
19 to 50 years old, pregnant/lactating	1,000	600

IU, international units; RDA, recommended dietary allowance.

Table 6.2 Available U.S. Food and Drug Administration–Approved Medications for the Prevention of Osteoporosis in Postmenopausal Patients

Drug Class	Medication	Dose
Estrogens	Many	Variable
Bisphosphonates	Alendronate	35 mg/week or 5 mg/day
	Risedronate	35 mg/week, 5 mg/day, or 150 mg/month
	Ibandronate	150 mg/month
	Zoledronic acid	5 mg IV once every 2 years
Selective estrogen receptor modulators	Raloxifene	60 mg/day
Conjugated equine estrogen	Bazedoxifene:	20 mg/0.45 mg daily

IV, intravenous.

▶ PREVENTION OF CARDIOVASCULAR DISEASE

Heart disease and stroke are two of the top causes of death in the United States every year. In the United States, cardiovascular diseases (CVDs) cause one in three deaths and account for over $260 billion in direct healthcare costs and $147 billion in lost productivity due to premature death.

Risk factors for heart disease are divided into two categories: nonmodifiable and modifiable. Nonmodifiable risk factors include age, sex, and family history of early coronary disease. The leading modifiable risk factors for heart disease and stroke are high blood pressure, high low-density lipoprotein (LDL) cholesterol, diabetes, smoking, secondhand smoke exposure, high BMI, poor diet, and physical inactivity (see later).

Screenings for risk and preventive therapies are integral components of the USPSTF, Centers for Disease Control and Prevention (CDC), American College of Cardiology (ACC), and American Heart Association (AHA) recommendations for prevention of CVD. Recommendations for primary prevention of heart disease are focused on promoting a healthy lifestyle and controlling modifiable risk factors throughout the life span. A collaborative team approach among clinicians and the patient considering social determinants of health is also essential. To facilitate decisions about preventive interventions, screening for traditional atherosclerotic CVD (ASCVD) risk factors and applying of race- and sex-specific pooled cohort equations (ASCVD Risk Estimator) to estimate 10-year ASCVD risk for asymptomatic adults age 40 to 75 years are recommended. The risk scoring models may under- or overestimate risk in some populations, so clinical judgment and knowledge of the patient's medical and family history are also critical. AGACNPs should engage in shared decision-making with patients in discussions of their ASCVD risk estimates and the benefits and risks of preventive strategies. Collaborative decisions are likely to address potential barriers to treatment options.

LIFESTYLE MODIFICATIONS

Tobacco use is the leading preventable cause of disease, death, and disability in the United States. Smoking and smokeless tobacco use increase the risk of all-cause mortality. Almost one third of CVD deaths are attributable to smoking and exposure to secondhand smoke. One of the focuses of Healthy People 2030 is prevention and cessation of the use of tobacco products. The first step in treating tobacco use and dependence is identifying tobacco users. Consistent identification of tobacco-use status provides an opportunity for successful interventions and guides clinicians to identify appropriate interventions based on patients' tobacco-use status and willingness to quit. Brief interventions in as little as 3 minutes can significantly increase cessation rates. These interventions apply to all populations, including adolescents, pregnant people, older smokers, smokers with medical comorbidities, smokers with mental illness, and smokers of racial or ethnic minorities.

The *5As model* represents the five significant steps in providing a brief intervention in the healthcare setting:

1. Ask the patient if they use tobacco.
2. Advise them to quit.
3. Assess readiness to make a quit attempt.
4. Assist those who are willing to make a quit attempt.
5. Arrange for follow-up contact to prevent relapse.

These strategies require 3 minutes or less of direct clinician time. After 6 months, tobacco users are more likely to quit when clinicians strongly advise them to quit using tobacco rather than give no advice or the usual care. When advising a patient to quit, it is critically important to use clear and strong, yet compassionate, nonjudgmental, and personalized language. Assessment of a patient's willingness guides the next steps in the process. If a patient is not ready to attempt to quit, clinicians should use a brief intervention designed to promote the motivation to quit. If they are willing to quit, U.S. Food and Drug Administration (FDA)–approved tobacco-cessation pharmacotherapy (Table 6.3) and behavioral interventions (even just 3 minutes of advice), alone or combined, in nonpregnant adults (≥18 years of age) who smoke have substantial effect. The benefits and harms of pharmacotherapy in pregnant patients are not determined, but behavioral interventions show benefits. Hospitalized adults who use tobacco should receive intensive counseling during hospitalization with supportive follow-up contacts for at least 1 month after discharge.

Table 6.3 Pharmacotherapy for Tobacco Cessation

First-Line Pharmacotherapy for Tobacco Cessation		
Nicotine Replacement Therapy[a]		
Drug	Dosage	Precautions
Patch (OTC)	21 mg, 14 mg, 7 mg Starting dose: 21 mg for ≥10 CPD[a]; 14 mg for <10 CPD	Local irritation possible; may be placed anywhere on the upper body, including arms and back. Rotate patch site each time a new patch is applied, remove for sleep if needed.

(continued)

Table 6.3 Pharmacotherapy for Tobacco Cessation (*continued*)

First-Line Pharmacotherapy for Tobacco Cessation		
Nicotine Replacement Therapy[a]		
Drug	Dosage	Precautions
Lozenge/gum (OTC)	2 mg or 4 mg Starting dose: 4 mg if first tobacco use is ≤30 min after waking; 2 mg if first tobacco use is >30 min after waking; maximum of 20 lozenges or 24 pieces of gum/day	Hiccups/dyspepsia possible; avoid food or beverages 15 min before and after use
Nasal spray	10 mg/mL Starting dose: 1–2 doses/hr (1 dose = 1 spray each nostril); maximum of 40 doses/day	Local irritation possible; avoid with nasal or reactive airway disorders
Nasal inhaler	10-mg cartridge Starting dose: Puff for 20 min/cartridge every 1–2 hr; maximum 16 cartridges/day	Cough possible; avoid with reactive airway disorders. Frequent puffing required, far more often than with a cigarette. Each cartridge is designed for 80 puffs. Patient does not need to inhale deeply to achieve an effect.
Other Drugs		
Bupropion (Zyban, Wellbutrin SR)	150 mg SR Starting dose: 150 mg daily (a.m.) for 3 days; then 150 mg twice daily; may use in combination with NRT. Can be used for as long as 12 months and may be effective for reducing relapse.	Avoid with history/risk of seizures, eating disorders, MAOI, or CYP 2D6 inhibitor
Varenicline (Chantix)	0.5 mg–1 mg Starting dose: 0.5 mg daily (a.m.) for 3 days; then 0.5 mg twice daily for 4 days; then 1 mg twice daily (use start pack followed by continuation pack) for 3–6 months	Nausea common, take with food. Renal dosing required. Very limited drug interactions.

Note: [a]Use caution with all nicotine replacement therapy (NRT) products for patients with recent (≤2 weeks) myocardial infarction (MI), serious arrhythmia, or angina; and patients who are pregnant or breastfeeding, adolescents, and patients undergoing microvascular surgery.
CPD, cigarettes per day; CYP 2D6, cytochrome pathway 450 2D6; MAOI, monoamine oxidase inhibitors; SR, sustained release.

Electronic nicotine delivery systems, often referred to as e-cigarettes, are a newer class of tobacco products that emit aerosol containing fine and ultrafine particulates, nicotine, and toxic gases. They are not recommended as a tobacco cessation method. Evidence of benefit is unclear. In addition, they may be harmful as chronic use is associated with persistent increases in oxidative stress and sympathetic stimulation, increasing risk of cardiovascular and pulmonary diseases.

In the United States, obesity among adults has increased from 30.5% to 42.4%. After four decades of decline, heart disease deaths rose in 2015 by 1%, and this trend may be associated with the obesity epidemic. Healthy nutrition and physical activity have an important impact on ASCVD and its risk factors and have the potential to reverse or reduce obesity, high cholesterol, diabetes, and hypertension (HTN). Recommendations include a diet emphasizing intake of vegetables, fruits, legumes, nuts, whole grains, and fish, and replacing saturated fat with dietary monounsaturated and polyunsaturated fats. Reducing processed meats, refined carbohydrates, sodium, cholesterol, trans fats, and sweetened beverages is also recommended. Regular physical activity has proven health benefits, including reduction of ASCVD. All adults should obtain at least 150 minutes per week of moderate-intensity physical activity or 75 minutes per week of vigorous-intensity physical activity (or a combination) to lower ASCVD risk. Shorter durations of exercise seem to be as beneficial as longer ones. Therefore, the focus of physical activity counseling should be on total accumulated amount of physical activity. For individuals unable to achieve this minimum, some moderate-to-vigorous physical activity among inactive individuals or an increase in the amount in those who are insufficiently active is still likely beneficial. These recommendations apply to all adults, including older adults.

Obesity is a substantial public health crisis in the United States and internationally, with the prevalence increasing rapidly in numerous industrialized nations. Multiple classification systems are used for obesity. The WHO designations are most commonly used:

- Grade 1 overweight (typically called overweight): BMI of 25 to 29.9 kg/m^2
- Grade 2 overweight (commonly called obesity): BMI of 30 to 39.9 kg/m^2
- Grade 3 overweight (typically called severe or morbid obesity): BMI $\geq$ 40 kg/m^2

Prevention of overweight and obesity is promoted by increasing physical activity and dietary modification to reduce caloric intake. Providers can facilitate the development of personalized eating plans to reduce energy intake by recognizing the contributions of fat, concentrated carbohydrates, and large portion sizes. Patients may underestimate calories, especially when consuming food away from home. Including caloric and nutritional information when counseling patients increases patient understanding of the importance of food choices and portion control. Clinically significant weight loss ($\geq$5% initial weight) is associated with moderate improvement in blood pressure, LDL cholesterol, triglycerides, and glucose levels among individuals with overweight/obesity.

Recommendations from the American College of Endocrinologists include a combination of diet, exercise, and behavioral modification for a BMI of 25 kg/m^2 or higher. Pharmacotherapy is recommended for a BMI of 27 kg/m^2 or higher with comorbidity or BMI over 30 kg/m^2. Bariatric surgical procedures such as adjustable gastric band, sleeve gastrectomy, and Roux-en-Y gastric bypass are reserved for patients with a BMI of 35 kg/m^2 with comorbidity or BMI over 40 kg/m^2, but they should be used in addition to behavioral modification when possible.

CHEMOPREVENTION

High LDL cholesterol and lower high-density lipoprotein (HDL) levels (i.e., *lipid disorders*) are associated with an increased risk of ASCVD. Measurement of lipid levels can help assess the degree of risk. However, the best age to start screening and the frequency are controversial. In determination of whether to initiate statin therapy, clinicians must first identify the risk of a future CVD event. A risk estimator tool using pooled cohort equations such as the ASCVD Risk Estimator should be used. For adults without a history of CVD, USPSTF recommends that they use a low- to moderate-dose statin for the prevention of CVD events and mortality when the following criteria are met:

- age 40 to 75 years
- one or more CVD risk factors (dyslipidemia, diabetes mellitus, HTN, or smoking)
- calculated 10-year risk of a cardiovascular event of 10% or greater

Although the benefit is not as clear, clinicians may offer a low- to moderate-intensity statin to patients without a history of CVD with an intermediate risk (7.5%–10%) if they are age 40 to 75 years and have one or more CVD risk factors. A coronary artery calcium score may be helpful to further refine risk in these populations. According to the USPSTF, there is insufficient evidence to assess the balance of benefits and harms of statin use for the primary prevention of CVD events and mortality in adults age 76 years and older if there is no history of heart attack or stroke. There are, however, specific recommendations for secondary prevention of CVD events. These strategies include lifestyle changes to reduce risk, intensive individualized medical management including antiplatelet therapy, and intensive management of dyslipidemia.

Aspirin reduces the risk of cardiovascular events but increases the risk for gastrointestinal bleeding, intracranial bleeding, and hemorrhagic stroke; therefore, low-dose *aspirin therapy* should be individualized. Adults who have a 10% or greater 10-year CVD risk and are not at increased risk for bleeding are more likely to benefit from a daily low-dose aspirin (81 mg). The USPSTF recommends against initiating low-dose aspirin for primary prevention of CVD in adults older than 60 years.

SCREENING

One-time screening for abdominal aortic aneurysm (AAA) by ultrasonography is recommended by the USPSTF in men age 65 to 75 years who have ever smoked. Women who have no family history of AAA and have never smoked do not appear to benefit from such screening. The current evidence for women who have never smoked or have a family history of AAA is insufficient to assess the balance of risks versus benefits.

According to the AHA, over 133 million U.S. adults have HTN, of which approximately 83 million are eligible for pharmacologic treatment. Of these 83 million, HTN is treated in only about 66% and well-controlled in only about 30%. More CVD events are attributable to HTN than any other modifiable CVD risk factor. Because HTN is usually asymptomatic, screening is strongly recommended to identify patients for treatment. The USPSTF recommends screening for HTN in adults age 18 years or older with an office blood pressure measurement. They also recommend obtaining additional blood pressure measurements outside the clinical setting to confirm before starting treatment. Categories of blood pressure ranges are shown in Table 6.4. Recommended frequency of screening is every year in adults 40 years or older and in adults at increased risk for HTN (see later in this chapter). Screening every 3 to 5 years for adults age 18 to 39 years not at increased risk for HTN and with prior normal blood pressure readings is recommended.

Table 6.4 Blood Pressure Categories and Pressure Ranges

BP Category	Pressure Ranges
Normal BP	<120/<80 mmHg
Prehypertension	120–129/<80 mmHg
Stage1 Hypertension	130–139/80–89 mmHg
Stage 2 Hypertension	≥140/≥90 mmHg

BP, blood pressure.

Primary prevention of HTN consists of strategies aimed at both the general population and special high-risk populations. High-risk populations include persons with high-normal blood pressure or a family history of HTN, Black patients, and patients with behavioral risk factors, such as physical inactivity; excessive consumption of salt, alcohol, or calories; and deficient potassium intake. Proven interventions for primary prevention of HTN include reduced sodium consumption, weight loss, and regular exercise. Potassium supplementation lowers blood pressure modestly, and a diet high in fresh fruits and vegetables and low in fat, red meat, and sugar-containing beverages also reduces blood pressure. Pharmacologic therapies are key, and recommendations for pharmacologic treatments are outlined in the Eighth Joint National Committee (JNC-8) guidelines.

▶ INJURY AND VIOLENCE PREVENTION

Injury is a leading cause of death for children and adults between ages 1 and 45 years in the United States and is an essential cause of loss of potential years of life before age 65 years.

OPIOID OVERDOSE

Opioid overdose, which has increased significantly in recent years, is the leading cause of injury death in the United States. Therefore, a significant focus of injury prevention in the United States is now prevention of opioid overdose through education related to risks of opioid use, polysubstance abuse, and use of naloxone to reverse opioid overdose. Patients should be educated on safe storage and disposal of unused controlled substances/medications and keeping medications secure from family and friends who may seek to obtain them.

The USPSTF recommends screening for unhealthy drug use in adults age 18 years or older. Unhealthy drug use is defined as use of substances (not including alcohol or tobacco products) obtained illegally or nonmedical use of prescription psychoactive medications. Screening refers to asking one or more questions about drug use or drug-related risks (not checking biologic specimens for the presence of drugs). A tool such as the National Institute on Drug Abuse Quick Screen, which asks four questions about the use of alcohol, tobacco, prescription drugs, and illegal drugs in the past year, may be used in busy care settings. More extended tools, such as the eight-item ASSIST (Alcohol, Smoking, and Substance Involvement Screening Test), which assesses risks associated with unhealthy drug use or comorbid conditions, may reveal information signaling the need for prompt diagnostic assessment. The recommendations for drug use disorders depend on type of drug used, severity of drug use, and type of use disorder.

MOTOR VEHICLE INJURIES

The second leading cause of death from unintentional injuries in the United States is motor vehicle injuries. Interventions to increase seat belt and car seat use; reduce impaired driving, distracted driving, and speed-related crashes; and protect pedestrians can reduce deaths from motor vehicle crashes.

FALLS

Falls are a significant cause of death and injury in older adults in the United States. Interventions to help older adults increase physical activity and exercise are recommended by the USPSTF to decrease the risk of injury or death from falls. The USPSTF also recommends that clinicians provide multifactorial interventions to prevent falls in adults age 65 years or older who are at increased risk for falls in the community. These interventions include initial assessment of modifiable risk factors for falls and individualized interventions for each patient based on issues identified in the initial assessment. The components of the initial assessment may include balance, gait, vision, postural blood pressure, medication, environment, cognition, and psychological health.

FIREARM INJURIES

In 2020, firearm-related injuries were among the five leading causes of death for people age 1 to 44 years in the United States. Men have the highest risk for death or injury from a firearm, accounting for 86% of firearm deaths and 87% of nonfatal firearm injuries. Firearm deaths and violence also vary by age and race/ethnicity. Homicide rates from firearms are highest among teens and young adults age 15 to 34 years. Having a gun in the home increases the likelihood of homicide nearly threefold and suicide fivefold. Firearm suicide rates are highest in adults age 75 years and older. Since having a firearm in the home is strongly associated with suicide, strategies to mitigate firearm suicides should include depression screening and asking anyone with depression if they have a gun in the home.

DEPRESSION/SUICIDE SCREENING

The risk for suicide varies according to age, sex, and race/ethnicity. Risk factors for suicide include:

- prior attempt of suicide
- presence of a mental health disorder
- serious childhood adverse events
- family history of suicide
- prejudice or discrimination associated with sexual and gender identity
- access to lethal means
- history of being bullied

Socioeconomic factors such as low income and unemployment are also associated with an increased risk of suicide. However, there are limited data to assess the benefits and harms of screening, and screening tools for suicide have variable accuracy; therefore, there is no current specific recommendation for screening.

Depression screening using the Patient Health Questionnaire-2 or the longer Patient Health Questionnaire-9 is recommended. In addition, it is crucial to counsel individuals with firearms to store them safely when not in use, including using gun locks, keeping weapons stored unloaded in a gun safe, and storing ammunition separately from weapons. Putting a gun out of sight or reach is not safe storage and is not adequate to prevent use by children or unauthorized adults. The American Foundation for Suicide Prevention and the National Shooting Sports Foundation has released a toolkit (Suicide Prevention is Everyone's Business: A Toolkit for Safe Firearm Storage) that describes methods for safe storage and provides guidance to enhance safe storage practices.

INTIMATE PARTNER VIOLENCE

Intimate partner violence (IPV) and abuse of older or vulnerable adults are frequent occurrences in the United States with significant risks of morbidity and mortality. IPV includes physical violence, sexual violence, psychological aggression (e.g., limiting access to financial resources), or stalking by a romantic or sexual partner. Severe physical violence includes being hit with a fist or a hard object, kicked, hurt by pulling hair, slammed against something, hurt by choking or suffocating, beaten, burned on purpose, or threatened with a knife or gun. The USPSTF recommends screening women of childbearing age for IPV. The inclusion of a single question in the medical history ("At any time, has a partner ever hit you, kicked you, or otherwise physically hurt you?") can increase the identification of this problem. There are also screening instruments to detect IPV in the past year among adult women accurately: Humiliation, Afraid, Rape, Kick (HARK); Hurt, Insult, Threaten, Scream (HITS); Extended–Hurt, Insult, Threaten, Scream (E-HITS); Partner Violence Screen (PVS); and Woman Abuse Screening Tool (WAST).

If IPV is detected, offering referrals to community resources has the potential to interrupt and prevent recurrence of domestic violence. Active follow-up with patients by clinicians whenever possible is recommended since IPV screening with passive referrals to services may not be sufficient.

ELDER MISTREATMENT

Elder abuse occurs when a trusted person's or caregiver's acts or neglect causes or creates the risk of harm to an adult age 60 years or older. Risk factors for elder abuse include isolation, lack of social support, functional impairment, and poor physical health. For older adults, lower income and shared living environment with many household members (other than a spouse) are also associated with an increased risk of financial and physical abuse. Although there are no validated screening tools for elder abuse, there are clues. These include an unkempt appearance, missed appointments, recurrent urgent care visits, suspicious physical findings, and implausible explanations for injuries.

▶ PREVENTION OF HOSPITAL-ACQUIRED CONDITIONS

Hospital-acquired conditions (HACs) are diagnoses that a patient develops while in the hospital receiving treatment for an unrelated illness. The Agency for Healthcare Quality and Research (AHRQ) monitors these conditions using a National Scorecard on Hospital-Acquired Conditions. The most recent report from 2014 to 2017 shows HACs fell by 13%, saving about 20,700 lives and about $7.7 billion in healthcare costs. However, it is estimated that a HAC impacts 10% of hospitalized patients during a hospital stay.

Hospitals and healthcare providers should prioritize reduction of specific HACs that occur frequently, can cause significant harm, and are often preventable based on existing evidence. The AHRQ has focused attention on 10 of these conditions and provides tools for healthcare providers and organizations tomitigate the risk of these conditions, which include:

- adverse drug events (ADEs)
- catheter-associated urinary tract infections (CAUTIs)
- central line–associated bloodstream infections (CLABSIs)
- *Clostridium difficile* infections (CDIs)
- falls
- obstetric adverse events
- pressure injuries
- surgical site infections
- venous thromboembolism (VTE)
- ventilator-associated events (VAEs)

PREVENTION OF ADVERSE DRUG EVENTS

An ADE is any adverse clinical effect resulting from a drug. These include effects ranging from minor drug rashes to significant reactions such as bone marrow suppression or anaphylaxis. Medication errors, such as dosing errors or ordering a medication for the wrong patient resulting in harm to the patient, are included in this definition. Prevention of ADEs—both side effects and those due to errors—is important to ensure safety. An ADE can reflect factors arising at any stage of the medication use process, including prescribing, dispensing, or administration. Many ADEs can be prevented.

PREVENTION OF HOSPITAL-ACQUIRED INFECTION

Nosocomial or hospital-acquired infections (HAIs) are infections that were not present or incubating at the time of hospital admission. They affect 1 in 31 hospitalized patients annually and increase morbidity and mortality. HAIs also have a major financial impact on organizations and individuals. HAIs in U.S. hospitals have direct medical costs of at least $28.4 million annually, accounting for an additional $12.4 billion in costs to society from early deaths and lost productivity. Up to 65% to 70% of the two most common HAIs, CLABSI and CAUTI, are preventable. Other pathogens common in HAIs have a reservoir and predictable transmission routes and require a susceptible host. These characteristics make them amenable to surveillance and prevention strategies. Measures such as hand hygiene and minimizing invasive procedures and catheters are key primary prevention strategies. Isolation and transmission-based precautions are also primary prevention strategies. In addition, evidence-based bundled interventions with toolkits that mitigate are available through AHRQ. The conditions with toolkits are CAUTI, CLABSI, ventilator-associated pneumonia (VAP), CDI, and surgical site infection.

PREVENTION OF VENOUS THROMBOEMBOLISM

VTE, which includes deep venous thrombosis (DVT) of the legs or pelvis and pulmonary embolism (PE), is a frequent complication in hospitalized patients. This complication contributes to increased length of stay and is the leading cause of preventable hospital death in the United States and globally. Evidence from multiple randomized clinical trials supports primary thromboprophylaxis in high-risk hospitalized medical and surgical patients as safe, clinically effective, and cost-effective for reducing VTE. Conducting a thorough history and physical to gauge the risk of VTE and bleeding is necessary before prescribing thromboprophylaxis. Recommendations for acutely ill patients from the American Society of Hematology (ASH) suggest use of unfractionated heparin (UFH), low-molecular-weight heparin (LMWH), or fondaparinux for thromboprophylaxis. Among these, ASH especially suggests using LMWH or fondaparinux. In critically ill patients, ASH recommends using UFH or LMWH. In both acutely and critically ill patients who are not candidates for pharmacological VTE prophylaxis, ASH recommends use of pneumatic compression devices or graduated compression stockings for VTE prophylaxis.

STRESS ULCER PROPHYLAXIS

Stress ulcer prophylaxis is often considered benign. However, its lack of proven benefit, additional cost, and risk of adverse events preclude using it routinely for all hospitalized patients. Pharmacologic therapy for stress ulcer prophylaxis is *not* recommended for adult patients in non-ICU settings. Drugs commonly used to treat or prevent stress ulcers, such as histamine-2 receptor antagonists (H2RAs) and proton pump inhibitors (PPIs), are associated with ADEs, increased medication costs, and enhanced susceptibility to community-acquired nosocomial pneumonia and CDI.

Prophylaxis with a PPI or H2RA is indicated in specific conditions, such as peptic ulcer disease, gastroesophageal reflux disease, chronic nonsteroidal anti-inflammatory drug therapy, and Zollinger–Ellison syndrome, and to eradicate *H. pylori* infection. Prophylaxis is also recommended in patients in critical care units with a higher risk of gastrointestinal bleeding. Guidelines from the American Society of Health-System Pharmacists suggest stress ulcer prophylaxis should be limited to patients at high risk of gastrointestinal bleeding. These include patients with respiratory failure (mechanical ventilation greater than 48 hours), coagulopathy (international normalized ratio [INR] greater than 1.5 or platelet count less than 50,000/μL), or more than two of the following risk factors: sepsis, ICU admission lasting more than 1 week, occult gastrointestinal bleeding lasting 6 or more days, head injuries, and glucocorticoid therapy (more than 250 mg of hydrocortisone or the equivalent daily). Cost and patient considerations should guide the selection of either an H2 blocker or a PPI. Pharmacologic prophylaxis should be discontinued when risk factors resolve or when patients transfer out of the ICU.

▶ SUMMARY

AGACNPs play an important role in disease prevention and health maintenance. Honest dialogue and a relationship built on trust between the patient and AGACNP can empower patients to make choices about their healthcare and lifestyle habits that are essential for improving their quality of life and health outcomes. The role of the AGACNP may also extend beyond the patient relationship into the community, where they can advocate for disease prevention and health maintenance strategies on a systems level.

KNOWLEDGE CHECK: CHAPTER 6

1. A 64-year-old male patient has received pneumococcal 13-valent conjugate vaccine (PCV 13) immunization. This is an example of which kind of prevention?

   A. Primary
   B. Secondary
   C. Tertiary
   D. Definitive

2. A 58-year-old patient has undergone a mastectomy to remove and control localized breast cancer. This is an example of which kind of prevention?

   A. Primary
   B. Secondary
   C. Tertiary
   D. Definitive

3. Domains of the social determinants of health are:

   A. Economic stability, education access and quality, healthcare access and quality, neighborhood and built environment, and social and community context
   B. Economic stability, education access and quality, income level and potential, availability of tobacco products, and social and community context
   C. Economic stability, education access and quality, transportation access and quality, neighborhood and built environment, and social and community context
   D. Economic stability, education access and quality, healthcare access and quality, neighborhood and built environment, and readily available transportation

4. The 5As model for treating tobacco use and dependence consists of:

   A. (1) Asking the patient if they use tobacco, (2) allocating funds for tobacco cessation products, (3) assessing readiness to seek counseling, (4) assisting those willing to make a quit attempt, and (5) arranging for follow-up contact
   B. (1) Asking the patient if they use tobacco, (2) advising them to quit, (3) assessing patient readiness to quit, (4) assisting those who are willing to make a quit attempt, and (5) arranging for follow-up contact
   C. (1) Asking the patient if they use tobacco, (2) advising the patient to call a quitline, (3) allocating funds for tobacco cessation products, (4) assisting those willing to make a quit attempt, and (5) arranging for transportation to healthcare provider follow-up visits
   D. (1) Asking the patient if they use tobacco, alcohol, or any other drugs; (2) advising the patient to call a tobacco cessation counselor; (3) assessing financial resources; (4) assisting those willing to make a quit attempt; and (5) arranging for follow-up contact

5. The starting dose in milligrams for nicotine replacement therapy in the form of a nicotine patch for someone who smokes 1½ packs of cigarettes per day is:

   A. 7
   B. 5
   C. 14
   D. 21

(See answers next page.)

1. A) Primary

Primary prevention aims to remove or reduce risk factors for disease (e.g., immunizations), secondary prevention strategies promote early detection of disease (e.g., Pap screening to detect carcinoma or dysplasia of the cervix), and tertiary prevention measures are aimed at limiting the impact of an established disease (e.g., mastectomy for breast cancer).

2. C) Tertiary

Tertiary prevention measures are aimed at limiting the impact of an established disease (e.g., mastectomy for breast cancer). Primary prevention aims to remove or reduce risk factors for disease (e.g., immunizations). Secondary prevention strategies promote early detection of disease (e.g., Pap screening to detect carcinoma or dysplasia of the cervix).

3. A) Economic stability, education access and quality, healthcare access and quality, neighborhood and built environment, and social and community context

The five domains of social determinants of health are economic stability, education access and quality, healthcare access and quality, neighborhood and built environment, and social and community context.

4. B) (1) Asking the patient if they use tobacco, (2) advising them to quit, (3) assessing patient readiness to quit, (4) assisting those who are willing to make a quit attempt, and (5) arranging for follow-up contact

The 5As model for treating tobacco use and dependence consists of (1) asking the patient if they use tobacco, (2) advising them to quit, (3) assessing patient readiness to quit, (4) assisting those who are willing to make a quit attempt, and (5) arranging for follow-up contact.

5. D) 21

The starting dose for the nicotine patch in anyone who smokes more than 10 cigarettes per day is 21 mg. It is 14 mg for anyone who smokes fewer than 10 cigarettes per day.

6. Which is *not* recommended at this time by the United States Preventive Services Task Force (USPSTF) as a tobacco cessation tool?

    A. Nicotine inhaler
    B. Bupropion
    C. E-cigarettes
    D. Varenicline

7. The AGACNP is advising a 68-year-old female patient on physical activity to decrease risk of atherosclerotic cardiovascular disease (ASCVD). Which statement from the AGACNP is correct?

    A. "You should get at least 150 minutes of moderate exercise or 75 minutes of vigorous exercise weekly, but it is only beneficial if you exercise for at least 30 minutes in one session."
    B. "You should get at least 150 minutes of moderate exercise and 75 minutes of vigorous exercise weekly, and there is no benefit to amounts less than this."
    C. "You should get at least 150 minutes of moderate exercise and 150 minutes of vigorous exercise weekly, and the focus should be on accumulated time, not duration."
    D. "You should get at least 150 minutes of moderate exercise or 75 minutes of vigorous exercise weekly, and shorter durations seem to be as beneficial as longer ones."

8. Pharmacotherapy for treatment of obesity is indicated in a patient with a body mass index (BMI) of:

    A. 30 kg/m^2
    B. Greater than 27 kg/m^2 with comorbid conditions
    C. Greater than 25 kg/m^2
    D. Greater than 20 kg/m^2

9. The United States Preventive Services Task Force (USPSTF) recommends use of a low- to moderate-intensity statin to manage lipid disorders if which criteria are met?

    A. Age 40–85 years; one or more cardiovascular disease (CVD) risk factors; and calculated 10-year risk of a cardiovascular event of 10% or greater
    B. (1) age 40–75 years; one or more CVD risk factors; and (3) calculated 10-year risk of a cardiovascular event of 5% or greater
    C. (1) age 40–75 years; (2) one or more CVD risk factors; and (3) calculated 10-year risk of a cardiovascular event of 10% or greater
    D. (1) age 40–75 years; (2) one or more CVD risk factors; and (3) calculated 10-year risk of a cardiovascular event of 15% or greater

10. The United States Preventive Services Task Force (USPSTF) recommends against initiating low-dose aspirin for primary prevention of cardiovascular disease (CVD) in adults older than how many years?

    A. 30
    B. 40
    C. 50
    D. 60

11. The leading cause of injury in the United States is:

    A. Opioid overdose
    B. Firearm injury
    C. Motor vehicle crash
    D. Drowning

(*See answers next page.*)

6. C) E-cigarettes

Electronic nicotine delivery systems, often referred to as e-cigarettes, are a newer class of tobacco products that emit aerosol containing fine and ultrafine particulates, nicotine, and toxic gases. Electronic nicotine delivery systems are not recommended as a tobacco cessation method. The evidence of benefit is unclear. In addition, they may be harmful as chronic use is associated with persistent increases in oxidative stress and sympathetic stimulation, increasing risk of cardiovascular and pulmonary diseases.

7. D) "You should get at least 150 minutes of moderate exercise or 75 minutes of vigorous exercise weekly, and shorter durations seem to be as beneficial as longer ones."

All adults, regardless of age, should obtain at least 150 minutes per week of moderate-intensity physical activity or 75 minutes per week of vigorous-intensity physical activity (or a combination) to lower ASCVD risk. Shorter durations of exercise seem to be as beneficial as longer ones. Therefore, the focus of physical activity counseling should be on the total accumulated amount of physical activity.

8. B) Greater than 27 kg/m² with comorbid conditions

Recommendations from the American College of Endocrinology include a combination of diet, exercise, and behavioral modification for a patient with a BMI of 25 kg/m² or higher. Pharmacotherapy is recommended for a BMI of 27 kg/m² or higher with comorbidity or BMI *over* 30 kg/m². Bariatric surgical procedures such as adjustable gastric band are reserved for patients with a BMI of 35 kg/m² with comorbidity or BMI over 40 kg/m² but should be used in addition to behavioral modification when possible.

9. C) (1) age 40–75 years; (2) one or more CVD risk factors; and (3) calculated 10-year risk of a cardiovascular event of 10% or greater

The USPSTF recommends use of a low- to moderate-intensity statin to manage lipid disorders if these criteria are met: (1) age 40–75 years; (2) one or more CVD risk factors (dyslipidemia, diabetes mellitus, hypertension [HTN], or smoking); and (3) a calculated 10-year risk of a cardiovascular event of 10% or greater. A low- to moderate-intensity statin may be considered if the risk is 7.5% to 10%, but it is a weaker recommendation.

10. D) 60

The USPSTF recommends against initiating low-dose aspirin for primary prevention of CVD in adults older than 60 years.

11. A) Opioid overdose

Opioid overdoses, which have increased significantly in recent years, are the leading cause of injury deaths in the United States.

12. Increased physical activity has which effect on risk of falls in older adults?

    A. It decreases risk of falls.
    B. It increases risk of falls.
    C. It maintains current risk of falls.
    D. The effect on risk of falls is not known.

13. Asking a female patient of childbearing age, "At any time, has a partner ever hit you, kicked you, or otherwise physically hurt you?" is aimed at detecting:

    A. Elder abuse
    B. Firearms safety
    C. Substance use
    D. Intimate partner violence

14. Which characteristics may be consistent with elder mistreatment?

    A. Well-kept appearance
    B. Reasonable explanation for injuries
    C. Missed appointments
    D. Occasional urgent care appointments

15. Which statement is accurate for screening for abdominal aortic aneurysm (AAA)?

    A. Screening by ultrasonography (US) should be performed annually on men older than 65 years.
    B. Screening by US should be performed biannually on men and women older than 65 years.
    C. One-time screening by US should be performed in men age 65 to 75 years who have ever smoked.
    D. One-time screening by US should be performed in men and women age 65 to 75 years who have ever smoked.

16. The AGACNP educates the patient that tobacco use is:

    A. A moderate risk factor for lung cancer
    B. The lowest risk factor for lung cancer
    C. The most important preventable cause of cancer
    D. Not harmful if used in moderation

17. The AGACNP educates the 72-year-old female patient that the recommended dietary allowance of calcium per day, in milligrams, is:

    A. 1,000
    B. 1,200
    C. 1,300
    D. 700

18. The AGACNP educates the 60-year-old female patient that the recommended daily dietary allowance of vitamin D, in milligrams, is:

    A. 600
    B. 800
    C. 1,200
    D. 900

(See answers next page.)

12. A) It decreases risk of falls.

Falls are a significant cause of death and injury in older adults in the United States. Interventions to help older adults increase physical activity are recommended by the United States Preventive Services Task Force (USPSTF) to decrease the risk of injury or death from falls. The USPSTF also recommends that clinicians provide multifactorial interventions to prevent falls in adults 65 years or older who are at increased risk for falls in the community.

13. D) Intimate partner violence

The inclusion of this question in the medical history can increase the identification of intimate partner violence. Screening instruments can also detect intimate partner violence accurately, including Humiliation, Afraid, Rape, Kick (HARK); Hurt, Insult, Threaten, Scream (HITS); Extended–Hurt, Insult, Threaten, Scream (E-HITS); Partner Violence Screen (PVS); and Woman Abuse Screening Tool (WAST).

14. C) Missed appointments

Even though there are no validated screening tools for elder mistreatment, there are clues, which include an unkempt appearance, missed appointments, recurrent urgent care visits, suspicious physical findings, and implausible explanations for injuries.

15. C) One-time screening by US should be performed in men age 65 to 75 years who have ever smoked.

One-time screening for AAA by US is recommended by the United States Preventive Services Task Force (USPSTF) for men age 65 to 75 years who have ever smoked. Women with no family history of AAA or who have never smoked do not appear to benefit from screening.

16. C) The most important preventable cause of cancer

Tobacco use is the most important preventable causes of cancer and accounts for 21% of total cancer death worldwide. Tobacco use is the highest risk factor for lung cancer.

17. B) 1,200

The recommended daily intake of calcium for women older than 70 years is 1,200 mg.

18. A) 600

The recommended daily vitamin D dietary allowance for women age 60 years is 600 mg.

19. The AGACNP is educating the patient on lifestyle recommendations to prevent cancer and suggests that the patient:

    A. Avoid tobacco
    B. Reduce physical activity
    C. Eat a diet high in saturated fat
    D. Visit tanning beds

20. The AGACNP is caring for a patient with *Clostridioides difficile* infection. The AGACNP understands that:

    A. Alcohol should be used to wash hands.
    B. Lotions should be used to wash hands.
    C. Soap and water should be used to wash hands.
    D. There is no need to wash hands if the AGACNP wears gloves.

(See answers next page.)

19. A) Avoid tobacco

Lifestyle recommendations include the following: avoid tobacco; engage in physical activity; maintain a healthy weight; eat a diet rich in fruits, vegetables, and whole grains that is low in saturated/trans fat, red meat, and processed meat; limit alcohol intake; protect against sexually transmitted infections such as human papillomavirus by getting vaccinated; protect against the sun and avoid tanning beds; and obtain regular screening for breast, cervical, colorectal, and lung cancer.

20. C) Soap and water should be used to wash hands.

Handwashing with soap and water should be used when caring for patients with known or suspected norovirus or *C. difficile* infection because alcohol does not kill *C. difficile* spores or norovirus.

● KEY BIBLIOGRAPHY

Only key resources appear in the print edition. Access the full bibliography for this chapter on ExamPrepConnect.com.

AHRQ tools to reduce hospital-acquired conditions. (n.d.). Author. Content last reviewed February 2023. https://www.ahrq.gov/hai/hac/tools.html

Anderson, D. J. (2022). Infection prevention: Precautions for preventing transmission of infection. *UpToDate.* Retrieved from https://www.uptodate.com/contents/infection-prevention-precautions-for-preventing -transmission-of-infection

Arnett, D. K., Blumenthal, R. S., Albert, M. A., Buroker, A. B., Goldberger, Z. D., Hahn, E. J., Himmelfarb, C. D., Khera, A., Lloyd-Jones, D., William McEvoy, J., Michos, E. D., Miedema, M. D., Muñoz, D., Smith, S. C., Virani, S. S., Williams, K. A., Yeboah, J., & Ziaeian, B. (2019). 2019 ACC/AHA guideline on the primary prevention of cardiovascular disease: A report of the American College of Cardiology/American Heart Association Task Force on Clinical Practice Guidelines. *Circulation, 140,* e596–e646. https://doi .org/10.1161/CIR.0000000000000678

Centers for Disease Control and Prevention. (n.d.). Firearm violence prevention. https://www.cdc.gov/ violenceprevention/firearms/index.html

Centers for Disease Control and Prevention. (n.d.). *Healthcare associated infections (HAI).* https://www.cdc .gov/policy/polaris/healthtopics/hai/index.html

Colditz, G. A. (2022). Overview of cancer prevention, *UpToDate.* Retrieved from https://www.uptodate.com /contents/overview-of-cancer-prevention

Evans, L., Rhodes, A., Alhazzani, W., Antonelli, M., Coopersmith, C. M., French, C., Machado, F., Mcintyre, L., Ostermann, M., Prescott, H. C., Schorr, C., Simpson, S., Wiersinga, W. J., Alshamsi, F., Angus, D., Arabi, Y., Azevedo, L., Beale, R., Beilman, G., … Levy, M. (2021, November). Surviving sepsis campaign: International guidelines for management of sepsis and septic shock 2021. *Critical Care Medicine, 49*(11), e1063–e1143. https://doi.org/10.1097/CCM.0000000000005337

Guirguis-Blake, J. M., Evans, C. V., Webber, E. M., Coppola, E. L., Perdue, L. A., & Weyrich, M. S. (2021). *Screening for hypertension in adults: A systematic evidence review for the U.S. Preventive Services Task Force.* Evidence Synthesis No. 197. Agency for Healthcare Research and Quality. AHRQ publication 20-05265-EF-1.

Lewiecki, E. M. (2022). Prevention of osteoporosis, *UpToDate.* Retrieved from https://www.uptodate.com/ contents/prevention-of-osteoporosis

Mercier, E., Nadeau, A., Brousseau, A.-A., Émond, M., Lowthian, J., Berthelot, S., Costa, A. P., Mowbray, F., Melady, D., Yadav, K., Nickel, C., & Cameron, P. A. (2020). Elder abuse in the out-of-hospital and emergency department settings: A scoping review. *Annals of Emergency Medicine, 75,* 181. https://doi.org/10 .1016/j.annemergmed.2019.12.011

National Organization for Nurse Practitioner Faculties. (2017). *Nurse practitioner core competencies content.* https://cdn.ymaws.com/www.nonpf.org/resource/resmgr/competencies/2017_NPCoreComps_with_ Curric.pdf

Office of Disease Prevention and Health Promotion. (2020). *Healthy people 2030 framework.* U.S. Department of Health and Human Services.

Office of Disease Prevention and Health Promotion. (n.d.). *Healthy people 2030* U.S. Department of Health and Human Services. https://health.gov/healthypeople

Papadakis, M. A., McPhee, S. J., Rabow, M. W., & McQuaid, K. R. (2022). *Current medical diagnosis and treatment 2022.* McGraw Hill. https://accessmedicine.mhmedical.com/content.aspx?bookId=3081&sectionId =258579240

Schünemann, H. J., Cushman, M., Burnett, A. E., Kahn, S. R., Beyer-Westendorf, J., Spencer, F. A., Rezende, S. M., Zakai, N. A., Bauer, K. A., Dentali, F., Lansing, J., Balduzzi, S., Darzi, A., Morgano, G. P., Neumann, I., Nieuwlaat, R., Yepes-Nuñez, J. J., & Wiercioch, W. (2018). American Society of Hematology 2018 guidelines for management of venous thromboembolism: Prophylaxis for hospitalized and nonhospitalized medical patients. *Blood Advances, 2*(22), 3198–3225. https://doi.org/10.1182/bloodadvances.2018022954

Tsao, C. W., Aday, A. W., Almarzooq, Z. I., Alonso, A., Beaton, A. Z., Bittencourt, M. S., Boehme, A. K., Buxton, A. E., Carson, A. P., Commodore-Mensah, Y., Elkind, M. S. V., Evenson, K. R., Eze-Nliam, C., Ferguson, J. F., Generoso, G., Ho, J. E., Kalani, R., Khan, S. S., Kissela, B. M., … Martin, S. S. (2022). Heart disease and stroke statistics—2022 update: A report from the American Heart Association. *Circulation, 145,* e153–e639. https://doi.org/10.1161/CIR.0000000000001052

U.S. Preventive Services Task Force. (2018). Interventions to prevent falls in community-dwelling older adults: U.S. Preventive Services Task Force recommendation statement. *JAMA, 319*(16), 1696–1704. https://doi.org/10.1001/jama.2018.3097

U.S. Preventive Services Task Force. (2018). Vitamin D, calcium, or combined supplementation for the primary prevention of fractures in community-dwelling adults: U.S. Preventive Services Task Force recommendation statement. *JAMA, 319,* 1592. https://doi.org/10.1001/jama.2018.3185

U.S. Preventive Services Task Force. (2018). Screening for intimate partner violence, elder abuse, and abuse of vulnerable adults: U.S. Preventive Services Task Force final recommendation statement. *JAMA, 320*(16), 1678–1687. https://doi.org/10.1001/jama.2018.14741

U.S. Preventive Services Task Force. (2020). Screening for unhealthy drug use: U.S. Preventive Services Task Force recommendation statement. *JAMA, 323*(22), 2301–2309. https://doi.org/10.1001/jama.2020.8020

Whelton, P. K., Carey, R. M., Aronow, W. S., Casey, D. E., Collins, K. J., Himmelfarb, C. D., DePalma, S. M., Gidding, S., Jamerson, K. A., Jones, D. W., MacLaughlin, E. J., Muntner, P., Ovbiagele, B., Smith, S. C., Spencer, C. C., Stafford, R. S., Taler, S. J., Thomas, R. J., Williams, K. A., … Wright, J. T. (2018). ACC/AHA/AAPA/ABC/ACPM/AGS/APhA/ASH/ASPC/NMA/PCNA guideline for the prevention, detection, evaluation, and management of high blood pressure in adults: A report of the American College of Cardiology/American Heart Association Task Force on Clinical Practice Guidelines. *Hypertension, 71,* 1269. https://doi.org/10.1161/HYP.0000000000000066

World Health Organization. (n.d.). *Constitution.* https://www.who.int/about/governance/constitution

Geriatric Review

Gail Lis

▶ INTRODUCTION

As the number of individuals age 65 years and older continues to grow, so does the rate at which those individuals seek healthcare and are ultimately hospitalized. Furthermore, patients age 85 years and older are twice as likely to be admitted to the hospital than persons between the ages of 65 and 84 years. In addition to increased risk of hospitalization, older adults are more likely to experience poor health-related outcomes secondary to increased complications, longer length of stay, and higher mortality. Additional influences within these factors include multiple comorbidities, delayed treatment secondary to vague presentation of illness, and concurrent geriatric syndromes that often include psychosocial elements. Data suggest that almost 50% of those 80 years and older have three chronic conditions, and one third of those have four or more chronic conditions.

Sepsis has surpassed cardiovascular illnesses as the principal diagnosis for inpatient stays according to the Agency for Healthcare Research and Quality (AHRQ) 2018 United States National Inpatient Stay Report. Furthermore, sepsis and acute respiratory distress syndrome are the most common reason for ICU admission among older adults. Additionally, persons age 64 years and older had a five times greater incidence of intubation and need for mechanical ventilation. It is not surprising that the mortality rates from these two illnesses are highest among the older adult population. Table 7.1 highlights the top five most common inpatient diagnoses for patient age 65 to 74 years and 75 years and older.

Table 7.1 Most Common Inpatient Diagnoses for Older Adults

Ages 65–74 Years	Ages 75+ Years ICU
Sepsis	Sepsis
Osteoarthritis	Heart failure
Heart failure	Pneumonia
Acute myocardial infarction	Cardiac dysrhythmias
Cardiac dysrhythmias	Osteoarthritis

Source: Data from Agency for Healthcare Research and Quality (AHRQ), Healthcare Cost and Utilization Project (HCUP), National Inpatient Sample (NIS), 2018, Clinical Classifications Software Refined (CCSR) for ICD-10-CM default categorization scheme for the principal diagnosis.

▶ GERIATRIC ASSESSMENT

Caring for the hospitalized older adult is a complicated endeavor that involves excellent communication skills, a comprehensive assessment, and an interdisciplinary approach. Communication is essential to relationship building and becomes even more important when working with older adults. Healthcare providers need to understand effective communication barriers that are often present among older adults, in particular, sensory and cognitive impairments. In order to compensate for these barriers, it is important to involve family and caregivers as part of the assessment and plan of care.

While assessment is key for all patients who are admitted to the hospital, it becomes even more important when caring for the older adult. A thorough assessment of even nonmedical factors will assist the provider to understand the "entire context of the patient." Clearly, the patient's presenting issue becomes the priority; however, the healthcare provider must understand that there may be additional elements that contribute to the presenting problem, complicate the hospital stay, or impact the discharge plan. These additional elements should be included as part of a geriatric inpatient assessment and are identified in Table 7.2. Functional measures encompass mobility, cognition, and sensation; are significant predictors of mortality even over comorbidities; and have an increased impact on overall hospital prognosis. These elements of geriatric assessment also can be the predictors for or result of geriatric syndromes (Table 7.3). It is through an interdisciplinary approach that all of the elements identified in Table 7.2 can be addressed throughout a hospital stay.

Table 7.2 Assessment Indicators for the Older Adult Hospitalized Patient

Element	Indicators	
Medical	Current presentation of illness Comorbidities, medication reconciliation	
Mobility	Functional status, sensory deficits	
Cognitive status	Ability to make own decision	
Psychosocial	Mental health/substance use Social support	Living environment Financial resources

Table 7.3 Common Geriatric Syndromes, Assessment Tools, Diagnostic Workup, and Management

Syndrome	Assessment Tool	Workup	Management
Delirium	CAM, CAM ICU	CBC, CMP, oxygen saturation, UA	Nonpharmacologic first: ■ Reorientation ■ Behavioral influences: family, sitter, move location ■ Personal contact ■ Low lights, decrease noise Pharmacologic ■ Haloperidol 0.25–0.5 mg orally or parenterally; repeat dose after vital signs rechecked and sedation reached; no more than 3–5 mg ■ Atypical antipsychotics; risperidone, quetiapine (have fewer sedative and extra pyramidal side effects); warning of increased mortality in patients with underlying dementia ■ Benzodiazepines: not recommended
Falls	Clinical judgment is best over screening tools; St. Thomas Risk Assessment History of Previous Falls	Gait/balance/mobility/ functional assessment Muscle strength Cognition, peripheral nerves, proprioception, reflexes, extrapyramidal, cerebellar HR, rhythm, postural changes, BP Visual acuity Feet examination Depression screen Vitamin D levels	Best approach incorporates interventions to target risk factors and workup findings PT/OT Cardiology, psychiatry, neurology, podiatry, and ophthalmology consults Medication adjustment Vitamin D supplements

(continued)

Table 7.3 Common Geriatric Syndromes, Assessment Tools, Diagnostic Workup, and Management (*continued*)

Syndrome	Assessment Tool	Workup	Management
Incontinence	History: focus on characteristics of incontinence, past medical/surgical history, medication history (anticholinergics), hospital related	UA, blood sugar, bladder scan, postvoid residual, mobility issues, prostate exam, gynecologic exam	Depends on type of incontinence: ■ Stress: pelvic muscle strengthening, bladders suspension ■ Urgency: bladder training, bladder relaxants (antimuscarinics, alpha antagonists) ■ Functional: remove barriers, scheduling ■ High postvoid residual: removal of obstruction, straight or indwelling catheter
Malnutrition	Mini Nutritional Assessment—Short Form: useful for those at risk for malnutrition	BMI less than 18.5, unintentional weight loss greater than 10% in last 3–6 months, albumin, prealbumin	Identify the cause Dietary consult Oral supplements Enteral feedings: useful for those with reversible deficit, or those cognitively intact that have a nonreversible mechanical issue (*Note:* Tube feedings do not improve the quantity or quality of life in those with dementia)
Depression	Geriatric Depression Scale Prior history of depression Sequelae of current illness	Somatic symptoms Symptoms associated with depression	SSRI Psychiatry consult
Pain	Numeric Rating Scale Wong–Baker Faces Pain Rating PAINAD: for those with advanced dementia		Mild to moderate pain/first-line chronic pain: ■ Acetaminophen ($\leq$4 g q24h with normal hepatic/renal function) ■ NSAIDs: more adverse side effects; should not be prescribed long term ■ Topical Moderate to severe pain: ■ Opioids: start low, titrate slowly Neuropathic pain: ■ Post herpetic neuralgia (tricyclic, anticonvulsant [gabapentin], corticosteroids) ■ Diabetic neuropathy (tricyclic, SNRI)

BMI, body mass index; BP, blood pressure; CAM, Confusion Assessment Method; CBC, complete blood count; CMP, comprehensive metabolic panel; HR, heart rate; NSAID, nonsteroidal anti-inflammatory drug; OT, occupational therapy; PAINAD, Pain Assessment in Advanced Dementia; PT, physical therapy; SNRI, serotonin-norepinephrine reuptake inhibitor; SSRI, selective serotonin reuptake inhibitor; UA, urinalysis.

PHYSIOLOGICAL CHANGES ASSOCIATED WITH AGING

An important aspect of geriatric assessment and providing effective care is for AGACNPs to differentiate between normal changes that occur with aging and pathological changes. Knowing these changes will assist the provider in discerning expected from unexpected findings, determining risk factors for potential hospital complications and increased mortality, and developing pertinent differential diagnoses. In addition, the changes that occur with aging contribute to geriatric syndromes. Geriatric syndromes are multifactorial conditions that are believed to be a result of accumulated impairments in multiple systems that impact their ability to compensate (see Table 7.3). Table 7.4 highlights physiological changes associated with aging, the consequences to particular body systems, and the potential disease processes or complications that could result from a disease process and/or geriatric syndrome.

Table 7.4 Physiologic Changes That Occur With Aging, Consequences, and Disease Processes

Body System	Physiologic Changes	Consequences	Diseases Processes/ Geriatric Syndrome
Integumentary			
Skin	▪ Thinning of epidermis ▪ Dermal thickness decreases ▪ Decreased elasticity	▪ Increased fragility, skin tears, skin sagging, prolonged healing time, atrophy	▪ Skin breakdown ▪ Pressure ulcers ▪ Infection
Hair	▪ Hair follicle atrophy, melanocytes decrease	▪ Hair density and color decrease; hair turns gray; eyebrow, ear, and nasal hairs coarsen	
Nails	▪ Linear nail growth slows, nail thickness decreases	▪ Nails become brittle, dull, opaque, yellowish	
Musculoskeletal			
Muscle	▪ Lean body mass decreases, increased fat deposited in muscle tissue	▪ Decreased tone, contractility, and strength ▪ Increased drug distribution to fat	▪ Falls ▪ Medication adverse reaction
Bone	▪ Loss of bone mass, cartilage degeneration, loss of tissue elasticity in joints	▪ Bones become brittle, fluid in joint may decrease, cartilage rub together and erode, joints become stiffer/less flexible, minerals may deposit in some joints, narrowing of central or spinal canal; intervertebral discs lose fluid, become thinner	▪ Fall, fracture, immobility ▪ Arthritis, bursitis, tendinitis ▪ Pain syndromes ▪ Lumbar spinal stenosis ▪ Degenerative disc disease
Nervous	▪ Number of functioning sensory neurons declines ▪ Decreased nerve conduction velocity: slower action potential ▪ Decreased production of neurotransmitters ▪ Reduced dopamine uptake sites ▪ Decline in production of neurohormones, response to nervous system signaling	▪ Decreased muscle innervation, increased muscle atrophy ▪ Decreased fine motor control ▪ Increased risk of illnesses/ syndromes dependent on neurotransmitter ▪ Autonomic dysregulation, decreased aortic arch and carotid sinus baroreceptors	▪ Weakness, fall, fracture ▪ Impaired nutrition, activities of daily living ▪ Insomnia, Parkinson disease, depression ▪ Orthostatic hypotension, syncope, falls
Cardiovascular			
Heart	▪ Increased size and weight ▪ Increased left ventricular stiffness ▪ Increased myocardium thickness ▪ Increased endocardium thickness	▪ Increased afterload ▪ Valves become thickened and calcified ▪ Impacts conduction system	▪ HFpEF ▪ Valvular heart disease; aortic stenosis most common ▪ Atrial fibrillation, sinus arrest, tachy–brady syndrome

(continued)

Table 7.4 Physiologic Changes That Occur With Aging, Consequences, and Disease Processes (*continued*)

Body System	Physiologic Changes	Consequences	Diseases Processes/ Geriatric Syndrome
Vascular	▪ Fibrosis, myocyte hypertrophy, calcium deposition, loss of pacemaker cells over time ▪ Vessels become dilated and stiff ▪ Intimal sclerosis ▪ Lose sensitivity to receptor-mediated agents	▪ Vascular stiffness ▪ Increased afterload ▪ Decreased blood flow ▪ Impaired responsiveness to carotid baroreceptors to acute changes in blood pressure	▪ Systolic hypertension ▪ Atherosclerosis ▪ Arterial and venous insufficiency ▪ Myocardial infarction ▪ Orthostatic hypotension, syncope, falls
Respiratory	▪ Loss of elasticity in airways; decreased recoil ▪ Loss of muscle/weakening of respiratory musculature	▪ Decreased intrathoracic negative pressure, airway collapse ▪ Surface area of lung decreases ▪ Residual volume increases ▪ Vital capacity decreases ▪ Forced expiratory volume decreases ▪ Forced vital capacity decreases ▪ A-a gradient increases ▪ Decreased exercise tolerance	▪ Increased exacerbation of existing lung diseases: COPD, ILD ▪ Pneumonia ▪ Acute respiratory distress syndrome ▪ Immobility
Gastrointestinal	▪ Decreased olfactory neurons ▪ Decreased saliva production ▪ Altered intestinal absorption ▪ Atrophy of GI mucosa ▪ Atheroma in vessels	▪ Altered taste ▪ Dry mouth ▪ Altered protein metabolism ▪ Altered nutrient and drug absorption ▪ Prolonged transit time ▪ Decreased blood supply	▪ Poor nutrition ▪ Oral infections ▪ Malnutrition ▪ Iron and vitamin B_{12} deficiency anemias ▪ Adverse drug reactions ▪ Constipation/diverticula/ diverticulitis ▪ Mesenteric ischemia
Urinary	▪ Decreased kidney size, number of functioning renal tubules and glomeruli ▪ Decreased renal blood flow ▪ Loss of muscle tone, ureters, urethra, poor vaginal support, prostate enlargement	▪ Decreased glomerular filtrate rate ▪ Concentrating ability of kidney declines ▪ Decline in functional bladder capacity, increased prevalence of involuntary bladder contractions and detrusor overactivity	▪ Acute/chronic kidney disease ▪ Fluid and electrolyte imbalances (sodium, hydrogen ion, ammonia) ▪ Dehydration ▪ Metabolic acidosis ▪ Urinary tract infections ▪ Urinary incontinence
Immunology (a key contributor to atypical presentation of conditions)	▪ Atrophy of thymus ▪ Impaired macrophage function ▪ Increased autoimmune antibodies	▪ Reduces function and production of T lymphocytes ▪ B-cell function decreases ▪ Requires more stimulus and time to be activated ▪ Increased autoimmune antibodies	▪ Delayed symptoms of infections ▪ Increased risk for infection; sepsis ▪ Decreased response to vaccines

(*continued*)

Table 7.4 Physiologic Changes That Occur With Aging, Consequences, and Disease Processes (*continued*)

Body System	Physiologic Changes	Consequences	Diseases Processes/ Geriatric Syndrome
Endocrine	■ Pineal gland ■ Thyroid gland atrophies ■ Adrenal gland increased fibrous tissue ■ Pancreas (minimal changes to organ) ■ Heart ■ Renal	■ Reduces diurnal melatonin ■ T_4 production declines with very old age but blood concentration may be normal secondary to decreased clearance ■ Moderate decrease in aldosterone secretion ■ Decline in insulin signaling, decreased receptors and cellular glucose transporters ■ Atrial natriuretic peptide levels increase, renal response decreases ■ Response of vasopressin to volume changes decrease ■ Circulating renin levels decrease	■ Altered sleep pattern ■ Hypothyroidism; Graves' disease ■ Contribute orthostatic hypotension ■ Diabetes mellitus ■ Hypotension ■ Hypotension, syncope
Sensory Vision	■ Decreased tear production ■ Lens increases in size, more rigid	■ Dry eyes ■ Farsightedness ■ Decreased peripheral vision ■ Increased intraocular pressure ■ Decreased pupil diameter	■ Depth perception: falls ■ Contribute to falls ■ Glaucoma ■ Slow adaptation in dark ■ Increased accidents, especially if driving or riding a bicycle
Hearing	■ Increased thickening of tympanic membrane ■ Decreased elasticity and efficiency of ossicular articulation	■ Hearing loss	

COPD, chronic obstructive pulmonary disease; GI, gastrointestinal; HFpEF, heart failure with preserved ejection fraction; ILD, interstitial lung disease.

The AGACNP must also be aware that the physiologic changes that occur with aging are the baseline goals for common comorbidities that older adults experience. Avoid aggressive management of these comorbidities because there is an increased risk for adverse effects; it may also be an opportunity to de-prescribe medications if they are not necessary. The AGACNP should consider a person-centered approach to each situation and understand that there will likely be variance among individuals. Table 7.5 identifies common comorbidities with suggested baseline targets (when applicable) for older adults, adverse effects from aggressive treatment, and treatment considerations.

PRESENTATION OF ILLNESS

One of the challenges that AGACNPs face when caring for the older adult patient is the vague and/or atypical presentation of illness. Older adults and their families will often underreport symptoms, as they associate these occurrences with normal aging. Furthermore, these vague and atypical presentations often lead to delays in diagnosis and treatment, complications, and increased mortality. The physiologic changes associated with aging outlined in Table 7.3 can contribute to these factors. The key aging elements include changes in autonomic nervous system, volume regulation, immune dysregulation, and overall decreased physiologic reserve. Altered mentation (delirium and other cognitive changes), weakness, and falls are the most common presentation findings related to illness in the older adult population. Often, family members or caregivers recognize changes in mentation, prompting medical evaluation. Mentation symptoms will progress prior to the development of other more common symptoms.

Table 7.5 Common Comorbidities With Target Outcomes for Older Adults

Comorbidity	Treatment Considerations
Hypertension	▪ Adverse effect: postural hypotension ▪ BP target varies among guidelines: 140/90 to 150/90 ▪ Treatment should focus on systolic reduction ▪ If initiating treatment, begin at half usual dose and increase slowly ▪ If adverse effects cannot be avoided, aggressive therapy is not recommended. ▪ Beta-blockers should not be first-line choice in those age 60 years or older. ▪ ACEI, ARB, calcium channel blocker, and thiazide diuretic are first-line choices
Diabetes mellitus	▪ Adverse effect of aggressive treatment: hypoglycemia; these episodes can increase cognitive decline, especially in those with current cognitive impairment. ▪ HbA1C target of less than 7.5% among older adults with intact cognitive function, functional capacity, and few comorbidities ▪ HbA1C target of less than 8.0% among older adults with mild to moderate cognitive impairment, complex, multiple comorbidities ▪ HbA1C target of less than 8.5% among older adults with moderate to severe cognitive impairment, very complex end-stage comorbidities, limited life expectancy ▪ Metformin medication of choice (without renal compromise); sodium-glucose cotransporter-2 ▪ Short-acting sulfonylureas (glipizide) preferred over long-acting (glyburide)
Hyperlipidemia	▪ No specific adverse effect ▪ Continuation remains controversial. ▪ Initiation of statins after age 80 years may not be necessary ▪ Consideration for de-prescribing if patient has end-stage illness
Anemia	▪ A low hemoglobin or hematocrit is not a normal age-related change. ▪ Those with anemia should have a complete hematologic workup (red blood cell smear count, reticulocyte count, iron studies). ▪ The threshold for transfusion should be based on symptoms and associated conditions. ▪ Acute blood loss post orthopedic procedure may need transfusion for Hgb less than 8 mg/dL. ▪ Anemia associated with active cardiovascular disease may require a transfusion for Hgb less than 8 or 9 mg/dL.

ACEI, angiotensin-converting enzyme inhibitor; ARB, angiotensin-receptor blocker; Hgb, hemoglobin.

The AGACNP must also be aware that other physical assessment findings and laboratory results may also be atypical for an underlying illness. Older adults may not have a fever or elevated white blood cell count with an infection; they may not experience the typical chest pain associated with a myocardial infarction or may not verbalize abdominal pain with an acute abdomen. Table 7.6 identifies common illness presentation in older adults for specific disease processes. In reviewing the symptoms that older adults present with, the AGACNP can recognize the importance of a comprehensive geriatric assessment that includes cognition and function. To improve care outcomes for the older adult patient, AGACNPs must understand the changes associated with aging, recognize subtle symptoms, enhance history through communication with family, and initiate treatment as early as possible.

Table 7.6 Common Illness Presentation in Older Adults

Specific Disease Process	Common Presentation
Infections, prone to urinary tract infections, pneumonia, sepsis	Change in mentation, appetite, anorexia, functional status, falls, one third do not experience fevers, 20% to 45% of patients with bacteremia do not experience leukocytosis; will have elevated lactic acid if septic
Myocardial infarction	May not experience chest pain, some may experience dyspnea only, fatigue, appetite changes, functional changes, syncope, weakness, confusion
Heart failure	Sleeping upright, using more than one pillow, fatigue, changes in function, appetite, and confusion
Diverticulitis	History of constipation, benign abdominal exam (no symptoms of peritonitis), mild tachypnea, vague respiratory symptoms, some no fever, or leukocytosis, changes to functional status

(continued)

Table 7.6 Common Illness Presentation in Older Adults (*continued*)

Specific Disease Process	Common Presentation
Cholecystitis	Benign abdominal exam, changes to appetite, normal biliary/liver studies
Mesenteric ischemia	Benign abdominal exam, mentation changes, high lactic acid
Thyroid disease	Hyperthyroidism: fatigue, slowing down Hypothyroidism: confusion, agitation
Depression	Lack of sadness, appetite changes, vague GI symptoms, sleep disturbances, hyperactivity

GI, gastrointestinal.

▶ MEDICATION RECONCILIATION AND POLYPHARMACY

Medication reconciliation is an important aspect of the geriatric assessment. The larger the number of comorbidities an individual has, the more medications they are likely to be prescribed. Polypharmacy is defined as taking five or more prescription medications and is responsible for increased adverse drug effects (ADEs), falls, mortality, and decreased cognitive function. In addition to prescription medications, the healthcare provider must assess for nonprescription medications and herbal supplements that may be interacting with the current prescribed medication to cause ADE. Polypharmacy is a risk factor for hospitalization in the older adult population and is a contributing factor to the development of two common geriatric syndromes, falls and delirium.

ADEs are the result of several factors, one being potential side effects of the medication that are often exacerbated in the older adult population. The physiologic changes associated with aging often contribute to the development of ADE and are typically the result of impaired pharmacokinetics. As persons age, medication absorption, distribution, metabolism, and elimination are decreased, thus increasing the bioavailability of many medications.

Several tools are available to assist the healthcare provider in prescribing medications and evaluating current therapy. The American Geriatrics Society (AGS) Beers Criteria is one tool that has been adopted by the AGS for medication evaluation in the older adult population. Table 7.7 identifies the different categories within the AGS Beers Criteria along with some examples. Please note that the examples provided are not all-inclusive.

Table 7.7 AGS Beers Criteria PIM Categories

AGS Beers Criteria PIM Category	Examples	
General Inappropriate Use in Older Adults (have side effects that could potentiate geriatric syndrome or multiple toxicities that would make it difficult for older adult to manage)	Anticholinergics or drugs with anticholinergic properties Nitrofurantoin Alpha-1 blockers Amiodarone Benzodiazepines Antipsychotics	Sulfonylureas Insulin sliding scale Proton-pump inhibitors Non-cyclo-oxygenase–selective NSAIDs Skeletal muscle relaxants
Inappropriate Use Secondary to Drug-Disease or Drug Syndrome Interaction That May Exacerbate the Disease or Syndrome	Heart failure: nondihydropyridine calcium channel blockers Syncope: nonselect alpha-1 blockers Delirium/dementia: anticholinergics, benzodiazepines History of falls: anticholinergics, antidepressants, antipsychotics, opioids Parkinson disease: prochlorperazine, all antipsychotics except quetiapine, clozapine	
Potentially Inappropriate Medications to Be Used With Caution	Aspirin for primary prevention of cardiovascular disease and colorectal cancer Dabigatran: increased risk of GI bleeding Antipsychotics—may cause hyponatremia Trimethoprim-sulfamethoxazole—may cause hyperkalemia	

(*continued*)

Table 7.7 AGS Beers Criteria PIM Categories (*continued*)

AGS Beers Criteria PIM Category	Examples	
Potentially Clinically Important Drug–Drug Interactions That Should Be Avoided in Older Adults	RAS inhibitor with another RAS inhibitor Opioid with benzodiazepine Corticosteroid with NSAID Lithium with ACE inhibitor or loop diuretic Phenytoin with trimethoprim-sulfamethoxazole Warfarin with amiodarone, ciprofloxacin	
Medications That Should Be Avoided or Have Their Dosage Reduced With Varying Levels of Kidney Function	Ciprofloxacin Trimethoprim-sulfamethoxazole Dabigatran Enoxaparin	Gabapentin Spironolactone Cimetidine Probenecid

ACE, angiotensin-converting enzyme; AGS, American Geriatrics Society; GI, gastrointestinal; NSAIDs, nonsteroidal anti-inflammatory drugs; PIM, potentially inappropriate medication; RAS, Renin angiotensin system.

There may be circumstances in which medications that have been identified as potentially inappropriateare to be used, but this should be done only with careful assessment and monitoring. Best practice in prescribing medications for older adults is to use the AGS Beers Criteria or other screening tools as a guide for appropriate prescribing, consider de-prescribing in certain circumstances, and start low and go slow when starting a new medication. Table 7.8 highlights screening tools to assist healthcare providers in prescribing medications for older adults. In addition, the following principles should be considered related to de-prescribing: duplicate medications, drug–drug interactions, drugs causing adverse effects, complexity of regimen, pill burden, and life expectancy. Use caution when de-prescribing as certain medications may need to be tapered off as opposed to suddenly stopped.

Table 7.8 Screening Tools for Prescribing

Screening Tools
AGS Beers Criteria
STOPP: Screening Tool of Older Persons' Prescriptions
START: Screening Tool to Alert to Right Treatment
MAI: Medication Appropriateness Index

▶ GERIATRIC SYNDROMES

Geriatric syndromes are a group of health conditions that occur most commonly in the older adult population, predominantly the frail older adult. These syndromes place the older adult at risk for hospitalization, complications during hospitalization, and overall mortality. Examples of geriatric syndromes include delirium, falls, incontinence, malnutrition, depression, and pain. As noted with the physiologic changes associated with aging, there is a decrease in the "homeostatic reserve capacity" of all organ systems (see Table 7.4). This reduction in reserve capacity not only places older adults at risk for disease but also places them at risk to develop additional conditions that further complicate their care. Furthermore, a geriatric syndrome is often the initial condition that an older adult presents with. Common presenting symptoms in the older adult population are cognitive changes, falls, and poor appetite. These conditions could further result in incontinence, malnutrition, and depression. The key assessment indicators identified in Table 7.2 relate back to the importance of screening for common geriatric syndromes. Common geriatric syndromes are discussed in the following sections, and a summary of assessment tools, additional diagnostic workup, and management strategies for each geriatric syndrome are found in Table 7.3.

DELIRIUM

In addition to falls, delirium is a common occurrence in the older adult population and can go unrecognized in about 70% of older adults. Delirium is often a chief complaint for underlying illnesses, especially infections, and is a marker of functional decline that leads to loss of independence, institutionalization, and death. Delirium is defined as acute alteration in mental status, disorder of attention and global cognitive function, fluctuating course, and additional cognitive deficits (memory, orientation, language, visuo-perceptual ability). There are two classifications of delirium:

- *hypoactive:* more common in older adults and carries an overall poorer prognosis because it is often unrecognized; lethargy and reduced psychomotor functioning
- *hyperactive:* agitation, increased vigilance, hallucinations

FALLS

Falls, like other geriatric syndromes, can be a symptom of changes that occur with aging and underlying illness or can occur as a result of hospitalization and treatment. Fall assessment tools have been developed but are not able to predict the occurrence of falls with accuracy across various populations. Therefore, current literature suggests that the best approach to falls is to understand the risk factors and develop interventions to target those risk factors. Risk factors include age-related changes; diseases (Parkinson disease, stroke, dementia, incontinence, acute illness [infection], dizziness, arthritis, vestibular disorders, cardiovascular, orthostatic hypotension); adverse medication effects (psychoactive, antihypertensive medications); taking four or more medications; sensorimotor and balance systems becoming impaired; psychosocial issues; and demographics.

INCONTINENCE

Incontinence is also a major risk factor for falls. There are several factors that place an older adult patient at risk for incontinence (see Table 7.4). Additional factors include medications (anticholinergics, narcotics, calcium channel blockers, beta-adrenergic medications) and the hospital environment (immobility, bed rails, restraints, delirium, tubes, lines). Reversible causes of incontinence include urinary tract infections, post prostatectomy (will usually last for approximately 1 year post surgery), increased urine production (diabetes, increased fluid, venous insufficiency, congestive heart failure), immobility or difficult time to reach toilet, fecal impaction, and medication side effects.

MALNUTRITION

A significant number of older adults are considered to have poor nutrition status upon hospitalization. Causes are multifactorial and can be triggered by underlying illness (with development of poor appetite), geriatric syndromes (immobility: unable to prepare foods), difficulty swallowing, and economic factors. Older adults with malnutrition have increased length of stay, increased likelihood of transfer to extended care facility, and higher mortality. The Joint Commission mandates nutrition screening in this population.

DEPRESSION

Like the other geriatric syndromes, depression is highly prevalent in older adults. Depression should not be considered a natural part of aging, nor is it a normal reaction to acute illness with hospitalization. Depression has several untoward consequences that can amplify pain or disability, delay recovery, worsen side effects from medications, and contribute to the development of other geriatric syndromes like immobility, pain, and malnutrition. Older adults may not experience typical signs/symptoms associated with depression. The symptoms may be more somatic than those of a depressed mood.

PAIN

Most older adults have chronic medical conditions that are associated with pain; however, pain is often poorly assessed and managed. Furthermore, age-related changes in the nervous system can impact pain perception. Cognitive impairment represents a particular challenge to pain management. Appropriate pain assessment and management can improve function, mobility, and mood and therefore decrease the occurrence of geriatric syndromes. Conversely, lack of adequate pain management can lead to impaired immune functioning and healing, cognitive impairment exacerbation, and postoperative complications.

▶ MAJOR NEUROCOGNITIVE DISORDER (DEMENTIA)

There are four common types of dementia: Alzheimer, Lewy body, frontotemporal, and vascular. Alzheimer dementia (AD) is the most common. Age has been identified as the single most validated risk factor for dementia. Other risk factors include genetics, vascular issues (hypertension, diabetes, metabolic syndrome, hypercholesterolemia), traumatic brain injury, and depression. Dementia is the result of functional and structural abnormalities in the brain that can lead to progressive cognitive and behavioral deficits, in addition to functional decline. Cognitive and behavioral symptoms that may occur can have the following characteristics:

- interfere with ability to function at work or usual activities
- represent a decline from previous levels of function and performance
- are not explained by delirium or other cognitive disorders
- involve a minimum of two of the following domains:
  - inability to acquire or remember new information
  - impaired reasoning, judgment, and handling of complex tasks
  - impaired visuospatial abilities
  - impaired language function
  - changes in personality

It is through careful assessment that dementia is diagnosed. Past medical history should focus on the following: cardio-/cerebrovascular disease, Parkinson disease, obstructive sleep apnea with hypoxia, depression (Geriatric Depression Scale), anxiety, other mood disorders, medication review, risk factors for delirium, hearing/visual loss, family history, and social history—alcohol.

Cognitive assessment can be evaluated by:

- Mini-Mental State Examination (MMSE): measures concentration, language, orientation, memory, attention; score of less than 24 indicates dementia
- Montreal Cognitive Assessment (MoCA)

The review of systems (ROS) should further evaluate for signs/symptoms related to depression, tremors, falls, hallucinations, stroke, transient ischemic attack, ataxia, dysphagia, urinary incontinence, waxing and waning of consciousness, and personality changes. Diagnostics include:

- complete blood count (CBC), comprehensive metabolic panel (CMP), thyroid, vitamin B_{12}, vitamin D
- noncontrast head CT or MRI

The different types of dementia are highlighted in Table 7.9, and AD is further defined in Table 7.10. It is possible that the diagnosis of dementia could be made during a patient's hospitalization. Older adults may also have what is classified as mild cognitive impairment (MCI). MCI is often recognized by a family member who notes that there is a change in cognitive level from baseline. The patient is likely to experience a decreased performance in one or more cognitive domains but does not meet the criteria for dementia. Persons with MCI and memory impairment or memory impairment plus an additional cognitive impairment are more likely to progress to AD. It is important for the healthcare provider to be able to identify and differentiate symptoms related to cognitive changes that include MCI, dementia, and delirium. Delirium is possible in a patient with underlying dementia, and this often complicates patient care. Avoidance of restraints and invasive devices may decrease worsening of cognition that occurs in patients with dementia or those who develop delirium in addition to dementia. Table 7.11 differentiates delirium and dementia.

Table 7.9 Types of Dementia

AD	Vascular	Lewy Body	Frontotemporal
■ Gradual onset ■ Progressive decline in cognitive function ■ Memory impairment with progression to learning difficulties, aphasia, apraxia, impaired judgment, and executive dysfunction	■ Suspicious in patients with history of vascular issues ■ Ischemic damage to multiple areas within cortex and subcortical structures; evidence of ASHD ■ Abrupt onset, stepwise progression with preservation of personality ■ Emotional lability, depression, nighttime confusion	■ Fluctuation in cognition, visual and auditory hallucinations ■ Mild spontaneous extrapyramidal symptoms ■ Shares symptoms with delirium but much worse ■ Associated with Parkinson disease	■ Common in those younger than 60 years ■ Executive and language dysfunction with significant behavioral changes ■ Memory deficits not as profound

ASHD, atherosclerotic heart disease.

Table 7.10 AD: Symptoms and Treatment

Symptoms	Treatment
Insidious onset of months/years Impairment in learning and recall of recently learned information and one of the following: ■ Word finding ■ Visuospatial ■ Impaired reasoning, judgment, and problem-solving Disease progression results in: ■ Personality changes ■ Increased passivity ■ Lack of interest ■ Agitation/restlessness ■ Alteration in appetite ■ Difficulty concentrating/ making decisions Late stages: ■ Increased confusion ■ Dysphagia ■ Impaired gait/repeat falls ■ Aggression/agitation ■ Physical/verbal hostility ■ Incontinence	Nonpharmacologic: ■ Physical activity ■ Behavioral support ■ Safety ■ Caregiver support ■ Palliative care Pharmacologic cognition related: ■ ACHeIs ■ Enhance cholinergic activity; patient reaches plateau or slowing of cognitive rate of decline ■ Donepezil (Aricept) 5 to 10 mg mild to moderate; 10 to 23 mg moderate to severe ■ Galantamine (Razadyne) 4 to 12 mg BID with meals (start at 4 mg) ■ Rivastigmine (Exelon) 1.5 mg BID for 2 weeks, then 3 mg for 2 weeks; also available as patch ■ NMDA receptor antagonist ■ Memantine (Namenda): moderate to severe AD ■ For those unable to tolerate ACHeIs Pharmacologic behavioral issues: ■ SSRIs: for agitation/depression/inappropriate sexual behavior ■ Antipsychotic medication should be used for the treatment of agitation only when symptoms are severe or dangerous and/or cause significant distress to the patient. ■ Haloperidol is not recommended as first-line drug. ■ Long-acting injectable antipsychotics (risperidone) are recommended.

ACHeIs, acetylcholinesterase inhibitors; AD, Alzheimer dementia; NMDA, N-methyl-D-aspartate; SSRIs, selective serotonin reuptake inhibitors.

Table 7.11 Differentiating Delirium and Dementia

Delirium	Dementia
■ Acute onset ■ Fluctuation ■ Duration: hours to weeks ■ Alertness: low to high ■ Illusion and hallucination ■ Memory: immediate and recent impaired ■ Disorganized thought ■ Incoherent speech ■ Physical illness: present ■ Treatment for agitation: conventional antipsychotics (haloperidol)	■ Insidious onset ■ Stable course ■ Duration: months to years ■ Alertness: normal ■ Perception: normal ■ Memory: recent and remote impaired ■ Impoverished thought ■ Word-finding difficulty ■ Physical illness: may be absent ■ Treatment for agitation: SSRI for mild to moderate or with depression; long-acting second-generation antipsychotic (risperidone, quetiapine)

SSRI, selective serotonin reuptake inhibitor.

▶ CARING FOR THE OLDER ADULT IN THE ICU

Sepsis and acute respiratory failure are the primary admission diagnoses for older adult patients in the ICU. Older adults are more susceptible to multiorgan failure secondary to comorbidities, injuries, environmental exposures, and changes in aging that occur, resulting in diminished physiologic reserves and capacity to maintain homeostasis. Areas of multiorgan failure include:

■ *respiratory failure:* decreased ability to compensate for increased respiratory demands. Reduced lung compliance leads to decreased vital capacity and increased ventilation-perfusion mismatch. Early use of incentive spirometry and use of positive end expiratory pressure (PEEP) help.

■ *cardiovascular failure:* systolic and diastolic function decline, reducing stroke volume and ventricular filling:
- inability to enhance stroke volume without atrial kick if older adult has atrial arrhythmia
- decreased beta-adrenergic response: decreases heart rate response to alterations in blood pressure
  - ❏ With shock, the aging heart maintains cardiac output by relying more on increasing preload than on increasing heart rate. Fluid resuscitation with stiff ventricles may result in pulmonary edema. It is a fine balance to maintain homeostasis in the older adult patient.
  - ❏ Management may require higher filling pressures to maintain adequate stroke volume; however, overhydration should also be avoided because it can lead to systolic failure, poor organ perfusion, and hypoxemia, resulting in diastolic dysfunction.
■ *renal failure:* loss of glomeruli, decreased renal blood flow, and regulation of fluid and electrolytes:
- diminished regulation in hyper- and hypotensive states
- reduction in glomerular filtration rate (GFR)

ICU healthcare providers must complete a comprehensive assessment of the geriatric patient once stabilization has occurred. This includes preadmission cognitive ability, medication history, psychosocial factors, functional ability, nutrition status, and geriatric syndromes as discussed earlier. The ABCDE bundle assists providers in improving care outcomes for older adults in critical care settings (see Chapter 19).

▶ POSTOPERATIVE CONSIDERATIONS FOR THE OLDER ADULT PATIENT

The odds of developing postoperative complications increase with aging. Postoperative complications are often associated with use of anesthesia and inability of the body to respond efficiently secondary to the changes that occur with aging. Table 7.12 indicates key systemic manifestations that occur in older adults secondary to surgery and use of anesthesia.

Table 7.12 Systemic Manifestation Secondary to Anesthesia and Surgery

System	Manifestation	Monitor
Cardiovascular	Hemodynamic instability intra- and postoperatively ■ Intubation: transient hypertension ■ Anesthesia: hypotension	Arrhythmias EKG changes for ischemia
Pulmonary	Decreased pulmonary function: ventilation-perfusion mismatch	Duration of mechanical ventilation may be prolonged Use of neuromuscular blocking agents Mobility as soon as possible Preoperative pulmonary toileting if able Opioids dosed carefully; benzodiazepines avoided if possible
GI	Risk for aspiration Risk for ileus	H_2 blocker preoperatively, especially if history of GERD Bowel sounds, abdominal distention Minimize use of opioids/anticholinergics
GU	Progression of renal disease Decreased urinary output Urinary retention	GFR, avoid nephrotoxic medications if possible Adequate fluids and perfusion Avoid anticholinergic Straight catheter if necessary; avoid indwelling Foley unless necessary
Nervous	Postoperative delirium, especially if history of dementia Autonomic dysfunction	CAM Sleep/wake cycles Minimize use of opioids/anticholinergics Avoid use of benzodiazepines Monitor for safety if using beta-blockers (at risk for orthostatic hypotension)

CAM, confusion assessment method; GERD, gastroesophageal reflux disease; GFR, glomerular filtration rate; GI, gastrointestinal; GU, genitourinary; H_2, Histamine H_2 blocker.

▶ TRANSITIONAL CARE

Transitional care is a set of actions that are created to ensure the coordination and continuity of healthcare as patients transfer from different levels of care within the same institution or different locations altogether. The older adult patient is often subject to transitional care because of the changes that may occur in required healthcare needs since admission (different levels of care) or the complexity of care required at the time of discharge. Transition of care from one area or facility to another is often a time of vulnerability to patient safety issues because of inadequate care coordination. More than 50% of all avoidable events following discharge from the hospital are related to poor communication. Another 30% to 50% is related to poor medication reconciliation. Effective, high-quality care coordination includes:

- involvement of patient and family or caregiver
- patient and caregiver empowerment
- complete and accurate communication
  - past medical history and remarkable events during hospital stay
  - functional status
  - psychosocial/family contact information
  - elimination/nutritional status
  - follow-up care
  - treatments
  - laboratory results, including pending results
- high-quality medication reconciliation
  - diagnoses, related medications, and rationale for current medications
  - significant medication changes
  - opioid prescriptions
  - allergies and intolerances

▶ PALLIATIVE AND HOSPICE CARE

Palliative and hospice care should be incorporated in their care of older adults. Palliative care should be considered in patients with diagnoses of dementia, frailty, and multiple comorbidities. The symptom burden that occurs in the progression of these illnesses supports the need for an interdisciplinary approach to care that can be provided with palliative and hospice care (see Chapter 19).

▶ SUMMARY

AGACNPs will care for hospitalized older adults on a daily basis. Care of this population requires the AGACNP to differentiate between normal aging and pathologic changes and differentiate between acute and chronic illnesses. Appropriate medication management in this population is key to improving outcomes and preventing adverse drug events. De-prescribing and avoiding medications on the AGS Beers Criteria will aid in maintaining cognitive and physical functioning. These skills can be applied across the spectrum of populations AGACNPs will care for in practice.

⬤ KNOWLEDGE CHECK: CHAPTER 7

1. An 82-year-old patient is admitted to the surgical unit after open cholecystectomy. The patient has a past medical history of hypertension and hypothyroidism. The AGACNP writes which of the following orders to prevent a postoperative complication?

   A. Buspirone 10 mg orally PRN for anxiety
   B. Incentive spirometry every 1 to 2 hours while awake
   C. Bedrest for 24 hours postsurgery
   D. 0.9 normal saline, 1 L per 6 hours

2. The AGACNP is completing an assessment on a 70-year-old patient who presented to the hospital with shortness of breath and dizziness with exertion. What finding would the AGACNP anticipate, indicating a cardiovascular condition that often develops in the older adult population secondary to changes associated with aging?

   A. High-pitched holosystolic murmur auscultated left lower sternal border
   B. Systolic murmur auscultated left midclavicular line
   C. High-pitched mid-systolic murmur auscultated right second intercostal space
   D. Early diastolic blowing murmur auscultated third to fourth intercostal space

3. The AGACNP is caring for an 86-year-old patient admitted to the hospital status post hip fracture repair. The patient's past medical history includes arthritis, benign prostatic hypertrophy, and colon cancer. The patient takes acetaminophen for arthritis. The patient's blood pressure readings have been consistently in the 140/85 to 150/90 range. The patient's body mass index (BMI) is 18. What is the best intervention for the AGACNP to take?

   A. Continue to monitor and provide instructions to follow up with primary care provider at discharge.
   B. Provide the patient with strict dietary sodium and fluid intake instructions.
   C. Discontinue the acetaminophen and add ibuprofen.
   D. Prescribe metoprolol, 100 mg orally daily.

4. A 75-year-old patient is brought to the hospital by family for increased fatigue, weakness, and confusion. The patient's family indicates that they have noticed the patient experiencing intermittent episodes of confusion over the past several months. The family noticed that the confusion worsened when fatigue and weakness occurred. Upon exam, the patient is lethargic, oriented to person only, with lung computed tomography angiography, heart rate 98, and blood pressure 90/52. What diagnostics indicate the best workup for this patient?

   A. Complete blood cell count (CBC), comprehensive metabolic panel, thyroid studies, Geriatric Depression Scale
   B. CBC, comprehensive metabolic panel, urinalysis, confusion assessment method (CAM)
   C. CBC with differential, comprehensive metabolic panel, urinalysis with culture and drug screen
   D. CBC with differential, comprehensive metabolic panel, urinalysis with culture, blood cultures, Mini-Mental State Examination (MMSE)

(See answers next page.)

1. **B) Incentive spirometry every 1 to 2 hours while awake**
The patient is at risk for postoperative pneumonia secondary to surgery and changes associated with aging. Preventive measures, especially incentive spirometry, should be encouraged. Buspirone is used for anxiety. The patient should be mobilized as soon as possible rather than placed on bedrest. Although it is important to ensure the patient is hydrated postoperatively, 4 L in a 24-hour period may place the patient at risk for pulmonary edema.

2. **C) High-pitched mid-systolic murmur auscultated right second intercostal space**
Older adults are at highest risk to develop aortic stenosis; this is a high-pitched mid-systolic murmur best heard at the right intercostal space with radiation up to the carotid. High-pitched holosystolic murmur auscultated left lower sternal border is tricuspid regurgitation. A systolic murmur auscultated left midclavicular line is mitral regurgitation. Early diastolic blowing murmur auscultated at the third to fourth intercostal space is aortic regurgitation.

3. **A) Continue to monitor and provide instructions to follow up with PCP at discharge.**
Continue to monitor the patient. These readings are in accordance with what is recommended for blood pressure in the older adult patient. The patient could be informed regarding sodium restriction, but it is important for this patient to eat foods that are palatable because the BMI is 18. Fluid restriction is not necessary. Acetaminophen is safe to prescribe in the older adult population. Ibuprofen is a nonsteroidal anti-inflammatory drug and may worsen blood pressure. Beta-blockers should not be used as first-line antihypertensives in older adults.

4. **D) CBC with differential, comprehensive metabolic panel, urinalysis with culture, blood cultures, Mini-Mental State Examination (MMSE)**
It is important to obtain a CBC with differential to determine the presence of bands. The patient's presenting symptoms could indicate an underlying infection along with the presence of dementia. Urinalysis and blood cultures would help to evaluate for infectious disease etiologies. An MMSE is useful to evaluate for dementia. The CAM evaluates for delirium, which is unlikely because the symptoms have been ongoing for 3 months. A comprehensive metabolic panel will evaluate electrolyte status that could also be the cause of cognitive changes.

5. An 85-year-old patient is brought to the hospital via emergency medical services secondary to sustaining a fall. The family indicates that the patient has been acting sluggish the past several days and has had a poor appetite. The patient denies pain and states that they are a bit tired but see no reason to be in the hospital. The patient denies nausea, vomiting, chest pain, and shortness of breath; they had their last bowel movement 3 days ago. Physical exam is normal. Vital signs are temperature 98.2°F, blood pressure 100/50, heart rate 92, respiratory rate 16, pulse oximetry 95% on room air. Laboratory results available are white blood cell (WBC) 6.8; hemoglobin (Hgb) 11.4; hematocrit (HCT) 34.2; platelets 205,000; 3% bands on differential; blood urea nitrogen (BUN) 36, creatinine 1.0; lactic acid 3.2. Urinalysis is normal, blood cultures preliminary gram-negative bacilli one bottle. What additional diagnostics should the AGACNP order?

   A. Chest x-ray
   B. Abdominal CT with contrast
   C. Abdominal MRI
   D. Head CT with contrast

6. A 77-year-old patient is admitted to the hospital status post fall. The patient has a history of Alzheimer dementia. The patient's spouse states that the patient was just started on a medication to help with memory. The AGACNP anticipates that the patient is taking:

   A. Risperidone (Risperdal)
   B. Benztropine mesylate (Cogentin)
   C. Levodopa–carbidopa (Sinemet)
   D. Donepezil (Aricept)

7. The AGACNP is called to evaluate a 92-year-old patient who has developed confusion. The patient has been in the hospital for 4 days and was alert and oriented on admission. The patient has been receiving treatment for community-acquired pneumonia. Vital signs are stable, including oxygen saturation. The chest x-ray shows improvement. Upon assessment, the patient is alert but confused as to place and time. The patient does not appear agitated but does move from bed to chair frequently. The *best* action the AGACNP should take at this time is to order:

   A. A psych consult
   B. Haloperidol
   C. A bedside sitter
   D. Buspirone

8. The AGACNP is caring for a 70-year-old patient who was admitted to the hospital with exacerbation of congestive heart failure. The patient also has a history of Alzheimer dementia. The patient was brought to the hospital by their family member, who tells the AGACNP that the patient has become quite agitated lately and difficult to handle. Upon assessment, the AGACNP notes the patient to be confused and restless and trying to get out of bed. The patient is also combative to the staff. The best action for the AGACNP to take is to prescribe:

   A. Risperidone (Risperdal)
   B. Haloperidol (Haldol)
   C. Diazepam (Valium)
   D. Buspirone (Buspar)

9. The AGACNP is beginning the discharge process for an older adult patient who has been in the hospital for 2 weeks. It is recommended that the patient be transferred to a rehabilitation center to continue their recovery. The patient remains weak but is alert and oriented. What should the AGACNP consider to achieve the best outcome in planning for transitional care?

   A. Have the family make the decisions so as not to increase the patient's stress.
   B. Include the patient and family in the decision-making process.
   C. Minimize collaboration among services to streamline the process.
   D. Provide the patient with limited placement options to simplify the decision.

(See answers next page.)

5. B) Abdominal CT with contrast

The patient has atypical presentation, high lactic acid supports sepsis, and the patient has positive blood cultures with gram-negative bacillus. Gram-negative pathogens are common intra-abdominal pathogens. The urinalysis (UA) is negative. It is likely the patient has some type of intra-abdominal infection. They have not had a bowel movement for the past 3 days, which could be related to diverticulitis. Abdominal CT will assist to rule in or out several different intra-abdominal pathologies. It is likely not a gram-negative pneumonia. Head CT would be warranted if the patient had confusion without gram-negative sepsis. Meningitis in the older adult is likely strep pneumonia or listeria.

6. D) Donepezil (Aricept)

Donepezil is an acetylcholinesterase inhibitor and the drug of choice for patients with Alzheimer disease. This medication will not decrease the symptoms but may decrease the progression. Risperidone is an atypical antipsychotic, and Cogentin is an anticholinergic used in the treatment of Parkinson disease. Levodopa–carbidopa increases dopamine levels and is used in the treatment of Parkinson disease.

7. C) A bedside sitter

The patient likely has delirium, and nonpharmacologic therapy is recommended if the patient is not overly agitated and presents no harm to self. Haloperidol can be used if the patient is agitated and at risk for harming self or others. Buspirone is an antianxiety drug that takes about 2 to 4 weeks to begin working and is not indicated in the treatment of delirium.

8. A) Risperidone (Risperdal)

Long-acting atypical antipsychotics are indicated in the treatment of agitation in the context of dementia. First-generation antipsychotics (haloperidol) are not recommended as they can increase mortality. Diazepam is a benzodiazepine and is not recommended for older adults (see AGS Beers Criteria). Buspirone is prescribed for anxiety but is long-acting.

9. B) Include the patient and family in the decision-making process.

A key element to successful transition is to include the patient and family in the decision-making process. Collaboration is also important among all providers to enhance outcomes. It is important for the patient to understand all placement options so they can make the best decision.

10. A patient is being transferred to another level of care in the hospital. What is the most important element that impacts patient safety in relation to care transition?

    A. Patient empowerment
    B. Family involvement
    C. Complete and accurate communication
    D. Medication reconciliation related to current medication use

11. The AGACNP is caring for an older adult patient with a history of advanced Alzheimer dementia. The patient has frequent hospital admissions for aspiration pneumonia. The family asks the AGACNP if a feeding tube would be a good option. What is the best response by the AGACNP?

    A. "Yes, a feeding tube would be a good option. I will order a gastrointestinal consult to have a feeding tube surgically placed, and I will also order a hospice consult."
    B. "Yes, a feeding tube would be a good option. I can have one placed that will go through the patient's nose. I will also order a palliative care consult."
    C. "No, a feeding tube is not a good option. We can work to strengthen the swallow reflex to prevent aspiration from occurring. I will order a speech therapy consult."
    D. "No, a feeding tube is not a good option. Studies suggest that there is no improvement in outcomes. I will order a palliative care consult."

12. The AGACNP is caring for an 85-year-old patient in the ICU who is admitted with sepsis and acute respiratory failure secondary to community-acquired pneumonia. The patient is currently intubated with mechanical ventilation support. Blood pressure is 118/80 without the use of pressor support. Lactic acid has normalized. What actions by the AGACNP will assist to enhance patient outcomes?

    A. Using lorazepam (Ativan) for sedation
    B. Advocating for early weaning trials
    C. Continuing aggressive hydration to minimize renal toxicity
    D. Avoiding enteral nutrition to prevent aspiration

13. An 84-year-old patient is brought to the hospital by his family because of increased weakness, fatigue, and poor appetite. The patient states that they have been feeling poorly for the past few days and started to develop shortness of breath last evening. The patient denies chest pain, abdominal pain, nausea, vomiting, diarrhea, constipation, fever, chills, and diaphoresis. The patient's vital signs are stable, oxygen saturation level is 94% on room air, and physical assessment findings are normal. Along with complete blood cell count with differential and comprehensive metabolic panel, what diagnostic studies reflect the best workup the AGACNP should order?

    A. Troponin, B-type natriuretic peptide (BNP), chest x-ray, EKG, urinalysis
    B. Chest x-ray, blood cultures, urinalysis
    C. Echocardiogram, chest x-ray, urinalysis
    D. Chest CT angiography (CTA), arterial blood gases, urinalysis

14. The AGACNP is caring for a 72-year-old patient diagnosed with acute myocardial infarction. The patient underwent a heart catheterization and developed complications post procedure, requiring an extended hospital stay. The patient has a prior history of coronary artery disease, hyperlipidemia, atrial fibrillation, diabetes mellitus, and anxiety. The patient has no history of cognitive changes. On day 4 of admission, the patient is noted to be confused and agitated, with hallucinations. What does the AGACNP evaluate *first* to differentiate potential etiology of these symptoms?

    A. Pain
    B. Presence of infection
    C. Medications
    D. Mental state

(See answers next page.)

10. C) Complete and accurate communication

Communication is the most important element in ensuring good patient outcomes with care transitions. It is important to empower the patient and family, but unless the healthcare provider communicates what the process is and the options, empowerment will likely not occur effectively. It is important for the healthcare provider to provide complete and accurate information related to all aspects of care, including medication reconciliation. Medication reconciliation should include information about all medication use during the hospital stay, not only what is current.

11. D) "No, a feeding tube is not a good option. Studies suggest that there is no improvement in outcomes. I will order a palliative care consult."

Studies have indicated that there is no improvement in outcomes in persons who are at advanced stages of Alzheimer disease; these individuals would remain at risk for aspiration pneumonia. Palliative care or even hospice consult would be appropriate for this patient. The patient has advanced dementia and therefore is unlikely to work with a speech therapist to strengthen swallowing.

12. B) Advocating for early weaning trials

Because of the changes that occur in the respiratory system with aging, the patient is at risk for longer ventilator days and increased complications. Lorazepam is a benzodiazepine that is contraindicated in older adults. The patient may not be able to tolerate aggressive fluids at this point in their recovery; they could lead to worsening respiratory compromise and longer ventilator days. Patients should always receive nutrition as soon as possible to assist with overall recovery.

13. A) Troponin, BNP, chest x-ray, EKG, urinalysis

The patient has vague atypical presentation. In addition to obtaining a urinalysis to screen for urinary tract infection, the healthcare provider should consider cardiovascular compromise. This would best be evaluated by troponin, BNP, and EKG. A chest x-ray is appropriate at this time in the evaluation as the oxygenation level does not support a CTA. An echocardiogram would be appropriate once the troponin and EKG are completed or if a murmur was auscultated and the patient has lower extremity swelling.

14. C) Medications

It is likely that the patient has delirium because this is an acute onset of symptoms. Medications are typically the number one cause of delirium. It would be best for the AGACNP to review the medications first and then evaluate if the patient is having pain or is at risk for infection (both are possible). Evaluation of mental state would be useful if dementia was suspected.

15. The AGACNP is caring for a 76-year-old patient who is post colon resection for diverticulitis. The patient has a medical history of hypertension, hyperlipidemia, and hypothyroidism. The patient's current medications include metoprolol, atorvastatin, and levothyroxine. What would be an important action to prevent a geriatric syndrome postoperatively?

A. Order opioids around the clock so patient can rest comfortably.

B. Check patient for orthostatic changes prior to ambulating.

C. Maintain bedrest until bowel sounds resume.

D. Hold the atorvastatin because it can contribute to delirium postoperatively.

(See answers next page.)

15. B) Check patient for orthostatic changes prior to ambulating.

The patient is receiving a beta-blocker, which can cause orthostatic hypotension, especially in older adults. Ambulation should not be restricted but done carefully to prevent falls. Older adults should not remain on bedrest because this will place them at risk for further complications. Atorvastatin is a safe medication, does not contribute to confusion, and is not known to cause delirium. It is important to medicate the patient for pain, but this does not need to be done around the clock unless the patient requires it.

KEY BIBLIOGRAPHY

Only key resources appear in the print edition. Access the full bibliography for this chapter on ExamPrepConnect.com.

American Geriatrics Society. (2019). 2019 update AGS Beers Criteria. *Journal of the American Geriatrics Society*, *67*, 674–694. https://doi.org/10.1111/jgs.15767

Halter, J. B., Ouslander, J. G., Studenski, S., High, K. P., Asthana, S., Supiano, M. A., & Ritchie, C. (Eds.). (2017). *Hazzard's geriatric medicine and gerontology* (7th ed.). McGraw Hill.

Jameson, J., Fauci, A. S., Kasper, D. L., Hauser, S. L., Longo, D. L., & Loscalzo, J. (Eds.). (2018). *Harrison's principles of internal medicine* (20th ed.). McGraw Hill. https://accessmedicine.mhmedical.com/content.aspx?bookid=2129&sectionid=159213747

Kennedy-Malone, L. (2019). Changes with aging. In L. Kennedy-Malone, L. Martin-Plank, & E. Duffy (Eds.), *Advanced practice nursing in the care of older adults* (2nd ed., pp. 2–5). F.A. Davis.

Resnick, B. (2022). *Geriatric nursing review syllabus: A core curriculum in advanced practice geriatric nursing* (7th ed.). American Geriatric Society.

Part III: Systems Review

Nervous System Review

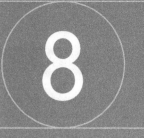

James Brinson, Jennifer Fisher, Alexander Menard, and Dawn Carpenter

▶ INTRODUCTION

The nervous system is complex, and the AGACNP must have a good understanding of the topics covered in this chapter. Neurologic pathologies require the AGACNP to incorporate physical exam findings and patterns learned in the advanced health assessment course to decipher what pathologies might be present.

▶ STROKE

DISEASE OVERVIEW
Stroke, cerebral vascular accident, or "brain attack" are broad, synonymous terms that can be further classified as ischemic or hemorrhagic in origin. Acute stroke results in loss of or decrease in blood flow to a certain area of the brain. Decreased blood flow decreases delivery of oxygen and nutrients, which can result in neurologic deficits. Early recognition, treatment, and rehabilitative programs have been shown to maximize meaningful recovery. In the United States, it is reported that nearly 800,000 new strokes are diagnosed annually.

CLASSIC PRESENTATION
A 74-year-old male patient presents with acute onset of dysarthria and right-sided weakness. The patient has a past medical history of hypertension and atrial fibrillation and is not on anticoagulation. The family notes that the patient's symptoms started 1 hour prior to presentation.

ISCHEMIC STROKE
Acute *ischemic stroke* occurs when a blood clot occludes blood flow to the brain, resulting in ischemia and tissue death. Acute ischemic strokes account for 90% of all strokes in the United States. The TOAST classification denotes five subtypes of ischemic stroke: (a) large-artery atherosclerosis, (b) cardioembolic, (c) small-vessel occlusion, (d) stroke of other determined etiology, and (e) stroke of undetermined etiology.

DIAGNOSTIC CRITERIA
Diagnosis of an acute ischemic stroke is, in the initial period, based largely on the patient's neurologic exam that is objectively scored by the National Institutes of Health Stroke Scale (NIHSS). Establishing the patient's last time known well, defined as the last time the patient was seen in their baseline state of health, is critical to determine eligibility for thrombolytic therapy.

Initial evaluation involves ruling out diagnoses that mimic strokes. Immediately assess blood glucose, as the most common diagnosis to mimic stroke is hypoglycemia. Next, a stat noncontrast head CT is obtained to rule out intracranial hemorrhage, which can also exhibit similar signs and symptoms of an ischemic event. Importantly, ischemic changes on a head CT will not appear until 24 hours post stroke, so if a hypodensity is appreciated on a head CT, it is indicative of a subacute event. A brain MRI will give more detailed insight into the infarct size, whereas a CT perfusion scan can define areas of hypoperfusion.

TREATMENT/MANAGEMENT

The initial treatment of acute ischemic stroke, if indicated, is an intravenous (IV) thrombolytic. The NIHSS score, last known well, and head CT findings will affect the decision to give an IV fibrinolytic. Current guidelines state that an IV fibrinolytic can be administered safely up to 3 to 4.5 hours from the time last known well.

Based on the patient's NIHSS score and neurologic exam, a head CT angiography (CTA) may be needed if the infarct is suspected to be caused by a large vessel occlusion. A large vessel occlusion is an occlusion of one of the large intracerebral arteries, including the internal carotid arteries, middle cerebral arteries, and basilar artery. The results of the CTA brain and CT perfusion imaging will determine whether the patient is a candidate for mechanical thrombectomy to extract the clot.

COMPLICATIONS

For patients with large infarcts, as in a complete middle cerebral artery (MCA) territory stroke, the patient may develop malignant cerebral edema, which can lead to increased intracranial pressure (ICP) and brain compression. This swelling peaks at poststroke day 3 to 5 and can be life threatening. In the instance of malignant cerebral edema, the patient's airway, breathing, and circulation must be assessed and secured. After hemodynamic stability is obtained, hyperosmolar therapy may be considered. Neurosurgical evaluation must be considered for decompressive hemicraniectomy.

Additional ischemic stroke complications include hemorrhagic conversion into large territory infarcts, dysphagia, aspiration, pneumonia, and deep vein thrombosis (DVT) in immobile extremities.

HEMORRHAGIC STROKE

Acute intracerebral hemorrhage (ICH) is a type of stroke defined by acute blood extravasation into the brain parenchyma from a ruptured intracranial blood vessel. Acute ICH accounts for approximately 10% of strokes per year in the United States and is associated with a 30% to 40% early-term mortality rate, with many survivors having long-term disability. Early identification, diagnosis, and intervention of acute ICH is essential. Older age, hypertension, cerebral amyloid angiopathy, and oral anticoagulant use are some of the most significant risk factors for acute ICH. The etiologies of ICH are outlined in Table 8.1.

Table 8.1 Etiologies of Intracerebral Hemorrhage

Type of ICH	Etiologies
Primary ICH	■ Uncontrolled hypertension ■ Cerebral amyloid angiopathy
Secondary ICH	■ Arteriovenous malformation ■ Ruptured aneurysm ■ Brain tumors ■ Hemorrhagic conversion of ischemic stroke ■ Cavernous malformation ■ Coagulopathies ■ Sinus venous thrombus ■ Vasculitis ■ Trauma ■ Medication ■ Illicit drug use

ICH, intracerebral hemorrhage.

DIAGNOSTIC CRITERIA

The diagnosis of an acute ICH is based on the patient's neurologic exam and brain imaging. Initially, a hemorrhagic stroke may present with similar signs and symptoms to an ischemic stroke, including focal neurologic symptoms such as visual changes, motor weakness, dysarthria, facial droop, and paresthesia. The key diagnostic criterion to differentiate an acute ICH from an acute ischemic stroke is the presence of hemorrhage noted on a noncontrast head CT. In addition to hematoma size and location, the head CT also gives further diagnostic criteria, including degree of mass effect, presence of vasogenic edema, midline shift, and intraventricular extension of the hemorrhage. Further diagnostic imaging, such as head CTA, brain MRI, and cerebral angiogram, may be indicated to give further insight into etiology.

TREATMENT/MANAGEMENT

Initial emergent management in the treatment of an acute ICH is the patient's airway, breathing, and circulation. After hemodynamic stability is achieved, the next intervention focuses on preventing hematoma expansion. ICH hematoma expansion is associated with worse neurologic outcomes. In the acute period, blood pressure control should achieve a systolic blood pressure goal of less than 40 mmHg. Correction of coagulopathy is also a high priority. Reversal of anticoagulation is critical.

Workup focuses on determining the underlying etiology of the acute ICH. Identifying the etiology determines the treatment plan. CTA of the brain may show a ruptured intracranial aneurysm, and the aneurysm must be secured with emergent intravascular coiling or surgical clipping. If the ICH is possibly due to a brain tumor or lesion, an MRI would help diagnose, and then resection is needed.

If intraventricular extension and midline shift or hydrocephalus are identified, the patient may require extraventricular drain (EVD) placement to monitor ICP and drain cerebrospinal fluid (CSF). In the event of elevated ICP hyperosmolar treatment, mannitol or hypertonic saline may be initiated. Depending on the hemorrhage size and location, surgical hematoma evacuation done by craniotomy or hemicraniectomy may be considered. Other supportive measures include seizure prophylaxis, maintenance of normothermia, blood glucose control, and ongoing blood pressure control. Hyperthermia and hyperglycemia are associated with poorer neurologic outcomes in ICH patients.

COMPLICATIONS

Early complications in the first 24 to 48 hours include rebleeding. Additionally, secondary brain injury can occur from hypoglycemia, hypoxia or hypotension, or herniation. Cerebral aneurysm rupture may develop vasospasm that commonly occurs 3 to 14 days post rupture but may occur up to 21 days after. Subsequently, blood products may block the flow of CSF through the ventricles, causing hydrocephalus. An EVD may be needed to drain excess CSF. If hydrocephalus persists after EVD weaning, a ventriculoperitoneal catheter (VP shunt) may be needed.

▶ HYDROCEPHALUS

DISEASE OVERVIEW

Hydrocephalus is defined as an accumulation of CSF in the cerebral ventricles. This accumulation may be due to CSF flow obstruction or issues with CSF absorption and can be acute or chronic in nature. In adults, there are four different types: obstructive, communicating, hypersecretory, and normal pressure hydrocephalus (NPH; Table 8.2).

Table 8.2 Types of Hydrocephalus

Type	Pathogenesis	Etiology
Obstructive hydrocephalus	Develops from a block in CSF pathways	Intracranial hemorrhage, space-occupying lesion, vasogenic or cytotoxic edema
Communicating hydrocephalus	Impaired CSF absorption	Posthemorrhagic and postinflammatory changes
Hypersecretory hydrocephalus	Overproduction of CSF	Plexus papilloma or carcinoma
Normal pressure hydrocephalus	Type of communicating hydrocephalus seen in older adults with poorly understood pathogenesis	Impaired CSF dynamics cause it with slight or no increase in intracranial pressure

CSF, cerebrospinal fluid.

CLASSIC PRESENTATION

Forty-three-year-old female patient presented 3 days ago with an aneurysmal subarachnoid hemorrhage. The patient is evaluated by the AGACNP on morning rounds and is noted to be somnolent. When evaluating pupillary responses, the AGACNP notes a downward gaze.

DIAGNOSTIC CRITERIA

Diagnosis is made from a combination of physical exam findings and diagnostic imaging. Clinical exam findings typically prompt the ordering of diagnostic tests; most commonly, head CT is done first, followed by a brain MRI. Brain MRI is the diagnostic test of choice in the diagnosis of hydrocephalus; however, a head CT is a quicker and more accessible diagnostic test in the case of acute hydrocephalus and to rule out bleeding as a cause of mental status changes. Both types of brain imaging will show CSF accumulation, typically resulting in ventriculomegaly.

TREATMENT/MANAGEMENT

The hallmark in the treatment of hydrocephalus is treating the underlying etiology. Chronic hydrocephalus typically presents with more efficient compensatory mechanisms due to the chronicity in its nature; therefore, treatment is done on a less emergent basis. Acute hydrocephalus is a medical emergency that can result in intracranial hypertension and brain herniation. Emergent measures must be taken, which include the placement of an EVD for CSF diversion.

Long-term treatment options for hydrocephalus include VP shunt placement and endoscopic third ventriculostomy placement. Choroid plexus coagulation can be used for cases of overproduction of CSF. Repeat lumbar punctures (LPs) can be done in cases of communicating hydrocephalus if it is considered that spontaneous resorption is likely to occur.

▶ NEUROLOGIC INFECTIONS

DISEASE OVERVIEW

Infections of the brain and the spinal cord cause a cascade of inflammatory events that activate the immune system and produce a wide variety of neurologic symptoms that, if not recognized and treated, can result in irreversible neurologic injury or death. Inflammation of the meninges is referred to as meningitis; inflammation of the actual brain tissue is referred to as encephalitis. This inflammation can be caused by a variety of pathologies including bacteria, viruses, fungi, and parasites.

CLASSIC PRESENTATION

A 33-year-old female patient presents with fever, chills, headache, and confusion. The patient has a past medical history of hydrocephalus, status postshunt revision 7 days ago.

DIAGNOSTIC CRITERIA

Classic signs of meningitis and encephalitis include fever, headache, nausea, vomiting, visual changes, photophobia, and neck stiffness. Other clinical findings include flu-like symptoms, altered mental status, and new-onset seizure activity. The diagnostic tool of choice for diagnosis of meningitis and encephalitis is an LP with CSF analysis and culture. CSF analysis can give insight into the etiology of the infection prior to receipt of culture results (Table 8.3). Brain imaging with head CT or brain MRI may also be considered to identify inflammatory or infectious changes. Electroencephalogram may be considered to assess seizure activity or specific discharges suggestive of an infectious or inflammatory process.

Table 8.3 Cerebrospinal Fluid Interpretation

	Appearance	Opening Pressure	WBC (cell/uL)	Protein (mg/dL)	Glucose (mg/dL)
Bacterial	Turbid	Elevated	>1,000	>200	<40
Viral	Clear	Normal	<300, lymphocyte predominance	<200	Normal
Fungal	Clear	Normal to elevated	<500	>200	Normal to low

WBC, white blood cell.

TREATMENT/MANAGEMENT
MENINGITIS

Bacterial meningitis is a life-threatening medical emergency, and prompt treatment is required. Pending preliminary workup, proper antimicrobial agents that can cross the blood–brain barrier must be initiated as soon as possible. Initially, it may be difficult to differentiate bacterial from viral meningitis, so it is reasonable to start empiric coverage for bacterial meningitis if highly suspected. First-line treatment for suspected bacterial meningitis includes vancomycin plus a third-generation cephalosporin. If the patient is older than 50 years or immunocompromised, vancomycin plus a third-generation cephalosporin plus ampicillin should be initiated. Adjunct therapy such as corticosteroids to control inflammation and seizure prophylaxis may also be considered. Viral and fungal meningitis are often treated with supportive care and close neurologic monitoring. In some instances, IV antiretroviral or antifungal agents may be considered.

ENCEPHALITIS

Most cases of encephalitis are viral in nature; however, approximately 60% of cases in the United States do not identify a pathogen. The most common causes of viral meningitis include herpes simplex 1 and 2, arboviruses such as West Nile Virus, and Lyme disease. If there is a strong clinical suspicion for viral encephalitis, empiric coverage with an IV antiretroviral such as acyclovir should be initiated.

COMPLICATIONS

Complications include seizures, hearing loss, limb weakness, and difficulties with speech, vision, language, communication, and memory. Severe cases can result in limb amputation and/or death.

▶ SPACE-OCCUPYING LESIONS

DISEASE OVERVIEW

Space-occupying lesions is a broad term that generally means tumors but can include abscesses. *Brain tumors* include both benign and malignant primary lesions and secondary lesions, which are commonly metastasis. Metastasis is most common in lung cancer (adenocarcinoma and small cell), breast cancer (HER2+ and triple negative), renal cell carcinoma, melanoma, ovarian carcinoma, colon cancer, choriocarcinoma, and sarcoma. Hemorrhage into brain metastases occurs more frequently in melanoma, renal cell carcinoma, and choriocarcinoma. Symptoms of space-occupying lesions vary by size, location in the brain, and presence of surrounding vasogenic edema.

CLASSIC PRESENTATIONS
PRIMARY TUMOR

A female patient in her mid-fifties presents with complaints of headache over the last few months. The headache is increasing in intensity and frequency. Migraine treatments are no longer effective. She is now complaining of progressive weakness in her right hand and has been dropping things. She presents today because her right leg has started dragging. CT scan is negative for bleeding. MRI shows a ring-enhancing lesion with surrounding edema in the left posterior frontal lobe.

METASTASIS

An older adult male patient with a history of small cell lung cancer presents with persistent headache and malaise and reports that 2 days ago he started vomiting. Family reports that his gait is "wobbly" when he walks and that he has fallen twice in the last week.

DIAGNOSTIC CRITERIA

Presenting symptoms can vary widely depending on the area of the brain that is affected, the size of the tumor, and the presence and amount of edema. Symptoms commonly include weakness, confusion, and seizures. CT is typically the initial diagnostic test done to assess for neurologic symptoms to look for intracerebral bleeding. However, the gold standard to identify brain tumors is an MRI. Tissue samples via biopsy will differentiate the specific type of tumor. For patients with neurologic symptoms and fevers or leukocytosis, an LP for glucose, cell count, gram stain, and culture should be done to assess for central nervous system (CNS) infection or abscess.

TREATMENT/MANAGEMENT

Initially, vasogenic edema can be treated with IV steroids, typically dexamethasone (Decadron) to reduce edema and improve symptoms. Treatment depends on the type of tumor and usually requires surgical resection. Radiation, chemotherapy, and immunotherapy supplement the treatment regimen depending on type and location of tumor. Abscess requires IV antibiotics that cross the blood–brain barrier. Consultation with infectious disease is recommended. Chemotherapy, antibiotics, and antifungals can be given intravenously or intrathecally into the ventricle of the brain via an Ommaya reservoir.

Supportive therapies, including physical therapy (PT), occupational therapy (OT), swallow therapy, and cognitive therapies should be used based on the patient's symptoms. Nutritional support is important, as it is with all oncology patients.

COMPLICATIONS

Patients with space-occupying lesions can be left with permanent neurologic deficits that are dependent on the size and location. Loss of function, dysphagia and aspiration, depression, and seizures are common complications of brain tumors.

▶ SPINAL CORD INJURY

DISEASE OVERVIEW

Spinal cord injury (SCI) is most commonly caused by blunt or penetrating injury; however, direct compression by tumors or vascular insufficiency from thromboembolism or aortic surgeries can cause spinal cord symptoms and injuries as well. Common causes of blunt SCIs include motor vehicle crashes (MVCs), falls, and diving. Penetrating injuries from knives or bullets more commonly cause incomplete injuries.

About 10% of all cervical spine fractures have a second, noncontiguous spinal fracture requiring full spinal immobility until ruled out. Injuries follow a dermatomal pattern and depend on which spinal tracts are injured. C3, C4, and C5 innervate the diaphragm; these injures commonly require intubation to support respiratory function. Injuries below C5 can also cause respiratory failure due to subsequent ascending edema and de-innervation of the intercostal muscles. Complete cord injuries above T6 result in neurogenic shock. Table 8.4 shows key terminology.

Table 8.4 Key Terminology for Spinal Cord Injury

Term	Description
Neurogenic shock	Loss of vasomotor tone and sympathetic innervation to the heart, resulting in bradycardia and hypotension
Spinal shock	Loss of sensory and/or motor tone and function, including reflexes below the level of the lesion immediately following the injury
Complete cord injury	Total loss of all motor and sensory function below the level of injury
Partial cord injury	Some function remaining below the level of the injury
Bony level of injury	The level of vertebral injury or fracture
Neurologic level of injury	The highest segment of the spinal cord that has normal sensory and motor function. Subsequent edema can cause a bony injury to have a more proximal neurologic level.

CLASSIC PRESENTATIONS

CERVICAL INJURY

A young female patient presents after diving into a pool. Vital signs are T 37.5°C, heart rate (HR) 44, respiratory rate (RR) 12, O_2 sat 94%, blood pressure (BP) 70/40. She is unable to move or feel her upper and lower extremities. Digital rectal exam reveals loss of tone, and anal and abdominal reflexes are absent.

LOWER THORACIC AND LUMBAR INJURY

A young adult male patient jumped off the roof of a second-story house while intoxicated and landed on his feet. He presents with severe lower pain in his thoracic spine and reports numbness in and inability to move his legs. He can move his arms fully; sensation in bilateral upper extremities is intact.

DIAGNOSTIC CRITERIA

Maintain a high index of suspicion for anyone who experiences a dangerous mechanism of injury (fall greater than 5 steps; axial load to the head; MVC with high rate of speed, rollover, or ejection; bicycle or all terrain vehicle (ATV) crash), is older than 65 years, and has neurologic deficits. These patients require a CT scan to diagnose fractures. Patients with ongoing pain with a negative CT should receive an MRI to assess for ligamentous injuries. Spinal cord syndromes have classic etiologies and physical exam findings (see Table 8.5).

Table 8.5 Spinal Cord Syndromes

Pattern	Etiology	Deficits
Central cord	Hyperextension injury commonly occurs in elderly patients with preexisting cervical canal stenosis; may or may not have a fracture	Loss of motor strength in the upper extremities more so than the lower extremities ("can dance but can't play the piano")
Anterior cord	Cord ischemia	Paraplegia and bilateral loss of pain and temperature sensation
Posterior cord	Compression or spinal artery occlusion leading to cord ischemia	Loss of proprioception and vibration, motor is preserved
Brown–Sequard	Hemi-transection of the spinal cord	Ipsilateral loss of motor, proprioception, and vibration; with contralateral loss of pain and temperature
Conus medullaris	L1-L2 injuries, tumors, vascular injuries	Normal motor function, no pain, saddle anesthesia, symmetric abnormalities, severe bowel, bladder, and sexual dysfunction; bulbocavernous and anal reflex preserved
Cauda equina	L2 to sacral injuries, pelvic ring fractures, sacral fracture	Flaccid paralysis of involved lumbar roots, areflexic lower extremities, asymmetric sensory loss in root distribution, pain present, higher lesions spare bowel and bladder, urinary and/or fecal incontinence, bulbocavernous and anal reflex absent

TREATMENT/MANAGEMENT

Initial treatment when an injured patient presents is to stabilize the spine until assessment and imaging (if needed) can be completed. All traumatically injured patients should have a hard cervical collar, and full spine alignment should be instituted until cleared. All fractures and ligamentous injuries require consultation with a spine surgeon. Depending on the institution, the consultation could be with neurosurgery or orthopedics. They will deem an injury stable or unstable. For stable injuries, a cervical, cervical–thoracic spine orthotic (CTSO), or thoracic–lumbar spine orthotic (TLSO) may be needed for 4 to 6 or more weeks. Unstable fractures require surgical fixation and may need traction for an initial period.

Much of the AGACNP role is aimed at prevention and treatment of complications of SCIs, including acute respiratory failure, infections (urinary tract infection [UTI], pneumonia), venous thromboembolism (VTE), pressure injuries, constipation, and urinary retention. Rehabilitation services with PT, OT, and speech and swallow therapies (S&S) and integration of adaptive devices are central to the recovery of the patient.

▶ INTRACRANIAL HYPERTENSION

DISEASE OVERVIEW

The Monro–Kellie doctrine explains that the cranium is a closed nondistensible system in which brain parenchyma, CSF, and intracranial blood exist in equilibrium. Physiologically, cranial components consist of 80% brain parenchyma, 10% CSF, and 10% intracranial blood. Because the skull is considered a closed compartment with a finite volume, any increase in the volume of components within the skull or addition of a pathologic element will result in increased pressure within the skull. When there is a disruption in the equilibrium of one component, a certain degree of compensation can occur; however, compensation is limited.

CLASSIC PRESENTATION

A 55-year-old male patient with a history of lung cancer with metastasis to the brain presents with headache and vision changes and, most recently, ataxia. The patient reports that the headache and vision changes started the day prior, and he came in for evaluation when he had difficulty walking this morning.

DIAGNOSTIC CRITERIA

Intracranial hypertension is defined as ICP within the skull elevated at greater than 22 mmHg for more than 5 minutes. It may be idiopathic or caused by a primary or secondary etiology. It can also be an acute or a chronic process. Primary or intracranial etiologies include head trauma (see section titled "Traumatic Brain Injury"), brain tumors, ischemic stroke, hydrocephalus, and meningitis. Secondary or extracranial etiologies include hypoxemia, hypercarbia, edema, hypertension, airway obstruction, seizures, hyperpyrexia, and high-altitude cerebral edema. It can also be drug induced. Any time there is an elevation in ICP, there is a risk of subsequent injury from direct brainstem compression or from reduction in cerebral blood flow. This is measured clinically by cerebral perfusion pressure (CPP). CPP is calculated as ICP subtracted from mean arterial pressure (MAP):

$$MAP - ICP = CPP$$

Normal CPP is 50 to 70. CPP of less than 50 mmHg can lead to secondary brain injury, herniation, and brain death.

Physical signs of acute intracranial hypertension and elevated ICP are directly related to brain compression and herniation syndromes. Physical exam findings include a deterioration of the neurologic exam, including focal neurologic symptoms; nausea; vomiting; and vision and pupillary changes. As ICP goes up and CPP falls, low CPP causes further ischemia, prompting worsening edema. The patient's neurologic exam will continue to deteriorate until abnormal posturing is noted, including decorticate and decerebrate/extensor posturing. Initial vital signs will demonstrate the "fight-or-flight" response as the body tries to perfuse the brain. Tachycardia and severe hypertension are noted if ICPs are not controlled or interventions fail to reverse the increasing ICPs. Subsequent vital sign changes are noted as herniation occurs. Cushing triad is a widened pulse pressure, bradycardia, and agonal or absent breathing suggestive of brainstem herniation. Physical signs of chronic intracranial hypertension are typically more subtle than acute and can include gait imbalances, dizziness, and symptoms associated with normal pressure hydrocephalus.

TREATMENT/MANAGEMENT

Acute intracranial hypertension is a medical emergency, and treatment is done in a stepwise approach ranging from Tier 0 to Tier 3 (Table 8.6). Due to the rapid increase in ICP resulting in neurologic deterioration, the patient's airway, breathing, and circulation must first be stabilized. After hemodynamic stability is achieved, any exacerbating factors such as pain, agitation, and fever must be closely controlled. Keep the head of the bed at 30 degrees with the neck in a midline position. Brain imaging is typically deferred during the emergent period, as the transfer to supine position to obtain the scan can exacerbate elevation of ICP. Maintain $PaCO_2$ at approximately 33 to 35, and avoid $PaCO_2 \geq 40$ or hypercarbia. Treatment measures in the emergent period focus on hyperosmotic therapy. Hyperosmolar agents such as mannitol and/or hypertonic saline may be given to decrease the ICP. With the administration of mannitol, it is important to note that the osmolality and osmolar gap must be trended. An osmolality of greater than 320 mOsm/kg or an osmolar gap greater than 20 mOsm/kg are unlikely to offer clinical benefit.

Table 8.6 Intracranial Pressure: Tiered Management Strategies

Tier	Management Strategies
Tier 0	■ Head of bed 30 degrees ■ Maintain neck in midline position ■ Decrease noxious stimuli ■ Maintain normothermia (avoid fevers) ■ PRN analgesics
Tier 1	■ Mannitol 0.5–1 g/kg bolus PRN up to Q6 hours (hold for osmolar gap >20, or serum osmo >320) ■ Hypertonic saline bolus 30 mL of 23.4% NaCl, bolus PRN up to Q6 hours (hold for Na > 160)
Tier 2	■ Continuous and deeper sedation
Tier 3	■ Craniectomy (depending on etiology) ■ Burst suppression (Pentobarbital coma) ■ Moderate hypothermia (goal of 32°C –34°C)

ICP monitoring must also be considered, including EVD placement for CSF diversion and ICP monitoring. Hyperventilation for a short period of time, typically 2 to 3 hours, may also be considered to decrease cerebral blood flow and thus decrease ICP. Depending on the underlying etiology, surgical options such as craniotomy and hemicraniectomy must also be considered. For refractory ICP crisis nonresponsive to treatment, therapies including barbiturate-induced coma and hypothermia with targeted temperature management must also be considered.

Treatment of chronic intracranial hypertension includes treatment of the underlying etiology. Diagnosis is typically made from head CT scan or brain MRI. Due to the chronicity in its nature, compensation efforts in the brain are typically more effective; therefore, treatment options can often be done on a nonemergent basis.

COMPLICATIONS

Complications of increased intracranial hypertension include secondary brain injury from hypoxia, hypotension, herniation, and progression to brain death. Complications of EVDs include ventriculitis, meningitis, and catheter occlusion from coagulated blood in the ventricle/catheter. Complications from barbiturate coma include ileus with associated malnutrition and hypotension.

▶ TRAUMATIC BRAIN INJURY

DISEASE OVERVIEW

Traumatic brain injury (TBI) can range from a simple concussion to a devastating brain injury. Brain injury is the leading cause of trauma-related death. In the United States, the frequency of TBI is 2.5 to 4 million cases annually. The frequency of TBI has a bimodal distribution demonstrating higher risk for younger and older adult populations. MVCs are the most common cause of TBI in younger adults, while falls are the predominant cause in older adults.

TBI is defined as an alteration in brain function, or other evidence of brain pathology, caused by an external force; it has a wide range of injury types (Table 8.7).

Table 8.7 Types of Injuries

Type of Injury	Description
Concussion	Trauma induced transient disturbance of brain function
Hematoma	A blood clot within or on the surface of the brain ■ Epidural hematoma is a collection between the dura mater and the inside of the skull (classic presentation/sign of epidural hematoma = loss of consciousness followed by a brief lucid interval followed by rapid decline in mental status, unresponsiveness). ■ Subdural hematoma is a collection between the dura mater and the arachnoid layer.

(continued)

Table 8.7 Types of Injuries (*continued*)

Type of Injury	Description
Contusion	Bruising of brain tissue
Intracerebral hemorrhage	Bleeding within brain tissue
Subarachnoid hemorrhage	Bleeding within the subarachnoid space
Diffuse injuries	▪ Diffuse axonal injury—refers to impaired function and loss of axons ▪ Ischemia—resultant of insufficient blood supply to parts of the brain

CLASSIC PRESENTATION

Twenty-three-year-old male patient who was the unrestrained driver in an MVC presents to the ED with a Glasgow Coma Scale (GCS) score of 11 (eye = 3, verbal = 3, motor = 5). Emergency medical services (EMS) report "starring" of the driver's side windshield. Head CT reveals contusion to the anterior frontal lobe.

DIAGNOSTIC CRITERIA

TBI can be evidenced by visual inspection of a patient and by neuroradiologic findings. TBI is most often diagnosed based on clinical criteria. The standard head CT is the test of choice in the diagnosis of TBI.

TBI is classified by severity, ranging from mild to moderate to severe. The GCS is needed to classify severity (Table 8.8).

Table 8.8 Glasgow Coma Scale

Evaluation	Documented Response	Points
Eye opening	▪ Spontaneous ▪ To voice ▪ To pain ▪ No response	4 3 2 1
Best verbal response	▪ Oriented to person, place, time ▪ Confused ▪ Inappropriate words ▪ Incomprehensible sounds ▪ No response	5 4 3 2 1
Best motor response	▪ Obeys commands ▪ Localizes pain ▪ Withdraws from pain ▪ Flexion to pain (decorticate posturing) ▪ Extension to pain (decerebrate posturing) ▪ No response	6 5 4 3 2 1
	TOTAL	3–15
Interpretation	Mild TBI Moderate TBI Severe TBI	13–15 9–12 <9

TBI, traumatic brain injury.

TREATMENT/MANAGEMENT

Acute treatment and management require early recognition and diagnosis. Airway, breathing, and circulation must be initially addressed, and any coagulopathy must be corrected. TBIs can be complicated by increases in ICP because of cerebral edema or other factors that disrupt the Monro–Kellie doctrine. The Monro–Kellie doctrine states that the total intracranial volume (brain tissue, CSF, venous blood, and arterial blood) should always remain constant given that the cranium is a rigid/fixed container. Sustained increases to ICP will result in further brain injury.

TBI guidelines inform care of the patient with such an injury. Treatment/management involves monitoring, thresholds, and treatments as outlined later in this chapter.

MONITORING

ICP monitoring is indicated in all salvageable patients with a severe TBI (GCS score of 3 to 8 after resuscitation) and an abnormal head CT scan (defined as a head CT that reveals hematomas, contusions, swelling, herniation, or compressed basal cisterns). ICP monitoring is also indicated in all patients with severe TBI with a normal head CT scan if two or more of the following features are present at admission: age older than 40 years, unilateral or bilateral posturing, or systolic blood pressure less than 90 mmHg. Additionally, patients should have CPP monitored.

THRESHOLDS

For severe TBI, certain thresholds should be monitored (Table 8.9). If defined thresholds are not met, treatments must be enlisted to meet suggested thresholds.

Table 8.9 Traumatic Brain Injury Thresholds

Parameter	Suggested Threshold
BP	Systolic blood pressure goal of 100 mmHg or greater age 60–69 years Systolic blood pressure goal of 110 mmHg or greater age 15–49 years or >70 years
ICP	Treating ICP >22 mmHg
CPP	Target CPP between 60 and 70 mmHg

BP, blood pressure; CPP, cerebral perfusion pressure; ICP, intracranial pressure.

TREATMENTS

Treatments are targeted at maintaining the thresholds shown in Table 8.9.

ANESTHETICS, ANALGESICS, AND SEDATIVES

Anesthetics, analgesics, and sedatives are used to control intracranial hypertension and seizures in the setting of TBI. Barbiturate administration is recommended to control elevated ICP that cannot be controlled through maximal use of medical and surgical therapies.

HYPEROSMOLAR THERAPY

Hyperosmolar therapy is an effective option for treatment of increased ICP and cerebral edema. It comes in the form of mannitol and hypertonic saline. Mannitol and hypertonic saline work to reduce ICP through reducing blood viscosity, which leads to improved microcirculatory flow of blood constituents and resultant constriction of pial arterioles, which ultimately results in decreased cerebral blood volume and ICP.

TEMPERATURE MANAGEMENT

Hypothermia has been well studied in the preservation of cells and tissues during an extreme metabolic challenge. Hypothermic interventions come with risks, which include and are not limited to coagulopathy and immunosuppression. For treatment of TBI, prophylactic hypothermia is not recommended; targeting normothermia is. It can be achieved with antipyretics, topical cooling methods, and infusion of cooled fluids.

NEUROSURGICAL INTERVENTION

Decompressive craniectomy can be considered for refractory ICP elevations despite optimal medical management. This decision will be made in consultation with a neurosurgeon. Surgical evacuation of subdural and epidural hematomas can be considered in TBI and the decision to surgically evacuate is made by the neurosurgeon.

COMPLICATIONS

Complications vary widely and can include posttraumatic seizures, posttraumatic stress disorder, hydrocephalus, mood, and/or behavior changes, cognitive decline or deficits, spasticity, and brain death.

▶ SEIZURE DISORDER

DISEASE OVERVIEW

Seizures involve sudden, temporary bursts of electrical activity in the brain that change or disrupt the way messages are sent between neurons. These bursts have the potential to produce involuntary changes in body movement, sensation, and awareness. When witnessing or recalling a seizure, inquire about the onset, duration, and characteristics that describe the seizure; urinary incontinence; and tongue biting.

Types of seizures are as follows:

- *Generalized onset seizures*: affect both sides of the brain at the same time and include tonic-clonic, absence, and atonic seizures
- *Focal onset seizures*: can start in one area or group of cells in one side of the brain and include focal onset awareness seizures and focal onset impaired awareness seizures
- *Unknown onset seizure*: When the beginning of a seizure is not known, it is called an unknown onset seizure. A seizure can also be called unknown onset if it is not witnessed by anyone.

Seizures are often associated with rhythmic facial twitching or body jerking and/or twitching. However, subclinical seizures, also referred to as absence seizures, must be considered in patients with an unexplained encephalopathic state. This type of seizure does not have any visible symptoms such as convulsions or twitching but may produce neurologic changes and a postictal state.

CLASSIC PRESENTATION

A 27-year-old patient with no past medical history is brought in by EMS after being found outside a bar with reported generalized tonic-clonic seizure. Friends report that the patient ingested an unknown substance earlier in the night. EMS reports cessation of seizure activity after administration of 2 mg IV Ativan.

DIAGNOSTIC CRITERIA

First-line seizure treatment, to abort an active seizure, includes administration of a short-acting benzodiazepine and monitoring for resolution of seizure activity. The initial workup should focus on determining the etiology of the seizure. Consider both acute and chronic etiologies. Nonmetabolic etiologies include electrolyte abnormalities, hypoglycemia, uremia, and sepsis. Central nervous etiologies include meningitis, encephalitis, autoimmune encephalitis, ischemic stroke, hemorrhagic stroke, head trauma, and subarachnoid hemorrhage. Drug toxicity, drug overdose, alcohol withdrawal, and hypoxemia are also possible underlying etiologies. For patients with a history of seizures and epilepsy, assess for noncompliance with antiepileptic drugs. Additional testing with brain imaging, LP, and electrographic monitoring may be considered.

TREATMENT/MANAGEMENT

Based on the etiology, initiation and maintenance doses of antiepileptic drugs may be considered. The choice of levetiracetam or fosphenytoin is provider dependent. Phenytoin levels must be monitored post administration. Phenytoin binds to albumin; thus, in hypalbuminemia, corrected serum levels must be calculated or free phenytoin levels obtained. Levetiracetam is less sedating and may be a better choice for older adults:

- *First line*: lorazepam 0.1 mg/kg IV, midazolam 0.2 mg/kg IV, or diazepam 0.15 mg/kg IV
- *Second line*: levetiracetam 1,000 mg to 3,000 mg IV, fosphenytoin 20 mg/kg IV

If first- and second-line treatment offer no resolution of seizure activity, consult an epileptologist and/or neurologist for further seizure management for possible status epilepticus.

▶ STATUS EPILEPTICUS

DISEASE OVERVIEW
Status epilepticus is defined as 5 minutes or more of continuous and/or electrographic seizure activity or recurrent seizure activity without returning to baseline between seizures. Types of status epilepticus include generalized convulsive status epilepticus, focal motor status epilepticus, and nonconvulsive status epilepticus. In the initial evaluation, it is important to assess the patient's circulation, airway, and breathing to ensure that hemodynamic stability is maintained. Considerations for the underlying etiology are also crucial.

CLASSIC PRESENTATION
A 45-year-old male patient presents after being found down by family, confused, and incontinent of urine and stool. The patient is admitted to the hospital where he remains confused and is having intermittent bouts of unresponsiveness. EEG monitoring is initiated and displays persistent seizure activity.

DIAGNOSTIC CRITERIA
Continuous EEG monitoring is needed to ensure that seizure activity is aborted/suppressed so possible subclinical seizures do not persist.

TREATMENT/MANAGEMENT
A bolus of short-acting benzodiazepines is the agent of choice for emergent initial treatment in status epilepticus. IV administration is preferred. However, benzodiazepines can be administered via intramuscular, rectal, nasal, or buccal routes when IV therapy is not feasible. Followed by the administration of a short-acting benzodiazepine, a loading dose to obtain a rapid therapeutic level followed by a maintenance dose of an antiepileptic drug should be initiated. The patient should then be connected to continuous electrographic monitoring and the dose and class of antiepileptic titrated up and added until the seizures have resolved by both clinical and electrographic evidence.

Refractory status epilepticus is defined as clinical or electrographic seizures that continue after adequate doses of an initial benzodiazepine followed by a second acceptable antiepileptic drug. At this stage, after attempts to control status epilepticus with bolus intermittent therapy fail, treatment recommendations are to use continuous infusion antiepileptic drugs to suppress seizures. This process is referred to as burst suppression. The antiepileptic drugs most often recommended for a continuous infusion are midazolam, propofol, and pentobarbital. These agents are titrated up based on electrographic findings. An important consideration for burst suppression is that mechanical ventilation is required due to the use of continuous infusion antiepileptic drugs. Mechanical ventilation weaning can begin when status epilepticus has resolved and the continuous antiepileptic drugs have been tapered off.

▶ ENCEPHALOPATHY

DISEASE OVERVIEW
Encephalopathy is any process affecting the functioning of the brain and can be either a structural or a nonstructural etiology. Encephalopathy is the formal term for an alteration in mental status or brain failure and can be either reversible or irreversible. AGANCPs are involved with diagnosing and treating patients with encephalopathy. To determine how to treat these patients, AGANCPs must use excellent history taking and diagnostic tools to determine contributing factors.

STRUCTURAL ETIOLOGIES OF ENCEPHALOPATHY
Structural changes in the brain result in dysfunction, which can be dramatic or subtle. It can occur with stroke, tumor, traumatic injury, or hypoxic ischemic brain injury. Sometimes, structural problems can result in nonstructural causes of encephalopathy, as with brain tumors and seizures (Table 8.10).

Table 8.10 Structural Etiologies of Encephalopathy

Etiology	Description
Stroke	In the setting mentioned in the text, the AGACNP may consider AIS as a differential. An acute blockage of a blood vessel in the brain results in immediate lack of function referable to the area of the hypoperfused brain. A noncontrast CT scan of the brain is performed showing no areas of hemorrhage. There is subtle hypodensity on the L frontal lobe and some edema and swelling of structures. A CT angiogram of the head and neck show no blockages of major vessels of the brain making AIS less likely a diagnosis.
Trauma	Falls, MVCs, or penetrating trauma can result in injury to the brain, directly or indirectly. There may be hemorrhagic contusions, subdural or epidural hemorrhages, or DAI related to rotation forces and tearing of connections within the brain. Additionally, shock states and hemorrhage may result in inadequate perfusion to the brain and other organs. Trauma is the leading cause of death in adults under age 45 years. Our patient had signs of minor external trauma, but CT scan of the brain did not show any acute injuries due to trauma.
CNS mass lesions	CNS mass lesions within the brain parenchyma, or lesions that are external to the brain itself but exert pressure upon the brain tissue, resulting in abnormal functioning. These include tumors (both primary and metastatic), infection, and demyelination. Our patient had an abnormal area in the left frontal lobe and right-sided weakness making further evaluation with MRI a reasonable next diagnostic step. This revealed a necrotic mass with vasogenic edema. On further investigation, it was noted our patient had subtle personality changes including pressured speech and short temper that may have been an early sign of brain dysfunction.
HIBI	HIBI is the diffuse injury that occurs to the brain after a global event such as a cardiac arrest, catastrophic hemorrhage, or poisoning. Improved efforts in cardiac resuscitation improve survival, and therapeutic hypothermia after cardiac arrest has led to improved neurologic recovery. CT scans may show diffuse swelling and edema and loss of gray–white differentiation after several days, though these are typically normal immediately following an acute event.

AIS, acute ischemic stroke; CNS, central nervous system; DAI, diffuse axonal injury; HIBI, hypoxic ischemic brain injury; MVCs, motor vehicle crashes.

NONSTRUCTURAL ETIOLOGIES OF ENCEPHALOPATHY

In the absence of abnormal imaging, there are a vast array of nonstructural causes of encephalopathy (Tables 8.11 and 8.12, Figure 8.1).

Table 8.11 Nonstructural Etiologies of Encephalopathy

Etiology	Description
Septic encephalopathy	Septic encephalopathy is due to systemic inflammation within or outside the CNS. Symptoms can range from mildly impaired consciousness to coma. Occurs in up to 70% of all patients admitted to adult ICU. Pathologic exam shows increased apoptosis in structures sensitive to stress. Treatment is supportive, though long-term cognitive impairments may occur.
HE	HE is a result of impaired brain function in the setting of liver failure due to accumulation of nitrogenous by-products and ammonia leading to astrocyte swelling in the brain. Ammonia is a by-product of protein digestion and is elevated in at least 90% of patients with hepatic encephalopathy. Treatment of patients with HE should first be avoidance of precipitant events. Subsequently, treatment is aimed at reducing serum levels of ammonia by enhanced transport through the colon by way of cathartic agents such as lactulose or rifaximin.

(continued)

Table 8.11 Nonstructural Etiologies of Encephalopathy (*continued*)

Etiology	Description
Meningitis	Inflammation of the meninges has classical features of fever, headache, nuchal rigidity, and altered consciousness. It can also cause seizures, focal deficits, and cranial nerve derangements. Etiology is viral, bacterial, fungal, or parasitic. Diagnostic workup includes CBC, blood cultures, coagulation studies and blood cultures. If CNS imaging, usually with CT, does not demonstrate a CNS mass lesion or diffuse cerebral edema, then LP (see Table 8.12 and Figure 8.1) to assess opening pressure, protein, glucose, cell counts, culture, and differential. CNS imaging should be obtained with any immunocompromised patient, those with known CNS mass lesions, seizures, papilledema, focal neurologic deficit, or abnormal LOC. With any clinical suspicion, antibiotics should not be delayed as this leads to worse outcomes. Dexamethasone should be given prior to antibiotic administration as it may reduce overall mortality and severe hearing loss in select patients with bacterial meningitis.
Encephalitis	Inflammation of the brain can be caused by bacteria or viral infections, autoimmune inflammation, and insect or tick-borne infections. Symptoms can vary from flu-like illness to seizures, confusion, focal neurologic symptoms, or language problems. Seasonal and geographic considerations may alter the risk of certain types of encephalitis. ■ *Herpes encephalitis* is due to herpes simplex type 1 and 2 viruses that can gain access to the CNS via the trigeminal nerve or olfactory tract. Infections are more commonly seen in the immunocompromised patient. Injury or edema is often seen in the medial temporal and orbitofrontal lobes and the insular cortex. Treatment should be initiated with any suspicion as delays are associated with increased morbidity and mortality. Treatment is with 10 mg/kg every 8 hours of IV Acyclovir for 14–21 days. ■ *Postinfectious encephalitis or ADEM* is more commonly seen in children but is an autoimmune disorder triggered by recent or acute infection resulting in CNS demyelination. Lesions are more discreet than those seen in MS. Treatment is supportive and often includes high-dose corticosteroids, IVIG, or plasma exchange. ■ *Autoimmune encephalitis* occurs when the body's own immune system mistakenly attacks healthy brain tissue leading to inflammation and dysfunction. Closely related, paraneoplastic encephalitis occurs when there is abnormal inflammation occurring in the brain due to cancer. In up to 50% of cases, a paraneoplastic syndrome may precede a diagnosis of cancer. ■ *Anti-NMDA receptor encephalitis* is a more recently identified paraneoplastic syndrome that is associated with a high incidence of ovarian teratoma and may present with anxiety, disordered thinking, hallucinations, and sleep disorders, and can progress to involve seizures and language disturbances. Treatment is aimed at immunosuppression and removal and treatment of the underlying cancer, if identified.
Seizures	Seizures may be provoked in the setting of drug or alcohol withdrawal and with structural abnormalities like tumor or stroke. They may be unprovoked in the setting of epilepsy or precipitated by low levels of antiepileptic drugs. Seizures may be underdiagnosed, so have a low clinical suspicion to obtain an EEG in selected patients without an overt cause of encephalopathy.
Toxic metabolic encephalopathy	Toxic metabolic encephalopathy refers to the presence of exogenous toxins or metabolic derangements resulting in confused states. These are often reversible unless not intervened upon quickly, in which case permanent structural injury may occur. ■ *Acute alcohol intoxication or alcohol withdrawal* may result in alteration in consciousness with clinical symptoms including dysarthria, nystagmus, incoordination, and behavioral disturbances. Many of these symptoms overlap vertebrobasilar stroke syndromes leading to late identification, treatment, and worse outcomes.

(*continued*)

Table 8.11 Nonstructural Etiologies of Encephalopathy (*continued*)

Etiology	Description
	▪ *Wernicke encephalopathy* is a syndrome due to deficiency of thiamine occurring in patients with excessive alcohol consumption resulting in confusion, ataxia, and ophthalmoplegia. Symptoms of ataxia, hypothermia, and hypotension can overlap alcohol overuse syndromes. Prolonged ICU admissions, recovery from GI surgery, periods of starvation, and prolonged parenteral nutrition are all less commonly identified risk factors for Wernicke encephalopathy. In early instances, prompt treatment may reverse the syndrome, but studies suggest that the incidence far exceeds its identification. ▪ *Intoxication* includes hallucinogens, sympathomimetics, anticholinergics, opiates, sedatives, cholinergic agents, and serotonin toxicity. All can result in altered consciousness, seizures, and significant changes in vital signs. ▪ *Uremic encephalopathy* clinically may result in lethargy, disorientation, and hallucinations, and can progress to coma. It accompanies elevated BUN levels in renal failure. Tremor, asterixis, and myoclonus also may be present. ▪ *Hypo- or hypernatremia* may be present due to other disorders including SIADH, cerebral salt wasting, or exogenous administration of water or solutes. Rapid correction of low sodium levels that are chronic can lead to osmotic demyelination. ▪ *Hypercarbia* can cause increased somnolence, cause confusion, and progress to coma. ▪ *Hypoglycemia and hyperglycemia* can result in altered consciousness and seizures to coma and may include focal deficits. Hypoglycemia is known to be a mimic of AIS.
Hypertensive encephalopathy	Hypertensive encephalopathy may result in altered consciousness and seizures, and can also result in decreased vision or cortical blindness.

ADEM, acute disseminated encephalomyelitis; AIS, acute ischemic stroke; BUN, blood urea nitrogen; CBC, complete blood count; CNS, central nervous system; GI, gastrointestinal; HE, hepatic encephalopathy; IVIG, intravenous immunoglobulin; LOC, level of consciousness; LP, lumbar puncture; MS, multiple sclerosis; NMDA, N-methyl-D-aspartate; SIADH, syndrome of inappropriate antidiuretic hormone.

Table 8.12 Lumbar Puncture

Indications
▪ Suspected CNS infection
▪ Subarachnoid hemorrhage with negative CT
▪ Nonurgent indications: MS, cancer, GBS, NPH
Contraindications
▪ Raised ICP
▪ Coagulopathy
▪ Thrombocytopenia
▪ Suspected spinal epidural abscess
Preparation
▪ Obtain consent, check coagulation studies, platelet levels
▪ CNS imaging is indicated if suspected ICP elevation
▪ Administer antibiotics without delay if suspected CNS infection
Positioning
▪ Lateral recumbent: curled into fetal position with neck flexed and knees pulled into chest; keep spine horizontal with bed
▪ Sitting: sit on edge of bed maximally flexed forward onto a table
▪ Prone: typically in IR settings
▪ See Figure 8.1
Procedure
1. Set up LP kit on bedside table. Clean area with alcohol or disinfectant such as chlorhexidine; drape the patient.
2. Perform time out.
3. Identify iliac crest. The imaginary line that connects the most superior portion of the iliac crest will intersect the L4-L5 interspace.
4. Inject local anesthesia (lidocaine) into the intervertebral space (L4-L5 usually chosen but can be one space above or below).

(*continued*)

Table 8.12 Lumbar Puncture (*continued*)

5. Use a 20-g or 22-g spinal needle in the chosen space, advancing slowly with the bevel turned toward the patient's flank (to prevent cutting of dural sac fibers).

6. Advance slowly, periodically removing the stylet to check for CSF flow toward the patient's umbilicus.

7. Once CSF flow is obtained, replace stylet; once ready, attach a manometer to measure opening pressure.

8. Obtain fluid for sampling; approximately 2–4 mL per each four tubes collected.

9. Replace stylet prior to removal of spinal needle, and apply dressing.

Complications

▪ Post-LP headache
▪ Pain
▪ Bleeding
▪ Spinal fluid leak
▪ Herniation

CNS, central nervous system; CSF, cerebrospinal fluid; GBS, Guillain-Barré syndrome; ICP, intracranial pressure; IR, interventional radiology; LP, lumbar puncture; MS, multiple sclerosis; NPH, normal pressure hydrocephalus.

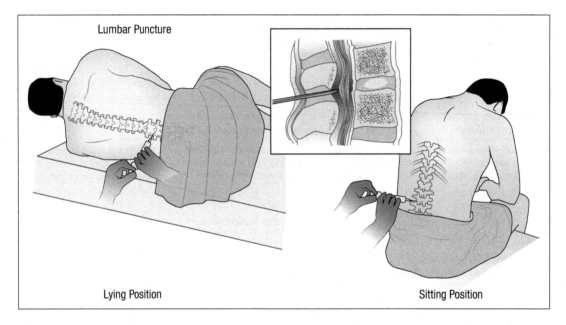

Figure 8.1 Lumbar puncture positioning.

Source: Courtesy of Blausen.com staff. https://commons.wikimedia.org/wiki/

CLASSIC PRESENTATION

A 55-year-old male patient who works as a bank manager and has a prior history of cigarette smoking, hypertension, hyperlipidemia, and gout was last seen well the day before presentation. He failed to show up to work, and at a wellness check he was found in the bathroom, supine with a small abrasion to the forehead. He was not moving the right side of his body as well as the left and was drowsy and mildly confused. He had urinary incontinence and was taken by EMS to the ED for evaluation.

The differential diagnosis is quite broad. He undergoes routine laboratory studies that are significant only for mild leukocytosis of 11.5. Review of home medications shows he takes hydrochlorothiazide 25 mg, atorvastatin 40 mg, and allopurinol 300 mg, all daily. Toxicology screening is negative for illicit substances or alcohol. Vital signs: temperature 37.8°C, HR 110 sinus rhythm (SR), BP 142/52, and O_2 sat 95% on room air.

DIAGNOSTIC CRITERIA

See Tables 8.11 and 8.12.

TREATMENT/MANAGEMENT

Excellent history taking, laboratory assessment, and clinical examination by the AGACNP can result in early identification of treatable causes of encephalopathy. In the case of the patient in the Classic Presentation, he is placed on video EEG and discovered to have nonconvulsive seizures. With appropriate treatment, he improves and is referred to a neurosurgeon for evaluation of a left frontal necrotic lesion.

COMPLICATIONS

Complications from encephalopathy are broad and can range from sleep disturbances, malnutrition, and seizures to coma and death.

▶ NEUROMUSCULAR DISORDERS

DISEASE OVERVIEW

Neuromuscular disorders encompass a wide range of diseases that affect the peripheral and central nervous system. Myasthenia gravis (MG), multiple sclerosis (MS), Guillain-Barré syndrome (GBS), Parkinson disease (PD), and amyotrophic lateral sclerosis (ALS) are the most common neuromuscular disorders and are commonly confused with each other. Additionally, MS has four subtypes: progressive relapsing multiple sclerosis (PRMS), secondary progressive multiple sclerosis (SPMS), primary progressive multiple sclerosis (PPMS), and relapsing/remitting multiple sclerosis (RRMS). These neuromuscular disorders can be difficult to diagnose as there are few definitive tests.

CLASSIC PRESENTATIONS
MYASTHENIA GRAVIS

A 47-year-old patient presents with fatigue, diplopia, and ptosis. The patient reports progressive weakness that worsens with activity and improves with rest, but it is out of proportion to their usual response to activity.

MULTIPLE SCLEROSIS

A 39-year-old female patient presents with unilateral (left) vision loss and pain with eye movement. On exam, the patient has reduced visual acuity. On fundoscopic exam, the left optic disc appears swollen. The patient reports these symptoms for approximately 1 day.

GUILLAIN-BARRÉ SYNDROME

A 55-year-old male patient presents with acute onset of lower extremity bilateral weakness. On exam, the patient has decreased reflexes in the lower extremities. The patient reports an upper respiratory infection that has resolved within the last week.

PARKINSON DISEASE

A 69-year-old male patient with a past medical history of hypertension and coronary artery disease presents for evaluation of a head and hand tremor, slow shuffling gate, muscular rigidity, and imbalance resulting in numerous falls.

AMYOTROPHIC LATERAL SCLEROSIS

A 58-year-old male patient who is a veteran with no past medical history presents with reports of a mechanical fall. The patient and family endorse several falls within the past 6 months. On exam, the patient has foot drop and bilateral upper extremity weakness. The patient notes that he has had progressive upper extremity weakness despite increased activity.

DIAGNOSTIC CRITERIA

Neuromuscular disorders can be difficult to diagnose as these disorders can often be diagnoses of exclusion. They do not have a single laboratory, imaging, or other diagnostic investigation that can be done to confirm a diagnosis. Diagnosis is often made based on a high level of suspicion and is supported with clinical findings (Table 8.13).

Table 8.13 Diagnostics for Neuromuscular Diseases

Neuromuscular Disease	History and Physical Exam Findings	Testing/Investigation
MG	▪ Fluctuating muscle weakness, worse after physical activity ▪ Proximal > distal muscles ▪ Upper extremity > lower extremity ▪ Diplopia ▪ Ptosis ▪ Bulbar muscle weakness	Diagnosis is made largely on clinical presentation and positive tests for specific antibodies: ▪ Anti-acetylcholine receptor antibodies ▪ Muscle-specific kinase ▪ LRP4
MS	▪ Vision loss, optic neuritis ▪ Vertigo, gait disturbances ▪ Dysarthria, dysphagia ▪ Tremor, spasticity, fatigue ▪ Inconvenience, retention ▪ Memory impairment ▪ Sensory disturbances	No single test to confirm diagnosis. The diagnosis is made based on a history and physical exam combined with other investigations: ▪ MRI ▪ CSF evaluation ▪ Visual evoked potentials
GBS	▪ Ascending paralysis	A clinical diagnosis but can be further investigated with: ▪ Electromyography ▪ Nerve conduction studies ▪ CSF evaluation ▪ MRI
PD	▪ Bradykinesia ▪ Resting tremor ▪ Rigidity ▪ Gait disturbance	No specific lab or imaging study. Diagnosis is clinically based. Additional testing can include an MRI.
ALS (Lou Gehrig disease)	**Upper motor neuron** ▪ Hyperreflexia ▪ Spasticity ▪ Rigidity ▪ Late progression of weakness **Lower motor neuron** ▪ Muscle atrophy ▪ Fasciculations ▪ Early progression of weakness ▪ Hyporeflexia	No specific lab or imaging study to diagnose. Diagnosis is clinically based on upper and motor neuron findings in three of the four body areas: ▪ Cranial/bulbar ▪ Upper extremities ▪ Truck ▪ Lower extremities

ALS, amyotrophic lateral sclerosis; CSF, cerebrospinal fluid; GBS, Guillain-Barré syndrome; LRP4, lipoprotein receptor-related protein 4; MG, myasthenia gravis; MS, multiple sclerosis; PD, Parkinson disease.

TREATMENT/MANAGEMENT

Treatment varies depending on diagnosis (Table 8.14). In the case of an acute exacerbation or flare, it is important to identify and address the precipitating factor/event. All disease states require standard supportive care as part of treatment/management.

Table 8.14 Treatment/Management of Respective Neuromuscular Diseases

Neuromuscular Disease	Treatment/Management
Myasthenia gravis	Stepwise process; if symptoms persist, move to next step. **1.** Acetylcholinesterase inhibitor (consider thymectomy) **2.** Prednisolone and azathioprine **3.** Mycophenolate (mild/moderate symptoms), Rituximab (severe symptoms) Severe exacerbations: ▪ ICU admission ▪ IV immune globulin or plasma exchange ▪ Treat/remove precipitating event

(continued)

Table 8.14 Treatment/Management of Respective Neuromuscular Diseases (*continued*)

Neuromuscular Disease	Treatment/Management
Multiple sclerosis	Mainstay of therapy: ■ Disease-modifying therapies (e.g., glatiramer acetate, natalizumab, mitoxantrone, fingolimod) Acute relapse treatment: ■ Pulse-dose corticosteroids
Guillain-Barré syndrome	■ IVIG ■ Plasma exchange
Parkinson disease	■ Levodopa ■ Pramipexole or ropinirole ■ Anticholinergics or amantadine ■ Deep brain stimulator
ALS	■ Symptomatic management is the mainstay of treatment.

ALS, amyotrophic lateral sclerosis; IV, intravenous; IVIG, intravenous immunoglobulin.

COMPLICATIONS

Complications include muscle atrophy, depression, respiratory failure, and death.

▶ SUMMARY

The neurologic system is complex and has several overlapping pathologies that share clinical characteristics, making primary diagnosis challenging. Clinical investigation including a through history and physical with additional investigative studies (e.g., CT, MRI, EEG, electromyelography [EMG]) will narrow the differential diagnosis and inform treatment.

KNOWLEDGE CHECK: CHAPTER 8

1. A 47-year-old female patient with prior history of anxiety and rheumatoid arthritis on Humira injections presents to the ED with a 2-day history of fever, headache, and myalgias including neck stiffness. She is confused but remains alert. Vital signs: T 38.7°C, heart rate (HR) 112 sinus rhythm (SR), respiratory rate (RR) 25, SpO$_2$ 97% on room air. She is given 2 L of intravenous (IV) fluids, and blood cultures are obtained. What is the next step?

   A. Obtain MRI of the brain to assess for infection
   B. Obtain a CT of the brain to assess for edema or mass lesions before lumbar puncture
   C. Start broad-spectrum antibiotics with vancomycin and Zosyn
   D. Wait to start antibiotics until lumbar puncture is obtained

2. The AGANCP is preparing for lumbar puncture (LP) to evaluate for meningitis or encephalitis in a patient. What is the appropriate next step?

   A. Wait to start antibiotics until LP is obtained to ensure the yield is higher on culture
   B. Start broad-spectrum antibiotics now
   C. Obtain a stat MRI to evaluate for cerebral edema
   D. Administer dexamethasone and then broad-spectrum antibiotics and acyclovir

3. A 65-year-old patient with a remote history of breast cancer presents with persistent headache for the last week. She mentions she has had clumsiness with her right leg. What should the AGANCP order?

   A. MRI breast
   B. CT head
   C. Complete blood count (CBC) and basic metabolic profile (BMP)
   D. Lumbar puncture (LP)

4. The AGACNP is preparing for a lumbar puncture (LP) at the bedside. What position should the AGACNP ask the nurse to place the patient in?

   A. Prone
   B. Standing
   C. Sitting, minimally flexing forward onto an over-bed table
   D. Curled in fetal position, neck flexed, knees pulled to chest

5. A 36-year-old female patient who is post Cesarean section is transferred to the ICU for severe headaches. Her C-section was uncomplicated. She was awake with an epidural for pain management. Estimated blood loss (EBL) was 100 mL. Vital signs: T 37.6°C, heart rate (HR) 110, respiratory rate (RR) 20, blood pressure (BP) 140/78, O$_2$ Sat 99% on 2 liters nasal cannula. What is the most likely cause of her headache?

   A. Eclampsia
   B. Preeclampsia
   C. Spinal fluid leak
   D. Hypovolemic shock

(See answers next page.)

1. **B) Obtain a CT of the brain to assess for edema or mass lesions before lumbar puncture**

In the setting of altered mentation and immunocompromised state, the AGANCP should obtain imaging to assess for mass lesions or edema that are a contraindication for lumbar puncture. CT is the initial scan. MRI may be needed if the CT is negative, but it is not the first diagnostic test. Antibiotics are not indicated at this time as a lumbar puncture (LP) has not been performed yet. A CT should be done before an LP to avoid herniation if edema is present.

2. **D) Administer dexamethasone and then broad-spectrum antibiotics and acyclovir**

The AGANCP must not delay therapy for possible meningitis or encephalitis as morbidity and mortality are worse. Dexamethasone should also be started prior to antibiotics in the setting of possible meningitis. If herpes simplex virus (HSV) encephalitis is suspected, acyclovir at 10 mg/kg should be administered every 8 hours as this is a treatable viral encephalitis.

3. **B) CT head**

A CT head is the first-line diagnostic to assess for head bleed or metastasis. MRIs are useful in diagnosing breast cancer but are not needed at this time. Labs are commonly obtained in almost all patients but are not always needed. Contrast is not needed for the CT scan, thus obtaining blood urea nitrogen (BUN)/creatinine is not needed. The "Choosing Wisely campaign" recommends against routinely checking CBCs if the patient is clinically stable. A CT must be done prior to an LP.

4. **D) Curled in fetal position, neck flexed, knees pulled to chest**

Lateral recumbent position with the patient curled into fetal position with neck flexed and knees pulled into chest and keeping spine horizontal with bed is one option for a bedside procedure. Alternatively, Sitting on edge of bed maximally flexed forward onto a table is an option. Prone positioning is typically reserved for interventional radiology settings. Standing is not an option.

5. **C) Spinal fluid leak**

A common complication from spinal anesthesia is spinal fluid leak that manifests as a severe headache. While this patient is of an advanced maternal age, she has no history of high-risk symptoms such as hypertension, preeclampsia, or eclampsia. Her blood pressure is high-normal but may be attributed to acute pain. She is tachycardic, which is expected due to maternal changes and pain. Her EBL is 100 mL; thus, hemorrhagic shock is less likely.

6. The AGACNP is called to evaluate a 35-year-old male patient admitted with diabetic ketoacidosis (DKA) who now has a change in mental status. His past medical history is significant for type I diabetes and hypertension. Social history is significant for drinking a fifth of vodka a day. Vital signs: T 36.4°C, heart rate (HR) 70, respiratory rate (RR) 16, blood pressure (BP) 136/72, O_2 sat 96% on 2 liters nasal cannula. Glucose is 168. On exam, he is lethargic but still able to follow simple commands. When asked to hold up his arms, there is no pronator drift, but he does repetitively flutter his fingers when asked to flex his wrists while his arms are outstretched. What is the most likely cause of his encephalopathy?

   A. Hepatic encephalopathy
   B. Diabetic coma
   C. Hypertensive emergency
   D. Sepsis

7. A male victim of a motor vehicle crash in which he was rear-ended at a high rate of speed presents with complaints of neck pain. He can move his lower extremities but has minimal movement and decreased sensation in his upper extremities. What type of injury does he likely have?

   A. Brown–Sequard syndrome
   B. Anterior cord syndrome
   C. Central cord syndrome
   D. Conus medullaris

8. An 82-year-old male patient who is a farmer presents after a tractor rolled over him. He complains of severe back pain, is unable to move his left leg, and is unable to sense deep painful stimuli in the right leg. What is the most likely diagnosis?

   A. Brown–Sequard syndrome
   B. Anterior cord syndrome
   C. Central cord syndrome
   D. Posterior cord syndrome

9. A 62-year-old man with a history of lung cancer currently undergoing chemotherapy presents with complaints of urinary incontinence and new erectile dysfunction that fails to respond to sildenafil (Viagra). On exam, he has decreased sensation in the perianal area and an absent rectal reflex. What is the most likely diagnosis?

   A. Conus medullaris
   B. Central cord syndrome
   C. Anterior cord syndrome
   D. Posterior cord syndrome

10. A 19-year-old male patient presents to the ED as an unrestrained passenger in a motor vehicle crash. The patient's Glasgow Coma Scale (GCS) score is 7 (eyes = 2, verbal = 1, motor = 4). Imaging reveals an abnormal head CT. What severity classification for traumatic brain injury (TBI) does this patient have?

    A. Mild
    B. Moderate
    C. Mild/moderate
    D. Severe

(See answers next page.)

6. A) Hepatic encephalopathy

The patient has a medical history of vodka use. Asterixis is a sign of toxic metabolic encephalopathy predominantly seen in hepatic failure but also in renal disorders. Blood sugar is 168 and stable, so diabetic coma is less likely. Hypertensive urgency or emergency would have a higher BP to cause target organ damage. This patient is afebrile, not tachycardic; normotensive; and not hypoxic; thus, his quick Sepsis Related Organ Failure Assessment (qSOFA) score is 1, and he is not likely to be septic. The quick Sepsis Related Organ Failure Assessment (qSOFA) allocates one point each for RR greater than 22, systolic blood pressure (SBP) less than 100, and altered mental status. A quick Sepsis Related Organ Failure Assessment (qSOFA) score of 2 or higher is suggestive of sepsis with significant in-hospital mortality.

7. C) Central cord syndrome

Central cord syndrome is commonly a result of hyperextension injuries and presents as loss of motor strength in the upper extremities, more so than in the lower extremities. Anterior cord syndrome presents as paraplegia and bilateral loss of pain and temperature sensation. Brown–Sequard syndrome presents as ipsilateral loss of motor control, proprioception, and vibration, with contralateral loss of pain and temperature. Conus medullaris exhibits perineal and perianal paresthesia, absent bulbocavernous and anal reflex, incontinence, and erectile dysfunction.

8. A) Brown–Sequard syndrome

Brown–Sequard syndrome presents as ipsilateral loss of motor control, proprioception, and vibration, with contralateral loss of pain and temperature. Central cord syndrome commonly presents as loss of motor strength in the upper extremities, more so than the lower extremities. Anterior cord syndrome presents as paraplegia and bilateral loss of pain and temperature sensation. Posterior cord syndrome presents with loss of proprioception and vibration with preserved motor function.

9. A) Conus medullaris

Conus medullaris presents with perineal and perianal paresthesia, absent bulbocavernous and anal reflex, incontinence, and erectile dysfunction, but normal motor function. Bone metastasis is common in breast, kidney, lung, prostate, and thyroid cancers and multiple myeloma and lymphoma. Other causes of conus medullaris include trauma, use of anticoagulation, and intravenous drug use.

10. D) Severe

TBI severity is based on GCS. A score of 3 to 8 = severe; 9 to 12 = moderate, and 13 to 15 = mild.

11. A 78-year-old female patient who sustained a fall down six stairs 1 day ago now presents for evaluation of confusion and headache. Head CT reveals a subdural hematoma measuring 1 cm in thickness. A repeat head CT 6 hours later reveals expansion of the subdural hematoma, now measuring 2 cm in thickness with associated midline shift. The AGACNP reexamines the patient after reviewing the most recent head CT and notes the patient to be somnolent. What is the next *best* step?

    A. Order a repeat head CT stat
    B. Consult neurosurgery for potential subdural hematoma evacuation
    C. Reevaluate the patient in 4 hours
    D. Initiate the normothermia protocol

12. A 22-year-old female patient presents as a helmeted driver involved in a motorcycle crash. The patient presents with a Glasgow Coma Scale (GCS) score of 7 (eyes = 2, verbal = 1, motor = 4). Imaging reveals an abnormal head CT. What monitoring modality is indicated for this patient?

    A. Intracranial pressure (ICP) monitoring
    B. Central venous pressure monitoring
    C. Lumbar drain
    D. Train of four

13. The AGACNP is evaluating a patient with bilateral lower extremity weakness that appears to be ascending in nature. The patient reports a rapid onset of symptoms following recovery from an upper respiratory illness. What will the AGACNP consider for initial therapy for this patient?

    A. Broad-spectrum antibiotics
    B. Intravenous immunoglobulin (IVIG)
    C. High-dose prednisone
    D. MRI of the cervical spine

14. A 42-year-old female patient with a past medical history of hypertension, diabetes, and multiple sclerosis (MS) now presents with acute weakness and lower extremity ataxia. On exam, the patient has hyperreflexia. The AGACNP knows the acute management of this patient will include:

    A. Low-dose corticosteroids
    B. Pulse-dose corticosteroids
    C. Baclofen
    D. Tolterodine

15. The AGACNP is caring for a patient in myasthenic crisis in the ICU. The patient has displayed increased bulbar weakness and diaphragm weakness despite initiation of intravenous immunoglobin (IVIG) therapy. What is the AGACNP's primary concern with these exam findings?

    A. Respiratory failure requiring intubation
    B. Reaction to IVIG therapy
    C. Nutritional status
    D. Worsening chronic pulmonary disease

16. The AGACNP is caring for a patient with amyotrophic lateral sclerosis (ALS) who is admitted with respiratory failure and is requiring high-flow nasal canula. The AGACNP understands the disease progression of ALS and has what discussion with the patient and family?

    A. Advance directives, mechanical ventilation, and tracheostomy
    B. Investigative medications for the treatment of ALS
    C. Genetic testing and counseling for the patient
    D. Genetic testing and counseling for the family

(See answers next page.)

11. B) Consult neurosurgery for potential subdural hematoma evacuation

The patient presents with a subdural hematoma, and imaging indicated expansion of the subdural hematoma with an associated change in neurologic exam. To address the subdural hematoma, the neurosurgical team must be consulted. Repeating a head CT will delay ultimate treatment, subdural evacuation, for this patient. Reevaluating in 4 hours is not appropriate as the patient is likely to continue to decline. Initiating a normothermia protocol does not address the underlying cause for the decline in neurologic status.

12. A) Intracranial pressure monitoring

The patient with a severe traumatic brain injury (TBI) and aGCS score of 8 or lower should have an ICP monitor to aide in management. Central venous pressure monitoring is not indicated, nor is a lumbar drain. Train of four is indicated when a patient is on paralytics.

13. B) Intravenous immunoglobulin (IVIG)

The patient has a classic finding consistent with Guillain-Barré syndrome (GBS). There are only two therapies: IVIG and plasma exchange. These therapies are recommended to be initiated at the start of symptoms. Broad-spectrum antibiotics play no role in the treatment of GBS, and steroids are only shown to have benefit when combined with IVIG. An MRI of the cervical spine may be part of the workup, but it is not a therapy.

14. B) Pulse-dose corticosteroids

The patient is presenting with an acute MS relapse, and treatment will include pulse dose corticosteroids. Low-dose corticosteroids would be insufficient dosing. Baclofen and tolterodine are common treatments for spasticity and urinary urgency, which are commonly seen in patient with MS.

15. A) Respiratory failure requiring intubation

A concern with myasthenic crisis is respiratory failure. Increased bulbar weakness and, particularly, evidence of diaphragmatic weakness raise concern for respiratory failure.

16. A) Advance directives, mechanical ventilation, and tracheostomy

ALS is a progressive disease, and commonly patients suffer from respiratory failure due to diaphragmatic weakness and weakness of intercostal muscles. Early discussions of advance care directives and particularly tracheostomy are recommended to be discussed early after diagnosis. It is most important for the AGACNP to know what the patient's wishes are. Discussing investigative medications and genetic testing in this acute phase is not a priority.

17. A 45-year-old patient presents for evaluation for headache, confusion, and fever. The AGACNP elicits Kernig sign during the physical exam. What will the AGACNP need to make a definitive diagnosis?

    A. EEG
    B. Lumbar puncture (LP)
    C. MRI brain with and without contrast
    D. Neurology consult

18. The AGACNP is caring for a 20-year-old patient who was the unrestrained passenger in a motor vehicle crash. The patient lost consciousness at the scene of the accident but is now able to provide past medical history to the AGACNP. During this time, the patient has a progressive decline in mental status, becoming unresponsive. Current vital signs: blood pressure (BP) 139/83, respiratory rate (RR) 15, heart rate (HR) 114, O_2 sat 97%. The AGACNP immediately orders:

    A. Stat MRI brain and cervical spine
    B. Stat noncontrast head CT
    C. Narcan
    D. Flumazenil

19. A 74-year-old female patient with a past medical history of diabetes, atrial fibrillation, and hypertension presents for evaluation of left-sided weakness. The family reports the symptoms started at 3 hours before arrival. A stat noncontrast head CT and CT angiography (CTA) of the head and neck were obtained and did not show hemorrhage or a large vessel occlusion. Vital signs: blood pressure (BP) 198/99, heart rate (HR) 92, respiratory rate (RR) 18, O_2 sat 93%. What should the AGACNP do next?

    A. Order an MRI of the brain
    B. Order labetalol 10 mg intravenous (IV) × 1
    C. Order tissue plasminogen activator (tPA)
    D. Order stat head CT

20. The AGACNP is caring for a 21-year-old patient who presents after a fall from a tree. The patient's physical exam reveals motor deficits in all four extremities, but the upper extremities are noticeably weaker than the bilateral lower extremities. What spinal cord syndrome does the AGACNP suspect?

    A. Anterior cord
    B. Posterior cord
    C. Brown–Sequard
    D. Central cord

(See answers next page.)

17. B) Lumbar puncture (LP)

Fever, headache, and confusion are signs of meningitis, and Kernig sign is indicative of meningeal irritation. An LP will allow sampling and evaluation of cerebrospinal fluid (CSF) to confirm the diagnosis of meningitis. EEG could be obtained to rule out seizures in the setting of meningitis, and imaging with an MRI will help support a diagnosis of meningitis, but CSF evaluation is diagnostic.

18. B) Stat noncontrast head CT

The mechanism of injury and presentation (loss of consciousness [LOC] followed by lucid period followed by unresponsiveness) is a classic presentation of an epidural hematoma. A head CT is needed to confirm this diagnosis. An MRI will take too much time to complete. Narcan and flumazenil are reversal agents for opioids and benzodiazepines; the patient's current vital signs do not support opioid or benzodiazepine overdose.

19. B) Order labetalol 10 mg intravenous (IV) × 1

The patient has evidence of an acute stroke without evidence of hemorrhage on a CTA. The patient would be a candidate for tPA, but their BP is too high, making labetalol 10 mg IV the best choice. A stat head CT will be of little value; one was just completed and there is no report of change to the neurologic exam.

20. D) Central cord

Central cord syndrome deficits present as loss of motor strength in the upper extremities more so than the lower extremities. Anterior cord syndrome presents as paraplegia and bilateral loss of pain and temperature sensation. Posterior cord syndrome presents as loss of proprioception and vibration; motor control is preserved. Brown–Sequard syndrome presents as ipsilateral loss of motor control, proprioception, and vibration, with contralateral loss of pain and temperature.

KEY BIBLIOGRAPHY

Only key resources appear in the print edition. Access the full bibliography for this chapter on ExamPrepConnect.com.

American College of Surgeons. Committee on Trauma (2018) *Advanced Trauma Life Support ATLS: Student course manual.* Author.

Arokszallasi, T., Balogh, E., Csiba, L., Fekete, I., Fekete, K., & Olah, L. (2019). Acute alcohol intoxication may cause delay in stroke treatment—Case reports. *BMC Neurology, 19,* 14. https://doi.org/10.1186/s12883-019-1241-6

Carney, N., Totten, A. M., O'Reilly, C., Ullman, J. S., Hawryluk, G. W., Bell, M. J., Bratton, S. L., Chesnut, R., Harris, O. A., Kissoon, N., Rubiano, A. M., Shutter, L., Tasker, R. C., Vavilala, M. S., Wilberger, J., Wright, D. W., & Ghajar, J. (2017, January 1). Guidelines for the management of severe traumatic brain injury, fourth edition. *Neurosurgery, 80*(1), 6–15. https://doi.org/10.1227/NEU.0000000000001432

Glauser, T., Shinnar, S., Gloss, D., Alldredge, B., Arya, R., Bainbridge, J., Bare, M., Bleck, T., Dodson, W. E., Garrity, L., Jagoda, A., Lowenstein, D., Pellock, J., Riviello, J., Sloan, E., Treiman, D. M ., & American Heart Association/American Stroke Association. (2016). Evidence-based guideline: Treatment of convulsive status epilepticus in children and adults: Report of the Guideline Committee of the American Epilepsy Society. *Epilepsy Currents, 16*(1), 48–61. https://doi.org/10.5698/1535-7597-16.1.48

Greenberg, S. M., Ziai, W. C., Cordonnier, C., Dowlatshahi, D., Francis, B., Goldstein, J. N., Hemphill, J. C., Johnson, R., Keigher, K. M., Mack, W. J., Mocco, J., Newton, E. J., Ruff, I. M., Sansing, L. H., Schulman, S., Selim, M. H., Sheth, K. N., Sprigg, N., Sunnerhagen, K. S. (2022). 2022 guideline for the management of patients with spontaneous intracerebral hemorrhage: A guideline from the American Heart Association/American Stroke Association. *Stroke, 53*(7). e282–e361. https://doi.org/10.1161/str.0000000000000407

Mazeraud, A., Righy, C., Bouchereau, E., Benghanem, S., Bozza, F. A., & Sharshar, T. (2020, April). Septic-associated encephalopathy: A comprehensive review. *Neurotherapeutics, 17*(2), 392–403. https://doi.org/10.1007/s13311-020-00862-1

McKean, S. C., Ross, J. J., Dressler, D. D., & Scheurer, D. B. (2017). *Principles and practice of hospital medicine.* McGraw-Hill Education.

Cardiovascular System Review

Jamie Gooch, Paula McCauley, and Elizabeth Singh

▶ INTRODUCTION

The AGACNP must have a solid understanding of the cardiovascular system to be able to provide safe and competent care to patients. This review chapter encompasses many of the critical areas that will be tested on board certification and will be required knowledge for an entry-level AGACNP.

▶ HYPERTENSION

DISEASE OVERVIEW

Hypertension (HTN) is a disease marked by chronic elevated blood pressure (BP) resulting from both pathologic/physical and neurohormonal changes over time. It can be classified as either primary/essential HTN or secondary HTN (related to another condition). This disease has both genetic and lifestyle factors associated with it. Modifiable risk factors for HTN include smoking, physical inactivity, a diet high in saturated fat and sodium, chronic alcohol consumption, and obesity. Nonmodifiable risk factors for HTN include race, age, male sex, family history, and diagnosis of diabetes. HTN is classified into stages by the American Heart Association and the American College of Cardiology. These are described as elevated 120 to 129/less than 80; stage 1 BP greater than 130 to 139 or 80 to 89; stage II BP ≥140 or ≥90.

CLASSIC PRESENTATION

A 55-year-old male executive at a local marketing firm has a history of smoking half a pack of cigarettes a day for 35 years. He drinks a "large" scotch in the afternoon and before bed. He is overweight and does not see a healthcare provider regularly. He tells the AGACNP that his father died "young" of a heart attack. Today while evaluating the patient in the orthopedics clinic for a "clicking shoulder," the AGACNP discovered his BP measurement is 158/84. He denies current discomfort or anxiety but does report that he has a "very type A personality." After allowing him to sit quietly for 15 minutes, the AGACNP retakes his BP, which is 156/84.

DIAGNOSTIC CRITERIA

HTN is an insidious disease. Symptoms only begin to appear after disease has been present for many years and results in end-organ damage. While symptoms may develop acutely in the setting of hypertensive urgency/emergency, the subtler symptoms that indicate longer-standing chronic HTN may not be obvious until severe irreversible damage has occurred. These may include impotence/sexual dysfunction, decrease in visual acuity from retinal damage, headaches, nose bleeds, angina, and potentially heart failure (HF).

DIAGNOSTIC TESTING

Lab testing seeks to uncover evidence of secondary causes as well as target organ damage. A urinalysis, creatinine, lipid profile, serum potassium, sodium, and calcium is required to evaluate etiologies of hypertention. HbgA1C, complete blood count (CBC), and thyroid-stimulating hormone (TSH). An EKG and echocardiogram may be obtained to screen for ventricular hypertrophy and other HTN-associated myocardial changes.

TREATMENT/MANAGEMENT

Treatment varies based on stage of HTN, race, age, and presence of comorbid conditions. People at any stage of HTN, however, should be treated with nonpharmacologic therapy and benefit from lifestyle modifications including increased physical activity, decreasing their saturated fat and sodium intake, avoiding smoking and alcohol, and maintaining a healthy weight. People with Stage I HTN with an estimated 10-year atherosclerotic cardiovascular disease (ASCVD) risk of ≥10% and those with Stage II HTN should also receive treatment with an appropriate antihypertensive medication (Table 9.1). Angiotensin-converting enzyme inhibitor (ACEI) or angiotensin-receptor blocker (ARB) have compelling indications for the treatment of coronary artery disease (CAD), post myocardial infarction (MI), HF, diabetes, and chronic kidney disease (CKD).

Table 9.1 HTN Treatment

Non-Black Patient	Black Patient	Patient with DM or CKD
BP goal: greater than 60, less than 150/90	BP goal: less than 60, less than 140/90	BP goal: all ages less than 140/90
Lifestyle Modifications		
Initiate and titrate thiazide, ACEI, ARB, or CCB	Initiate and titrate thiazide or CCB	Initiate and titrate ACEI or ARB
Titrate drug 1 to achieve BP goal or maximal dosing, then add a second class from above.		
If not at goal BP, add a beta-blocker, aldosterone antagonist (eplerenone [Inspra] or spironolactone [Aldactone]), or another agent, and titrate to achieve BP goal or maximal dose.		
Refer to HTN specialist.		

ACEI, angiotensin-converting enzyme inhibitor; ARB, angiotensin-receptor blocker; BP, blood pressure; CCB, calcium channel blocker; CKD, chronic kidney disease; DM, diabetes mellitus; HTN, hypertension.

COMPLICATIONS

Complications include left ventricular hypertrophy, retinal damage, cardiovascular disease (CVD), stroke, impotence, MI, and aneurysm. Hypertensive urgency and hypertensive emergency can also occur.

▶ HYPERTENSIVE URGENCY AND EMERGENCY

DISEASE OVERVIEW

Hypertensive urgency/emergency are syndromes characterized by a severely elevated BP that can result in damage to target organs. The defining characteristics between hypertensive urgency and emergency are the degree of BP elevation along with the presence of target organ damage. In a hypertensive urgency, the BP must be greater than 180/90. In hypertensive emergency, pressures of greater than 200/100 may be observed and have evidence of end-organ damage.

Organ damage differs by system. Evidence of brain, kidney, and cardiac dysfunction are common. Hypertensive encephalopathy, headache, and blurred vision may be reported, along with dizziness. Renal injury is often noted on the basic metabolic panel (BMP) where elevations in blood urea nitrogen (BUN) and creatinine are suspicious for acute kidney injury. Elevated BP may also result in acute HF, pulmonary edema, and MI. Retinal hemorrhages and nosebleeding may be observed. Hypertensive crisis is a medical emergency, and prompt identification and treatment are required to avoid potentially life-threatening sequelae.

CLASSIC PRESENTATION

A 49-year-old female patient, who works as a certified nursing assistant (CNA) at the local rehabilitation hospital, has a past medical history (PMH) significant for essential HTN. She is the primary wage earner for her family and struggles to make ends meet. Today she was driven to the clinic by her friend with complaints of new-onset, severe, tearing-type back pain, headache, shortness of breath, and feelings of persistent anxiety. Her friend reports that she appears somewhat confused but did tell her that she has not taken her prescribed antihypertensives for over a month due to inability to afford them. Her vital signs (VS) are as follows: heart rate (HR) 122, respiratory rate (RR) 28, BP 205/110. On exam, the AGACNP notes crackles bilaterally, tachypnea, and mild confusion.

DIAGNOSTIC CRITERIA

The physical exam may be notable for a lateral displacement of the point of maxillary impulse (PMI) indicating left ventricular hypertrophy (LVH), as well as the presence of S4. Other exam findings are related to end-organ damage and may include both the subjective complaints and objective findings of headache, confusion, retinal hemorrhage, slurred speech, dyspnea and shortness of breath, angina, pulmonary edema, and blurred or double vision.

DIAGNOSTIC TESTING

Obtain cardiac enzymes, B-type natriuretic peptide (BNP), BMP to assess for hyperkalemia, and elevated BUN and creatinine and an EKG to assess for target organ damage. The EKG may show LVH or possibly ischemia.

TREATMENT/MANAGEMENT

Several intravenous (IV) medications may be employed including beta-blockers like labetalol, and Esmolol, vasodilators including nitroglycerin (Nipride), the calcium channel blockers (CCBs) nicardipine or clevidipine, or ACEIs like enalaprilat. A mainstay of treatment is to slowly bring the BP back toward normal. Too quick of a drop in the BP can result in catastrophic cerebral edema or ischemic stroke. In patients with severe sequelae (pheochromocytoma crisis or eclampsia), the goal is to bring systolic BP (SBP) to less than 140 in the first hour of treatment, and less than 120 if aortic dissection is present. For all others, BP should be reduced no more than 25% over the first hour, then toward 160/100 within the following 2 to 6 hours. BP can be safely brought toward normal over the next 1 to 2 days. Hypertensive emergency should be admitted to the ICU for continuous BP monitoring and treatment with IV antihypertensive agents.

COMPLICATIONS

Complications include end-organ damage including encephalopathy, delirium, hemorrhagic stroke, MI, HF, retinal hemorrhage, and aortic aneurysm.

▶ DYSLIPIDEMIA

DISEASE OVERVIEW

Dyslipidemia involves an imbalance in the lipids required for normal body functioning, including high-density lipoprotein (HDL) and low-density lipoprotein (LDL) cholesterol, as well as triglycerides. Pathogenesis of primary dyslipidemia is related to lifestyle factors like diet (high intake of saturated fat, low intake of fiber) and activity level, as well as hereditary causes (familial hypercholesterolemia). Other risks include tobacco use and obesity. Secondary dyslipidemia is also seen co-occurring with conditions like hypothyroidism, alcohol use disorder, and obesity.

CLASSIC PRESENTATION

A 47-year-old female patient has been admitted for observation after complaining of substernal pressure. She has a body mass index of 31 and a history of hypothyroidism. During her interview, she tells the AGACNP that she has not been taking her levothyroxine as prescribed due to losing her health insurance. Exam reveals several scattered xanthomas around her eyelids and that her fingers have a yellow discoloration. When asked about the yellow staining, she reports that she smokes 20 cigarettes a day and has done so for the past 15 years.

DIAGNOSTIC CRITERIA

Physical manifestations of dyslipidemia are limited to the presence of xanthomas, which may be seen on the eyelids. These most often appear as a small yellow outpouching of skin. Other findings consistent with secondary dyslipidemia may be present and include obesity, coarse hair, telangiectases, and a cushingoid appearance.

DIAGNOSTIC TESTING
Laboratory testing includes a fasting lipid panel as the gold standard for evaluation of dyslipidemia and includes LDL, HDL, very low-density lipoprotein (VLDL), and triglyceride testing.

TREATMENT/MANAGEMENT
Dyslipidemia treatment is aimed at either primary prevention in those without CAD, or secondary prevention (+ history of CAD). All people diagnosed with dyslipidemia should be counseled to adopt lifestyle modification including limiting saturated fat intake and increasing their intake of fresh fruits and vegetables, whole grains, and heart-healthy fats. Physical activity goals include three to four sessions of at least 40 minutes of moderate to vigorous aerobic activity each week. The determination to start medication is based on age, the presence of cardiovascular risk factors, and the calculated 10-year CVD risk. For adults aged 40 to 75 years who have one risk factor and a calculated CVD risk score of greater than 10%, a statin is recommended. Diabetes is a high-risk condition to develop CAD. In patients with diabetes mellitus (DM; type I or II), adults age 40 to 75 years, regardless of 10-year risk, should receive moderate intensity statin. In adults with diabetes and CAD or multiple risk factors for CAD, prescribe high-intensity statins to lower low-density lipoprotein cholesterol by 50% or more.

COMPLICATIONS
Complications of dyslipidemia include atherosclerosis-related diseases, including ASCVD, including but not limited to CAD, MI, peripheral arterial disease (PAD), carotid stenosis, chronic mesenteric ischemia, aortic aneurysm, and stroke.

▶ CORONARY ARTERY DISEASE

DISEASE OVERVIEW
CAD is a complex, chronic, and progressive disease associated with inheritable traits and environmental and lifestyle factors. The primary feature of CAD is development of an atherosclerotic plaque that evolves over time. The resultant arteriosclerosis reduces the intraluminal diameter of the coronary artery. This process begins with injury to the endothelial lining of the coronary wall resulting in development of a fatty streak. Wall damage is related to many factors, including hyperglycemia, HTN, smoking, and a high-fat diet. Once a fatty streak develops, leukocyte aggregation occurs along with proliferation of smooth muscle cells within the vessel wall. Foam cell development follows, and the atherosclerotic plaque grows. Plaques are unstable and over time may rupture leading to potential acute occlusion of downstream vessels and subsequent acute coronary syndrome (ACS). Growing plaques may also lead to critical narrowing of the vessel over time. These may be asymptomatic or result in the development of angina. Angina is classified as stable, unstable, or variant/Prinzmetal (Table 9.2).

CAD development is influenced by the presence of modifiable and nonmodifiable risks. Nonmodifiable risk factors include male sex, post menopause, advancing age, and family history of CAD. Modifiable risks are tobacco use, dyslipidemia, HTN, diabetes, obesity, and sedentary lifestyle.

Table 9.2 Angina Types

Type of Angina	Description
Unstable	A medical emergency. Can occur at rest, is new, or is more severe and frequent if angina has typically been chronic. May signal acute coronary syndrome.
Stable	Predictable pattern of exacerbation with physical or emotional stress caused by a supply–demand mismatch. Lasts several minutes and is relieved by rest.
Variant/Prinzmetal	Rare. Occurs in the presence of arterial spasm and is unrelated to CAD. More common in women.

CLASSIC PRESENTATION

An AGACNP finds an older, overweight white man sitting at the top of the stairs and appearing unwell. He reports that upon reaching the top of the stairs, he started to feel a sense of impending doom, nausea, and a crushing heaviness in the center of his chest. On exam he is pale, diaphoretic, and appears breathless. He denies palpitations or recent illness but tells the AGACNP he is 65 years old, has diabetes type 2, and takes a small blue pill for his cholesterol. He has recently quit smoking. The AGACNP notices the color return to his face and his breathing return to normal. He thanks the AGACNP for their concern and says his chest discomfort has improved since he sat down and is now almost completely resolved after several minutes.

DIAGNOSTIC CRITERIA

Physical exam may be unremarkable in those not experiencing active angina. Signs of comorbid illness like hypercholesterolemia and HTN may be evident, including xanthelasma, decreased peripheral pulses, cool lower extremities, hemosiderin staining, bilateral lower extremity (LE) edema, and bruits of the carotid or femoral arteries. Yellowed, nicotine-stained fingers may reveal a tobacco history, and the presence of obesity may also be noted.

Obtain the following labs: CBC, creatinine, lipid panel, HgA_{1c}, and thyroid panel, plus cardiac enzymes if angina reported. An EKG and echo should be obtained. In patients with high suspicion of CAD, a coronary CT angiography (CTA) should be obtained. Coronary angiography is considered the gold standard for diagnosing CAD.

TREATMENT/MANAGEMENT

In patients with chronic CAD, initial treatment includes statin, beta-blockers, or CCBs, in addition to a short-acting nitrate if symptoms of angina are present, plus aspirin (ASA) or clopidogrel (Plavix) for secondary prevention. Routine use of aspirin in primary prevention of CAD is no longer recommended.

COMPLICATIONS

Complications include ACS, non-ST-segment elevation myocardial infarction (non-STEMI), ST-segment elevation myocardial infarction (STEMI), HF, and arrhythmias.

▶ ACUTE CORONARY SYNDROME

DISEASE OVERVIEW

ACS occurs when one or more of the coronary arteries acutely becomes completely or partially occluded resulting in decreased perfusion to the portion of the myocardium supplied by that vessel. It may happen abruptly as in the case of an occluding embolus or atherosclerotic plaque rupture with clot formation. The resultant ischemia leads to myocardial dysfunction within minutes, resulting in decreased contraction, worsening ischemia, and eventual tissue death if the obstruction is not relieved. Dysrhythmia and cardiac arrest may follow if perfusion is not rapidly restored. ACS is a medical emergency and can result in STEMI or NSTEMI. Typically, an NSTEMI that can be identified by ST depressions and T-wave inversions on EKG involves only a portion of the endocardium and myocardium. STEMI, on the other hand, is a transmural infarction involving all layers of the heart and presents with ST-segment elevation on EKG. STEMI has the worst prognosis and complications of the two.

CLASSIC PRESENTATION

A 73-year-old postmenopausal woman presents with a PMH of hyperlipidemia, HTN, and hypothyroidism. While sitting at church today, she began to experience sudden-onset severe jaw and substernal chest pain. Her daughter noticed that she was sweating profusely and looked nauseous. She took two Tylenol and waited for the service to end. After 45 minutes, her pain had not decreased, and she vomited. Emergency medical services (EMS) was called to transport her to the hospital. En route, she was given sublingual nitroglycerin without effect. A STAT EKG revealed 4-mm ST elevations in leads II, III, and aVF. On arrival to the hospital, she was diagnosed with acute STEMI, the cardiac catheterization lab was activated, and she was sent for emergent percutaneous coronary intervention (PCI).

DIAGNOSTIC CRITERIA

Classic unstable angina occurs at rest, is of new onset, or demonstrates significant worsening in intensity if chronic stable angina has been present. Angina pectoralis, diaphoresis, jaw or neck pain, a feeling of impending doom, and nausea and vomiting may be present. The pain is often described as dull or aching. A new heart murmur may be detected if papillary rupture has occurred. Tachycardia or bradycardia may be present along with hyper- or hypotension and extra heart sounds including an S4 indicating ventricular dysfunction.

Women and patients with diabetes may have atypical presentations. Vague or difficult-to-describe symptoms in these patients co-occurring with a history suspicious for CVD should be reviewed carefully and be assumed to be ACS until proven otherwise.

In addition to the labs indicated when chronic CAD is suspected, cardiac enzymes including troponin T or troponin I should be obtained. Creatine kinase (CK) and serum creatine kinase, myocardial-bound (CK-MB) may also be collected. A BNP may give useful information about the presence of HF.

EKG confirms acute myocardial ischemia or infarction and identifies the culprit artery (Table 9.3). In suspected ACS, coronary angiography is the gold standard for diagnosis and treatment with PCI and should not be delayed.

Table 9.3 Location of MI by EKG Pattern

Leads with ST-Segment Elevation	Artery	Type of MI
II, III, aVF	RCA	Inferior wall MI
V1–V6	LAD	Anterior wall MI
I, aVL, V3–V6	LAD + RCA or LCX	Anterio–lateral MI
V7–V9 (posterior EKG)	RCA	Inferio–basal/posterior MI

LAD, left anterior descending; LCX, left circumflex; MI, myocardial infarction; RCA, right coronary artery.

TREATMENT/MANAGEMENT

Interventions for ACS include aspirin, oxygen if O_2 saturation ≤90%, opioids for pain control, and continuous telemetry monitoring. NSTEMIs require anticoagulation and antithrombotics or PCI. STEMI is a medical emergency requiring immediate intervention with fibrinolytics or PCI. Do not delay treatment to collect more data or await the return of cardiac enzymes. STEMI requires emergent primary PCI within 2 hours of diagnosis (12 hours of symptom onset), fibrinolytics if not able to have primary PCI within this window. Current guidelines recommend a door-to-needle time of 30 minutes or less from presentation of STEMI in the ED to receiving fibrinolytic therapy, or 90 minutes door-to-balloon time if receiving primary PCI.

Medications include ASA + P2Y12 inhibitor, and anticoagulation with unfractionated heparin (UFH) or enoxaparin. Long-term treatment of post-STEMI patients should include smoking cessation, cardiac rehab, BP control, diet, weight control, and moderation of alcohol consumption. Long-term treatment post-STEMI should include dual antiplatelet therapy (DAPT) with indefinite low-dose ASA, + Ticagrelor or Prasugrel 12 months post PCI, long-term beta-blocker, statin, and ACEI. Patients presenting with inferior wall MI (ST elevations in leads II, III, and aVF) may be extremely preload dependent. Avoid nitrates and consider IV fluid boluses if hypotension occurs. Bradycardia may also be seen.

COMPLICATIONS

Complications include arrhythmia, pericarditis, shock, HF, and cardiac arrest.

▶ NONSURGICAL/PERCUTANEOUS CORONARY INTERVENTIONS

DISEASE OVERVIEW

Immediate reperfusion is the hallmark treatment for ACS by either fibrinolytic medications or mechanical intervention and must be made within minutes of the presentation of the patient with

ACS. Door-to-needle or door-to-balloon time benchmarks have documented outcomes with significant impact and improvement on morbidity and mortality. PCI is the preferred intervention, and healthcare systems have developed programs to provide PCI either within their respective facility or through a collaborative agreement with a tertiary care facility that can provide rapid access to PCI. Fibrinolytic therapy is considered if in a remote location without the ability to provide PCI or if there is a delay in transport to a tertiary center.

DIAGNOSTIC CRITERIA

Physical exam is the first step. Those presenting with STEMI are taken for emergent left heart catheterization (LHC); those with NSTEMI may be less urgent and typically are admitted and treated with systemic anticoagulation and guideline-directed medical therapy (GDMT). If positive enzymes, a LHC is performed; if negative, a stress test may be considered. In an asymptomatic or mildly symptomatic patient, objective evidence of a moderate to large area of viable myocardium or moderate to severe ischemia on noninvasive testing is an indication for PCI.

Needed labs include cardiac enzymes. (See "Acute Coronary Syndrome" section.) EKGs are trended. Stress testing may be performed.

TREATMENT/MANAGEMENT

Systemic anticoagulation therapy includes either heparin or enoxaparin sodium (Lovenox), a high-intensity statin, and DAPT. Beta blockade should be considered unless contraindicated by bradycardia, heart block, or cardiogenic shock.

FIBRINOLYTIC THERAPY

Fibrinolytic therapy or thrombolysis includes lysis of intracoronary thrombus with "clot busting" medication. Recombinant tissue-type plasminogen activator (alteplase, tPA), reteplase (rPA), and tenecteplase (TNK-tPA) are all fibrinolytic drugs that act by stimulating the natural fibrinolytic mechanism. Current guidelines recommend use of fibrinolytic therapy for ACS if symptoms have begun within 12 hours of presentation and PCI is not available within 120 minutes of first medical contact in patients with no contraindications for thrombolytics. The greatest benefit from fibrinolytics is when they are administered within 2 to 3 hours after initial symptoms. Attempts to start should occur within 10 minutes of diagnosis.

PERCUTANEOUS CORONARY INTERVENTION

PCI or *angioplasty* is described as enlargement of the vessel lumen through compression. PCI is accomplished primarily by balloon catheters, atherectomy, and intracoronary stents. Atherectomy devices permit drilling or grinding of the atheroma and calcium. Aspiration thrombectomy extracts thrombus or provides distal embolic protection during PCI.

Current stents include bare metal stent (BMS) and drug-eluting stent (DES):

- BMSs are used for patients with a high bleeding risk who are unable to be treated with DAPT or likely to undergo invasive or surgical procedures within the next year.
- DES contains a polymer coating with an antiproliferative drug that reduces restenosis. The second-generation DESs are currently used in the United States and have more favorable outcomes with lower need for target vessel revascularization. DAPT therapy is necessary post placement to prevent in-stent restenosis.

Intravascular ultrasound (IVUS) was developed to provide intraluminal information including level of plaque, degree of luminal narrowing, and vessel wall integrity. It is used to evaluate stent deployment and indeterminate lesion assessment. Intracoronary Doppler pressures are used to estimate lesion severity. Fractional flow ratio (FFR) is obtained, comparing pressure distal to a lesion to determine if there is hemodynamic significance. In an angiographically intermediate (40%–70%) stenosis, an FFR lower than 0.80 is consistent with hemodynamic or ischemic significance, indicating higher need for intervention. Both IVUS and FFR assist in decision-making for nonculprit lesions or staged interventions with multivessel disease.

MEDICATIONS

Medication management also includes DAPT, which reduces the risk of in-stent restenosis and further ischemic events. Current guideline recommendations are for DAPT for a 1-year duration. Historically, DAPT has been continued for 12 months with BMS and first-generation DES. With the newer second-generation stents, holding or stopping DAPT earlier may be considered if bleeding is encountered or if there is need for other interventions with a high risk of bleeding (Table 9.4).

Table 9.4 DAPT Options

Drug	Loading Dose	Maintenance Dose
Aspirin	325 mg	81 mg daily
P2Y12 receptor inhibitors	Clopidogrel: 300 or 600 mg Prasugrel: 60 mg Ticagrelor: 180 mg	Clopidogrel: 75 mg daily Prasugrel: 10 mg daily Ticagrelor: 90 mg twice daily

DAPT, dual antiplatelet therapy.

GPIIb-IIIa inhibitors such as abciximab, tirofiban, and eptifibatide were used with aspirin prior to P2Y12 inhibitors to prevent thrombotic complications. They inhibit GPIIb-IIIa receptors, which bind fibrinogen and mediate platelet aggregation. They may be used short term immediately after the procedure if a large burden of thrombus is present, there is distal occlusion of small vessels, or there is inadequate P2Y12 loading prior to the procedure. Due to an increased risk of bleeding, these agents have largely been removed as standard treatment with PCI.

COMPLICATIONS

Complications of fibrinolytic therapy include increased risk of bleeding and stroke. Hemorrhage is most frequently associated with the gastrointestinal tract followed by intracerebral hemorrhage (ICH). Postprocedure care includes baseline EKG following the procedure, frequent VS and vascular exams, and evaluation of the access site immediately after completion. A new thrill or bruit raises concern for pseudoaneurysm and requires ultrasound evaluation. Complications of PCI are listed in Table 9.5.

Table 9.5 Complications of PCI

Complications		
Dissection/perforation	Hemorrhage	Stroke
Thrombosis	Hematoma	Contrast-induced nephropathy
Vasospasm	Pseudoaneurysm	Anaphylaxis to contrast
Restenosis	AV fistula	Thrombosis
In-stent thrombosis	Dissections	Coronary vasospasm

AV, arteriovenous; PCI, percutaneous coronary intervention.

▶ SURGICAL INTERVENTIONS

CORONARY ARTERY BYPASS GRAFTING

OVERVIEW

Coronary artery bypass grafting (CABG) is used to revascularize narrowed or occluded coronary arteries and to restore reperfusion to the myocardium. The surgery involves one of two approaches, either the "on pump" method, which uses a cardiopulmonary bypass (CPB) machine to circulate the blood while the patient's own heart is in cardiac arrest, or the "off pump" method where the heart continues to contract.

The Society of Thoracic Surgeons (STS) score should be calculated for risk stratification of mortality and morbidity, and to assist in shared decision-making. There are several indications and considerations for patients undergoing CABG (Box 9.1).

Box 9.1 Indications and Considerations for CABG

Indications for CABG include but are not limited to:
- people with DM and triple vessel disease or involvement of the LAD
- CAD of the left main artery
- previous CABG, with angina refractory to GDMT and involving the LAD

CABG, coronary artery bypass grafting; CAD, coronary artery disease; GDMT, guideline-directed medical therapy; LAD, left anterior descending.

At the outset of the surgery, the patient is sedated and intubated. A radial arterial line for accurate BP monitoring may be placed along with a large-bore central line, and sometimes a pulmonary artery catheter is placed in the internal jugular vein. These assist with administration of medications, blood products, venous sampling, and management of hemodynamics during and after the surgery.

The chest is prepped and opened via an incision known as a median sternotomy. Anticoagulation is given to allow for the patient to be placed on CPB in an "on pump" procedure. The aorta and the heart are then cannulated and bypassed to allow continuous circulation of blood during the procedure. After being placed on the CPB, cardioplegia is then induced. This involves the use of a potassium-rich solution and may also involve the physical cooling of the heart itself with an iced slush to induce cardiac arrest. The culprit vessels are then surgically bypassed using either vein or arterial grafts, and sometimes a combination of both. Examples of grafts commonly used in CABG include the saphenous veins and arteries like the left internal mammary artery (LIMA), right internal mammary artery (RIMA), and radial artery. The grafts are attached by the surgeon distal to the site of coronary narrowing or blockage and then brought up to be attached at the aorta, creating an alternate pathway around the lesion, and restoring blood flow to the ischemic area. Once the grafts have been placed, the potassium solution is drained, and the heart will begin to contract. The sternum is then closed and secured using sternal wires, and the soft tissues of the chest are closed.

Other devices support the recovery of the patient including chest and mediastinal tubes that are placed to drain blood and serous fluid to keep from accumulating in the pleural and mediastinal spaces. Retained clot in the pericardial sac can cause cardiac tamponade. Temporary pacemaker wires are inserted directly through the chest wall to the pericardium in the event bradyarrhythmia or high-grade heart blocks develop. Patients often remain intubated after CABG for management, recovery, and extubation by the ICU team.

COMPLICATIONS

CABG is a major surgery and thus has a variety of expected postoperative issues that may arise. Patients commonly experience brief periods of hemodynamic instability immediately postoperatively. Intravenous fluid (IVF) boluses, vasopressors, and/or inotropes may be required to support recovery. Hypotension can be managed with boluses or vasopressors depending on the hemodynamic parameters. Pulmonary artery catheters are commonly used; thus, the AGACNP must be able to interpret results and recognize cardiogenic shock and cardiac tamponade. (See Chapter 19.) Electrolyte imbalances must be aggressively managed to prevent arrhythmias and cardiac arrest. Atelectasis is the most common complication after CABG; thus, early mobility and use of incentive spirometer are key. The AGACNP must also be alert to the presence of life-threatening bleeding from vascular anastomoses, the presence of coagulopathy, cardiogenic shock, and heart block. Additional complications include MI, stroke, prolonged need for mechanical ventilation, acute kidney injury, bleeding requiring transfusion and/or reoperation, wound infection, and death.

TRANSCATHETER AORTIC VALVE REPLACEMENT
OVERVIEW

Transcatheter aortic valve replacement (TAVR) is a minimally invasive surgical option for patients with severe or critical aortic stenosis who would benefit from an aortic valve replacement. This is a suitable option for any patient who requires an aortic valve replacement but is a safer option, particularly for patients who are at moderate to high surgical risk and an STS score with a predicted mortality of 3% or greater.

The procedure is completed with a flexible catheter in the arterial system to reach the heart and aortic valve. The most common approach/access is transfemoral. It is possible for patients to be discharged within 24 to 48 hours after the procedure depending on patient-specific characteristics and needs.

COMPLICATIONS

AGACNPs must be able to recognize postprocedural complications, which include cardiac conduction disturbances, stroke, paravalvular leak, bleeding, annular rupture, aortic dissection, left ventricular perforation, cardiac tamponade, access site hematoma or pseudoaneurysm, MI, infection, and death.

▶ CARDIOMYOPATHIES: HYPERTROPHIC, DILATED, IDIOPATHIC, RESTRICTIVE

DISEASE OVERVIEW

The cardiomyopathies are a group of illnesses that affect the myocardium; this group includes hypertrophic, dilated, idiopathic, and restrictive cardiomyopathies. While their etiologies are varied, all result in impaired cardiac function and can ultimately result in HF if not treated.

HYPERTROPHIC CARDIOMYOPATHY

Hypertrophic cardiomyopathy (HCM) is an inherited disease characterized by hypertrophy/thickening of the left ventricle, which impairs cardiac contractility and eventually results in obstruction of flow from the left ventricle (LV) to the rest of the body. As HCM progresses, diastolic dysfunction, mitral regurgitation, and ischemia develop. It is the most common cardiomyopathy and occurs more often in men, typically presenting in people in their 30s. It is associated with sudden cardiac death sometimes occurring in athletes during exertion.

IDIOPATHIC DILATED CARDIOMYOPATHY

Idiopathic dilated cardiomyopathy (IDCM) is a progressive disease that occurs when one or both ventricles become enlarged impairing their contractility and resulting in a decrease in their ability to eject blood. Genetics plays a role, and up to 50% of family members of someone diagnosed with IDCM will have an associated gene mutation. Despite this, IDCM is usually idiopathic or due to secondary causes including myocarditis, alcohol abuse, cocaine, medication effects, HIV, and infiltrative disease. IDCM is more common in men and is the leading cause of heart transplant. It commonly presents with arrhythmia and may result in sudden cardiac death.

RESTRICTIVE CARDIOMYOPATHY

Restrictive cardiomyopathy (RCM) is the least common among the cardiomyopathies and is related to multiple pathologies including radiation, some medications, infiltrative processes, malignancy, and inherited storage diseases, among others. All etiologies result in diastolic dysfunction and stiffening of the ventricular walls with atrial dilation. The most common causes of RCM are the infiltrative diseases amyloidosis and sarcoidosis, and the storage disorder hemochromatosis. RCM has the poorest prognosis of all the cardiomyopathies, with most cases being fatal.

CLASSIC PRESENTATION

An AGACNP is volunteering at the medical tent during an annual soccer championship when medics approach carrying an unconscious patient on a stretcher. The patient is an otherwise healthy-appearing man in his mid-thirties without overt signs of illness. The medics report that he had been playing soccer on the field when he suddenly collapsed and was unresponsive. The AGACNP notes that he is apneic and pulseless. Subsequently, the AGACNP calls for the automated external defibrillator and begins CPR for presumed sudden cardiac death.

DIAGNOSTIC CRITERIA

Symptoms and exam vary between types of cardiomyopathies. Diagnostic workup is aimed at differentiating between the types of cardiomyopathies. All types of cardiomyopathies require an EKG and echocardiogram.

HYPERTROPHIC CARDIOMYOPATHY

Most people have no symptoms of hypertrophic cardiomyopathy. When present, they may complain of fatigue, dyspnea, chest pain on exertion, and syncope. A double apical impulse, prominent A wave in jugular venous pulsation (JVP), double carotid pulse, or systolic ejection murmur may be present.

IDIOPATHIC DILATED CARDIOMYOPATHY

Idiopathic dilated cardiomyopathy is nonspecific and similar to other causes of cardiomyopathy resulting in HF (crackles, jugular venous distention [JVD], S3, elevated JVP, lateral displacement of PMI). Orthopnea, bilateral LE edema, paroxysmal nocturnal dyspnea, and shortness of breath may also be present.

RESTRICTIVE CARDIOMYOPATHY

RCM has poor exercise tolerance, atrial fibrillation (AF), S4, and Kussmaul's sign. Manifestations of underlying amyloidosis (carpal tunnel), sarcoidosis (bilateral hilar infiltrates), or bronze skin and arthralgias associated with hemochromatosis may be present.

DIAGNOSTIC TESTING

EKG can assess for LVH, ST abnormalities, T-wave inversion, and presence of Q waves. Echocardiogram is diagnostic for the cardiomyopathies and helps to distinguish them from one another. Exercise stress testing is useful to evaluate symptoms and monitor response to therapy. Cardiac magnetic resonance (CMR) imaging can produce three-dimensional images that can provide detailed description of HCM and can aid in diagnosing phenotypes and offering prognostic information.In patients with RCM, thyroid function, electrolytes, HIV serology, and iron studies are useful to differentiate the etiology of RCM. An endomyocardial biopsy or aspirate is definitive to diagnose cardiac amyloidosis in RCM.

TREATMENT/MANAGEMENT
HYPERTROPHIC CARDIOMYOPATHY

Conservative management includes avoiding hypovolemia and pursing weight loss if indicated. Strenuous exercise is discouraged. If symptoms are present, these may be treated with negative inotropes: beta-blockers, nondihydropyridine CCBs, and disopyramide. Other interventions include myomectomy, mitral valve replacement, and septal ablation with alcohol. Use diuretics with extreme caution in patients with HCM as they may result in volume depletion and decreased stroke volume, which worsens left ventricular outflow tract (LVOT) obstruction and precipitate hypotension. Many people with HCM are asymptomatic and may present initially with arrhythmia-induced sudden cardiac death.

IDIOPATHIC DILATED CARDIOMYOPATHY

Treatment addresses HF symptoms with recommended medications and is aimed at preventing/treating arrhythmia, which may include an automatic implantable cardioverter defibrillator (AICD) or biventricular pacemaker (PM). Patients may benefit from a left ventricular assistance device (LVAD) or be candidates for heart transplantation.

RESTRICTIVE CARDIOMYOPATHY

Treat the underlying cause of HF. Antiarrhythmics are indicated if sarcoidosis is the etiology, along with corticosteroids. Therapeutic phlebotomy is used when hemochromatosis is present.

COMPLICATIONS

Complications of all types of cardiomyopathies include HF, arrhythmia, stroke, and sudden cardiac death.

▶ HEART FAILURE

DISEASE OVERVIEW

Heart failure is a syndrome characterized by the inability of the heart to meet the metabolic needs of the body. Its causes are varied, ranging from structural defects involving the heart tissue (valvular disease, hypertrophic cardiomyopathy), to the sequelae of acquired illnesses (CAD, HTN, pulmonary arterial hypertension [PAH]), and autoimmune conditions (amyloid). HF may begin abruptly (in the presence of acute MI or hypertensive emergency) or develop slowly as the consequence of another chronic disease/illness (amyloid, HTN). HF is considered a life-long chronic relapsing pathology with a poor overall prognosis. HF can be characterized as systolic (heart failure with reduced ejection fraction [HFrEF]), indicating an inability of the heart to contract appropriately, or diastolic (heart failure with preserved ejection fraction [HFpEF]), which is associated with the inability of the LV to fully relax and fill.

CLASSIC PRESENTATION

A 62-year-old male patient presents with a history significant for metabolic syndrome, coronary artery disease, STEMI × 2 with DES to his RCA and LAD, HFrEF, and HTN. His most recent MI occurred last year, and on discharge home, echocardiogram revealed an ejection fraction (EF) of 35%. Today, he reports that he has noticed an increased weight gain of 7 lb this week, worsened LE edema, and increased abdominal girth. He is now sleeping sitting up in his recliner due to orthopnea. He is comfortable only at rest. On exam, the AGACNP notes that he has crackles throughout, his JVP is measured at 14 cm above the angle of Louis. He has positive hepatojugular reflux. He is tachycardic with an oxygen saturation of 88%, and his BP is 94/50. The AGACNP assesses him as being New York Heart Association (NYHA) classification III and Stevenson classification of warm and wet.

DIAGNOSTIC CRITERIA

Diagnostic criteria include shortness of breath, pulmonary edema, LE edema, anasarca, abdominal edema, positive hepatojugular reflux, and engorged jugular veins with an elevated JVP. Subjective complaints of weight gain, exercise intolerance, fatigue, anorexia, and orthopnea may be present. The patient's functional status can be classified by the NYHA Functional Classifications system (Table 9.6).

Table 9.6 New York Heart Association Functional Classification

Class	Description
NYHA Class I	Normal functional status, ordinary physical activity without symptoms
NYHA Class II	Mild symptoms with activity, none at rest, slight limitations
NYHA Class III	Moderate symptoms with less than normal activity, comfortable only at rest, marked limitations
NYHA Class IV	Severe symptoms, any activity results in discomfort, severe functional limitations

NYHA, New York Heart Association.

DIAGNOSTIC TESTING

Obtain BNP, cardiac enzymes, CBC, BMP, thyroid function tests, HbA1C, lipids, iron studies. Transthoracic echocardiogram, EKG, chest x-ray (CXR).

TREATMENT/MANAGEMENT

HF treatment is guided by the current EF, the NYHA classification (see Table 9.6), and the Stevenson classification. These assessments provide important information about real-time symptoms and functional status. While no medications have been shown to reduce morbidity or mortality in those with HFpEF, a treatment strategy aimed at reducing volume overload and ameliorating symptoms should be targeted. Early palliative care consult has been shown to reduce readmission and improve quality of life for patients with HF.

DIASTOLIC HEART FAILURE/HEART FAILURE WITH PRESERVED EJECTION FRACTION

EF is greater than 50%. No current therapies have proven to reduce morbidity and mortality in this group of patients. If there is evidence of volume overload, this should be treated with diuretics. If the BNP is elevated, a sodium-glucose cotransporter-2 (SGLT2) inhibitor may be added followed by a mineralocorticoid receptor antagonist (MRA). Both medications decrease rehospitalization and improve quality of life.

HEART FAILURE WITH MILDLY REDUCED EJECTION FRACTIONS (HFMREF)

EF is 41% to 49%. Diuretics are recommended. Other medications that may be considered include an ACEI, ARB, beta-blockers, MRAs, and sacubitril/valsartan (Entresto).

HEART FAILURE WITH REDUCED EJECTION FRACTION

EF is less than 40%. It is treated with GDMT, which includes an MRA, beta-blocker, sodium-glucose cotransporter-1 (SLGT-I), ACEI, or angiotensin receptor-neprilysin inhibitor (ARNI) and loop diuretics. An AICD is also indicated for those patients with an EF less than 20% due to the risk of sudden cardiac death. Other options include cardiac resynchronization therapy (CRT).

▶ MECHANICAL CIRCULATORY SUPPORT

OVERVIEW

Cardiogenic shock and severe cases of HF may require additional supportive therapies, referred to collectively as mechanical support devices, to prevent death. Mechanical support devices include intra-aortic balloon pump (IABP) counterpulsation, intravascular microaxial blood pump, ventricular assistance device (VAD), and extracorporeal membrane oxygenation (ECMO). ECMO can also be used for severe cases of hypoxic respiratory failure.

INTRA-AORTIC BALLOON PUMP

An IABP is a mechanical circulatory support device that helps the heart by decreasing afterload and augmenting diastolic aortic pressure resulting in better perfusion to peripheral organs and improvement in coronary blood flow. Indications for placement of an IABP include acute HF exacerbation with hypotension, prophylactic or adjunctive treatment in high-risk PCI, MI with reduced left ventricular function and hypotension, MI with cardiogenic shock, or low cardiac output post CABG. IABPs are contraindicated with uncontrolled infection or bleeding diathesis, moderate to severe aortic regurgitation, aortic aneurysm, or dissection.

Complications of IABP include bleeding from insertion site, balloon rupture, limb ischemia from thrombosis or emboli, aortic dissection, renal failure and/or bowel ischemia, stroke, heparin-induced thrombocytopenia (HIT), and infection.

INTRAVASCULAR MICROAXIAL BLOOD PUMP

The intravascular microaxial blood pump, also known as an Impella device, is a percutaneous catheter-based, miniature pump to assist the LV to pump blood from the LV into the ascending aorta and into systemic circulation. An Impella can augment cardiac output at a flow between 2.5 and 5.0 L/min.

VENTRICULAR ASSIST DEVICE

A VAD is a pump that supports selected patients with HF (Table 9.7). A VAD can be implanted into the LV (LVAD), right ventricle (RVAD), or both ventricles (biventricular; BiVAD). Approximately a third of patients who are placed on LVAD develop right ventricle failure. Thus, the addition of an RVAD to support the right ventricle improves survival rates and has fewer adverse events, leading to increased hospital discharges.

Table 9.7 LVAD Indications and Contraindications

LVAD	
Indications	Eligible for VAD when if despite optimal pharmacotherapy and electrotherapy symptoms persist for 2 or more months and patient has two or more of the following: ■ three or more HR exacerbations requiring hospitalization in the last 12 months ■ necessity of using IV positive inotropes ■ significant impairment of LVEF (less than 25%) and VO_2max < 12 mL/kg b.w./min ■ kidney or liver impairment form perfusions disturbance from low cardiac output (CO) ■ progressive impairment of right ventricular function These hemodynamic parameters constitute criteria for VAD: ■ systolic arterial BP less than 80 mmHg ■ cardiac index less than 2 L/min/m² ■ central venous pressure greater than 20 mmHg ■ pulmonary wedge pressure greater than 20 mmHg
Absolute Contraindications	■ Irreversible injury to the central nervous system ■ Generalized neoplastic disease
Relative Contraindications	■ Severe organ lesions and infections refractory to treatment

BP, blood pressure; CO, cardiac output; HR, heart rate; IV, intravenous; LVAD, left ventricular assist device; LVEF, left ventricular ejection fraction; VAD, ventricular assist device.

VAD therapies are most commonly utilized as temporary therapies as a bridge to transplant, decision, or recovery, or can be destination therapy. Bridge to transplant is intended to provide circulatory support to a transplant-eligible patient awaiting a donor. The bridge to decision application of a VAD, for patients with relative contraindications to transplant, is to attempt to stabilize hemodynamics, improve renal function, nutritional status, or pulmonary HTN to get a patient to a transplant-eligible status. Bridge to recovery is temporary support in select HF patients to allow time for myocardial function to improve and recover. Finally, VADs can be used as destination therapy, such that an ineligible transplant patient receives a VAD knowing transplant is not an option.

EXTRACORPOREAL MEMBRANE OXYGENATION

Adult ECMO is also referred to as extracorporeal life support (ECLS). ECMO therapy is defined as the use of mechanical circulatory support (MCS) where a pump in combination with an oxygenator are used to achieve extended (hours to weeks) but temporary support of heart and/or lung function. This is a lifesaving, temporary supportive therapy and NOT a disease-modifying treatment. ECMO therapy can be used as a bridge to decision, recovery, short-term/long-term MCS, and/or transplant. Indications for ECMO therapy include viable patients with potentially reversible acute heart and/or lung failure with high mortality risk despite optimal conventional therapy. ECMO can be used to support pulmonary, cardiac, or cardiopulmonary dysfunction. Different configurations of ECMO exist, depending on the clinical indication for therapy, including respiratory failure, cardiac failure, or both.

Adult Respiratory Indications for Extracorporeal Membrane Oxygenation Therapy

Respiratory indications for ECMO include a high predicted risk of mortality that is unresponsive to optimal conventional therapies. The most common indication for ECMO is acute respiratory distress syndrome (ARDS). Mortality risk is calculated based on the Murray lung injury score (Table 9.8).

For acute hypoxemic respiratory failure, ECMO is considered at 50% predicted mortality risk and is indicated at 80% risk:

■ 50% mortality risk is associated with a PaO_2/FIO_2 less than 150 on FIO_2 greater than 0.9 and/or Murray Lung Injury Score 2 to 3.
■ 80% mortality risk is associated with a PaO_2/FIO_2 less than 100 on FIO_2 greater than 0.9 and/or Murray Lung Injury Score ≥3.

Table 9.8 Murray Lung Injury Score

Parameter	Possible Points					Patient Points
	0	1	2	3	4	
P/F ratio	300	225–299	175–224	100–174	Less than 100	
PEEP (cmH$_2$O)	5	6–8	9–11	12–14	15	
Infiltrate(s) on CXR (number of quadrants)	none	1	2	3	4	
Compliance (mL/cmH$_2$O)	80	60–79	40–59	20–39	Less than 20	
Total Points:						
Total points/number of categories = Score						
Interpretation: Murray score range: 0 and 4. To obtain score: divide the total points by the number of criteria scored (e.g., if three criteria are answered, the total sum of points is divided by three to obtain the final score). 0 points: no lung injury; 1 to 2.5 points: mild to moderate lung injury; ≥3 (≥2.5 with rapid deterioration) points indicate severe lung injury and is an indication for ECMO.						

CXR, chest x-ray; ECMO, extracorporeal membrane oxygenation; P/F, PaO$_2$/FIO$_2$; PEEP, positive end-expiratory pressure.
Source: Modified from Hong Kong Society of Critical Care Medicine. (2010, March 20). *Murray score calculator.* https://www.hksccm.org/index.php/professional/useful-resources/70-respiratory-medicine-and-thoracic-surgery/1444-2010-mar-20-murray-score-calculator

For acute hypercapnic respiratory failure:

■ pH less than 7.20 despite best-practice ventilatory strategies

A combination of both acute hypoxic and hypercapnic respiratory failure is also considered for ECMO.

Adult Cardiac Indications for Extracorporeal Membrane Oxygenation Therapy

Several etiologies contribute to cardiac indications for ECMO (Box 9.2). Indications for cardiac ECMO include refractory cardiogenic shock and refractory cardiac arrest. Refractory cardiogenic shock is defined as cardiogenic shock requiring more than two vasoactive drugs with escalating care or mechanical support with more than one vasoactive drugs and escalating care. Refractory cardiac arrest is defined as no return of spontaneous circulation (ROSC) within 10 minutes, end-tidal carbon dioxide (ETCO$_2$) greater than 20, and ECMO CPR. Additional indications for ECMO include a bridge to recovery, device placement, or cardiac transplant.

Box 9.2 Etiologies of Adult Cardiac Diseases Supported With ECMO

Postcardiotomy cardiogenic shock/inability to wean from CPB
Preoperative support
Acute myocarditis
Decompensated cardiomyopathy: dilated, hypertrophic, restrictive
Ischemic cardiogenic shock
Massive PE
Acute graft failure after heart transplantation
Peripartum cardiomyopathy
Severe pulmonary HTN
Arrhythmias
Anaphylactic shock
Sepsis with profound cardiac depression
Accidental hypothermia
Medication overdose with potential for reversal

CBP, cardiopulmonary bypass; ECMO, extracorporeal membrane oxygenation; HTN, hypertension; PE, pulmonary embolism.

Contraindications for Extracorporeal Membrane Oxygenation Therapy

Most contraindications are relative, and each patient case should be considered uniquely by the multidisciplinary team. Contraindications include, but are not limited to, those in Box 9.3.

Box 9.3 Contraindications to Adult ECMO Therapy

Irreversible cardiac and/or respiratory conditions when patient is not a transplant candidate
Uncontrolled bleed or contraindication to anticoagulation therapy
Patient too large or too small for adequate vessel cannulation
Significant irreversible end-stage neurological disorder
Futility (end-stage malignancy or terminal diagnosis)
Patient and/or family directives limit escalation of invasive therapy
Brain death

ECMO, extracorporeal membrane oxygenation.

ECMO Configurations

ECMO configurations depend on the need for veno-venous (VV ECMO), veno-arterial (VA ECMO), or veno-arterial-venous ECMO. The type of configuration will also determine whether peripheral or central cannulation is needed and whether single cannula or multiple cannulas are needed. An understanding of adult vasculature and blood flow through the heart is critical in understanding ECMO physiology. In an ECMO, circuit blood is drained from the patient to an external pump. The external pump sends the blood through a membrane oxygenator where gas is exchanged, blood is oxygenated, and CO_2 is removed. The blood can be warmed or cooled by the circuit and is then returned to the patient. Additionally, ventricular assistance (LVAD, RVAD, or BiVAD) may be needed to support a failing ventricle.

Veno-Venous Extracorporeal Membrane Oxygenation Scheme

VV ECMO drains the venous system and returns oxygenated blood to the venous system. Critically ill patients in severe respiratory failure are at risk for right ventricular (RV) failure in the setting of increased pulmonary vascular resistance as well as biventricular failure.

Peripheral veno-venous cannulation uses a short cannula via the left femoral vein that drains the inferior vena cava (IVC) to the blood pump and then the oxygenator. Oxygenated blood is returned to the right atrium (RA) via a long right femoral cannula. The most common peripheral veno-venous cannulation scheme is where blood is drained via the right femoral cannula in the IVC, sent to the blood pump, then oxygenator and oxygenated blood is returned via a cannula in the right internal jugular vein. Alternatively, a single bicaval dual lumen cannula can be placed under fluoro and echo guidance. The single cannula is placed in the right internal jugular vein and drains blood from the superior vena cava (SVC) and IVC simultaneously to the blood pump and oxygenator and has an outflow port that delivers oxygenated blood directly to the RA. This single cannula is only used for VV ECMO therapy. VV ECMO does not typically have a central cannulation scheme.

Veno-Arterial Extracorporeal Membrane Oxygenation Scheme

VA ECMO provides complete cardiovascular support. VA ECMO drains the venous system and returns oxygenated blood to the arterial system. Deoxygenated blood is taken from the venous system (femoral vein, internal jugular, or RA). Oxygenated blood is returned to the arterial system (femoral, axillary, or subclavian artery, aorta). The goal is cardiac and respiratory rest.

Configurations: In VA ECMO, there can be either peripheral or central cannulation, both of which require multiple cannulas:

- Peripheral veno-arterial cannulation includes a drainage cannula via the right femoral vein that drains the IVC, sends the blood to the blood pump and then the oxygenator, and returns oxygenated blood via the right common femoral artery.
- In central cannulation, cannulas are surgically implanted and drain the RA to the blood pump and then the oxygenator and returns oxygenated blood to the ascending aorta. These cannulas are sutured directly onto the RA and aorta. Alternatively, a peripheral axillary configuration drains the

blood from the RA via the right internal jugular (RIJ), is sent to the blood pump and oxygenator, and returns blood to the right axillary artery.

The VA ECMO setup has two situations that require special consideration.

■ A weak, poorly contracting LV may be unable to unload the blood that reaches the left ventricle. Coupled with increased afterload from an antegrade flow of blood to the aorta by the ECMO circuit, left ventricular distention and stasis of blood increases the risk of myocardial ischemia, pulmonary edema, and thrombus formation. Thus, the LV can be "vented" by using either an IABP or a percutaneous LVAD.

■ Distal perfusion of the extremity where the femoral arterial cannulas are placed may become impaired causing limb ischemia. Specific cannulas can be used to create a vascular conduit into the superficial femoral artery to avoid the obstruction of distal arterial blood flow by the ECMO cannula and ensure perfusion of the limb. This requires pedal saturation monitoring, therapeutic anticoagulation, hourly monitoring of circulation, motor, and sensation, as well as monitoring the thigh and calf compartment for increased fullness and pain.

Veno-Arterial-Venous Extracorporeal Membrane Oxygenation Scheme
In veno-arterial-venous ECMO, an uncommon cannulation scheme occurs when a third cannula is added to the circuit for additional oxygen delivery. In VA ECMO, a cannula is added if additional oxygen delivery to the head vessels is needed. In VV ECMO, it is added if the patient progresses to cardiogenic shock and needs full cardiovascular support.

COMPLICATIONS
Complications of mechanical circulatory support include bleeding, thromboembolism, coagulopathy, infection, limb ischemia, stroke, liver failure, kidney failure seizures, and death.

▶ CARDIAC TRANSPLANTATION

OVERVIEW
Heart transplant rates have been increasing since the first successful transplant in 1967 by Christiaan Barnard. In an ideal patient, a cardiac transplant can be the treatment of choice for advanced heart failure. AGACNPs must know indications for heart transplant to facilitate timely referral to a transplant center (Table 9.9). Cardiac transplantation has contraindications, which include advanced irreversible renal, liver, pulmonary disease (forced expiratory volume in first 1 second [FEV_1] less than 1 L/min), PAH, and a history of solid organ or hematologic malignancy within 5 years.

Table 9.9 Indications for Cardiac Transplant

Refractory cardiogenic shock requiring IABP or LVAD
Cardiogenic shock requiring continuous intravenous inotropic therapy
Peak VO_2 (VO_2max) less than 10 mL/kg per min
NYHA class III or IV heart failure, despite maximized medical and resynchronization therapy
Recurrent, life-threatening left ventricular arrhythmias despite an AICD, antiarrhythmic therapy, or catheter-based ablation
End-stage congenital HF with no evidence of pulmonary HTN
Refractory angina without potential medical or surgical therapeutic options

AICD, implantable cardiac defibrillator; HF, heart failure; HTN, hypertension; IABP, intra-aortic balloon pump; LVAD, left ventricular assistance device; NYHA, New York Heart Association; VO_2, oxygen consumption; VO_2max, maximum oxygen consumption.

COMPLICATIONS
Complications include primary graft dysfunction, rejection, cardiac allograft vasculopathy, infection, chronic kidney disease, and malignancy.

▶ STRUCTURAL HEART DISORDERS

DISEASE OVERVIEW

Structural heart defects occur in various sizes and may be small and asymptomatic and are often not repaired; those that are moderate to large size with symptoms are monitored and more often require repair. They include atrial septal defects, ventricular septal defects (VSDs), and patent ductus arteriosus (PDA).

ATRIAL SEPTAL DEFECT

An *atrial septal defect* (ASD) is a communication between the right and left atrium. They can occur in conjunction with other congenital anomalies or in isolation. Long-term issues include right HF, atrial arrhythmias, and PAH. Shunting of blood from the left atrium (LA) to the RA causes right-sided heart enlargement and RV dysfunction over time. They may be asymptomatic if size is small; moderate to larger defects may develop symptoms that include dyspnea, fatigue, right HF, and atrial arrhythmia. Physical exam findings include fixed split-second heart sound and systolic murmur in the pulmonic area. Diagnostic testing includes EKG, CXR, and echocardiogram. Treatment depends on the size and age at diagnosis. Closure may be done surgically or percutaneously. Complications include PAH.

VENTRICULAR SEPTAL DEFECT

Physical exam reveals a holosystolic murmur. Larger VSDs may present with dyspnea, exercise intolerance, and cyanosis. Diagnostics include EKG that may reveal biventricular hypertrophy and echocardiogram. Treatment of VSD is based on size; small VSDs may be monitored over time without intervention. Moderate to large VSDs can be treated with surgical or transcatheter closure.

PATENT DUCTUS ARTERIOSUS

PDA is a fetal connection between the aorta and pulmonary artery that normally closes shortly after birth. Moderate to large PDAs will present with exercise intolerance, dyspnea, and atrial arrhythmias. Treatment includes catheter, or surgical closure is indicated if there is left-sided hypertrophy.

ARRHYTHMOGENIC RIGHT VENTRICULAR CARDIOMYOPATHY

Arrhythmogenic right ventricular cardiomyopathy (ARVC) is an inherited disease with fibrous or fibrofatty myocardium with global hypertrophy leading to ventricular arrhythmias. Physical exam reveals palpitation, syncope, chest pain, dyspnea, and HF.

▶ CONGENITAL HEART DISEASE

DISEASE OVERVIEW

Adult *congenital heart disease* (CHD) encompasses several structural abnormalities that are present at birth. While these may be diagnosed in utero, or shortly thereafter, some patients may not receive a diagnosis until adulthood. Common defects include tetralogy of Fallot, VSD, ASD, and bicuspid aortic valve. CHD is a chronic disease that has implications for the person throughout their life. These include the need for repeated interventions, ongoing medication, development of HTN, increased risk for endocarditis, pregnancy complications, and reduced life expectancy.

DIAGNOSTIC CRITERIA

Subjectively, patients may report palpitations and exercise intolerance. Heart murmur may be auscultated. There may be lateral displacement of the PMI in LVH. Crackles are found in the lung fields or there is elevated JVP. The exam is focused on identifying new signs that may indicate development of heart failure. Obtain a BNP to assess for development of heart failure. Elevations of C-reactive protein (CRP) are associated with poorer outcomes. Evaluation of cardiac size, pressures, and function is key. While echocardiogram is the primary diagnostic utilized, CXR, and cardiac MRI are also beneficial. Cardiopulmonary exercise testing (CPET) is also used to provide insight into a patient's functional abilities.

TREATMENT/MANAGEMENT

Treatment strategies vary based on the type of CHD present and may include both surgical and pharmacologic interventions. One important feature of the treatment of CHD patients is a focus on improving functional capacity and maintaining quality of life. Development of PAH is one particularly problematic pathology that may be seen in those with CHD and is of special concern for patients who become pregnant. Treatment of PAH in this population is targeted at avoiding physical stress, maintaining current vaccinations, and providing social and psychological support. For a subset of patients with CHD and PAH, the outcome of pregnancy may be catastrophic. These patients should be encouraged to have open conversations with their CHD specialist to help them understand the risks and recommendations.

COMPLICATIONS

Complications of CHD include the development of HF, arrhythmia, and sudden cardiac death. All surgical procedures in those with CHD are higher risk because a delicate hemodynamic balance is required. People with CHD are at higher risk of developing infective endocarditis; therefore, patient teaching should include an emphasis on good hygiene practices including oral care, hand washing, and the discouraging of receiving tattoos and piercings.

▶ VALVULAR HEART DISEASE

DISEASE OVERVIEW

Valvular heart disease includes damage or destruction of any of the four valves leading to incompetence or narrowing. Major causes include rheumatic heart disease, congenital abnormalities, calcification, endocarditis, connective tissue disorders, or progressive HF and ischemic heart disease.

AORTIC VALVE

The tricuspid valve can develop aortic regurgitation (AR) and/or aortic stenosis (AS):

- AR results from abnormalities of the leaflets or the aortic root or both. The leaflets do not close properly resulting in regurgitation back into the ventricle during systole; this can lead to LV failure due to increased stroke volume, HTN, and increased afterload.
- AS is usually caused by degenerative calcification or progressive stenosis with a bicuspid aortic valve that has only two leaflets. This leads to reduced systemic perfusion and LV dysfunction.

PULMONIC VALVE

- Pulmonic stenosis (PS) is generally benign and may be found with other cardiac structural disease.
- Pulmonic regurgitation (PR) can lead to right ventricular overload with remodeling and deterioration.

MITRAL VALVE

Mitral valve dysfunction is most often due to leaflet disorder but also due to the structures surrounding the valve:

- Mitral regurgitation (MR) can result from leaflet dysfunction, chordae tendineae, or papillary muscle dysfunction, or LV dilation with HF, all which allow backflow of blood into the atrium and impact cardiac output.
- Mitral stenosis (MS), most often caused by rheumatic fever, results in obstruction of flow through the valve leading to increased volume and dilation of the atrium.

TRICUSPID VALVE

Tricuspid valvular disease is often related to IV drug use and endocarditis:

- Tricuspid regurgitation (TR) can occur from valvular injury from a pacemaker or implantable cardioverter-defibrillator leads.
- Tricuspid stenosis (TS) is most often caused by rheumatic heart disease.

CLASSIC PRESENTATION

Valvular abnormalities are often asymptomatic and found incidentally on noninvasive testing or diagnosed after murmur detection on physical exam. Symptoms are usually gradual and progressive and include exercise intolerance, dyspnea, arrhythmias, or HF. Syncope, angina, and HF are ominous symptoms.

DIAGNOSTIC CRITERIA

Comprehensive physical exam commonly reveals murmurs:

- *AS:* harsh crescendo-decrescendo systolic ejection murmur, is heard best R to L upper sternal boarder, may radiate to neck
- *AR:* diastolic murmur is heard best at left upper sternal border
- *MR:* harsh holosystolic murmur that may radiate to the axilla
- *MS:* apical low-pitched rumbling during diastole heard best at apex
- EKG, transthoracic echocardiogram, MRI

TREATMENT/MANAGEMENT

Treatment is based on severity of disease, which is staged as A, B, C, or D as defined in Box 9.4. Medical treatment may include medical management of HF and other comorbidities such as diabetes and HTN. Close follow-up and surveillance of symptoms and valve pathology progression are done with serial transthoracic echo (TTE) or MRI.

Box 9.4 Staging of Valvular Dysfunction

A: Risk for VSD
B: Progressive disease with moderate severity, asymptomatic
C: C1 asymptomatic/severe without ventricular decompensation; C2 asymptomatic severe with ventricular decompensation
D: Symptomatic/severe

VSD, ventricular septal defect.

The purpose of surgical treatment and transcatheter repair is to improve symptomatology, prolong survival, and minimize risk of ventricular dysfunction. Surgical treatment is based on pathology, patients' comorbidities, preoperative risk, and frailty. Surgical repair includes leaflet or cusp repair or annuloplasty with a ring reinforcement. Replacement is necessary if tissue is too damaged for repair. Mechanical versus bioprosthetic valve will dictate need for anticoagulation. Transcatheter replacement includes transcatheter aortic implantation (TAVI) and TAVR.

COMPLICATIONS

Complications include stoke, arrhythmia, wound infection, perivalvular dysfunction, and endocarditis and aortic dissection.

▶ ACUTE INFLAMMATORY DISEASE: MYOCARDITIS, ENDOCARDITIS, PERICARDITIS

DISEASE OVERVIEW

Acute inflammatory disease is a broad term to characterize inflammation of heart tissues and can be caused by bacteria, viruses, other pathogens, and even the effects of some drugs. They are classified by the cardiac tissue that is affected: myocardium, endocardium, or the pericardial sac.

MYOCARDITIS

Myocarditis is an inflammation of myocytes and primarily occurs when inflammatory cells invade the myocardium. This most commonly occurs following a viral infection, but other etiologies are also seen, including bacterial, autoimmune, protozoal, and effects of certain drugs. The COVID-19 viral infection can cause myocarditis. Left untreated, myocarditis can develop into inflammatory cardiomyopathy/dilated cardiomyopathy.

CLASSIC PRESENTATION

A 42-year-old male patient with no past medical history presents for evaluation of syncope and is noted to have new dyspnea and leg swelling. The patient has never experienced this before and states he is relatively healthy except for fever and arthralgias that the patient attributed to an upper respiratory illness 1 week prior to presenting.

DIAGNOSTIC CRITERIA

Myocarditis has a variable presentation of illness. If precipitated by a viral infection, then fatigue, fever, and malaise may be reported. There may be a history of recent upper respiratory infection. Often there are no obvious signs of myocarditis on PE. If advanced, signs/symptoms of new-onset HF may be evident.

Laboratory testing includes an erythrocyte sedimentation rate (ESR) and CRP, which will be elevated. CBC will demonstrate leukocytosis and possibly eosinophilia. Cardiac enzymes are elevated in fulminant myocarditis, but normal values do not rule out the disease.

Diagnostic testing includes EKG, echocardiogram, and endocardial biopsy. EKG commonly show sinus tachycardia with nonspecific ST-T-wave changes. Echocardiogram can show wall motion abnormalities and both systolic and/or diastolic dysfunction. Definitive diagnosis is made by endocardial biopsy.

TREATMENT/MANAGEMENT

In asymptomatic individuals, it may self-resolve; however, in severe cases, inotropic or mechanical support may be necessary. Goals of treatment involve supporting pump function and alleviating congestion. Standard heart failure treatment with beta-blockers, ACEI, diuretics, and vasodilators may be required.

COMPLICATIONS

Poor prognosis depends on whether the left ventricle is affected, HF develops, or arrhythmia are present. Atrioventricular (AV) block may develop. In some, ventricular arrhythmia and sudden cardiac death can occur.

PERICARDITIS

Pericarditis is an inflammation of the pericardial sac that surrounds the heart. As with other acute inflammatory diseases of the heart, this may be precipitated by viral or bacterial infection, autoimmune disease, or other etiologies including malignancy. Pericarditis can also co-occur with myocarditis.

CLASSIC PRESENTATION

A 63-year-old woman with recent history of "flu-like" upper respiratory illness presents complaining of acute onset anterior chest pain. She is afebrile and mildly tachycardic. On exam her lungs are clear, and she has no lymphadenopathy. A pericardial friction rub can clearly be heard across the precordium. She is hunched forward and when you ask her to sit up straight she refuses "because it hurts too much." Her discomfort is relieved by leaning forward.

DIAGNOSTIC CRITERIA

Classic findings include acute onset chest pain that is relieved by leaning forward, and the presence of a pericardial friction rub. ESR and CRP are elevated in almost 80% of cases. CBC will demonstrate leukocytosis. Cardiac enzymes should be obtained to rule out STEMI. EKG will show global concave-shaped ST elevations; PR depressions may be present on the EKG. Echocardiogram may reveal a pericardial effusion. Diagnosis is made if two of the following are present: typical chest pain, pericardial friction rub, EKG changes as described, and a new or worsening pericardial effusion.

TREATMENT/MANAGEMENT

Most cases of pericarditis in the United States are related to a viral infection. Symptoms are treated with nonsteroidal anti-inflammatory drugs (NSAIDs) and colchicine. Glucocorticoids may be substituted if NSAIDs are contraindicated.

ENDOCARDITIS

Infective endocarditis (IE) is an infection of the inner lining of the heart including the valves (the endocardium). IE may be viral, fungal, or bacterial in nature. The most common cause of bacterial endocarditis is *Staphylococcus aureus,* though other organisms including strep and enterococcus are also involved. An important group of organisms known as the HACEK group (Box 9.5) are less common but are important not to miss. These can take several weeks to grow in culture. Endocarditis may develop in those who are immunocompromised, have a history of IV drug abuse, have rheumatic heart disease, have a recently placed prosthetic valve, and have poor dentition.

Box 9.5 HACEK Organisms

H = *Hemophilus* A = *Actinobacillus* C = *Cardiobacterium* E = *Eikenella* K = *Kingella*

DIAGNOSTIC CRITERIA

Presentation is often nonspecific and commonly presents as sepsis, with a fever of unknown origin, chills, and fatigue. Physical exam may reveal a new or worsening murmur, Osler nodes, splinter hemorrhages, and Janeway lesions. CBC reveals leukocytosis and anemia. ESR and CRP will be elevated. Blood cultures will be positive.

The Modified Duke Criteria is the standard for diagnosis (Table 9.10). Two major criteria, or one major and three minor, or five minor criteria are needed to confirm the diagnosis. Major criteria include (two major): two separate blood cultures positive for one of the expected organisms without another locus of infection and positive sonographic evidence of infection (transthoracic echo [TTE] showing vegetation). The five minor criteria are (a) predisposing conditions (e.g., intravenous drug abuse [IVDA]); (b) fever greater than 38°C; (c) evidence of vascular involvement (Janeway lesions, septic infarct, ICH); (d) immunologic manifestations (Osler nodes, Roth spots); and (e) positive blood cultures of atypical infective endocarditis (IE) organisms.

Imaging for evaluation of endocarditis can include any of the following: TEE or TTE, or CT or CT/PET.

Table 9.10 Modified Duke Criteria

Major Criteria	Minor Criteria
▪ Positive blood culture for organisms known to be associated with IE (for at least two different blood cultures) ▪ Proof of endocardial involvement (mass/vegetation on TEE or TTE)	▪ IE risk factor or IVDA ▪ Fever greater than 38°C ▪ Vascular involvement (arterial emboli, ICH, Janeway lesions) ▪ Immunologic involvement (Roth's spots, Osler nodes) ▪ Blood culture positive for atypical IE organism

IE, infective endocarditis; ICH, intracerebral hemorrhage; IVDA, intravenous drug abuse; TTE, transthoracic echo.

TREATMENT/MANAGEMENT

Treatment of bacterial and fungal IE varies by organism and degree of infection, but all involve prolonged IV antibiotic regimens. Obtain infectious disease (ID) consult and two blood cultures should be drawn every 24 to 48 hours until clear. The most common reasons that valve repair/replacement may be indicated include acute HF, arterial embolization, AV block or perivalvular abscess, and mobile large valve vegetations.

COMPLICATIONS

Complications include stroke, meningitis, acute decompensated HF, septic shock, arterial emboli, empyema, pneumonia, and death.

Clinical Pearls

- People with prosthetic valves, CHD, previous endocarditis, and valvular insufficiency, and those undergoing high-risk dental procedures should receive antibiotic prophylaxis to reduce the risk of developing endocarditis.
- Antibiotic therapy should be initiated after blood cultures are obtained, not before.
- Patients with drug abuse and IE should be referred for addiction treatment/recovery and opioid substitution therapy.

▶ DYSRHYTHMIA

DISEASE OVERVIEW

Dysrhythmia refers to a group of rhythm disorders occurring within the conduction system of the heart at the cellular level of the myocardium. These range from benign as in the case of sinus arrhythmia to rapidly lethal in the setting of untreated ventricular fibrillation (VF) or pulseless electrical activity (PEA). Pathological dysrhythmias interfere with the normal cardiac conduction pathway of the heart. These may affect the heart's natural pacemaker, the rate of origin of impulse conduction, or the ability of conducted impulses to be transmitted effectively. All patients who develop dysrhythmia should be worked up for cardiac ischemia and electrolyte abnormalities. The dysrhythmias vary in presentation, diagnosis, treatment recommendations, and potential complications.

CLASSIC PRESENTATION

A 72-year-old man presents with a history significant for moderate alcohol use, CKD, and diabetes type II. During a scheduled appointment in the renal clinic, he reports that he has been feeling increasingly fatigued and is concerned about "extra heartbeats." He reports that at times he notices a fluttering in his chest and becomes light-headed. These episodes have been occurring three to four times a week and are associated with shortness of breath. He decided to take his BP with his home monitor during the latest episode, and it showed that his heart rate was 136. On exam today he has an irregular pulse, is tachycardic with a heart rate of 124, and is having five- to six-word dyspnea. His lung exam reveals scattered crackles, and he has new trace bipedal edema.

DIAGNOSTIC CRITERIA

The subjective symptoms associated with dysrhythmia are characterized by insufficient perfusion to the myocardium and the rest of the body. These may manifest as complaints of palpitations, pre-syncope, syncope, dyspnea, chest heaviness or tightness, hot flashes, or feelings of impending doom. Anginal symptoms may be present along with pallor and diaphoresis. Physical manifestations may also include alterations in pulse speed (brady or tachycardias), regularity, and strength. Patients may also report activity intolerance and fatigue.

DIAGNOSTIC TESTING

The gold standard for diagnosing dysrhythmia is the 12-lead EKG. Thyroid function tests, BMP, serum calcium, serum magnesium, and cardiac enzymes should be obtained. A loop recorder or Holter monitor may also be used in the outpatient setting.

TREATMENT/MANAGEMENT

Treatment including interventions, and medication management is highly dependent on the type of dysrhythmia present and its cause. American Heart Association (AHA) advanced cardiac life support (ACLS) algorithms should be followed. Management of underlying ischemia, and heart disease when present, and correction of abnormal electrolyte levels play a part in management of all abnormal cardiac rhythms.

TREATMENT OF SELECTED DYSRHYTHMIAS

Asystole

Asystole is the absence of electrical activity (and consequently all mechanical activity/contraction) in the heart. It is classically described as a "flat line"—incompatible with life. Asystole is cardiac arrest and is often preceded by another dysrhythmia. It holds the poorest prognosis. Treatment includes emergent administration of epinephrine and vasopressin along with high-quality CPR. Defibrillation is not indicated. During CPR, a search for potentially reversible causes must take place. These are known as the H's and T's (Table 9.11).

Table 9.11 Potentially Reversible Causes of Asystole/PEA

H's	T's
Hypoxia	Tension pneumothorax
Hydrogen ions (acidosis)	Tamponade
Hypovolemia	Toxins
Hypothermia	Thrombosis
Hypo-/hyperkalemia	

PEA, pulseless electrical activity.

Pulseless Electrical Activity

PEA occurs when an EKG demonstrates an organized electrical rhythm, but cardiac contractility is not occurring. This can be detected through the absence of peripheral pulses or a flat line on the arterial catheter monitor. This is a particularly ominous finding, and with asystole is among the dysrhythmias with the poorest prognosis. Treatment is aimed at restoring contractility and a perfusing rhythm. Epinephrine and CPR are the recommended treatment. A search for correctible causes identified by the H's and T's should be undertaken (see Table 9.11).

Ventricular Tachycardia

Ventricular tachycardia (VT) is a wide complex ventricular rhythm that can be classified as sustained (lasts more than 30 seconds or is accompanied by hemodynamic instability) or nonsustained. VT may be associated with ventricular rates of up to 200 bpm. It can also be described as monomorphic (having one QRS morphology throughout) or polymorphic as in torsades de pointes. Rapid ventricular contraction prevents adequate chamber filling, and cardiac output fails. This dysrhythmia is most commonly associated with myocardial ischemia but may also be associated with electrolyte derangements including hypomagnesemia. Treatment focuses on terminating the rhythm and restoring normal perfusion with rapid defibrillation. In those who are hemodynamically unstable defibrillation is indicated. In asymptomatic patients a medication strategy may be employed using IV amiodarone.

Torsades de Pointes

Torsades de pointes is a type of polymorphic VT associated with a prolonged QT interval and hypomagnesemia. It is characterized by a twisting pattern that oscillates around the isoelectric line on EKG. Torsades is treated with IV magnesium 2 mg IV and avoidance of QT-prolonging medications in those at risk.

Ventricular Fibrillation

VF represents a fully disorganized rhythm where the ventricles are incapable of contracting in a coordinated way. This dysrhythmia may follow VT that is uncontrolled and is an ominous sign. The goal of treatment is to restore normal electrical conduction via defibrillation. If not terminated, VF will devolve into asystole and lead to death. Treatment focuses on high-quality CPR, early defibrillation, and administration of epinephrine IV/intraosseous (IO) every 3 to 5 minutes, followed by 300 mg IV amiodarone or lidocaine IV 1 to 1.5 mg/kg. In an emergent situation, many antiarrhythmic medications can be given via the endotracheal tube if IV access is lost. These include epinephrine, lidocaine, and atropine.

Atrial Fibrillation

The most common arrhythmia, AF is characterized by multiple ectopic atrial foci (atrial rate may be up to 180) and becomes problematic when rapid ventricular depolarization (rapid ventricular response) occurs. This results in both a loss of time for atrial filling, a loss of atrial kick, as well as a reduced ventricular volume and ejection which ultimately leads to a decreased cardiac output. AF tends to occur in older individuals as well as in those with pulmonary disease. Goals of treatment involve rate control with beta-blockers or CCBs, as well as anticoagulation (AC), if indicated. AF results in chaotic and turbulent atrial blood flow that supports creation of clots in the atria. These may embolize, traveling to the lungs to become a PE or to the brain resulting in ischemic stroke. A rate versus rhythm strategy is considered for patients with ongoing A-fib. AF complications include emboli, stroke, HF, and exercise intolerance. Symptoms may include palpitations, light-headedness, fatigue, and dyspnea. The EKG is notable for multiple P waves that are described as irregularly irregular. While QRS complexes are present, there is no consistent communication between the P waves and QRS complexes. Treatment includes the use of beta-blockers and CCBs for rate control, and the addition of AC when indicated. In the hemodynamically unstable patient, emergent cardioversion is indicated.

Treatment strategy and the decision to prescribe AC are based on several factors. The CHA_2DS_2-VASc score in part guides the decision by calculating risk of ischemic stroke (Table 9.12). AC therapy is indicated for men with a score of ≥ 2 and women with a score of ≥ 3. It is also essential to ensure that AC has been addressed in stable patients with new AF present for more than 48 hours for at least 3 weeks before and 4 weeks after cardioversion (electrical or pharmacological). Novel oral anticoagulants (NOACs) are recommended over Coumadin unless a mechanical valve is present or in the case of moderate to severe mitral stenosis. Patients with AF and at risk of ischemic stroke and requiring AC must have their risk of bleeding assessed using a tool such as HAS-BLED. In patients with contraindications to AC or at high risk of stroke, a percutaneous left atrial appendage occlusion may be appropriate. Additionally, weight loss is recommended for all those with AF who are obese or overweight.

Table 9.12 CHA_2DS_2-VASc

CHF:	+1
HTN:	+1
Age ≥75 years:	+2
DM:	+1
Stroke, CVA, TIA:	+2
Vascular disease:	+1
Age 65 to 74 years:	+1
Female sex:	+1
TOTAL: _____	
Men scoring 0 and women scoring +1 do not need AC due to low stroke and mortality of less than 1%/year. Men scoring ≥1 and women scoring ≥2 should be initiated on AC.	

AC, anticoagulation; CHF, chronic heart failure; DM, diabetes mellitus; HTN, hypertension; CVA, cerebrovascular accident; TIA, transient ischemic attack.

Source: Hindricks, G., Potpara, T., Dagres, N., Arbelo, E., Bax, J. J., Blomström-Lundqvist, C., Boriani, G., Castella, M., Dan, G. A., Dilaveris, P. E., Fauchier, L., Filippatos, G., Kalman, J. M., La Meir, M., Lane, D. A., Lebeau, J. P., Lettino, M., Lip, G., Pinto, F. J., . . . ESC Scientific Document Group. (2021). 2020 ESC Guidelines for the diagnosis and management of atrial fibrillation developed in collaboration with the European Association for Cardio-Thoracic Surgery (EACTS): The Task Force for the diagnosis and management of atrial fibrillation of the European Society of Cardiology (ESC) Developed with the special contribution of the European Heart Rhythm Association (EHRA) of the ESC. *European Heart Journal, 42*(5), 373–498. https://doi.org/10.1093/eurheartj/ehaa612

Sinus Tachycardia

Sinus tachycardia (ST) is a rhythm originating from the sinus node at a rate greater than100 bpm. This is often a normal variant of rhythm and is considered a functional rhythm in the cases of exercise and emotional states (fear, anxiety) and in the presence of fever. ST may also be an indicator of underlying hypoxia, reduced cardiac output, hyperthyroidism, or pain. Attempts to alleviate ST should be focused at identifying and treating (if necessary) the underlying cause rather than attempting to reduce the heart rate.

Sinus Bradycardia

This rhythm originates from the sinus node and is characterized by a regular pattern with a HR less than 60. This may be a benign and normal variant in conditioned athletes. Sinus bradycardia (SB) is only treated if evidence of poor perfusion is present: hypotension, dizziness, pre-syncope/syncope, or acute kidney injury. Emergent treatment often involves the administration of IV atropine. If this is unsuccessful or the bradycardia persists, transcutaneous pacing may be required. All patients undergoing transcutaneous pacing must be given medication for pain as this is a painful and distressing procedure. New SB may also be associated with inferior wall MIs and so should prompt an evaluation with an EKG if a new finding or accompanied by other worrying signs.

Heart Block

Heart blocks are characterized by the slowing or absence of an action potential along the normal conduction pathway. This can occur at any point between the sinus and AV node, or between the AV and junctional node. Heart blocks are identified as first-degree, second-degree type I/Mobitz I/Wenckebach, second-degree type II/Mobitz II, or complete.

First-Degree Heart Block: A first-degree AV block occurs when the impulse between the sinoatrial (SA) and AV nodes is slowed. A PR interval greater than 0.2 msec is present. Although slowed, the impulse travels along the conduction pathway to depolarize the AV node resulting in a delay but no dropped beats. This dysrhythmia is asymptomatic, and each P wave communicates with a single QRS complex.

Second-Degree Heart Block: Second-degree heart block is further divided into either Mobitz type I/ Wenckebach or Mobitz type II.

- *Mobitz Type I (Wenckebach):* Mobitz type I is characterized by progressively longer delay through the AV node with longer PR intervals until the impulse is no longer conducted and a ventricular beat is dropped. It often has a predictable pattern of P waves to QRS complexes, that is, 2:1, 3:1. This is complete heart block.
- *Mobitz Type II:* Mobitz type II is defined by the presence of a stable first-degree AV block of greater than 2.0 msec along with a dropped beat over a predictable timeline (2:1, 4:1, etc.). It is often asymptomatic, but palpitations may be felt.

Complete Heart Block: Complete heart block is characterized by the complete dissociation between atrial and ventricular activity. Impulse is blocked at the AV node. P waves are greater than QRS complexes. There is no communication between the SA node and the AV node. In this case, the junctional pacemaker takes over resulting in a ventricular rate in the 30s. While the atrial rate will remain normal, QRS complexes widen and become bizarre looking. Patients are often symptomatic due to the ventricular bradycardia. Hypotension is common. Emergent transcutaneous pacing is indicated. Analgesia must be provided with any attempt to transcutaneously pace a patient. This procedure is distressing and painful.

PERMANENT PACEMAKERS AND IMPLANTABLE CARDIAC DEFIBRILLATORS

Advances in technology with permanent pacemakers (PPMs) and implantable cardiac defibrillators (ICDs) has concurrently increased the use of these devices. The primary role of a PPM is to control an abnormal rate, and an ICD primarily detects and internally defibrillates VF or VT. Combination PPM and ICD devices can monitor and control rate as well as sense and treat dangerous rhythms. The British Pacing and Electrophysiology Group (BPEG) and the North American Society of Pacing and Electrophysiology (NASPE) have standardized pacemaker codes for ease of understanding the functionality of the devices. An AGACNP must know this standard nomenclature associated with PPM (Table 9.13).

Table 9.13 BPEG and NASPE Pacemaker Codes

Letter	What the Letter Represents	Options
First letter	Chamber paced	O = None A = Atrium V = Ventricle D = Dual (A + V)

(continued)

Table 9.13 BPEG and NASPE Pacemaker Codes (*continued*)

Letter	What the Letter Represents	Options
Second letter	Chamber(s) sensed	O = None A = Atrium V = Ventricle D = Dual (A + V)
Third letter	Response to sensing	O = None T = Triggered I = Inhibited D = Dual (T = I)
Fourth letter	Rate modulation	O = None R = Rate modulation
Fifth letter	Anti-tachycardia pacing function	O = None A = Atrium V = Ventricle D = Dual (A + V)

BPEG, British Pacing and Electrophysiology Group; NASPE, North American Society of Pacing and Electrophysiology.

Indications for PPMs are often related to bradycardia caused by sinus and or AV node dysfunction (Table 9.14). PPM should be considered when a patient has sinus node dysfunction and is symptomatic due to the bradycardia. Symptoms include chest pain, light-headedness, dizziness, syncope, HF, hypotension, shock, or other signs of malperfused organs. PPM should be considered in the patient with third-degree AV block or type II (Mobitz II) AV blocks regardless of symptoms, as these arrhythmias can progress to symptomatic bradycardia.

Table 9.14 Frequently Seen Indications for PPM

Sinus Node Dysfunction	AV Nodal Dysfunction
▪ Symptomatic bradycardia ▪ Symptomatic sinus pauses ▪ Symptomatic chronotropic incompetence ▪ Required medications that causes symptomatic sinus node dysfunction	▪ Symptomatic type I second-degree AV block (Mobitz I or Wenckebach) ▪ Type II second-degree AV block ▪ High-grade complete AV block ▪ A-fib with symptomatic slow ventricular response ▪ AV block cause by ablation of AV node ▪ Required medications that causes symptomatic AV node dysfunction

AV, atrioventricular; PPM, permanent pacemaker.

Indications for ICDs focus on prevention of death due to ventricular tachyarrhythmia (Table 9.15).

Table 9.15 Frequently Seen Indications for ICD

Indication	Examples
Prevention of cardiac arrest	Ischemic cardiomyopathy with an EF less than 35% and NYHA class II–III, greater than 40 days after MI Ischemic cardiomyopathy EF less than 30% NYHA class I Nonischemic cardiomyopathy, EF less than 35% NYHA class II–III Survivors of cardiac arrest from VF or sustained VT without reversible cause Structural heart disease Syncope with inducible hemodynamic VT or VF during electrophysiology study
Special populations	Long QT syndrome with VT or syncope Brugada syndrome with VT or syncope Hypertrophic cardiomyopathy with risk for sudden cardiac arrest Arrhythmogenic right ventricular dysplasia with risk for sudden cardiac arrest

EF, ejection fraction; ICD, implantable cardiac defibrillator; NYHA, New York Heart Association; VF, ventricular fibrillation; VT, ventricular tachycardia.

ABLATION

Ablation is a treatment option for arrhythmias and can be direct surgical or catheter ablation of the cardiac tissue. Direct surgical intervention has fallen out of favor due to higher rates of complications and catheter-directed ablation the mainstay of therapy. Catheter ablation is done by an electrophysiologist who purposely induces tachycardia to facilitate mapping and identification of critical portions of the tachycardia cycle. Radiofrequency (RF) current is applied to cause thermal injury of the cardiac tissue causing the arrhythmia. Ablation is also a long-term treatment/management option for patients with accessory pathways and recurrent symptoms or asymptomatic patients with Wolff-Parkinson-White pattern on EKG and high-risk features at baseline or during electrophysiology study.

COMPLICATIONS

Complications of ablation and pacemakers include AV block, cardiac tamponade, and thromboembolic events, decreased exercise tolerance, syncope, stroke, HF, device malfunction, infection, bleeding, lead mispositioning or dislodgement, pneumothorax, and sudden cardiac death. Pacemakers can malfunction due to the device or the environment or can be patient specific. AGACNP must be able to identify these malfunctions (Table 9.16).

Table 9.16 Pacemaker Malfunctions

Malfunction	Description	Potential Cause
Failure to pace	Pacemaker dose not fire when pacing should occur	Pacemaker malfunction Wire fracture Lead dislodgement Disconnected wire/cable Generator failure
Failure to capture	Occurs when the generated pacing stimulus does not initiate a depolarization	Low battery Wire displacement or fracture Ischemia Medications Hyperkalemia
Failure to sense	*Oversensing:* The pacemaker senses electrical signals that it normally should not (does not pace when required). *Undersensing:* The pacemaker fails to sense patient cardiac activity (paces when they should not occur).	Wires have moved Inadequate QRS signal Ischemia or fibrosis Electrolyte abnormalities Sensitivity set too high or too low

▶ CARDIAC ARREST

DISEASE OVERVIEW

Cardiac arrest in the hospital setting most commonly presents as a nonshockable rhythm associated with a primary cardiac cause. Second only to this is respiratory insufficiency. The rhythms associated with cardiac arrest are the shockable rhythms VT and VF and the nonshockable rhythms PEA, and asystole. Individually, they are among the rhythms with the poorest overall prognosis of any described in the AHA ACLS. In the absence of an organized and functional cardiac rhythm, all forward flow of blood ceases, and cerebral perfusion fails. Without immediate resolution of the problem or implementation of assisted circulation, anoxic injury will commence, and death will follow. Current recognition and treatment of cardiac arrest are guided by implementation of the AHA's Cardiac Arrest ACLS Algorithm with an emphasis on early detection, and intervention with high-quality CPR, and treatments to address possible reversible causes.

CLASSIC PRESENTATION

The AGACNP is called to a patient room by the nurse. The patient is pale, grimacing, appears to be sweating profusely, and is clenching their fist in front of the chest. The AGACNP enters the room. The patient's eyes close, and they lose consciousness. The AGACNP examines the patient and finds the patient is apneic and pulseless. CPR is initiated.

DIAGNOSTIC CRITERIA

The person in cardiac arrest is apneic and pulseless. They may appear pale, diaphoretic, and have cool extremities and cyanotic lips and nail beds. While no labs are needed to confirm cardiac arrest, often labs will be drawn in the inpatient setting to determine reversible causes. These include CBC, comprehensive metabolic panel (CMP), magnesium, phosphorous, calcium, lactic acid, cardiac enzymes, BNP, and arterial blood gas (ABG). Cardiac arrest can be confirmed via echocardiogram, which demonstrates a nonbeating heart. Bedside echocardiogram results can be used to determine ongoing resuscitation or termination of resuscitation attempts. An EKG may be obtained; however, CPR should not be interrupted while attempting to get an EKG or echocardiogram.

TREATMENT/MANAGEMENT

Treatment of cardiac arrest follows the AHA's Adult Cardiac Arrest Algorithm. This includes activating a "Code Blue" to secure response team, attaching the patient to the defibrillator, and providing oxygen. After attaching the patient to the defibrillator, a rhythm check is conducted. If VF or pulseless VT is present, then a shock is delivered. CPR continues with an emphasis on minimizing interruptions, avoiding overventilation, and maintaining the quality of compressions. After 2 minutes have elapsed, CPR is paused for a rhythm check. This cycle continues until ROSC. Once ROSC is achieved, post-cardiac care begins.

Once CPR has begun, IV or IO access must be obtained. Epinephrine is administered every 3 to 5 minutes. For refractory VF or pulseless VT, amiodarone or lidocaine may also be administered. Additional interventions to consider include placement of an advanced airway, measurement of capnography, and search for reversible causes.

After ROSC is achieved, management of the person with cardiac arrest is guided by the AHA's Post–Cardiac Arrest Care Algorithm. This includes certain respiratory and hemodynamic parameters (Table 9.17). This care is divided into a stabilization phase and a continued management/emergent activities phase. During stabilization, the airway should be secured with an endotracheal tube if not already done. Respiratory and hemodynamic parameters are defined and attended to, and a 12-lead EKG is performed.

Table 9.17 Respiratory and Hemodynamic Parameters Post Cardiac Arrest

Respiratory Parameters	Hemodynamic Parameters
10 breaths/min SpO_2 92% to 98% $PaCO_2$ 35 to 45 mmHg	Systolic BP greater than 90 mmHg Mean arterial pressure greater than 65 mmHg

BP, blood pressure; $PaCO_2$, partial pressure of carbon dioxide; SpO_2, oxygen saturation.

After stabilization, cardiology consult should be obtained for possible intervention if STEMI or cardiogenic shock or to determine need for mechanical circulatory support. If the patient is awake after the arrest, additional needed care should be provided in the critical care unit. This includes continued evaluation and treatment of reversible causes and expert consultation for ongoing management. For the patient who does not regain consciousness after ROSC, a brain CT should be obtained, EEG ordered, and targeted temperature management may be initiated.

TARGETED TEMPERATURE MANAGEMENT

For the patient who does not regain consciousness after ROSC, targeted temperature management may be indicated to mitigate neurologic injury in these patients. The 2020 AHA guidelines recommend patients be cooled to 32°C to 36°C for at least 24 hours. Shivering can be managed with sedation and neuromuscular blocking medications, and the patient must be monitored closely as hypotension and bradycardia may develop due to hypothermia. Once cooling has been completed, passive rewarming commences until the person reaches normothermia. Fever is associated with negative outcomes and should be aggressively managed with antipyretics as well as cooling devices.

▶ SYNCOPE

DISEASE OVERVIEW

Syncope is a transient loss of consciousness related to another diagnosis/primary problem. Syncope is a symptom rather than a unique pathology. Fainting occurs due to a reversible disruption to cerebral perfusion resulting in loss of consciousness. It is characterized by spontaneous awakening and when symptoms are present may be preceded by dizziness, light-headedness, nausea, or visual changes. Severity of syncope can range from benign to life threatening.

Etiologies of syncope include vasovagal or neurocardiogenic syncope, orthostatic hypotension, hypovolemia, arrhythmia, and severe aortic stenosis. Cardiogenic causes of syncope are more common in older adults, while younger adults tend to suffer from neurocardiogenic syncope. Vasovagal syncope is often triggered by noxious stimuli (pain, stress, severe fatigue, crowded places), which causes depression in sympathetic and parasympathetic activity leading to the vasodilation and bradycardia that result in fainting.

CLASSIC PRESENTATION

A 32-year-old woman has been admitted after undergoing a previously scheduled uterine myomectomy for removal of fibroids. Her surgery went well, and she has been recovering as expected. Today while ambulating in her room with the nurse, she asked for help lifting her gown to examine her Pfannenstiel incision. The nurse assisted her; however, moments after visualizing the incision, the patient began to complain of light-headedness. She appeared pale and slightly diaphoretic and stated, "I feel woozy." At that time, her eyes rolled back, and she collapsed into the nurse's arms and was assisted to the floor. Her pulse was noted to be 42 bpm, and her RR was 18. A rapid response was activated; however, after several minutes and before the team arrived, the patient opened her eyes and was able to get up and into her bed without assistance. Her HR had returned to her normal rate of 76, and she was no longer pale or diaphoretic.

DIAGNOSTIC CRITERIA

History is most important; the events and timing surrounding the episode should be determined. VS should be ascertained and a medication history compiled. The cardiovascular and neurologic systems should be examined for evidence of vascular, valvular disease, or cerebrovascular disease.

Hemoglobin is needed to ensure the patient does not have hemorrhagic shock. Glucose is needed to ensure the patient is not hypoglycemic. Electrolytes should be obtained to assess for possible causes of arrhythmias. Diagnosis is typically made based on the history and physical exam. An EKG should be obtained to rule out cardiac ischemia/infarction. The remainder of testing is determined by the suspected underlying condition and may include cardiac enzymes, echocardiogram, telemetry, CT head, and carotid duplex. Tilt-table testing may be used if syncope is recurrent.

If urinary or fecal incontinence occurs, unconsciousness lasts more than a few minutes, or the syncopal episode is followed by a period of altered mental status, the clinician should be highly suspicious for possible seizure and not true syncope.

TREATMENT/MANAGEMENT

Treatment is dependent on the underlying etiology. Vasovagal syncope is the most common form, and treatment is conservative, focused on lifestyle modification, maintaining hydration, and utilizing counterpressure maneuvers (leg-crossing, hand gripping).

COMPLICATIONS

Injuries may occur due to mechanical falls if standing/walking. Degree of trauma may be significant if syncope occurred during driving.

▶ POSTURAL ORTHOSTATIC TACHYCARDIA SYNDROME

DISEASE OVERVIEW

Postural orthostatic tachycardia syndrome (POTS) is characterized by an inappropriate cardiovascular response to a sudden change in posture from the sitting or lying position to standing. POTS predominantly affects women of childbearing age and results in a sudden onset of tachycardia, hypotension, and symptoms of pre-syncope. Syncope may occur, although this is rare. A history of orthostatic intolerance (less than 6 months) and the presence of a HR increase ≥30 bpm within 10 minutes of standing must be seen. Orthostatic hypotension (BP decreased more than 20/10) is absent. Confounding causes of tachycardia or hypotension (medications, dehydration, bleeding) must be ruled out, and LV function must be normal.

CLASSIC PRESENTATION

A 22-year-old woman has been receiving IV antibiotics for a recent bout of cellulitis that occurred after sustaining an injury while gardening. She has been in good health and has no other documented PMH. Today while entering her room to evaluate her progress, the AGACNP observed her become pre-syncopal while standing up to work with the physical therapist. The AGACNP helped her return to her bed and immediately obtained her vital signs, which were as follows: HR 168, BP 110/60. Her BP is similar to her last recorded vital signs from an hour ago, although her HR is quite elevated. She tells the AGACNP that she feels "okay" but is a bit foggy. After 15 minutes in bed, her HR has returned to normal, and her brain fog has abated. She reports that she has been having similar episodes of light-headedness and a racing heartbeat when standing from sitting or lying down for the last 8 months. Her symptoms resolve quickly after returning to a recumbent position.

DIAGNOSTIC CRITERIA

The physical exam is notable for the presence of an abrupt increase in the HR along with multiple subjective symptoms that occur with standing and are alleviated with resuming a recumbent position. Paradoxically, the BP will often remain stable or increase with standing. Pre-syncope, light-headedness, palpitations, brain fog, dyspnea, and chest discomfort may be reported. Obtain CBC to rule out anemia, BMP to assess for dehydration, and plasma or urinary metanephrines to rule out pheochromocytoma. POTS can be diagnosed via tilt-table testing.

TREATMENT/MANAGEMENT

Physical therapy and cardiovascular conditioning are often prescribed. Patients are encouraged to keep well hydrated and to drink water throughout the day. They should maintain adequate dietary salt intake as well.

COMPLICATIONS

Complications include syncope, fatigue, and palpitations. Patients who do syncopize are at risk for injury.

▶ CARDIAC TRAUMA

DISEASE OVERVIEW

Cardiac trauma includes both blunt force and penetrating injuries and can result in rupture of one of the cardiac chambers, tearing of a coronary artery, or dissection of the great vessels. Although cardiac trauma makes up a small percentage of total body trauma, it has an outsized effect on mortality compared to traumatic injuries in other organ systems. Blunt force injuries to the chest such as those that occur in motor vehicle collisions, falls, and sudden deceleration may all result in myocardial contusion, aortic disruption, and development of aneurysm or acute pericardial effusion from bleeding. Most cases of myocardial contusion involve sudden deceleration injuries related to motor vehicle collisions. The speed at which a vehicle was traveling prior to a collision or the height from which a fall occurred can aid in determining the potential severity of injuries sustained.

Penetrating injuries involving gunshot wounds, stabbing, or impalement by foreign bodies can also result in direct cardiac trauma. These injuries are often life-threatening and require emergent surgical intervention. Treatment is indicated especially in the case of aortic damage or disruption of the integrity of the heart. Patients should be transferred to a level 1 trauma center where emergency specialist care is available on site.

CLASSIC PRESENTATION

A 15-year-old female patient presents after being involved in a car crash where she was a passenger. She was reportedly wearing a seat belt and experienced a sudden deceleration, slamming into the belt, when the car came to an abrupt stop. On arrival she is hypotensive with weak and thready pulses. There is severe bruising across her chest and overlying her sternum. She is placed on telemetry and is tachycardic with frequent runs of nonsustained ventricular tachycardia.

DIAGNOSTIC CRITERIA

Symptoms vary depending on the mechanism of injury. While a piercing injury will be associated with an obvious puncture or laceration, as well as bleeding both internal and external, the internal damage from blunt force trauma or an internal penetrating injury from a fractured rib may not be immediately apparent. The astute clinician should be on the lookout for symptoms of internal and external hemorrhage, cardiac failure, signs of tamponade, as well as other associated trauma that could portend acute decompensation. Shortness of breath, dizziness, tearing-type pain located at the back, dyspnea, bulging neck veins, and hypotension are all ominous signs and indicate the need for prompt evaluation. Bruising across the chest and sternum should raise suspicion for a blunt force chest injury. Stability of the sternum should be assessed as well as palpation for fractures and soft tissue crepitus. Skin should be examined for bruising and stippling associated with a close-range gunshot.

Patient history plays an integral role in determining the cause of the trauma, as does the primary and secondary survey. Laboratory testing includes hemoglobin and hematocrit, creatine kinase (CK), creatine kinase-myocardial band (CK-MB), troponin I, and BMP. These assessment techniques do not however negate the need for CT or CTA to ascertain the level of damage below the surface and possible involvement of the vasculature. EKG should be obtained, and if normal with a normal troponin I can rule out blunt cardiac trauma. Echocardiogram while not helpful for evaluating myocardial contusion may demonstrate a new pericardial effusion concerning for acute bleeding.

TREATMENT/MANAGEMENT

Always be sure to remove EKG leads and bandaging during the initial/primary survey as a stab wound or bullet entry or exit may be obscured by a sticker or tape. Do not attempt to remove objects that have pierced or impaled the heart or chest. This should only be done under the supervision of the trauma service in the operating room where immediate steps can be taken to repair life-threatening injuries. Treatment is supportive care with monitoring for arrhythmias. If hypotensive, a transthoracic echocardiogram can evaluate cardiac function.

COMPLICATIONS

Complications include cardiac tamponade, hemorrhagic shock, arrhythmias, rupture of the heart wall, and death.

▶ CARDIAC TAMPONADE

DISEASE OVERVIEW

Cardiac tamponade is typically associated with pericarditis, malignancy, and trauma. An enlarging pericardial effusion causes pressure within the pericardial sac, compressing the cardiac chambers and compromising their ability to fill. The result is decreased preload, leading to underfilling of the RV, LV, and ultimately the inability of the heart to maintain cardiac output. This results in obstructive shock and inability of the heart to maintain perfusion. Effusions that grow slowly over weeks to months may allow the heart to compensate, and so relatively larger volumes of fluid may be tolerated within the pericardial sac. Those that develop quickly over minutes or hours can acutely lead to cardiovascular collapse and death without emergent intervention

CLASSIC PRESENTATION
A 19-year-old man was brought to the ED after sustaining a fall from a ladder while hanging holiday lights. On his initial exam, he reported falling on his chest and complained of 6/10 verbal analog scale pain that was relieved with low-dose IV morphine. His chest x-ray was negative for rib fractures; however, the radiologist commented that the heart had a "water bottle" appearance. While being readied for discharge home, the patient reports that he is "not feeling so good." His BP is now 70/40, his heart sounds are muffled, and the AGACNP notices bilateral JVD.

DIAGNOSTIC CRITERIA
Cardiac tamponade classically presents with hypotension, JVD, and muffled heart sounds known as Beck triad. Patients may complain of sudden-onset chest pain that is relieved by leaning forward if pericarditis is present. Other findings including shortness of breath, crackles if heart failure is present, dyspnea, angina, and bulging neck veins may be present. Pulsus paradoxus, an inspiratory decrease in systolic BP greater than 10 mmHg may be noted as well as a narrow pulse pressure.

Laboratory workup should include CK-MB, and ESR may be useful to detect infection or myocardial damage. EKG may demonstrate tachycardia, electrical alternans, and a decrease in voltage. Diagnosis is made using echocardiogram which is the gold standard though CT or MRI may also confirm the presence of an effusion.

TREATMENT/MANAGEMENT
Emergent cardiothoracic surgery consult is required with a plan for relief of the tamponade via creation of a pericardial window, or placement of a pericardial drain. In some cases, bedside pericardiocentesis or emergent needle aspiration may be required. This is helpful to relieve the tamponade and to obtain fluid testing to determine etiology. In cases of recurrent effusion and tamponade, a pericardial window may be necessary. NSAIDs may also be administered to relieve the pain of inflammation from pericarditis.

COMPLICATIONS
Complications include pulmonary edema, HF, shock, and death.

▶ VASCULAR CONDITIONS

PERIPHERAL ARTERY DISEASE/ACUTE OCCLUSION
DISEASE OVERVIEW
PAD symptoms arise from the inability of the peripheral arteries to provide sufficient perfusion to the tissues of the extremities. This is most commonly caused by narrowing of the lumen of the peripheral arteries due to atherosclerotic accumulation of the arterial walls; however, injury from inflammatory processes and radiation can also be causative. Atherosclerotic changes are not limited to the peripheral arteries, and any of the larger arteries may be affected as well. As tissue oxygenation demand increases due to activity, ischemia develops from the inability of the arteries to supply sufficient blood volume. This ischemic pain is called intermittent claudication and is relieved with rest. Risks for PAD include HTN, DM, hyperlipidemia, age older than 50 years, family history, and smoking. Smoking is the most significant factor related to severity of PAD and multiplies the risk for developing the disease.

CLASSIC PRESENTATION
While monitoring a 64-year-old male patient who is POD 4 after CABG and is ambulating in the hall, the AGACNP observes that he suddenly stops while walking and requests that the physical therapist bring him a chair. He is visibly uncomfortable and grimacing and has begun to rub his right leg. After a chair is brought, he sits down. The AGACNP asks him what the trouble is. He reports that his legs "always cramp and hurt after I walk any distance." He shares that he can walk about 20 ft at a time but then must sit down and stop walking due to significant discomfort. He shares that his pain will abate after sitting for several minutes and that he can then continue walking a short distance.

DIAGNOSTIC CRITERIA

Criteria include subjective complaints of thigh or calf pain during activity, classically described as cramping; diminished or loss of pulses; pallor; pain with palpation; muscle atrophy; loss of hair; cool or cyanotic skin; and bruit. Ankle-brachial index (ABI) is a tool to assess lower extremity perfusion; it compares the systolic pressure in the upper extremities with systolic pressure in the ankle (see Table 9.18 for interpretation).

Table 9.18 ABI Interpretation

ABI value	Symptoms	Pulse Waveform	Interpretation
0.9–1.4	NA	Triphasic	Normal
0.7–0.9	Claudication	Biphasic	Mild to moderate arterial insufficiency
0.3–0.5	Ulcers	Monophasic	Severe peripheral arterial disease
Less than 0.3	Gangrene	Weak monophasic or absent	Critical peripheral arterial disease

ABI, ankle-brachial index.

Source: Adapted from Tenny, E. (2021). *How to calculate and interpret ankle-brachial index (ABI) numbers.* https://www.medmastery.com/guides/ultrasound-clinical-guide-arteries-legs/how-calculate-and-interpret-ankle-brachial-index-abi.

TREATMENT/MANAGEMENT

PAD treatment goals are aimed at reducing cardiovascular risk and aiding in ambulation without symptoms. Treatments include lifestyle modification, exercise, medications including aspirin, and consultation with vascular surgery for possible endovascular surgery. Currently, several surgeries are available for those who have PAD. These include arterial angioplasty and stenting and arterial bypass grafting.

COMPLICATIONS

Plaque from the aorta or other affected arteries may embolize causing an acute occlusion and ischemia. Infection and ulceration may ensue, as well as gangrene necessitating amputation.

CAROTID ARTERY STENOSIS
DISEASE OVERVIEW

Like the iliac arteries, abdominal aorta, and femoral arteries, the carotid arteries are also at risk of the effects of systemic atherosclerosis. When luminal narrowing is greater than 50% of carotid diameter, hemodynamically significant reductions in cerebral blood flow can occur. The most serious potential complication for those with carotid artery stenosis is stroke due to embolism of carotid plaque. Once a significant carotid plaque burden has developed, revascularization with carotid endarterectomy or carotid stenting may be indicated.

DIAGNOSTIC CRITERIA

Physical exam findings can include the presence of a carotid bruit. No specific lab is diagnostic for carotic artery stenosis (CAS); however, a lipid profile may demonstrate dyslipidemia, and CRP or D-dimer may be elevated. A duplex ultrasound of the carotids is the first-line imaging of choice; CTA head and neck may also be used to provide further information once ultrasound has been obtained.

TREATMENT/MANAGEMENT

Lifestyle modifications are indicated for all individuals with carotid stenosis. A "tri-therapy" strategy for medical management is employed that includes the use of statins, ACEI, and antiplatelet drugs. Revascularization may also be required and can be accomplished through either placement of a carotid stent, surgical carotid endarterectomy (CEA), or transcarotid artery revascularization (TCAR). TCAR with a flow diverter is a minimally invasive option to CEA for high-risk patients and has the lowest stroke rate for any carotid intervention. During endarterectomy, a surgical incision is made to the carotid artery allowing surgical removal of plaque. Post-endarterectomy care involves close monitoring of BP in order to avoid cerebral hyperperfusion syndrome. This rare complication occurs due to dysfunction of cerebral autoregulation post-endarterectomy and may manifest as unilateral headache, altered mental status, or seizure.

COMPLICATIONS

A complication of carotid artery stenosis is embolic stroke.

VENOUS CONDITIONS
DISEASE OVERVIEW

Venous insufficiency and the symptoms related to venous stasis, skin changes, edema, and discomfort are related to a progressive incompetence of valves in the venous system. This results in either reflux of venous blood or obstruction. Venous insufficiency is classified as primary, having no precipitating cause, or secondary, due to an inflammatory response caused by a deep venous thrombosis (DVT). Chronic venous insufficiency leads to venous HTN. Several modifiable risk factors have been identified including prolonged standing, smoking, obesity, sedentary lifestyle, and pregnancy. Nonmodifiable risks are older age, HTN, and a previous history of DVT.

DIAGNOSTIC CRITERIA

Criteria include pain, fatigue, pitting edema, pruritis, skin discoloration known as hemosiderin staining, varicosities, tenderness to palpation, ulcers of the medial malleolus, and subjective symptoms that may be relieved by rest or elevation. D-dimer may be elevated and indicates venous thrombosis. Duplex ultrasound is the diagnostic modality of choice. Chronic venous insufficiency (CVI) may also be measured using plethysmography. Venography with magnetic resonance venography (MRV) may also be performed.

TREATMENT/MANAGEMENT

Goals are to heal ulceration, protect skin integrity, reduce edema and discomfort, and remove varicosities. Long-term compression therapy with stockings is a mainstay of therapy. Treatment should also include leg exercises, elevation, and weight management. Ulcers should be treated with compression bandaging.

COMPLICATIONS

Complications include venous ulcers, which can be slow to heal and can result in DVT, and postphlebitic syndrome.

AORTIC SYNDROMES
DISEASE OVERVIEW

Aortic syndromes include acute aortic dissection, intramural hematoma, and penetrating aortic ulcer. Although these are considered distinct and separate pathologies, they may also coexist. All aortic syndromes involve the development of a defect of the wall of the aorta. The aortic wall is composed of three layers: from the innermost out they are the intima, media, and adventitia.

Aortic dissection involves the development of a tear in the intima resulting in the creation of a false lumen between the intimal and medial layers. Risk factors for dissection include HTN, connective tissue disorders such as Marfan syndrome, smoking, and male sex. Aortic dissections are described based on their location. Two systems commonly used for this are the Stanford and DeBakey classifications (Table 9.19).

Table 9.19 Aortic Dissection Classifications

Stanford	DeBakey
Type A: Involves the ascending aorta	*Type I:* Dissection begins in the ascending aorta and involves the aortic arch and descending aorta
Type B: Does not affect the ascending aorta but may involve the aortic arch	*Type II:* Only ascending aorta involved
	Type III: Involves the descending and thoracic aorta

An intramural hematoma (IMH) occurs when a disruption within the media forms allowing a collection of blood to accumulate without the presence of an intimal tear. These may resolve spontaneously or go on to become full aortic dissections with communication with the intima, whereas a penetrating aortic ulcer may form when an atherosclerotic plaque is destabilized and tears away from the aortic wall.

CLASSIC PRESENTATION

A 66-year-old man with a history of HTN has been brought to the ED with sudden-onset severe chest pain. He is hypertensive with a BP of 160/80 and tachycardic at 128. He reports that he had been working at his desk when he experienced a 10/10 ripping-type chest pain that has now moved to his back. Additionally, he now has left arm and hand tingling and numbness. Exam reveals he has a new murmur consistent with AR and that his left radial pulse is +1 and thready, while his right radial pulse is strong and +2. His pain is not reproducible and has changed in location since it first began. The BP in his left arm is 30 points lower than in his right.

DIAGNOSTIC CRITERIA

The history of presenting illness (HPI) may be notable for subjective complaints of sudden-onset severe pain. Pain may be described as tearing in nature and may be located along the back. The murmur of AR may be auscultated if the aortic valve is involved. Other findings may include muffled heart sounds, JVD, unilateral radial or femoral pulse changes, and evidence of ischemia of extremities such as cyanosis.

Obtain STAT and serial CBCs, BMP, BUN, and creatinine if renal arteries are involved, and cardiac enzymes. Although aortography had been standard imaging, it is now being replaced by CTA as the study of choice. CXR may show widened mediastinum, and echocardiogram may show the ascending aortic enlargement and dilated aortic root. If an aortic syndrome is present, obtain STAT type and screen and crossmatch for 4 units packed red blood cells (PRBCs) to be on hold.

TREATMENT/MANAGEMENT

Medical treatment with beta-blockers is the first-line approach for intralumenal hematomas and penetrating aortic ulcers. Treatment of aortic dissection on the other hand depends on the location of the dissection and other involved structures. Beta-blockers (esmolol or labetalol drips) are often prescribed to decrease HR and provide shear force reduction alongside other antihypertensives to ensure tight BP control. Consultation with cardiothoracic surgeons with emergent surgery is indicated in the case of an ascending thoracic aortic dissection (Stanford A; DeBakey 1 or 2). Aortic root involvement may necessitate the need for aortic valve replacement and coronary revascularization. Descending thoracic aortic dissections moving distally toward branching vessels of the abdominal aorta may result in compromised perfusion. Abdominal aortic aneurysms require vascular surgery consultation and can be managed by endovascular aortic repair (EVAR). Alternatively, if the aneurysm is not amenable to EVAR, then open abdominal aneurysm repair may be needed.

COMPLICATIONS

Complications include AV damage, acute kidney injury or mesenteric ischemia, ischemic stroke, hemorrhage, paralysis from cross clamping above the spinal arteries, and death. Subsequently, endovascular aortic aneurysm repair may develop endo leaks. There are five types of endo leaks. Type I leaks occur at the proximal, distal, or side graft attachment sites, allowing blood to flow into the aneurysm sac. Type II leak, the most common leak, has retrograde flow into the aneurysm sac from side branches of the lumbar, inferior mesenteric, or other arteries. Type III leaks are caused by a tear in the graft or graft misalignment. Type IV leak is caused by a porous graft. Type V leak is an expanding aneurysmal sac without identifiable etiology.

VENOUS THROMBOEMBOLISM
DISEASE OVERVIEW

Venous thromboembolic disease includes both DVT and pulmonary embolism (PE). Both processes involve the development of a blood clot in a distal vein, usually in the lower extremities; however, veins in the pelvis and proximal extremities may also develop venous thromboembolism (VTE). This clot may become mobile and travel through the body, ultimately becoming lodged in the pulmonary vascular system, where it is referred to as a pulmonary embolus. Clot development is thought to occur in the presence of three factors known as Virchow triad: endothelial injury, hypercoagulability, and venous stasis. DVTs are classified as being either provoked (develop in the presence of risk factors) or unprovoked (no inciting factor identified). Risks for DVT are both modifiable and nonmodifiable and include malignancy, recent surgery, immobility, male sex, obesity, pregnancy, smoking, heredity, antiphospholipid syndrome, and hormone-based medications such at oral contraceptive pills.

CLASSIC PRESENTATION

A 35-year-old female patient presents to the ED with right lower leg swelling and pain. She reports no recent injury to the right leg but is concerned as her right lower extremity has grown over the last couple of days.

DIAGNOSTIC CRITERIA

Symptoms may be absent, but when present unilateral pain, and the presence of warmth, tenderness, or edema in the calf are highly suspicious for DVT. Subjective complaints of shortness of breath may be present if the DVT has traveled and embolized to the lungs. The Wells Criteria for DVT (Box 9.6) are a useful clinical prediction tool used for assessing the probability of DVT.

Box 9.6 Wells DVT Criteria

Add: One point for each of the following criteria:
Active cancer treatment within 6 months, or palliative
Paralysis or paresis, or recent immobilization of lower extremities
Bedrest ≥3 days or after major surgery ≤12 weeks or general or regional anesthesia
Local tenderness along the deep vein system
Calf swelling greater than 3 cm larger than asymptomatic side
Pitting edema of the affected limb
Collateral superficial veins
Previous DVT
Subtract: Two points if an alternative diagnosis is equally likely as DVT
Interpretation: ≤1 point, DVT unlikely; ≥2 points, DVT likely

DVT, deep vein thrombosis.

Diagnostic Testing

D-dimer will be positive. False positives are common with D-dimer; therefore, the presence of DVT must be confirmed with venous duplex ultrasound for diagnosis.

TREATMENT/MANAGEMENT

VTE treatment is focused on the prevention of extension of the thrombus and embolism development, and avoidance of development of the postthrombotic syndrome. Anticoagulation with direct oral anticoagulants (DOACs) is the first-line treatment for outpatient management. DOACs are equally as effective as warfarin in the treatment of DVT and have the added benefit of a better safety profile and increased convenience for patients. Heparin infusion or enoxaparin are commonly used with hospitalized patients if invasive procedures are warranted. Enoxaparin dose adjustment is needed for those with renal impairment.

Where AC is contraindicated, placement of an inferior vena cava (IVC) filter may also be considered. For patients with large/extensive DVTs, thrombectomy may be warranted, or catheter-directed thrombolysis may also be required. The length of therapy depends on whether DVT/PE is provoked or unprovoked. Current recommendations include that AC be continued indefinitely for those with unprovoked DVT or a chronic risk factor.

Prophylaxis is required for all high-risk hospitalized patients. Both mechanical and chemical prophylaxis are needed. The preferred agent is low-molecular-weight heparin (LMWH) and sequential compression devices.

COMPLICATIONS

Postthrombotic syndromes are characterized by swelling, discomfort, and pain after the resolution of the original VTE. PE and DVT recurrence are also possible complications.

PULMONARY EMBOLISM

DISEASE OVERVIEW

A *PE* is most commonly a blood clot that forms as a DVT in the extremities and then embolizes traveling to the vasculature of the lungs where it becomes lodged, obstructing pulmonary arterial blood flow. Other forms of PE include air embolism and fat embolisms. Regardless of the makeup of the PE, the effect is the same, creation of a ventilation/perfusion mismatch (V/Q mismatch). This results in unoxygenated blood returning to the left side of the heart. If the V/Q mismatch is severe enough, PE can result in obstructive shock and may be fatal. Risk factors are similar for those of DVT and include pregnancy, immobility, obesity, malignancy, advancing age, and hormone-based medications like oral contraceptive pills.

CLASSIC PRESENTATION

A 57-year-old Australian man arrived to the United States after a long flight last week. He presents with complaints of shortness of breath, dyspnea, and right-sided calf pain and swelling. His past medical history (PMH) is significant for HTN, and a recent colon cancer diagnosis is now status post treatment 4 months ago. His VS are as follows: HR 125, BP 90/50, O_2 sat 86%. On exam, the AGACNP notes that he has engorged jugular veins, a loud S2, and unilateral swelling and edema of his right calf.

DIAGNOSTIC CRITERIA

Symptoms of PE are usually nonspecific. When present, subjective complaints include sudden acute pleuritic chest pain, palpitations, dyspnea, and shortness of breath. Hypoxia, tachycardia, and hemoptysis are hallmark signs of PE. Other findings on PE may include a loud S2 and parasternal heave. Signs of obstructive shock including JVD, hypotension, and rapid, thready pulse may also be present if the clot burden is large. CXR is of limited utility in patients with PE unless pulmonary infarction is present.

Obtain D-dimer, Lactate Dehydrogenase (LDH), ABG, BNP, and troponin. CTA of the chest is the gold standard for diagnosis of PE; however, a V/Q scan is an acceptable alternative if CTA is not available or the patient has contraindications to contrast. Echocardiogram should be obtained to evaluate for right heart strain. EKG may demonstrate an $S_1Q_3T_3$ pattern associated with acute PE. A lower extremity venous duplex ultrasound may demonstrate DVT. The Modified Wells Criteria (Table 9.20) is a clinical prediction tool that is used to evaluate probability of PE. The pulmonary embolism severity index (PESI) can be used to predict mortality.

Table 9.20 Modified Wells Criteria

Criteria	Points
Previous PE/DVT	+1.5
HR greater than 100	+1.5
Surgery/immobilization within the previous 30 days	+1.5
Clinical signs of DVT	+3
Alternative diagnosis less likely than PE	+3
Hemoptysis	+1
Cancer treated within the last 6 months	+1
Interpretation: Clinical probability of PE Low Intermediate High	 0–1 2–6 ≥6

DVT, deep vein thrombosis; HR, heart rate; PE, pulmonary embolism.

TREATMENT/MANAGEMENT

Treatment differs based on PE severity, which is classified as either low risk, intermediate risk/sub-massive, or high risk/massive. Treatment includes systemic AC (where not contraindicated). If suspicion for PE is high, systemic AC should begin even before the presence of PE is confirmed with CTA. In the case of patients with a low-risk PE per the PESI tool, treatment at home with anticoagulation may be appropriate. DOACs are first-line treatment in low-risk PE and stable intermediate and massive PE. Otherwise, UFH is recommended for those with intermediate and high risk along with systemic administration of thrombolytics. Systemic thrombolysis carries a high risk of bleeding, and the patient should be closely monitored for signs of significant bleeding including intracranial hemorrhage. Other treatments include catheter-directed thrombolysis, and surgical embolectomy. An IVC filter may be placed if contraindications to anticoagulation exist.

COMPLICATIONS

Complications include acute hypoxic respiratory failure, chronic thromboembolic pulmonary hypertension (CTEPH), obstructive shock, cardiac arrest, and death.

▶ SUMMARY

AGACNPs must completely understand all CVD processes, associated diagnostic testing, and specific treatments to pass the certification exam and be efficient in practice. Safe practice begins with foundational knowledge in the disease pathophysiology to understand how and why specific interventions are recommended. Review of clinical practice guidelines will supplement this chapter.

KNOWLEDGE CHECK: CHAPTER 9

1. Adults with a history of congenital heart disease (CHD) are at risk of what common complication?

   A. Deep vein thrombosis (DVT)
   B. Myocardial infarction
   C. Heart failure
   D. Stillbirth

2. When providing patient education for a patient diagnosed with dyslipidemia, the AGACNP demonstrates an understanding of treatment goals for this population by incorporating information about:

   A. Medication adherence
   B. Secondary causes of dyslipidemia
   C. Diagnostic tests
   D. Therapeutic lifestyle modification

3. An 18-year-old male patient has presented for workup of new-onset syncopal episodes. These episodes are preceded by the presence of an aura and are often accompanied by episodes of incontinence. What differential diagnosis is most consistent with this presentation?

   A. Vasovagal syncope
   B. Orthostatic hypotension
   C. Arrhythmia
   D. Seizure

4. Targeted temperature management of the patient who is post cardiac arrest requires that the person be cooled to what temperature post arrest?

   A. 30°C to 34°C for 12 hours
   B. 32°C to 36°C for 24 hours
   C. 30°F to 34°F for 24 hours
   D. 40°C to 44°C for 12 hours

5. Which interventions are prioritized during the stabilization phase of the American Heart Association's post–cardiac care algorithm?

   A. Place endotracheal tube, obtain EKG, monitor, and optimize respiratory and hemodynamic parameters
   B. Transfer to higher level of care, initiate sedation, and consult cardiology
   C. Administer high-quality CPR with an emphasis on quality of compressions and minimization of interruptions
   D. Call for help, and assess the scene for safety

6. What diagnostic is considered the test of choice when differentiating between the cardiomyopathies?

   A. Cardiac catheterization
   B. Echocardiogram
   C. EKG
   D. Cardiac CT

(See answers next page.)

1. C) Heart failure

Patients with a diagnosis of CHD are monitored frequently for the development of heart failure. While DVT can be a result of an unrepaired congenital heart defect, this is not considered a common complication in most adults. Myocardial infarction is not a frequent complication in CHD. Some women with a concurrent diagnosis of CHD and pulmonary arterial hypertension (PAH) are counseled against pregnancy due to the risk of maternal death; however, development of heart failure is of concern to a wider group of these patients.

2. D) Therapeutic lifestyle modification

All patients diagnosed with dyslipidemia should have counseling related to therapeutic lifestyle modification regardless of the cause of their disease. Lifestyle modification includes limiting saturated fat intake and increasing dietary fiber and intake of whole grains, fruits, and vegetables. While medication adherence is an important part of any pharmacologic intervention, therapeutic lifestyle modification is central to the care of those diagnosed with dyslipidemia, making it the most appropriate choice. Secondary causes of dyslipidemia and their treatment do not apply to everyone with a diagnosis of dyslipidemia. Lifestyle modification, however, is applicable universally. Diagnostic testing is not a treatment goal for those with dyslipidemia.

3. D) Seizure

Syncope that is preceded by an aura and that has fecal or urinary incontinence as a feature is highly suspicious for the diagnosis of a seizure disorder. Vasovagal syncope is associated with noxious stimuli including fear, anxiety, or pain. It is not preceded by an aura, and the person does not experience incontinence. Orthostatic hypotension uncommonly results in syncope and is preceded by a sudden change in position from sitting or lying to standing. This is inconsistent with this patient's presentation. Arrhythmogenic syncope may be preceded by palpitations, chest discomfort, diaphoresis, and a feeling of light-headedness. It is not notable for the presence of incontinence or aura.

4. B) 32°C to 36°C for 24 hours

To achieve optimal outcomes post cardiac arrest, the patient must be cooled to a temperature of 32°C to 36°C for at least 24 hours. Cooling below this threshold is associated with increased complications including bradyarrhythmia and hypotension. Cooling to 30°F to 34°F will result in hypothermic death. Cooling to 40°C to 44°C over 12 hours is insufficient to achieve improved outcomes.

5. A) Place endotracheal tube, obtain EKG, monitor, and optimize respiratory and hemodynamic parameters

The stabilization phase occurs after return of spontaneous circulation (ROSC) is achieved. During this time, the endotracheal tube (ETT) is placed, EKG is obtained, and respiratory and hemodynamic parameters are monitored and optimized. Transferring to a higher level of care and obtaining expert consultation occur in the emergent activities phase following the stabilization phase. High-quality CPR is the primary goal in achievingROSC. This occurs prior to the stabilization phase. Calling for help and securing the scene are the initial steps in performing advanced cardiac life support (ACLS) and occur before ROSC and the stabilization phase.

6. B) Echocardiogram

Echocardiogram provides a window to the structure of the heart and is diagnostic for the type of cardiomyopathy present. Cardiac catheterization can give detailed information about coronary perfusion, and intracardiac hemodynamics but is not considered the diagnostic of choice for cardiomyopathy. EKG gives information about the conductive system of the heart but does not allow for differentiation between the types of cardiomyopathies. Cardiac CT is not indicated for differentiating between types of cardiomyopathies.

7. Which class of medications must be used with extreme caution in patients with hypertrophic cardio-myopathy (HCM)?

   A. Beta-blockers
   B. Antibiotics
   C. Diuretics
   D. Calcium channel blockers

8. What characteristic findings on EKG are expected for the patient diagnosed with cardiac ischemia?

   A. ST depressions
   B. Global concave-shaped ST elevations
   C. T-wave elevations
   D. An $S_1Q_3T_3$ pattern

9. A 16-year-old female patient presents after having passed out after jumping up quickly to answer a knock at the door. This event was preceded by a feeling of warmth throughout. A bystander reports that the patient became "pale and sweaty." What differential diagnosis is most consistent with this presentation?

   A. Vasovagal syncope
   B. Orthostatic hypotension
   C. Arrhythmia
   D. Seizure

10. What is considered the intervention of choice to treat a ST-segment elevation myocardial infarction (STEMI)?

    A. Percutaneous coronary intervention (PCI)
    B. Echocardiogram
    C. EKG
    D. Coronary artery bypass grafting (CABG)

(See answers next page.)

7. C) Diuretics

Diuretics must be used with extreme caution in people with HCM as they may result in hypovolemia and reduced stroke volume that will further exacerbate a left ventricular outflow obstruction and may result in hypotension. Beta-blockers are not contraindicated in HCM and may be part of the treatment plan. Antibiotics are not indicated in the treatment of HCM. Calcium channel blockers may be used to treat HCM and do not carry any special precautions with their use for this illness.

8. A) ST depressions

ST depressions are indicative of myocardial ischemia. T-wave inversions may indicate ischemia but not elevations. Global concave-shaped ST elevations and PR depressions may be seen in patients with pericarditis. An $S_1Q_3T_3$ pattern may be seen in the presence of pulmonary embolism (PE).

9. B) Orthostatic hypotension

Orthostatic hypotension uncommonly results in syncope and is preceded by a sudden change in position from sitting or lying to standing. Arrhythmogenic syncope may be preceded by palpitations, chest discomfort, diaphoresis, and a feeling of light-headedness. Syncope that is preceded by an aura and that has fecal or urinary incontinence is highly suspicious for a seizure.

10. B) Echocardiogram

Echocardiogram provides a window to the structure of the heart and is diagnostic for the type of cardiomyopathy present. CABG is a suitable intervention, but not initially, unless other circumstances dictate need for immediate CABG. PCI gives detailed information about coronary perfusion and intracardiac hemodynamics and is the choice of intervention to reperfuse coronary vessels in patients without diabetes. EKG provides information about the ischemia of the heart but does not allow for intervention.

11. A 62-year-old male patient with a history of hypertension, hyperlipidemia, and diabetes presents with 3 hours of substernal chest pain. He is anxious, diaphoretic, and nauseous. His blood pressure (BP) is 90/70 mmHg, pulse 50 beats per minute, respirations 24 per minute. His lungs are clear, no murmurs, and there is ~10 cm of jugular venous distension (JVD). His EKG is shown below.

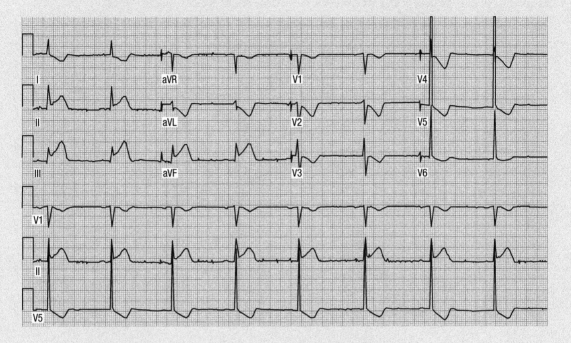

Based on these findings, which of the following diagnosis is most likely?

A. Inferior myocardial infarction with evidence of right ventricular involvement

B. Anterior myocardial infarction with lateral extension

C. Anterior myocardial infarction with aneurysm formation

D. Posterior myocardial infarction with lateral extension

(See answers next page.)

11. A) Inferior myocardial infarction with evidence of right ventricular involvement

This patient has ST-segment elevation in the inferior leads, II, III, and aVF indicating inferior wall involvement. He also has elevated jugular venous distension in the setting of clear lung fields, a sign for right ventricular involvement. Confirming right ventricular involvement would be noted by changes in the placement of right ventricular V3–V4 leads with noted ST-segment changes.

12. A 33-year-old patient with a recent history of viral infection is now presenting with acute onset of substernal chest pain that radiates to the left shoulder. The patient denies worsening chest pain with exertion, but the pain improves when leaning forward. Vital signs are stable; exam reveals clear lungs, a normal S_1 and S_2, and a scratchy sound heard at the left sternal border. EKG is shown below.

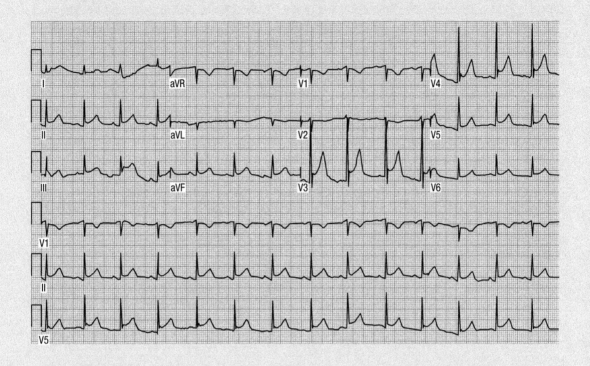

Treatment includes which of the following?

A. Nitroglycerin

B. Oral steroids

C. Indomethacin (Indocin)

D. Ibuprofen (Advil/Motrin)

13. A 53-year-old male patient with a history of hypertension presents with complaints of sudden, severe chest pain radiating to his back and headache. His blood pressure (BP) is 214/121, heart rate (HR) 58, and respiratory rate (RR) 20. EKG shows left ventricular hypertrophy (LVH) without ischemic changes. Which medication is most appropriate?

A. Sublingual nitroglycerin

B. Oral metoprolol

C. Nicardipine infusion

D. Esmolol infusion

(See answers next page.)

12. D) Ibuprofen (Advil/Motrin)

The patient presents with acute pericarditis. Her symptoms of substernal chest pain improved with sitting up, together with the friction rub on exam, support this diagnosis. The EKG in the first hours to days is characterized by diffuse ST-segment elevation with reciprocal ST depression in leads aVR and V1. Also, there may be an atrial injury, reflected by elevation of the PR segment in lead aVR and depression of the PR segment in other limb leads and in the left chest leads, primarily V5 and V6. The most likely cause in this otherwise healthy patient is viral or idiopathic. In many cases, acute pericarditis is self-limited and will resolve in 2 to 6 weeks. In the treatment of acute pericarditis, the goals of therapy are the relief of pain, resolution of inflammation, and prevention of recurrence. Acute pericarditis is painful, so acute therapy usually requires nonsteroidal anti-inflammatory agents. The patient should also be treated with colchicine concurrently because it is well tolerated, reduces symptoms, and decreases the rate of recurrent pericarditis. High-dose corticosteroids are reserved for individuals whose pericarditis is unresponsive to nonsteroidal agents and colchicine. Corticosteroids are not usually used as first-line therapy, because individuals treated with them have a higher rate of recurrent pericarditis. Nitroglycerin in not indicated for the treatment of pericarditis.

13. C) Nicardipine infusion

Severe, sudden, persistent chest pain radiating to the back is characteristic of aortic dissection. A medication that addresses BP is the most appropriate intervention currently, making nicardipine infusion the appropriate choice. Oral medications are not sufficient for BP control in the acute scenario. Esmolol is not appropriate due to the patient being bradycardic on presentation. Sublingual nitroglycerin is not indicated for aortic dissection.

14. A patient with known coronary artery disease, post myocardial infarction and preserved left ventricular function, presents to the office with the rhythm shown below. His only complaint is palpitations. Vital signs are stable, and he has not taken any medications for over a year because he cannot afford them. Which of the following medications should *initially* be prescribed?

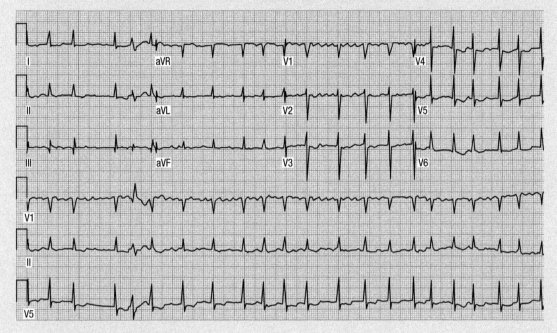

A. Amiodarone (Cordarone)

B. Metoprolol (Toprol/Lopressor)

C. Procainamide (Pronestyl)

D. Dofetilide (Tikosyn)

(See answers next page.)

14. B) Metoprolol (Toprol/Lopressor)

This patient is hemodynamically stable with a complaint of palpitations caused by atrial fibrillation and thus does not require hospitalization. Beta-blockers or calcium channel blockers are first-line treatment for rate control for a patient who is hemodynamically stable. Amiodarone has a relatively slow onset and is most useful as an adjunct when rate control with beta-blockers or calcium channel blockers is incomplete or contraindicated or when cardioversion is planned. Procainamide, due to multiple side effects, is rarely used, and dofetilide must be initiated in the hospital due to potential risk of torsades de pointes.

15. A 58-year-old man is seen in the ED for syncope. His spouse reports being in the kitchen and hearing him fall on the living room floor. The patient recalls feeling very light-headed but remembers nothing more. Upon further questioning, he recalls feeling dizzy on several occasions over the past few months. He has a history of hypertension and a myocardial infarction 10 years earlier. He has since been well and exercises on a daily basis. In the ED, he has a blood pressure (BP) of 95/55 mmHg and a heart rate of 30 beats/min. An EKG is obtained (see below). What is the most important initial step in managing this patient?

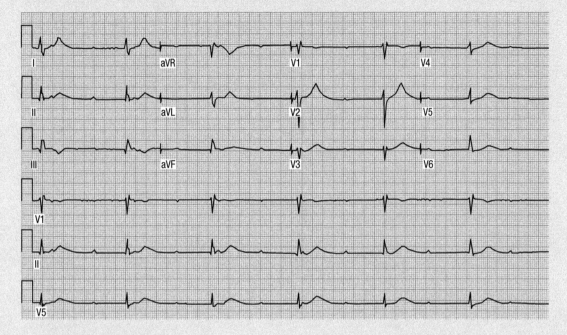

    A. Administer dopamine
    B. Admit for further monitoring
    C. Place a temporary pacemaker
    D. Administer isoproterenol

(See answers next page.)

15. C) Place a temporary pacemaker

This patient's EKG shows third-degree heart block. He is clearly symptomatic with syncope. In the ED, he is still not stable as his BP is very low and he remains light-headed. Urgent treatment is required, and a temporary pacemaker is the most important initial step. Management of the symptomatic patient can be with either medication and/or pacing. Nodal blocks (narrow QRS complex) may respond to atropine; infranodal blocks (wide QRS complex) are unlikely to respond to atropine or other medications that can enhance AV nodal conduction. Patients should have transcutaneous cardiac pacer pads applied in the ED. If there is no or incomplete response to atropine, use transcutaneous (temporary) cardiac pacing, recognizing that transvenous pacing is eventually necessary in most patients.

16. A 24-year-old woman presents to the ED, stating, "My heart is pounding out of my chest, and I've been short of breath for 4 hours." She has had similar episodes, but all have spontaneously stopped. She is in good health and takes no medications. Her blood pressure (BP) is 120/80 mmHg, and her pulse too rapid to count. Her rhythm is shown below.

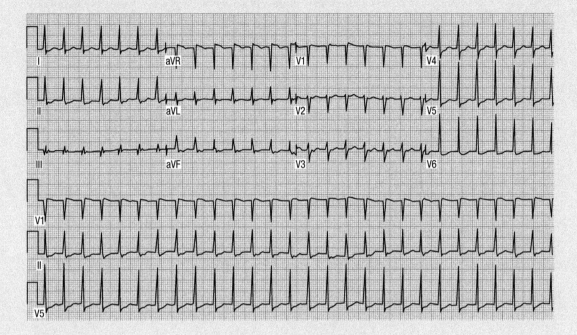

What is the *most appropriate* immediate management for this patient?

A. Administer verapamil orally

B. Immediate cardioversion after administration of a mild sedative

C. Elicit a vagal maneuver

D. Insert a temporary transvenous pacemaker

17. A 24-year-old male patient presents to the ED with a cocaine overdose. He is awake, with tachycardia, anxiety, diaphoresis, headache, confusion, and a blood pressure (BP) of 230/120. Which of the following is the most appropriate medication to treat his hypertension?

A. Isoproterenol (Isuprel)

B. Esmolol (Brevibloc)

C. N-Acetylcysteine (Mucomyst)

D. Phentolamine (OraVerse)

18. A 62-year-old male patient is 1 day post cardiac bypass surgery. He suddenly develops hypotension with pulsus paradoxus and has no urinary output for 2 hours. Point-of-care two-dimensional echocardiogram demonstrates right systolic collapse. AGACNP diagnosis is which of the following?

A. Cardiac tamponade

B. Dissecting thoracic aortic aneurysm

C. Hemorrhage

D. Barotrauma

(See answers next page.)

16. C) Elicit a vagal maneuver

Vagal maneuvers are often effective. If there is no response to vagal maneuvers, adenosine is recommended to convert to sinus rhythm. It is rare that the patient requires calcium channel blocker. If the patient becomes unstable, use of electrical cardioversion may be necessary for conversion. Overdrive pacing is rarely needed in young adults. Paroxysmal supraventricular tachycardia is seen more frequently in female patients, with a peak in the late teenage and young adult years. The majority of patients are without active cardiovascular disease. Patients may be able to describe the abrupt onset of this reentrant dysrhythmia and also note when it self-terminates. Palpitations, light-headedness, and dyspnea are common symptoms.

17. D) Phentolamine (OraVerse)

This patient presents with hypertensive emergency and thus requires parental treatment. In hypertensive emergencies that arise from catecholaminergic mechanisms such as cocaine use, beta-blockers can worsen the hypertension because of unopposed peripheral vasoconstriction. Calcium channel blockers or phentolamine are better choices in treating this patient.

18. A) Cardiac tamponade

The patient presents with classic signs of tamponade. There is no mention of bleeding, uncorrected coagulopathy, arrhythmia, or ventilator management. Thus, the patient has tamponade that requires emergent intervention.

19. The AGACNP is caring for a 38-year-old Black male patient who has no known medical history and was admitted to the hospital for management of newly diagnosed type II diabetes mellitus and renal dysfunction with proteinuria. Throughout the hospitalization, the patient has been noted to be persistently hypertensive, with blood pressure (BP) readings in the general range of 160/90. The *most appropriate first-line medication* for this patient would be:

    A. Metoprolol succinate (Toprol XL) 25 mg orally twice per day
    B. Amlodipine (Norvasc) 10 mg orally once per day
    C. Hydrochlorothiazide (Microzide) 25 mg orally once per day
    D. Lisinopril (Prinivil) 20 mg orally once per day

20. TheAGACNP is caring for a 58-year-old male patient who was recently diagnosed with coronary artery disease after having an ST-segment myocardial infarction. Based on the American College of Cardiology (ACC)/American Heart Association (AHA) Guidelines for Management of Cholesterol, which option for statin therapy would be most appropriate for this patient when planning for hospital discharge?

    A. Atorvastatin (Lipitor) 40 mg orally once per day
    B. Lovastatin (Mevacor) 40 mg orally once per day
    C. Pravastatin (Pravachol) 40 mg orally once per day
    D. Simvastatin (Zocor) 40 mg orally once per day

(See answers next page.)

19. D) Lisinopril (Prinivil) 20 mg orally once per day

According to guidelines for the management of hypertension by the Eighth Joint National Committee, patients of all ages who have evidence of kidney disease, with or without diabetes and regardless of race, should be treated with an angiotensin-converting enzyme inhibitor (ACEI) or angiotensin-receptor blocker (ARB), either alone or in combination with antihypertensive medications of other drug classes. For Black patients with proteinuria, the use of an ACEI or ARB is especially important given a higher likelihood of progression of renal disease to end stage. Hydrochlorothiazide is the recommended initial treatment of patients of all ages and races without kidney dysfunction.

20. A) Atorvastatin (Lipitor) 40 mg orally once per day

According to ACC/AHA Guidelines for Management of Cholesterol, patients with clinical evidence of atherosclerotic heart disease (such as coronary artery disease and myocardial infarction) should be treated with high-intensity statin therapy regardless of lipid levels unless they have a history of intolerance to the therapy or other contraindication. Examples of high-intensity statin therapy include atorvastatin (Lipitor) 40 to 80 mg orally once daily and rosuvastatin (Crestor) 20 to 40 mg daily. Daily dosing of lovastatin, pravastatin, or simvastatin is moderate-intensity statin therapy.

Only key resources appear in the print edition. Access the full bibliography for this chapter on ExamPrepConnect.com.

Chiabrando, J. G., Bonaventura, A., Vecchié, A., Wohlford, G. F., Mauro, A. G., Jordan, J. H., Grizzard, J. D., Montecucco, F., Berrocal, D. H., Brucato, A., Imazio, M., & Abbate, A. (2020). Management of acute and recurrent pericarditis: JACC State-of-the-Art Review. *Journal of the American College of Cardiology, 75*(1), 76–92. https://doi.org/10.1016/j.jacc.2019.11.021

Coagulation Cascade. (2019, January 18). *Medbullets.* https://step1.medbullets.com/hematology/111004/coagulation-cascade

Danchin, N., Popovic, B., Puymirat, E., Goldstein, P., Belle, L., Cayla, G., Roubille, F., Lemesle, G., Ferrières, J., Schiele, F., & Simon, T. (2020). FAST-MI investigators year outcomes following timely primary percutaneous intervention, late primary percutaneous intervention, or a pharmaco-invasive strategy in ST-segment elevation myocardial infarction: The FAST-MI programme. *European Heart Journal, 41*(7), 858. https://doi.org/10.1093/eurheartj/ehz665

Gregory, D., Badhwar, V., Bermudez, E., Cleveland, J., Cohen, M., D'Agostino, R., Ferguson, T., Hendel, R., Isler, M., Jacobs, J., Jneid, H., Katz, A., Maddox, T., & Shahian, D. (2020). AHA/ACC key data elements and definitions for coronary revascularization: A report of the American College of Cardiology/American Heart Association Task Force on Clinical Data Standards (Writing Committee to Develop Clinical Data Standards for Coronary Revascularization). *Journal of the American College of Cardiology, 75*(16), 1975–2088. https://doi.org/10.1016/j.jacc.2020.02.010

Grundy, S. M., Stone, N. J., Bailey, A. L., Beam, C., Birtcher, K. K., Blumenthal, R. S., Braun, L. T., de Ferranti, S., Faiella-Tommasino, J., Forman, D. E., Goldberg, R., Heidenreich, P. A., Hlatky, M. A., Jones, D. W., Lloyd-Jones, D., Lopez-Pajares, N., Ndumele, C. E., Orringer, C. E., Peralta, C. A., … Yeboah, J. (2019). 2018 AHA/ACC/AACVPR/AAPA/ABC/ACPM/ADA/AGS/APhA/ASPC/NLA/PCNA. Guideline on the management of blood cholesterol: Executive summary: A report of the American College of Cardiology/American Heart Association Task Force on Clinical Practice Guidelines. *Journal of the American College of Cardiology, 73*(24), 3168–3209. https://doi.org/10.1016/j.jacc.2018.11.002

Hindricks, G., Potpara, T., Dagres, N., Arbelo, E., Bax, J. J., Blomström-Lundqvist, C., Boriani, G., Castella, M., Dan, G. A., Dilaveris, P. E., Fauchier, L., Filippatos, G., Kalman, J. M., La Meir, M., Lane, D. A., Lebeau, J. P., Lettino, M., Lip, G., Pinto, F. J., … ESC Scientific Document Group. (2021). 2020 ESC Guidelines for the diagnosis and management of atrial fibrillation developed in collaboration with the European Association for Cardio-Thoracic Surgery (EACTS): The Task Force for the diagnosis and management of atrial fibrillation of the European Society of Cardiology (ESC) developed with the special contribution of the European Heart Rhythm Association (EHRA) of the ESC. *European Heart Journal, 42*(5), 373–498. https://doi.org/10.1093/eurheartj/ehaa612

Ibanez, J. S., Agewall, S., Antunes, M. J., Bucciarelli-Ducci, C., Bueno, H., Caforio, A. L. P., Crea, F., Goudevenos, J. A., Halvorsen, S., Hindricks, G., Kastrati, A., Lenzen, M. J., Prescott, E., Roffi, M., Valgimigli, M., Varenhorst, C., Vranckx, P., & Widimský, P. (2018). 2017 ESC Guidelines for the management of acute myocardial infarction in patients presenting with ST-segment elevation: The Task Force for the management of acute myocardial infarction in patients presenting with ST-segment elevation of the European Society of Cardiology (ESC). *European Heart Journal, 39*(2), 119–177. https://doi.org/10.1093/eurheartj/ehx393

January, C. T., Wann, L. S., Calkins, H., Chen, L. Y., Cigarroa, J. E., Cleveland, J. C., Jr., Ellinor, P. T., Ezekowitz, M. D., Field, M. E., Furie, K. L., Heidenreich, P. A., Murray, K. T., Shea, J. B., Tracy, C. M., & Yancy, C. W. (2019). 2019 AHA/ACC/HRS Focused Update of the 2014 AHA/ACC/HRS Guideline for the Management of Patients With Atrial Fibrillation: A Report of the American College of Cardiology/American Heart Association Task Force on Clinical Practice Guidelines and the Heart Rhythm Society in Collaboration With the Society of Thoracic Surgeons. *Circulation, 140*(2), e125–e151. https://doi.org/10.1161/CIR.0000000000000665

Knuuti, J., Wijns, W., Saraste, A., Capodanno, D., Barbato, E., Funck-Brentano, C., Prescott, E., Storey, R., Deaton, C., Cuisset, T., Agewall, S., Dickstein, K., Edvardsen, T., Escaned, J., Gersh, B., Svitil, P., Gilard, M., Hasdai, M., Hatala, R., … Bax, M. (2019). ESC Scientific Document Group, 2019 ESC Guidelines for the diagnosis and management of chronic coronary syndromes: The Task Force for the diagnosis and management of chronic coronary syndromes of the European Society of Cardiology (ESC). *European Heart Journal, 41*(3), 407–477. https://doi.org/10.1093/eurheartj/ehz425

McDonagh, T. A., Metra, M., Adamo, M., Gardner, R. S., Baumbach, A., Böhm, M., Burri, H., Butler, J., Čelutkienė, J., Chioncel, O., Cleland, J., Coats, A., Crespo-Leiro, M. G., Farmakis, D., Gilard, M., Heymans, S., Hoes, A. W., Jaarsma, T., … ESC Scientific Document Group. (2022). 2021 ESC Guidelines for the diagnosis and treatment of acute and chronic heart failure: Developed by the Task Force for the diagnosis and treatment of acute and chronic heart failure of the European Society of Cardiology (ESC). With the special contribution of the Heart Failure Association (HFA) of the ESC. *European Journal of Heart Failure, 24*(1), 4–131. https://doi.org/10.1002/ejhf.2333

Ortel, T. L., Neumann, I., Ageno, W., Beyth, R., Clark, N. P., Cuker, A., Hutten, B. A., Jaff, M. R., Manja, V., Schulman, S., Thurston, C., Vedantham, S., Verhamme, P., Witt, D. M., Florez, I. D., Izcovich, A., Nieuwlaat, R., Ross, S., Schünemann, H. J., … Zhang, Y. (2020). American Society of Hematology 2020 guidelines for management of venous thromboembolism: Treatment of deep vein thrombosis and pulmonary embolism. *Blood Advances, 4*(19), 4693–4738. https://doi.org/10.1182/bloodadvances.2020001830

Otto, C. M., Nishimura, R. A., Bonow, R. O., Carabello, B. A., Erwin, J. P., Gentile, F., Jneid, H., Krieger, E. V., Mack, M., McLeod, C., O'Gara, P. T., Rigolin, V. H., Sundt, T. M., Thompson, A., & Toly, C. (2021). 2020 ACC/AHA guideline for the management of patients with valvular heart disease: A report of the American College of Cardiology/American Heart Association Joint Committee on Clinical Practice Guidelines. *Circulation, 143*(5), e72–e227. https://doi.org/10.1161/cir.0000000000000923

Rivera-Lebron, B., McDaniel, M., Ahrar, K., Alrifai, A., Dudzinski, D. M., Fanola, C., Blais, D., Janicke, D., Melamed, R., Mohrien, K., Rozycki, E., Ross, C. B., Klein, A. J., Rali, P., Teman, N. R., Yarboro, L., Ichinose, E., Sharma, A. M., Bartos, J. A., … PERT Consortium. (2019). Diagnosis, treatment and follow up of acute pulmonary embolism: Consensus practice from the PERT consortium. *Clinical and Applied Thrombosis/Hemostasis, 25*, 1076029619853037. https://doi.org/10.1177/1076029619853037

Stout, K. K., Daniels, C. J., Aboulhosn, J. A., Bozkurt, B., Broberg, C. S., Colman, J. M., Crumb, S. R., Dearani, J. A., Fuller, S., Gurvitz, M., Khairy, P., Landzberg, M. J., Saidi, A., Valente, A. M., & Van Hare, G. F. (2018a). AHA/ACC guideline for the management of adults with congenital heart disease: A report of the American College of Cardiology/American Heart Association Task Force on Clinical Practice Guideline. *Journal of the American College of Cardiology, 73*, e81. https://doi.org/10.1016/j.jacc.2018.08.1028

Whelton, P. K., Carey, R. M., Aronow, W. S., Casey, D. E., Jr., Collins, K. J., Dennison Himmelfarb, C., DePalma, S. M., Gidding, S., Jamerson, K. A., Jones, D. W., MacLaughlin, E. J., Muntner, P., Ovbiagele, B., Smith, S. C., Jr., Spencer, C. C., Stafford, R. S., Taler, S. J., Thomas, R. J., Williams, K. A., Sr., … Wright, J. T., Jr. (2018). 2017 ACC/AHA/AAPA/ABC/ACPM/AGS/APhA/ASH/ASPC/NMA/PCNA Guideline for the prevention, detection, evaluation, and management of high blood pressure in adults: A Report of the American College of Cardiology/American Heart Association Task Force on Clinical Practice Guidelines. *Journal of the American College of Cardiology, 71*(19), e127–e248. https://doi.org/10.1016/j.jacc.2017.11.006

Pulmonary System Review

Donna Lynch-Smith, Dawn Carpenter, and Helen Miley

▶ INTRODUCTION

AGACNPs manage pulmonary disorders daily, including airway, parenchymal, pleural, and vascular disorders. AGACNPs must be astute diagnosticians, recognize urgent and emergent situations, and make rapid, lifesaving decisions. To do so, AGACNPs must fully comprehend the disease pathophysiology, interpret diagnostic findings, and know when to select appropriate interventions.

▶ UPPER AIRWAY OBSTRUCTION

DISEASE OVERVIEW
Airway obstruction has multiple etiologies, including but not limited to epiglottitis, angioedema, anaphylaxis, trauma, masses, and postsurgical hematoma compressing the trachea. Upper airway obstruction is an emergency and should trigger a code airway to mobilize a seasoned team to address. An anesthesiologist, trauma surgeon, thoracic surgeon, or otolaryngologist should be immediately available to perform advanced airway management interventions.

CLASSIC PRESENTATION
Upper airway obstruction presentation varies based on etiology but typically presents with stridor, patient in a tripod position, restlessness, anxiety, hoarse voice, and drooling/inability to manage oral secretions. Epiglottitis also has a viral prodrome of fever or chills, severe sore throat, and odynophagia. Angioedema and anaphylaxis typically also present with facial, tongue, and eye swelling, and the patient may have hives and recent exposures to triggering agents such as medications, specifically angiotensin-converting enzyme (ACE) inhibitors (which can trigger at any time during use), contrast, or insects.

DIAGNOSTIC CRITERIA
CT scans of the chest, neck, and face demonstrate soft tissue swelling, hematomas, tumors, abscesses, and other potential causes of the edema. Complete blood count (CBC) will demonstrate leukocytosis indicative of epiglottitis or abscess, while the differential may also reveal eosinophilia seen with allergic reactions.

TREATMENT/MANAGEMENT
Management of upper airway obstruction requires treatment of the underlying trigger and interventions to maintain airway patency. This can range from noninvasive methods or require advanced airway management techniques. Noninvasive options include keeping head of bed elevated 45 degrees, inhaled racemic epinephrine, application of cool mist oxygen, inhaled heliox mixture, continuous positive airway pressure (CPAP) or bilevel positive airway pressure (BiPAP), intramuscular (IM) epinephrine, intravenous (IV) antihistamine such as diphenhydramine (Benadryl), and H_2 blockers such as famotidine (Pepcid) for anaphylaxis.

Surgical intervention may be needed for incision and drainage of abscesses or hematoma. Intubation may be needed if these interventions fail to reverse the airway obstruction. Intubation is likely to be difficult, and adjunctive therapies should be available, including a variety of endotracheal tube sizes, a variety of laryngoscope types and sizes, glidescope, bronchoscope, bougie or tube exchanger, cricothyroidotomy kit, and open tracheostomy tray. Trauma patients may need surgical intervention and depending on the specific injury will need consultation with plastic and reconstructive surgery and oral, maxillofacial, otolaryngological, or thoracic surgery teams. Upper airway tumors may require an urgent or emergent tracheostomy in the operating room.

▶ EPIGLOTTITIS

DISEASE OVERVIEW

Epiglottitis is an acute infection of the epiglottis and nearby structures. Epiglottitis is a life-threatening condition causing significant edema of the upper airway that can lead to airway compromise and respiratory arrest. An upper respiratory infection can be a precursor. Symptoms may be mild and then dramatically worsen. Common pathogens include *Streptococcus pyogenes, Streptococcus pneumoniae, Staphylococcus aureus,* and *Haemophilus influenzae.* The 4D's of epiglottitis are dysphagia, dysphonia, drooling, and distress.

CLASSIC PRESENTATION

A 32-year-old man presents appearing very uncomfortable. He reports an upper respiratory infection that started 2 days ago and abruptly got worse. He is sitting upright with a hoarse voice. He is anxious, more so when lying back on the stretcher, and asks to sit on the edge of the stretcher. His arms are outstretched and resting on his knees (tripod position). Vital signs: temperature (T) 102°F, heart rate (HR) 120, respiratory rate (RR) 26, blood pressure (BP) 150/80, O_2 sat 98%. He reports dysphagia and inability to swallow saliva. Stridor is present, and he begins to have suprasternal retractions.

DIAGNOSTIC CRITERIA

Avoid oral and throat exam to avoid respiratory arrest. Epiglottitis is a clinical diagnosis. A lateral x-ray of the soft tissues of the neck may show a "thumbprint sign" but is not needed to confirm the diagnosis. CT scan of the neck is likely not to be tolerated by the patient as they may respiratory arrest in the scanner by lying flat.

TREATMENT/MANAGEMENT

The highest priority is to ensure the patient maintains a patent airway. Intubation, if needed, should be done by the most experienced providers in a controlled environment. Admit to the ICU for ongoing monitoring, and keep an open tracheostomy tray at the bedside. IV corticosteroids with dexamethasone (Decadron) are indicated to reduce airway edema. Antibiotic therapy with ceftriaxone is indicated to cover common respiratory and oral cavity flora.

COMPLICATIONS

Complications can include epiglottic abscess, cellulitis, empyema, meningitis, pneumonia, septic shock, respiratory failure, hypoxia, tracheostomy, prolonged ventilation, and death.

▶ OBSTRUCTIVE SLEEP APNEA

DISEASE OVERVIEW

Obstructive sleep apnea (OSA) is a complex and heterogeneous multisystem breathing disorder affecting 1 billion people worldwide. OSA increases with age, affecting twice as many males as females. Prevalence increases with increased body weight. OSA is present in 90% of patients with hypoventilation syndrome. Obesity hypoventilation is distinguished from OSA by the presence of hypercarbia. OSA results from narrowing of the upper airway causing diminished or cessation of airflow during sleep resulting in oxyhemoglobin desaturation and sleep fragmentation. The upper airway obstruction can be due to negative pressure during inspiration, expiratory narrowing in retropalatal area, or upper airway narrowing during sleep due to large body mass index (BMI). Multiple etiologies incrvease risk and predispose people to OSA (Table 10.1).

Table 10.1 Risk Factors for OSA

Risk Factors	Medical Diagnoses Predisposing to OSA
Older age	Congestive heart failure
Male sex	Atrial fibrillation
Obesity	Resistant hypertension
Craniofacial abnormalities	Diabetes mellitus
Upper airway abnormalities	Metabolic syndrome
Smoking	Myasthenia gravis
Family history of snoring or OSA	Pulmonary hypertension
Nasal congestion	End-stage renal disease
Alcohol use	Chronic lung disease (asthma, COPD, IPF)
Use of sedatives and hypnotics	TIA
Supine sleeping position	Spinal cord injury
Environmental exposure	Stroke
	Pregnancy
	Acromegaly
	Hypothyroidism
	Polycystic ovary syndrome
	Parkinson disease
	Obesity
	Fibromyalgia
	GERD and/or Barrett esophagus

COPD, chronic obstructive pulmonary disease; GERD, gastroesophageal reflux disease; IPF, idiopathic pulmonary fibrosis; OSA, obstructive sleep apnea; TIA, transient ischemic attack.

Symptoms of OSA can include some or all the following: loud snoring while sleeping, witnessed episodes of apnea, choking and/or gasping during sleep, excessive sleepiness in the daytime, drowsiness while driving with a near-miss or recent accident, frequent nocturnal awakenings with or without nocturia, morning headaches, decreased concentration, depressed mood, irritability, and decreased libido.

Physical exam findings suggestive of OSA include macroglossia, tonsillar hypertrophy, uvula enlargement or elongation, arched or high palate, nasal obstructions or polyps, deviation of septum, turbinate hypertrophy, significant nasal congestion, retrognathia, Friedman tongue position, and Mallampati class III or IV. The modified Mallampati classification score is an oropharyngeal assessment visualizing structures with mouth open and with tongue protruding. The Mallampati classification score predicts the difficulty in laryngoscopy and endotracheal intubation. Mallampati scores of III and IV are associated with higher risk of OSA (Table 10.2 and Figure 10.1).

Table 10.2 Mallampati Score and Description

Mallampati Score	Visible Structures
I	Tonsils, uvula, and soft palate fully visible
II	Hard palate, soft palate, upper portion of tonsils, and uvula are visible
III	Hard palate, soft palate, and base of uvula are visible
IV	Hard palate is only visible

Source: Adapted from Samsoon, G. L., & Young, J. R. (1987). Difficult tracheal intubation: A retrospective study. *Anaesthesia, 42,* 487. https://doi.org/10.1111/j.1365-2044.1987.tb04039.x

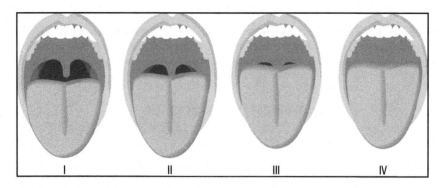

Figure 10.1 Mallampati score visual.

Source: Adapted from https://commons.wikimedia.org/wiki/File:Mallampati.svg.

CLASSIC PRESENTATION

A 65-year-old male patient who has a significant history of diabetes mellitus type 2 and gastroesophageal reflex presents to the ED with headaches during the day, fatigue, and inability to focus. The patient is a 20 pack/year cigarette smoker. On presentation, the patient is a well-nourished male sitting up in bed at 45 degrees, in no acute distress but appearing tired. His BMI is greater than 35 kg/m^2. His vital signs are T 37°C, BP 150/90, HR 80, and RR 18, with a pulse oximetry of 94% on room air. His labs are normal except for a glucose of 150 mg/dL. After further evaluation of the patient, the AGACNP finds out that he does not sleep throughout the night and wakes up with a headache most every morning. His spouse states that he snores loudly throughout the night and has witnessed him not breathing at least three times a night. The patient's Mallampati score is III (see Table 10.2 and Figure 10.1). The patient's neck size is 18 cm. The polysomnography findings show that this patient has moderate obstructive sleep apnea (OSA) with apnea–hypopnea index (AHI) of 20. The patient is sent home with a CPAP machine on 10 cm H_2O pressure, lifestyle modifications, prescriptions for smoking cessation, and a medical nutritional therapist to instruct on diet and exercise.

DIAGNOSTIC CRITERIA

Screening for OSA should be routinely done by primary care physicians. However, many patients are undiagnosed, and symptoms are frequently observed or exacerbated while hospitalized. Opioids, sedatives, conscious sedation, and general anesthetics exacerbate symptoms. Preoperative assessment should include screening and can be done with these tools:

- STOP-Bang questionnaire (Table 10.3)
- Epworth sleepiness scale (Table 10.4)
- Berlin score (Table 10.5)

Table 10.3 STOP-Bang Questionnaire

Answer		Description
Yes	No	*S = Snoring* Snore loudly that can be heard through closed doors or bed partner elbows you for snoring at night?
Yes	No	*T = Tired* Often feel tired, fatigued, or sleepy during the daytime such as falling asleep during driving?
Yes	No	*O = Observed* Anyone observe you stop breathing or choking/gasping during your sleep?
Yes	No	*P = Pressure* (Blood Pressure) Have HTN or being treated for HTN?

(continued)

Table 10.3 STOP-Bang Questionnaire (*continued*)

Answer		Description
Yes	No	*B = Body mass index* Body mass index greater than 35 kg/m²?
Yes	No	*A = Age* Older than 50 years old?
Yes	No	*N = Neck size* Measured at Adam's apple or shirt collar, greater than 16 inches
Yes	No	*G = Gender* Male (biologic sex)?
Interpretation: Yes to 0–2 questions: low risk of OSA; Yes to 3–4 questions: intermediate risk; Yes to 5–8 questions: high risk.		

HTN, hypertension; OSA, obstructive sleep airway.
Source: Adapted from http://www.stopbang.ca/osa/screening.php

Table 10.4 Epworth Sleepiness Scale

Rate Situations Associated With Sleepiness	
Sitting and reading No chance (0 points) Slight chance of dozing (1 point) Moderate chance of dozing (2 points) High chance of dozing (3 points)	Points ____
Watching television No chance (0 points) Slight chance of dozing (1 point) Moderate chance of dozing (2 points) High chance of dozing (3 points)	Points ____
Sitting inactive in public place No chance (0 points) Slight chance of dozing (1 point) Moderate chance of dozing (2 points) High chance of dozing (3 points)	Points ____
Sitting for an hour as a passenger in a car No chance (0 points) Slight chance of dozing (1 point) Moderate chance of dozing (2 points) High chance of dozing (3 points)	Points ____
Lying down in the afternoon to rest No chance (0 points) Slight chance of dozing (1 point) Moderate chance of dozing (2 points) High chance of dozing (3 points)	Points ____
Sitting and talking to another person No chance (0 points) Slight chance of dozing (1 point) Moderate chance of dozing (2 points) High chance of dozing (3 points)	Points ____

(*continued*)

Table 10.4 Epworth Sleepiness Scale (*continued*)

Rate Situations Associated With Sleepiness	
Sitting quietly after lunch (without consumption of alcohol) No chance (0 points) Slight chance of dozing (1 point) Moderate chance of dozing (2 points) High chance of dozing (3 points)	Points ____
Sitting in a car stopped for a few minutes due to traffic No chance (0 points) Slight chance of dozing (1 point) Moderate chance of dozing (2 points) High chance of dozing (3 points)	Points ____
Total Points:	

Points	Interpretation of Score
0–7	Unlikely you are abnormally sleepy
8–9	Have an average amount of daytime sleepiness
10–15	May be excessively sleepy depending on situation May want to consider seeking medical attention
16–24	Excessively sleepy and should consider seeking medical attention

Source: Adapted from Johns, M. W. (1991). A new method for measuring daytime sleepiness: The Epworth Sleepiness Scale. *Sleep, 14*(6), 540–545. https://doi.org/10.1093/sleep/14.6.540

Table 10.5 Berlin Score (Risk of Sleep Apnea)

Height (cm)_____ Weight (kg)_____ Age _____ Male/Female Please choose the correct response to each question	
Category 1	Item 1: Do you snore? _a. Yes _b. No _c. Do not know If you snore: Item 2: Your snoring is: _a. Slightly louder than breathing _b. As loud as talking _c. Louder than talking _d. Very loud as it can be heard in adjacent rooms Item 3: How often do you snore? _a. Nearly every day _b. Three to four times a week _c. One to two times a week _d. One or two times a month _e. Never or nearly never Item 4: Has your snoring ever bothered other people? _a. Yes _b. No _c. Do not know Item 5: Has anyone noticed that you quit breathing during your sleep? _a. Nearly every day _b. Three to four times a week _c. One to two times a week _d. One or two times a month _e. Never or nearly never

(*continued*)

Table 10.5 Berlin Score (Risk of Sleep Apnea) (*continued*)

Category 2	Item 6: How often do you feel tired or fatigued after your sleep?
	_a. Nearly every day
	_b. Three to four times a week
	_c. One to two times a week
	_d. One or two times a month
	_e. Never or nearly never
	Item 7: During your waking time, do you feel tired, fatigued, or not up to par?
	_a. Nearly every day
	_b. Three to four times a week
	_c. One to two times a week
	_d. One or two times a month
	_e. Never or nearly never
	Item 8: Have you ever nodded off or fallen asleep while driving a vehicle?
	_a. Yes
	_b. No
	Item: If Yes:
	How often does this occur?
	_a. Nearly every day
	_b. Three to four times a week
	_c. One to two times a week
	_d. One or two times a month
	_e. Never or nearly never
Category 3	Do you have high blood pressure?
	_a. Yes
	_b. No
	_c. Do not know

Note: High risk, two or more categories where the score is positive; Low risk, only one or no categories where the score is positive.
Source: Adapted from Netzer, N. C., Stoohs, R. A., Netzer, C. M., Clark, K., & Strohl. (1999). Using the Berlin Questionnaire to identify patients at risk for the sleep apnea syndrome. Annals of Internal Medicine, *131*, 485.

A patient with suspected OSA should undergo comprehensive evaluation by a provider with expertise in sleep medicine, including comprehensive history and physical exam that includes evaluation of the upper airway for nasal and oropharyngeal anatomical abnormalities. Polysomnography (PSG) is the gold standard for evaluation. PSG measures apnea–hypopnea index and respiratory disturbance index. Diagnosis of OSA is confirmed by the following:

- five or more predominantly obstructive respiratory events per hour of sleep:
  - obstructive and mixed apneas
  - hypopneas
  - respiratory effort–related arousals (RERAs)
- with one or more of the following:
  - sleepiness, nonrefreshed sleep, fatigue, or symptoms of insomnia
  - waking up with gasping or choking
  - habitual snoring, breathing interruptions witnessed by bed partner
  - medical conditions—hypertension (HTN), mood disorder, cognitive interruptions, coronary artery disease, stroke, congestive heart failure, atrial fibrillation, or type 2 diabetes mellitus
- assessment of AHI = (apneas + hypopneas/total sleep time in hours)
- respiratory disturbance index (RDI) = (apneas + hypopneas + RERA)/total sleep time in hours

Alternatively, a home sleep apnea test (HSAT) can be done. An HSAT often expresses AHI as the Respiratory Event Index (REI)—the number of respiratory events per hour of recording time. Positive results for OSA include:

- REI greater than 15 events per hour
- REI 5 to 14 per hour

Classification of severity of OSA is as follows:

- mild: AHI/RDI/REI 5 to 14 respiratory events per hour of sleep
- moderate: AHI/RDI/REI 15 to 30 respiratory events per hour of sleep
- severe: AHI/RDI/REI greater than 30 respiratory events per hour

TREATMENT/MANAGEMENT

Patients should be counseled on lifestyle modifications including avoiding alcohol, sedating medications, and sleeping in the supine position, as this can increase apneic episodes. The gold standard for treatment is CPAP. Adjunctive therapies include oral airway appliances such as tongue-retaining devices and mandibular advancement devices. Surgery may be needed for patients who fail CPAP and oral airway appliances. Patients who have anatomical upper airway obstructions such as hypertrophy of tonsils or adenoids may need tonsillectomy and adenoidectomy or uvulopalatopharyngoplasty (UPPP).

COMPLICATIONS

Complications of undiagnosed and unmanaged OSA include motor vehicle crashes, neuropsychiatric dysfunction, cardiovascular morbidity, cerebrovascular morbidity, pulmonary hypertension (PH), right ventricular failure, metabolic syndrome, diabetes mellitus type 2, and nonalcoholic fatty liver disease.

▶ ASTHMA

DISEASE OVERVIEW

Reactive airway disease is a nonspecific term, usually related to hyperreactive airways and very often related to asthma. Triggers for both syndromes include pets, dust, pollen, smoke, mold or mildew, exercise, stress, strong odors, and weather extremes.

CLASSIC PRESENTATION

An adult Black male patient with a 3-day history of an upper respiratory viral illness presents with reporting of wheezing, chest tightness, and shortness of breath. He has been using his albuterol inhaler two puffs every 2 hours for the last 16 hours and feels he is getting worse, not better. He has been regularly using his Advair 500/50 BID without missing any doses. He reports his peak flow is less than 40% of his personal best. On exam his breath sounds are significantly decreased throughout. Vital signs: T 37.6°C, HR 122, RR 30, BP 150/80, O_2 sat 94%. Arterial blood gases (ABG) reveal pH 7.46, $PaCO_2$ 28, PaO_2 95. He is placed on a continuous albuterol nebulizer and given methylprednisolone (Solu-Medrol) 60 mg IV × 1. Four hours later, he complains of severe fatigue and denies feeling better. The AGACNP notes near-absent breath sounds. ABG reveals pH 7.35, $PaCO_2$ 45, PaO_2 80. The AGACNP intubates the patient and initiates mechanical ventilation.

DIAGNOSTIC CRITERIA

A chest x-ray (CXR) should be done to exclude other diagnoses. In asthma, the CXR should be clear. An ABG will show respiratory alkalosis. Peak flow spirometry will be decreased. Pulmonary function tests will be normal with a positive methacholine challenge.

TREATMENT/MANAGEMENT

Asthma treatment includes avoidance of triggers, allergy testing, and management following a stepwise approach:

- step 1: short-acting beta-agonist (SABA)
- step 2: SABA plus low-dose intercostal space (ICS)
- step 3: low-dose ICS plus long-acting beta-agonist (LABA) or medium-dose ICS
- step 4: medium-dose ICS plus LABA
- step 5: high-dose ICS plus LABA *and* consider omalizumab for patients with allergies
- step 6: high-dose ICS plus LABA and oral corticosteroids *and* consider omalizumab for patients with allergies

Adjunctive therapies can include cromolyn, leukotriene modifiers, mast cell stabilizers, methylxanthines such as theophylline, or other immunomodulators (i.e., monoclonal antibodies). Acute exacerbations of asthma require IV corticosteroids and nebulized albuterol. In more severe cases, IV magnesium sulfate or inhaled heliox may be used as adjunctive therapy. Intubation may be required if these interventions fail to reverse the bronchospasm. Normalizing carbon dioxide levels signal impending respiratory failure in asthmatics, and they should be intubated immediately before they become hypercarbic and develop respiratory acidosis.

COMPLICATIONS
Complications of acute exacerbation of asthma include acute hypoxic and/or hypercarbic respiratory failure, acute respiratory distress syndrome (ARDS), pneumothorax, pneumomediastinum, and cardiac arrest.

▶ CHRONIC OBSTRUCTIVE PULMONARY DISEASE

DISEASE OVERVIEW
Chronic obstructive pulmonary disease (COPD) affects almost 400 million people and is the third leading cause of death globally. In the United States, it is the third leading cause of death. Ten percent of the patient population is age 40 years or older, which varies among countries. Since 2000, the number of women with COPD has surpassed that of men. The leading cause of COPD is cigarette smoking; however, 25% of patients have never smoked. Exposure to lung irritants such as secondhand smoke, chemical fuels, biomass fuels, and organic and inorganic dusts may contribute to COPD. Alpha-1 antitrypsin deficiency, a rare genetic condition, may also contribute to COPD. The hallmark of COPD is chronic expiratory flow limitation and hyperinflation.

Chronic lung inflammation that causes airway remodeling results in narrowing and loss of peripheral airways. Emphysema results in parenchymal destruction, loss of alveolar units causing gas trapping, resulting in hyperinflation. COPD is preventable and treatable. This pulmonary disease is characterized by respiratory symptoms and chronic airflow limitation documented on spirometry. The airflow obstruction is not fully reversible. COPD includes emphysema, chronic bronchitis, and chronic obstructive asthma. Clinical presentation includes pulmonary and extrapulmonary manifestations.

Pulmonary manifestations include dyspnea and cough, including chronic cough; those with chronic illness have associated frequent exacerbations. Extrapulmonary manifestations include cardiovascular comorbidities, systemic inflammation, muscle wasting, weight loss, and nutritional deficits. Risk factors include cigarette smoking, indoor air pollution (secondhand cigarette smoke, biomass fuel, and wood burning stoves), and occupational exposures (chemical fuels and organic and inorganic dusts).

EMPHYSEMA
Damage to airways distal to the terminal bronchioles, including the acinus (respiratory bronchiole alveolar sacs, alveolar ducts, and alveoli), causes permanent dilatation of airspaces and destruction of walls and decreases alveolar and capillary surface area. Emphysema is classified into three types. Centrilobular-proximal acinar is the most common and is associated with smoking. Panacinar occurs in alpha-1 antitrypsin deficiency. Paraseptal or distal acinar may occur alone or in combination with centrilobular-proximal acinar and panacinar. It is usually seen in pneumothorax when occurring alone.

CHRONIC BRONCHITIS
Chronic *bronchitis* manifests as airway inflammation, airflow obstruction, increased sputum production, inadequate mucus transport, pulmonary mucus accumulation, increased airway mucin concentration (MUC5AC and MUC5B), mucus plugging, mucus cell metaplasia, hyperplasia, and exacerbations in muco-obstructive disease.

ASTHMA/CHRONIC OBSTRUCTIVE PULMONARY DISEASE OVERLAP
Asthma and COPD can have overlapping symptoms. Asthma/COPD overlap has manifestations of chronic bronchitis and emphysema with chronic inflammation. However, airflow obstruction is partially reversible.

CLASSIC PRESENTATION

A 67-year-old male patient presents to the ED with complaints of shortness of breath and a productive cough of yellow sputum that has worsened over the week. He has a significant medical history of emphysema and HTN. The patient has a 40 pack-year history. On presentation, the patient is thin and pale, is sitting up with HOB at 45 degrees, and is purse-lipped breathing. He can speak in three-word sentences. Vital signs: T 37°C, HR 100, RR 28, BP 140/72, O_2 sat 84%. CXR shows flattened diaphragms without infiltrates. Spirometry results from last week show his FEV_1 (forced expiratory volume in 1 second) is 40% of predicted.

DIAGNOSTIC CRITERIA

Spirometry is the diagnostic test used with COPD. The Global Initiative for Chronic Obstructive Lung Disease (GOLD) classifies the severity of airflow limitation:

- GOLD 1: mild obstruction, FEV_1 is ≥80% predicted
- GOLD 2: moderate obstruction, FEV_1 is 50% to 79% predicted
- GOLD 3: severe obstruction FEV_1 is 30% to 49% predicted
- GOLD 4: very severe obstruction, FEV_1 is less than 30% predicted

Other spirometry results indicating COPD include post-bronchodilator FEV_1/forced vital capacity (FVC) less than 0.70, decline in FEV_1, and reduction in diffusing capacity. Reduction in single-breath diffusing capacity of the lungs for carbon monoxide (DLCO) is predictive of emphysema. Severe reduction in DLCO predicts exertional oxyhemoglobin desaturation associated with PH. Lung volume measurements can reveal air trapping, increase in residual volume (RV), and increased residual volume/total lung capacity.

An ABG may be normal in early stages of COPD and have an increased first alveolar-arterial gradient (A-aDO$_2$). In late stages of COPD, the ABG reveals hypoxemia with a compensated respiratory acidosis that increases in acidemia during acute exacerbations. CBC with differential should be obtained. Monitor hemoglobin to assess oxygen transport capacity. The hematocrit (HCT) should be assessed for secondary polycythemia. The differential may reveal eosinophils, which may demonstrate asthma/COPD overlap. Assess a basic metabolic profile to monitor for increased serum bicarbonate that occurs with chronic hypercarbia.

Further workup for acute exacerbations could include markers of chronic inflammation such as C-reactive protein (CRP), lactic acid level, procalcitonin, and respiratory viral panel including SARS-CoV-2 testing. Sputum cultures are useful to distinguish COPD from pneumonia. Common pathogens in patients with COPD are *S. pneumoniae, H. influenza,* and *Moraxella catarrhalis.*

Patients with COPD and/or acute exacerbations of COPD (AECOPD) may develop arrhythmias, thus ECGs should be obtained. Patients with AECOPD should be placed on telemetry to assess for supraventricular arrhythmias including sinus tachycardia, multifocal atrial tachycardia, atrial flutter, atrial fibrillation, and ventricular arrhythmias.

CXR may show hyperinflation and diaphragmatic flattening, barrel chest (widened anterior–posterior diameter), bullae, infiltrate/consolidation, and pneumothorax. Assess a noncontrast CT of the chest for emphysematous changes, mucus plugging in visible airways, or nodules or spiculated masses that may indicate a possible lung cancer.

TREATMENT/MANAGEMENT

The goal of management is to slow or prevent the progressive loss of lung function. Smoking cessation is critical, and education should be done at every encounter as well as offering nicotine replacement therapy.

Prevention of severe infections with vaccinations should be encouraged for all patients with COPD and include pneumococcal, influenza, and COVID-19 vaccinations. Additionally, pulmonary rehabilitation should be encouraged for stages B, C, and D.

Oxygen therapy is a mainstay intervention for chronic hypoxia. Continuous oxygen, classified as use longer than 15 hours, increases survival rate in patients with severe resting hypoxia. Initiate for PaO_2 less than 55 mmHg or O_2 Sat less than 88% or PaO_2 less than 59 mmHg in cor pulmonale. Supplemental oxygen is used for patients who desaturate with exercise to maintain oxygen saturation greater than 90% or to improve ventilation-perfusion mismatch caused by hypoxic vasoconstriction of pulmonary arteries.

Escalating treatment strategies are used to manage COPD (Table 10.6). Inhaled bronchodilators (short-acting and long-acting) are the cornerstone of medication treatment. Short-acting bronchodilators include SABA such as albuterol/levalbuterol and short-acting muscarinic antagonist (SAMA) such as ipratropium bromide. Long-acting bronchodilators include LABA such as salmeterol/formoterol/arformoterol/indacaterol and long-acting muscarinic antagonists (LAMA) such as tiotropium/aclidinium. Combination inhalers are helpful to enhance compliance and include albuterol/ipratropium (Combivent, DuoNeb, Respimat), fluticasone/salmeterol (Advair), budesonide/formoterol (Symbicort), and umeclidinium/vilanterol (Anoro). ICS such as AeroBid, Azmacort, Beclovent, Flovent, and Pulmicort are used in GOLD stages 3 and 4. Systemic steroids are used in acute exacerbations. Phosphodiesterase-4 (PDE4) inhibitors (Roflumilast) can be added for severe COPD. Theophylline is a last-line therapy. IV alpha-1 antitrypsin (A_1AT) can be used in A_1AT-deficient patients.

Table 10.6 Comparison of COPD Guidelines

GOLD Guidelines (Stepwise Approach)	American College of Physician Guidelines	European Respiratory Society/ American Thoracic Society Guidelines
COPD stage I (FEV$_1$ ≥ 80%) ■ Short-acting beta-agonists ■ Anticholinergics	FEV$_1$ less than 80% ■ Short-acting bronchodilators	Mild COPD/FEV$_1$ greater than 80% ■ Short-acting bronchodilators
COPD stages II–VI Add: ■ Long-acting beta-agonists	FEV$_1$ less than 60% ■ Long-acting bronchodilators ■ For patients who are symptomatic, add inhaled corticosteroid	Moderate COPD/FEV$_1$ less than 80% ■ Long-acting bronchodilators
COPD stages III–VI Add: ■ Oral or parenteral steroids ■ Inhaled steroids if had antibiotics in last 12 months (perform CRP and procalcitonin before antibiotics) ■ Theophylline		FEV$_1$ less than 50% or exacerbations ■ Oral steroids or antibiotics in the preceding 12 months
		FEV$_1$ less than 30%: theophylline

COPD, chronic obstructive pulmonary disease; CRP, C-reactive protein; FEV$_1$, forced expiratory volume in 1 second.

Empiric antibiotics can be used during AECOPD when concomitant community-acquired infection is suspected. Follow community-acquired pneumonia (CAP) guidelines. Suppressive antibiotic therapy, specifically azithromycin (250 mg or 500 mg daily three times a week) for 1 year, can reduce the number of acute exacerbations.

Adjunctive therapies include anti-IL-5 monoclonal antibody (mepolizumab) can be used for eosinophilic COPD, and anti-IL-5-receptor monoclonal antibody (benralizumab) can reduce the number exacerbations requiring admission to hospital.

Lung transplantation may be of benefit in patients with advanced COPD, emphysema due to A_1AT deficiency, pulmonary arterial hypertension, interstitial lung disease (ILD), and cystic fibrosis (CF). Lung volume reduction surgery, bullectomy, or endobronchial valves are treatments used for patients with large bullae. Patients with end-stage COPD with severe dyspnea should be offered palliative care and hospice and be provided opioid (oral morphine, oxycodone) and sedative-hypnotics (diazepam) for symptom management.

▶ ACUTE RESPIRATORY FAILURE

DISEASE OVERVIEW

Acute respiratory failure is a disorder by which the respiratory system is unable to perform the gas-exchanging functions, oxygenation, ventilation, or both. Acute respiratory failure is one of the most common diagnoses in the ICU. Acute respiratory failure is categorized according to pathophysiological disorders in respiratory function. There are four types of acute respiratory failure, which are outlined in the following sections.

RESPIRATORY FAILURE TYPE I: ACUTE HYPOXIC RESPIRATORY FAILURE

Acute hypoxic respiratory failure, the most common type of respiratory failure, characterized by severe arterial hypoxemia, is the most common type of respiratory failure that is refractory to supplemental oxygen, with a partial arterial oxygen (PaO_2) less than 60 mmHg or arterial oxygen saturation (SaO_2) less than 90% (Table 10.7). Type I respiratory failure may be combined hypoxia and hypercapnia with an arterial pH less than 7.25 and a partial pressure of carbon dioxide ($PaCO_2$) greater than 45 mmHg.

Table 10.7 Causes of Hypoxia

Etiology	Description
Low-inspired oxygen partial pressure	▪ Causes tachypnea and hyperventilation that occur due to low levels of inspired oxygen (occurs at high altitudes) ▪ Normal A-a gradient with decreased $PaCO_2$ due to hyperventilation ▪ A-a gradient = PAO_2–PaO_2. A-a gradient = (Age + 10)/4 ▪ Normal A-a gradient is 5–10 mmHg; A-a gradient increases by 1 mmHg per decade ▪ A-a gradient is used to assist in determining the cause of hypoxemia. ▪ A-a gradient assesses the alveolar-capillary gas exchange, indirectly quantifying the ventilation-perfusion defects. ▪ A-a gradient can assess whether the cause of hypoxemia is due to intrapulmonary or extrapulmonary causes. ▪ Elevated A-a gradient is due to alveolar-capillary dysfunction.
Alveolar hypoventilation	▪ Alveolar hypoventilation increases $PaCO_2$, causing a decrease in PAO_2. Normal A-a gradient with a decrease in both PAO_2 and PaO_2. ▪ Central nervous system depression as in coma, sleep apnea (central), obesity hypoventilation syndrome, hypothyroidism, and metabolic encephalopathy ▪ Decrease in chest wall compliance as in flail chest and kyphoscoliosis ▪ Neuromuscular diseases as in ALS, GBS, and MG
Diffusion impairment	▪ Increased A-a gradient ▪ Alveolar structure: decreased surface area or increased thickness ▪ Decrease time during alveolar-capillary level ▪ Diffusion defects occur in emphysema, interstitial lung disease, and during exercise
Ventilation-perfusion mismatch	▪ Increased A-a gradient ▪ Most common etiology of Acute Respiratory type I ▪ Occurs in acute respiratory distress syndrome, atelectasis, chronic obstructive pulmonary disease, pneumonia, pulmonary embolism, and congestive heart failure
Right to left shunt	▪ Increased A-a gradient ▪ Absence of gas exchange at alveolar-capillary level ▪ True shunt seen in atrial septal defect and patent foramen ovale ▪ Pulmonary right to left shunt seen in arteriovenous malformation, complete atelectasis, severe pneumonia, and severe pulmonary edema

ALS, amyotrophic lateral sclerosis; GBS, Guillain-Barré syndrome; MG, myasthenia gravis; $PaCO_2$, partial pressure of carbon dioxide; PaO_2, partial pressure of oxygen, arterial; PAO_2, partial pressure of oxygen, arterial blood.

Presenting signs and symptoms of acute hypoxic respiratory failure include those of the underlying disease along with symptoms of hypoxia, which include tachypnea causing hypocapnia (initially), dyspnea, anxiety, restlessness, bradycardia or tachycardia, arrhythmias, tremor, and confusion. Somnolence and cyanosis are late findings. Acute hypoxic respiratory failure accompanied by hypercapnia includes the previously mentioned signs plus signs of hypercarbia, such as headache, peripheral hyperemia, conjunctival hyperemia, papilledema, HTN, and asterixis.

CLASSIC PRESENTATION

A 55-year-old female patient presents to the ED with complaints of shortness of breath and a productive cough of yellow sputum for the past week. She has a past medical history of HTN for which she takes hydrochlorothiazide. The patient has never smoked or been exposed to smoking. On presentation, the patient is a well-nourished female sitting up with HOB at 45 degrees and is in acute respiratory distress as she is only able to speak in one-word sentences. Vital signs: T 38°C, BP 110/60, HR 110, RR 30, pulse oximetry 88% on room air. Trachea is midline. Normal anterior/posterior (AP) diameter and normal contour are noted. The patient has moderate use of accessory muscles. Equal excursion. No subcutaneous emphysema. Breath sounds heard throughout all lobes with crackles in bases. Cardiac monitor shows normal sinus rhythm. Normal S_1S_2. No murmurs, gallops, or rubs. Capillary refill less than 3 seconds. ABG shows pH 7.45, $PaCO_2$ 33, PaO_2 58, BICARB 23, oxygen saturation 90%, brain natriuretic peptide (BNP) less than 100, troponin 0.001; white blood cell (WBC) 12, red blood cell (RBC) HCT 38, hemoglobin (Hgb) 12. Radiographic studies: Ultrasound: B-lines (focal) with subpleural consolidations and bronchograms. CXR: bilateral pleural effusions. CT scan of thorax: consolidations in lower lobes.

DIAGNOSTIC CRITERIA

ABG are the gold standard. Assessment of A-a gradient, capnography, pulse oximetry can be substituted. Adjunctive diagnostics to identify etiology can include CBC with differential, cultures (blood, sputum, and urine), serum chemistry, BNP, troponin, inflammatory markers (CRP, creatinine phosphokinase, lactic acid level, and procalcitonin, respiratory viral panel, including SARS-CoV-2), urinary antigen test, thyroid function test (thyroid stimulating hormone [TSH], triiodothyronine [T_3], levorotatory thyroxine [T_4]), EKG, echocardiogram, bronchoscopy, pulmonary function studies (except in the acute phase of illness), CXR, and CT of thorax.

Ultrasound of thorax is increasingly being used to diagnose thoracic conditions. The BLUE protocol is the gold standard. Normal lungs have A-lines denoting the presence of aerated lungs. B-lines represent interstitial fluid. A pneumothorax will have a barcode sign indicating the absence of lung sliding, whereas pulmonary edema and ARDS will have diffuse B-lines.

RESPIRATORY FAILURE TYPE II: HYPERCAPNIC RESPIRATORY FAILURE

Respiratory failure type II is characterized by a partial pressure carbon dioxide greater than 45 mmHg causing respiratory acidosis with a pH less than 7.35. This condition does not include carbon dioxide retention. Hypercapnic respiratory failure is caused by alveolar hypoventilation resulting in the inability to effectively eliminate carbon dioxide. Hypoventilation can be caused by

- loss of central nervous system drive resulting in an impaired ventilator drive due to oversedation, brainstem injury, drug overdose, sleep apnea, and severely untreated hypothyroidism;
- impaired strength with failure of neuromuscular function in the respiratory system due to respiratory weakness secondary to decreased muscle due to neuromuscular diseases (amyotrophic lateral sclerosis [ALS], Guillain-Barré syndrome [GBS], myasthenia gravis [MG], poliomyelitis, and transverse myelitis), hypophosphatemia, and organophosphate poisoning;
- increased load on the respiratory system such as resistive loads due to bronchospasms, decreased lung compliance due to atelectasis, alveolar edema, and intrinsic positive and expiratory pressures, excessive dead space or mechanical load; and
- reduced chest wall compliance caused by abdominal distension, pleural effusion, and pneumothorax.

Clinical manifestations include mild dyspnea, headache, lethargy, hypersomnolence, delirium, confusion, coma, seizures, asterixis, papilledema, warm skin, and dilated superficial dilated veins. Differential diagnoses include cardiogenic shock, cor pulmonale, cyanosis, diaphragmatic paralysis, dilated cardiomyopathy, emphysema, myocardial infarction (MI), OBS, and pulmonary embolism.

RESPIRATORY FAILURE TYPE III: PERIOPERATIVE RESPIRATORY FAILURE

Respiratory failure type III is caused by a decrease in functional residual capacity due to atelectasis ultimately causing dependent lung units to collapse. Decreased functional residual capacity is caused by obesity, general anesthesia, and surgical procedures of the chest and abdomen. Clinical manifestations include dyspnea, hypoxia, and tachypnea. CXR will demonstrate loss of lung volumes/atelectasis.

RESPIRATORY FAILURE TYPE IV: HYPOPERFUSION OF RESPIRATORY MUSCLES DUE TO SHOCK STATES

Respiratory muscles normally consume up to 5% of cardiac output (CO). In shock conditions, the respiratory muscles consume up to 40% of CO. Signs and symptoms are related to specific shock state.

TREATMENT/MANAGEMENT

Management of acute hypoxic respiratory failure always begins by assessing airway, breathing, and circulation. The AGACNP needs to focus on reversing the underlying cause of acute respiratory failure. Hypoxia in COPD requires administration of low-flow oxygen by nasal cannula 1 to 3 L/min. Hypoxia in parenchymal lung diseases such as in ARDS and pneumonia may require higher levels of oxygen. Hypoxia due to acute respiratory failure may require humidified high-flow nasal cannula. High-flow oxygen settings are flow rate from 5 to 60 L/min and fraction of oxygen in the inspired air (FIO_2; 0.21–1.00). Set flow rate to start at 20 to 35 L/min and titrate to patient's work of breathing (WOB). Titrate FIO_2 to SpO_2 goal. As flow rates increase, wean the FIO_2.

Patients with respiratory failure type III, perioperative respiratory failure, should have the following to manage atelectasis: keep head of bed (HOB) up 30 to 45 degrees, reposition every 2 hours, use incentive spirometry, use positive expiratory pressure (PEP) therapy (also known as "flutter valve"), and manage incisional pain to facilitate use of incentive spirometer and chest physiotherapy. Patients may also require noninvasive positive pressure ventilation (high-flow nasal canula [NC], CPAP, or BiPAP) to augment inspiratory volumes.

Escalation to noninvasive positive pressure ventilation may be needed in patients with hypoxia in COPD and cardiogenic pulmonary edema, such as CPAP to prevent alveolar collapse during expiration starting at 5 cm H_2O up to 15 cm H_2O, and BiPAP that supports both inspiration and expiration with an inspiratory pressure of 5 to 10 cm H_2O and an expiratory pressure of 5 cm H_2O.

Invasive mechanical ventilation may be needed for moderate to severe acute hypoxic respiratory failure. Relative indications for intubation are as follows:

- depressed mental status (Glasgow Coma Scale [GCS] ≤ 8)
- inability to clear pulmonary or oral secretions
- shock states
- severe hypoxia or hypercarbia with pH less than 7.2
- metabolic acidosis with pH less than 7.2
- trauma to airway, mouth, face, or neck
- impending airway compromise

Once intubated, employ lung-protective and diaphragmatic protective strategies. Initial ventilator settings should include tidal volumes (TV) ≤8 mL/kg ideal body weight (IBW). For patients who meet criteria for ARDS, a low TV strategy should be targeted, 4 to 6 mL/kg IBW.

VENTILATOR MANAGEMENT

Initial ventilator settings can be determined through the following steps:

- Step 1: Calculate IBW.
  - For men, start at 50 kg and add 2.2 kg for each inch over 5 ft.
  - For women, start at 45 kg and add 2.2 kg for each inch over 5 ft.
  - Be sure to use a tape measure to obtain an actual height.
- Step 2: Select a mode of ventilation (Table 10.8). Names of specific ventilation modes vary by manufacturer.
- Step 3: Select a TV to either set or limit. Initially it should be set to ≤8 mL/kg IBW; for patients with ARDS, should be ≤6 mL/kg IBW.
- Step 4: Set rate. Try to match the patient's RR to minimize their WOB.
- Step 5: Set FIO_2. A good practice for patients with acute hypoxic respiratory failure is to start at 100% and then can wean rapidly if O_2 saturations remain greater than 92%.
- Step 6: Select positive end-expiratory pressure (PEEP) level. The minimal PEEP level is 5; for obese and morbidly obese patients, minimal PEEP needed is likely to be 7.5. Prior to and during intubation, patients will de-recruit alveoli; thus, starting with a PEEP level of 10 may be needed to re-recruit alveoli. Wean PEEP after FIO_2 is ≤50%.

Table 10.8 Ventilator Modes

Preferred Term	Intended Meaning Mechanical Ventilation With:
VC-CMV	Preset TV and inspiratory flow. Every breath is mandatory (i.e., inspiration is patient or machine triggered and machine cycled).
VC-IMV	Preset TV and inspiratory flow. Spontaneous breaths can exist between mandatory breaths.
PC-CMV	Present inspiratory pressure and inspiratory time. Every breath is mandatory.
PC-IMV	Preset inspiratory pressure and inspiratory time. Spontaneous breaths can exist between mandatory breaths.
CSV	Any mode of mechanical ventilation where every breath is spontaneous

CSV, continuous spontaneous ventilation; PC-CMV, pressure-controlled continuous mandatory ventilation; PC-IMV, pressure-controlled intermittent mandatory ventilation; TV, tidal volume; VC-CMV, volume-controlled continuous mandatory ventilation; VC-IMV, volume-controlled intermittent mandatory ventilation.
Source: Carpenter, D. (2022). *Fast facts for the adult-gerontology acute care nurse practitioner.* Springer Publishing Company.

Adjusting Ventilator Settings

▨ Step 7: Obtain ABG and adjust settings based on ABG.
  ● *To adjust the PaCO$_2$:* Adjust the rate or TV. Hypercarbia causes respiratory acidosis, whereas low PaCO$_2$ creates an alkalotic state.
  ● *To adjust the PaO$_2$:* Adjust the FIO$_2$ or PEEP. PEEP takes longer (2–4 hours to see an effect) to improve oxygenation, whereas O$_2$ can effect a change immediately. Both interventions may need to be employed initially, then wean PEEP after oxygenation is improved and FIO$_2$ is weaned to $\leq$50%.
▨ Step 8: Continue to monitor peak inspiratory pressure (PIP) and plateau pressures.
  ● PIP reflects the amount of pressure required for the ventilator to deliver each breath. PIP is increased depending on the amount of resistance (e.g., patient coughing or biting on tube, size of tube, secretions in tube, or decreased lung compliance).
  ● Plateau pressure reflects the amount of pressure remaining in the lungs at peak inspiration when airflow ceases; the goal plateau pressure is less than 30 cm H$_2$O. Be sure to trend and monitor plateau pressures. If plateau pressures are trending up toward 30 cm H$_2$O, then decrease the TV and increase the RR to keep the same minute ventilation.

Nonconventional mechanical ventilation may also be used as in pressure control ventilation and bilevel or airway pressure release ventilation (APRV). Last, veno-venous extracorporeal membrane oxygenation (VV ECMO) may be required for patients with the most severe and refractory acute hypoxic respiratory failure.

Patients who are intubated should have sedation titrated to a Richmond Agitation Sedation Score (RASS) of 0 to −1 or Riker Sedation-Agitation Scale (SAS) of 4. Avoidance of benzodiazepines, daily awakening trials (if not on paralytics), daily spontaneous breathing trials (once at or below 50% FIO$_2$ and 8 PEEP), and early mobilization (out of bed to chair, ambulation) improve outcomes. Analgesics should be titrated to a pain score or care pain observation tool (CPOT) score.

CRITERIA FOR EXTUBATION

Extubation can be considered when the reason (or reasons) the patient was intubated is reversed or significantly improved and when the following are met:

▨ not requiring paralytic agent
▨ adequate mental status (exception may be neurologically impaired patients)
▨ rapid shallow breathing index (RSBI) less than 105; RSBI = TV/RR
▨ Sat greater than 88%, RR greater than 8
▨ decreasing/minimal vasopressor support
▨ absence of cardiac arrhythmias and ischemia during spontaneous breathing trial (SBT)
▨ controlled intracranial pressure (ICP)
▨ reduced secretions and strong enough to cough/clear secretions

Although less predictive of successful extubation, some clinicians still like to know the following parameters: patient can lift head off bed and has a strong cough, negative inspiratory force (NIF) ≥20 cm H_2O (measures strength of respiratory muscles [the more negative the number, the stronger are the patient's muscles]); vital capacity greater than 10 mL/kg; and if an endotracheal tube (ETT) cuff leak is present.

COMPLICATIONS

Complications of acute respiratory failure include shock, iatrogenic effects from mechanical ventilation (intubation complications, ventilator-induced lung injury, oxygen toxicity, atelectrauma, barotrauma, volutrauma, ARDS, ventilator-associated pneumonia, and diaphragmatic weakness), nosocomial infections, sepsis, acute kidney injury, multiorgan system failure, deep venous thrombosis (DVT), stress ulcers, ICU-acquired weakness, anemia, and anoxic cerebral injury.

▶ RIB FRACTURES

DISEASE OVERVIEW

Rib fractures are most often associated with blunt trauma although they can be from penetrating trauma or pathologic from metastasis. Spontaneous rib fractures from coughing are most commonly noted in patients with osteoporosis. Pathologic rib fractures can occur due to metastasis. Rib fractures of two or more consecutive ribs in two or more locations is considered a flail section. The flail section moves paradoxically during respirations, increasing the risk for acute respiratory failure. Elderly patients have a high risk of mortality associated with even one or two rib fractures.

CLASSIC PRESENTATION

A frail elderly woman presents after reportedly falling. She cannot recall whether she tripped or passed out. She is complaining of right-sided chest pain and hip pain. Examination reveals an abrasion and ecchymosis of her right lateral chest wall. She is complaining of worse pain with deep inspiration.

DIAGNOSTIC CRITERIA

A CT scan is the most sensitive diagnostic test, but the initial test should be a CXR to assess for life-threatening injury such as a pneumothorax or widened mediastinum indicating an aortic injury. CXR can show rib fractures but are not the most sensitive.

TREATMENT/MANAGEMENT

Patients with rib fractures require aggressive multimodal pain management to allow for pulmonary hygiene. Pulmonary hygiene includes use of an incentive spirometer, PEP also known as a "flutter valve," and early mobility, which are key to preventing atelectasis. Should these measures fail, noninvasive ventilation should be instituted early. Use of high-flow nasal cannula (HFNC), CPAP, and BiPAP are all options. Use of these while patients sleep can passively prevent de-recruitment while allowing patients to sleep and can ease pain by internally splinting the ribs. Intubation may be needed if the previous interventions fail. Surgical stabilization of affected rib fractures remains controversial but may be needed for severe malalignment or angulation.

COMPLICATIONS

The greatest complication risk is atelectasis that, if not treated aggressively, can develop into pneumonia. Other complications include pneumothorax, hemothorax, shock, and death. Elderly with even one rib fracture are at grave risk of death and warrant admission to intermediate care units or even ICUs.

▶ PNEUMOTHORAX

DISEASE OVERVIEW

A *pneumothorax* (PTX) is air outside the lung but within the pleural space. PTXs are classified as simple, tension, or open. A simple PTX does not have mediastinal structure shift, as is seen with tension PTX.

An open PTX is also referred to as a "sucking" chest wound, where the atmosphere is open directly to the pleural space. PTX are commonly caused by trauma. PTX are categorized into four types:

- *Primary spontaneous PTX:* Occurs spontaneously without associated lung diseases. This type is common in younger tall, thin individuals, those with Marfan syndrome, those with familial PTX, individuals who are pregnant, and individuals who smoke. Patients may report shortness of breath and/or chest pain that is pleuritic or sharp in nature and may radiate to the ipsilateral shoulder.
- *Secondary spontaneous PTX:* Occurs due to underlying lung disease, such as COPD and bullous emphysema, ARDS, pulmonary fibrosis, bronchogenic carcinoma, CF, sarcoidosis, and others. Patients report chest pain and more severe dyspnea.
- *Traumatic:* Occurs with history of a recent trauma, commonly with rib fractures and penetrating injuries such as stabbings. Subcutaneous emphysema may be noted along with distended chest wall and absent breath sounds.
- *Iatrogenic PTX:* Occurs due to provider's interventions including but not limited to central venous catheterization in the subclavian or internal jugular veins, during biopsy, as a result of barotrauma from positive pressure ventilation, during bronchoscopy, during percutaneous tracheostomy or thoracentesis, during pacemaker insertion, during cardiopulmonary resuscitation, and during intercostal nerve blocks.

Any of these PTXs can progress into tension pneumothorax, whereby the pneumothorax increases in size, and pressure displaces intrathoracic contents, including trachea, heart, and great vessels to the contralateral side. Tension physiology is demonstrated by tachycardia, hypotension, and distended neck veins.

CLASSIC PRESENTATION
A patient with a history of severe COPD on 2 L home O_2 has just been intubated and due to hypoxia has had the PEEP increased to 10. He now complains of sharp chest pain and worsening dyspnea. Subcutaneous emphysema is noted on his anterior chest and ascending to his neck and jaw.

DIAGNOSTIC CRITERIA
CXR is the most used diagnostic test; however, ultrasound is increasingly being used to look for lung sliding. Lack of lung sliding is indicative of a PTX. A noncontrast CT scan of the chest will identify smaller PTXs. Tension physiology is denoted by tachycardia, hypotension, and JVD and requires immediate intervention.

TREATMENT/MANAGEMENT
Smaller PTXs can be managed conservatively. Tension PTX requires emergent needle decompression (at the ipsilateral second intercostal space [ICS] midclavicular line [MCL]) if the patient becomes hemodynamically unstable. Anyone who has been needle decompressed must follow with a chest tube to prevent recurrence. Small-bore chest tubes or pigtail catheters can be placed (second ICS MCL or fourth or fifth ICS mid-axillary line) for simple PTX. Larger chest tubes (28–36 Fr) are needed if a hemothorax is also present. Surgical intervention may be required if chest tubes fail. Surgical options include video-assisted thoracoscopic surgery (VATS) or open thoracotomy.

COMPLICATIONS
Complications depend on the etiology and extent of the PTX. Initially, for large PTX, pleural effusions or hemothorax, re-expansion pulmonary edema can occur immediately after lung re-expansion. Chest tubes should be clamped after a liter of output is noted. The most common complications are pain and skin infection at the site of tube thoracostomy. Recurrence of the PTX can also occur with changing to water seal or upon removal of the chest tube. Additionally, and less commonly, patients can develop acute possibly leading to chronic respiratory failure, cardiac arrest, pneumopericardium, bronchopulmonary fistula, and damage to the neurovascular bundle during tube thoracostomy.

▶ HEMOTHORAX

DISEASE OVERVIEW

Hemothorax is the collection of blood in the pleural space (space between the visceral and parietal pleura). Hemothorax is commonly a result of blunt chest trauma due to rib fractures. When vessels are lacerated by the fractured ribs, substantial bleeding can occur. Blood loss of greater than 1,500 mL is considered massive hemothorax.

CLASSIC PRESENTATION

A young adult male patient presents after a motorcycle crash where he was T-boned by a car. He complains of severe right-sided chest pain. His oxygen saturation is 90% on 6-L NC. CXR reveals severely displaced lateral rib fractures of ribs 6, 7, 8, and 9 with a large meniscus of fluid blunting the costophrenic angle collapsing the right lower lung field.

DIAGNOSTIC CRITERIA

CXR will identify a pleural effusion but cannot differentiate between blood, lung collapse, or other types of effusion. Ultrasound can demonstrate fluid and provide an estimation of volume but cannot distinguish between blood or other pleural effusion fluid. CT scan of the chest will identify fluid, and measuring the Hounsfield units (HU) can differentiate between blood and other types of tissues or effusions. HU of blood range from 45 to 65 HU, and hematomas can range from 40 to 90 HU.

TREATMENT

Most require thoracostomy tubes to prevent the hemothorax (HTX) from becoming infected and the lung becoming permanently collapsed. Be sure to reverse any anticoagulation. For massive hemothorax, ensure appropriate treatment of hemorrhage with a fixed ratio of transfusion (i.e., packed red blood cells [PRBC], fresh frozen plasma [FFP], platelets at 1:1:1 ratio).

COMPLICATIONS

Complications of HTX include infected hemothorax, chest tube site infections, trapped lung, solid organ injury from misplaced chest tubes, shock, organ failure, and death.

▶ PULMONARY CONTUSIONS

DISEASE OVERVIEW

Pulmonary contusions are most commonly a result of blunt force trauma to the lung parenchyma without laceration to the lung tissue or vascular structures. Contusions can also be caused by falls from substantial height, contact sports, shock waves associated with a penetrating injury to the chest cavity, or explosive injuries. A contusion results in bleeding and inflammation into the lung tissue causing reduced lung compliance, ventilation-perfusion mismatch, and intrapulmonary shunting.

CLASSIC PRESENTATION

A 45-year-old man presents after falling off a second-story roof onto his right side. He complains of right chest, hip, and arm pain. Workup reveals a right humerus fracture, right intertrochanteric fracture, and right rib fractures 4 to 10. He reports pain 10/10 and is unable to take deep breaths or cough. He is hemodynamically stable. His incentive spirometry (IS) is 500 mL. He is medicated with Tylenol, methocarbamol (Robaxin), and ketorolac (Toradol). A lidocaine patch is applied, and he has been given oxycodone. Six hours later, his pain is 6/10, and he complains of progressive shortness of breath. IS remains at 500 mL. His O_2 saturation has dropped to 88% on 6-L NC. CXR shows hyperdensities in the right lung fields.

DIAGNOSTIC CRITERIA

CXR is the most common diagnostic test; however, CT scans are the most sensitive diagnostic test to identify pulmonary contusions. Contusions may not be evident in the first 6 hours and become more evident over the first 24 to 48 hours.

TREATMENT

Treatment of pulmonary contusion is supportive in nature including IS, coughing, and deep breathing. CPAP and BiPAP can be used to prevent de-recruitment and to recruit alveoli and support respiration. Conservative fluid management, diuretics, and avoidance of blood transfusions (if able) minimize the inflammatory process and fluid sequestration into the lung tissues. Severe pulmonary contusions may require intubation and mechanical ventilation. VV ECMO may be employed in severe and refractory hypoxemia.

COMPLICATIONS

Complications of pulmonary contusions may result in acute hypoxic respiratory failure, pneumonia, and ARDS.

▶ ASPIRATION PNEUMONITIS

DISEASE OVERVIEW

Aspiration can result in an *aspiration pneumonitis* from the inhalation of gastrointestinal (GI) contents into one or both of the lungs. The right lung is most affected as the left mainstem bronchus is more acutely angulated to accommodate the heart. Typically, patients can cough and expectorate contents. Suctioning may be needed for the medically frail and/or intubated patients. Risk factors include impaired cognition or swallowing, vomiting, GI procedures (including placement of nasogastric tube or feeding tube), dental procedures, and gastroesophageal reflux disease (GERD). Patients with respiratory muscle weakness or strokes and older adult patients are at highest risk for aspiration.

Aspiration pneumonitis is an inflammation of the lung tissues caused by a chemical irritant, which does not need antibiotics. However, if gastric contents cannot be expectorated or suctioned out, then aspiration pneumonitis can progress into aspiration pneumonia over the next 48 to 82 hours. To qualify for aspiration pneumonia, patients need to develop classic signs of pneumonia including fever or chills, worsening hypoxia, productive sputum, leukocytosis, and infiltrate on CXR. Aspiration pneumonia can range from mild to severe illness, depending on the amount and the body's innate defense mechanisms. The most common pathogens are gram-negative enteric pathogens or oral anaerobes.

CLASSIC PRESENTATION

A patient who is admitted for a large middle cerebral artery (MCA) ischemic stroke is noted to be coughing, dyspneic, tachypneic, tachycardic, and progressively hypoxemic and now has a new fever and diffuse crackles.

DIAGNOSTIC CRITERIA

CXR will show an infiltrate in one or more of the lobes of the lungs, most commonly in the right lower lobe (RLL). The RLL is mostly affected due to the anatomy of the right mainstem bronchus being straighter, whereas the left mainstem is more acutely angulated. The AGACNP should obtain a CBC, comprehensive panel, lactate, ABG, and sputum and blood cultures.

TREATMENT/MANAGEMENT

Aspiration pneumonitis needs only supportive care (oxygen, pulmonary clearance) for the first 48 to 72 hours, whereas aspiration pneumonia requires antibiotics to cover gram negatives and anaerobes with beta-lactam/beta-lactamase antibiotic.

COMPLICATIONS

Complications include lung abscess, pleural effusion, ARDS, and septic shock.

▶ PNEUMONIA

DISEASE OVERVIEW

Pneumonia can be bacterial, viral, or fungal in nature. Viral pneumonia can develop into a superimposed bacterial pneumonia. Viral pneumonia has become more prevalent due to the COVID-19 virus. Fungal pneumonia is the least common and occurs in immunocompromised patients. The severity of pneumonia can range from mild to deadly, as occurs when patients experience multisystem organ failure. According to the Centers for Disease Control and Prevention (CDC), there are 1.5 million visits with pneumonia as the diagnosis. Mortality is 14.4/100,000, excluding COVID-19 deaths.

COMMUNITY-ACQUIRED PNEUMONIA

CAP is defined as being acquired prior to hospitalization or within 48 hours of admission. The most common bacterial pathogens for CAP are *S. pneumoniae, H. influenza, C. pneumoniae,* and *M. pneumoniae.* Viral pathogens include coronaviruses, respiratory syncytial virus (RSV), adenoviruses, influenza, human metapneumovirus, and parainfluenza. Common fungal infections include histoplasma capsulation, coccidioides immitis, and *Pneumocystis jiroveci.* Risk stratification of CAP uses the CURB65 or the pneumonia severity instrument (PSI) to determine the course and place of treatment.

HOSPITAL-ACQUIRED PNEUMONIA

HAP is classified as a pneumonia that develops ≥48 hours after hospital admission or within 48 hours after discharge from the hospital. Common pathogens include gram-negative bacilli and *S. aureus.* Resistant bacteria must be considered when the patient has had exposure to IV antibiotics within the last 90 days.

VENTILATOR-ASSOCIATED PNEUMONIA

VAP develops ≥48 hours after intubation or within 48 hours after extubations and has a similar presentation and treatment to HAP, whereas a ventilator-associated event (VAE) is a broader term that encompasses complications associated with ventilators and includes VAP as well as sepsis, ARDS, PE, barotrauma, and pulmonary edema.

CLASSIC PRESENTATION

An older adult presents with a new cough with yellow sputum production, fever, dyspnea, pleuritic chest pain, tachypnea, tachycardia, and general malaise. Physical exam reveals adventitious breath sounds, egophony, and use of accessory muscles.

DIAGNOSTIC CRITERIA

CXR is essential. CBC assesses for leukocytosis and differential assesses for neutrophilia (shift to left) to identify bacterial infection. ABG and lactate levels aid in determining the patient's acuity and need for noninvasive ventilation and/or intubation and mechanical ventilation. Sputum analysis is needed (may need bronchalveolar lavage (BAL) or bronchoscopy to obtain), *S. pneumoniae* antigen, legionella titer to identify the organisms, and sensitivities to tailor antibiotics. Chemistries assess for acidosis, renal function, hyponatremia, and other electrolyte disorders. Procalcitonin is done to differentiate between infectious versus noninfectious etiology and determine a baseline on when to stop antibiotics.

TREATMENT

Empiric antibiotics should be started immediately until culture results have been obtained (Table 10.9). Antiviral agents are indicated if suspicion of viral pneumonia is present. Supportive measures include administration of oxygen, fluids, and analgesics. If the patient requires intubation and mechanical ventilation, follow VAP bundles, and implement early mobilization.

Table 10.9 Treatment of Bacterial Pneumonia

CAP

Outpatient treatment of CAP

No comorbidities or risk factors for MRSA or pseudomonas
- Amoxicillin *or*
- Doxycycline *or*
- Macrolide (if local pneumococcal resistance is less than 25%)
- *Note*: Amoxicillin and doxycycline do not cover pseudomonas.

With comorbidities (chronic heart, lung, liver, or renal disease; diabetes mellitus; alcoholism; malignancy; or asplenia) or risk factors for MRSA or pseudomonas
- Combination therapy with amoxicillin/clavulanate or cephalosporin AND a macrolide or doxycycline

OR
- Monotherapy with respiratory fluoroquinolone

Inpatient treatment of CAP

Nonsevere inpatient CAP
- Standard therapy = Beta-lactam PLUS macrolide or respiratory fluoroquinolone
- Prior MRSA = Standard therapy PLUS MRSA coverage AND obtain MRSA nasal swab, de-escalate if negative.
- Prior *Pseudomonas aeruginosa* = Standard therapy PLUS add coverage for *P. aeruginosa*, obtain respiratory cultures, and de-escalate as able.

Severe inpatient CAP
- Standard therapy = Beta-lactam PLUS macrolide OR beta-lactam PLUS respiratory fluoroquinolone
- Prior MRSA = Standard therapy PLUS MRSA coverage and obtain MRSA nasal swab, de-escalate if negative.
- Prior *Pseudomonas aeruginosa* = Standard therapy PLUS add coverage for *P. aeruginosa*, obtain respiratory cultures, and de-escalate as able.

KEY	
Beta-lactam	Ampicillin + sulbactam 1.5–3 g every 6 hours OR Cefotaxime 1–2 g every 8 hours OR Ceftriaxone 1–2 g daily OR Ceftaroline 600 mg every 12 hours
Macrolide	Azithromycin 500 mg daily OR Clarithromycin 500 mg twice daily
Respiratory fluoroquinolone	Levofloxacin 750 mg daily OR Moxifloxacin 400 mg daily
MRSA coverage	Vancomycin (15 mg/kg every 12 hours, adjust based on trough goal 15–20) OR Linezolid (600 mg every 12 hours)
Pseudomonas coverage	Piperacillin-tazobactam (4.5 g every 6 hours) OR Cefepime (2 g every 8 hours) OR Ceftazidime (2 g every 8 hours) OR Imipenem (500 mg every 6 hours) OR Meropenem (1 g every 8 hours) Aztreonam (2 g every 8 hours)

Empiric Antibiotic Therapy for Hospital-Acquired Pneumonia

Not at high risk of mortalityand no factors increasing the likelihood of MRSA:
One of the following:
- Piperacillin-tazobactam 4.5 g IV q6h

OR
- Cefepime 2 g IV q8h
- Levofloxacin 750 mg IV daily

OR
- Imipenem 500 mg IV q6h
- Meropenem 1 g IV q8h

(continued)

Table 10.9 Treatment of Bacterial Pneumonia (*continued*)

CAP

Not at high risk of mortalitybut with factors increasing the likelihood of MRSA:

One of the following:
- Piperacillin-tazobactam 4.5 g IV q6h
- Cefepime or ceftazidime 2 g IV q8h

OR
- Levofloxacin 750 mg IV daily
- Ciprofloxacin 400 mg IV q8h

OR
- Imipenem 500 mg IV q6h
- Meropenem 1 g IV q8h

OR
- Aztreonam 2 g IV q8h

PLUS:
- Vancomycin 15 mg/kg IV q8–12h with goal to target 15–20 mg/mL trough level (consider a loading dose of 25–30 mg/kg × 1 for severe illness)

OR
- Linezolid 600 mg IV q12h

High risk of mortality or IV antibiotics within 90 days, prescribe two of the following while avoiding double beta-lactam coverage:
- Piperacillin-tazobactam 4.5 g IV q6h

OR
- Cefepime or ceftazidime 2 g IV q8h

OR
- Levofloxacin 750 mg IV daily
- Ciprofloxacin 400 mg IV q8h

OR
- Imipenem 500 mg IV q6h
- Meropenem 1 g IV q8h

OR
- Amikacin 15–20 mg/kg IV daily
- Gentamicin 5–7 mg/kg IV daily
- Tobramycin 5–7 mg/kg IV daily

OR
- Aztreonam 2 g IV q8h

PLUS:
- Vancomycin load with 25 mg/kg IV × 1 then 15 mg/kg IV q8–12h with target trough of 15–20 mcg/mL

OR
- Linezolid 600 mg IV q12h

If MRSA coverage is not needed, be sure to include coverage for MSSA including piperacillin-tazobactam, cefepime, levofloxacin, imipenem, and meropenem.

Empiric Treatment Options for Suspected HAP/VAP When MRSA and Double Antipseudomonal/ Gram-Negative Coverage Are Needed

---

Choose one from A, B, and C:

A. (*Gram + coverage with MRSA coverage*):
- Vancomycin load 25 mg/kg IV × 1 then 15–20 mg/kg q8–12h trough goal 15-20 mcg/mL OR
- Linezolid 600 mg IV or PO q12h

  AND

B. (*Gram − coverage with antipseudomonal coverage with beta-lactam–based agents*)
- Piperacillin-tazobactam 4.5 gm IV q6h or via extended infusions over 4 hours q8h

  OR
- Cefepime 2 g IV q8h
- Ceftazidime 2 g IV q8h

  OR
- Imipenem 500 mg IV q6h

(*continued*)

Table 10.9 Treatment of Bacterial Pneumonia (*continued*)

CAP

• Meropenem 1 g IV q8h
  OR
• Aztreonam 2 g IV q8h
AND:
C. *(Gram–coverage with antipseudomonal coverage with non-beta-lactam–based agents)*
• Ciprofloxacin 400 mg IV q8h
• Levofloxacin 750 mg IV q24h
  OR
• Amikacin 15–20 mg/kg IV q24h
• Gentamicin 5–7 mg/kg IV q24h
• Tobramycin 5–7 mg/kg IV q24h

Note: Be sure to renal dose based on patient's creatinine clearance. If in doubt, consult a pharmacist.

CAP, community-acquired pneumonia; HAP, hospital-acquired pneumonia; IV, intravenous; MRSA, methicillin-resistant *Staphylococcus aureus*; MSSA, methicillin-susceptible *Staphylococcus aureus*; VAP, ventilator-acquired pneumonia.

Source: Carpenter, D. (2022). *Fast facts for the adult-gerontology acute care nurse practitioner.* Springer Publishing Company.

COMPLICATIONS

Complications of pneumonia include acute hypoxic respiratory failure, mucous plugging, empyema, septic shock, multisystem organ failure, and death. Mucous plugging may present with hypoxia, recent history of pneumonia or COPD exacerbation, shallow breathing or high peak inspiratory pressures on ventilator, or low TV alarms; CXR will show total collapse of a lobe or lung with a narrowing of the bronchus. Management of mucous plugging involves multimodal therapies, including chest physiotherapy, albuterol, mucolytic agents such as inhaled Mucomyst, or hypertonic saline nebulizers, percussive vests, insufflation-exsufflation, and PEP therapy (also known as a flutter valve). Bronchoscopy may be required if conservative therapies fail.

▶ SARS-COV-2 (COVID-19)

Viral pneumonia is common and can progress to a superimposed bacterial pneumonia. Recently, COVID-19 has brought viral pneumonia to the forefront. Documenting whether an infection is bacterial or viral or fungal is important to guide the treatment regimen.

Exam Tip

Viral pneumonia may be on certification exams; however, COVID-19 viral pneumonia may be too recent to be on the exams yet. A lag time of 2 or more years exists between practice changes and information becoming mainstream knowledge to be tested on the exams. COVID-19 is presented here as it will likely be on the exam before the next edition of the book is published.

DISEASE OVERVIEW

SARS-CoV-2 (COVID-19) is a respiratory virus that caused a worldwide, severe pandemic. COVID-19 virus is a member of lineage B of the *Betacoronavirus* genus; MERS-CoV a lineage C virus; and lineage A common cold viruses CoV-OC43, CoV-HKU1, and MERS-CoV. These are RNA viruses. Coronaviruses are enveloped single-stranded RNA viruses that are found in humans and other mammals causing respiratory, neurologic, and GI diseases. Severe acute respiratory syndrome (SARS) in 2002 to 2003 resulted in the SARS-CoV pandemic. The second coronavirus was Middle East Respiratory Syndrome (MERS) in 2012. The third coronavirus is SARS-CoV-2, which resulted in COVID-19. Coronaviruses can adapt and infect new hosts by genetic combination and variation.

VARIANTS

At the time of publication, seven variants exist (Alpha, Beta, Gamma, Delta variant B.1.621, Delta plus variant, Lambda variant C.37, Omicron variant B.1.1.529). The omicron variant has several subvariants (BA1, BA1.1, BA.2, BA 2.1.2.1, XE [mutation of BA.1 and BA.2], BA.4, BA.5, BA 2.75, BA 5.2.1A). As the virus continues to mutate, other variants are expected to be identified.

TRANSMISSION

The principal mode of transmission is by respiratory droplets from person to person within 6 ft of each other. Infectious respiratory secretions (respiratory droplets and sputum) are inhaled by airborne transmission, which is increased during exercise or singing. Transmission can occur from an asymptomatic or presymptomatic persons.

REINFECTION

Reinfection with SARS-CoV-2 is possible and is not specific to any strain. The causes and risk factors of reinfection are not completely understood. Immune response may be inadequate to the first infection, and those with comorbid conditions are at higher risk.

BREAKTHROUGH INFECTION

Fully vaccinated persons are associated with reduced risk of COVID-19 breakthrough infections. Most breakthrough infections may be asymptomatic or with mild symptoms. Fully vaccinated persons with immune dysfunction are associated with a higher risk of COVID-19 breakthrough infections. Breakthrough infections are associated with neutralizing antibody titers during the peri-infection period. Completion of all SARS-CoV-2 vaccinations and continued preventive measures of masking in public places and maintaining social distancing are recommended.

CLINICAL MANIFESTATIONS

The onset of COVID-19 disease occurs typically 4 to 5 days after exposure. Symptoms vary between variants and individuals. Common symptoms include fever/chills, upper respiratory tract symptoms (rhinorrhea, congestion, pharyngitis), lower respiratory tract symptoms (shortness of breath, cough), GI symptoms (nausea, vomiting, diarrhea), dysgeusia, and anosmia (loss of taste and smell).

SEVERITY OF ILLNESS

Severity of illness can progress from mild to moderate to severe disease. Severe disease symptoms include dyspnea, hypoxia (oxygen saturation ≤94% on room air), or greater than 50% lung involvement on imaging. Elevated labs (D-dimer, ferritin, CRP, interleukin 6 [IL-6]) associated with severe COVID-19 D-dimer. Critical illness includes respiratory failure, shock, or multisystem dysfunction.

Severe manifestations include neurologic (microembolic stroke, encephalopathy). Severe GI symptoms include COVID-19–associated coagulopathy and the development of disseminated intravascular coagulation (DIC). Additionally, elevated serum alanine aminotransferase (ALT) and aspartate aminotransferase (AST) levels, and lactate hydrogenase (LDH) indicate hepatic dysfunction. COVID-19–associated cytokine release syndrome includes severe systemic inflammatory signs (fever, tachycardia, tachypnea, hypotension). Inflammatory markers of infection include high CRP and ferritin levels. The degree of elevated ferritin level is associated with greater severity of illness, with some patients deteriorating rapidly within 1 week. Hematologic manifestations of severe COVID-19 infection include lymphopenia and neutrophilia.

RISK FACTORS

COVID-19 has multiple risk factors, including age (children and advanced age). Men and Black Americans are affected more. Overweight and obesity, including severe obesity, are a significant risk factor. Those with chronic lung and cardiovascular diseases are at especially high risk. Pulmonary conditions include COPD, asthma (moderate to severe), CF, ILD, and PH. Additionally at high risk are those with cardiac conditions (HTN, coronary artery disease [CAD], cardiomyopathies, and heart failure) or cerebrovascular disease. Diabetes type 1 and type 2 and chronic liver disease are also risk factors. Immunosuppressed patients, including those with cancer and cancer treatments (hematologic malignancies, solid organ transplant, and stem cell transplant) and primary immunodeficiency and acquired immunodeficiencies (corticosteroids, immunosuppressive medications, and HIV type I), are at high risk of dying from COVID-19 pneumonia. Substance use, including alcohol, opioids, cocaine, and cigarettes, elevates the risk of being infected.

CLASSIC PRESENTATION

A 26-year-old male patient presents in transfer from an outside hospital having complained of fever, chills, and shortness of breath accompanied by dry cough for 3 days. The patient has no significant past medical history. The patient smokes one pack of cigarettes per day and admits to smoking marijuana and crack cocaine several times a week. On presentation, the patient is a thin male lying in bed on full ventilator support. The ventilator is set on volume control with the following settings: TV 400 cc, RR 20, FIO_2 1.0, PEEP 10 cm H_2O. Labs are positive for COVID-19 and elevated D-dimer, ferritin level, LDH, ALT, and AST. CXR shows multifocal pneumonia. CT of thorax shows diffuse pulmonary infiltrates. Vital signs: T 38°C, HR 110, BP 110/60, O_2 sat 88%. He is sedated on propofol RASS-2 and moves extremities to mild stimulation with minimal use of accessory muscles. There is no subcutaneous emphysema. Breath sounds are heard throughout all lobes with crackles in bases.

DIAGNOSTIC CRITERIA

Reverse transcriptase polymerase chain reaction (RT-PCR) assay is the standard for diagnosis of COVID-19. Nucleic acid amplification testing (NAAT) of respiratory tract secretions via nasopharyngeal swabs is less sensitive. Initial labs include CBC with differential, complete metabolic profile, CK, CRP, PT/INR, PTT, and fibrinogen. Systemic disease may manifest with lymphopenia, thrombocytopenia, elevated inflammatory markers (IL-6, tumor necrosis factor-α, and CRP), elevated liver enzymes, elevated LDH (repeat while elevated), elevated markers of acute kidney injury, elevated D-dimer, elevated PT, PTT, fibrinogen, elevated troponin, and elevated creatinine phosphokinase (CPK). Repeat these tests as clinically indicated. If not previously performed, consider hepatitis B serologies, hepatitis C virus antibody, and HIV antigen/antibody testing.

CXR will demonstrate multifocal infiltrates (bilateral distribution in lower lung regions). Confirmed COVID-19 infection confirms the diagnosis of COVID-19 viral pneumonia. CT shows multifocal ground glass opacity. Peripheral and linear consolidations may be observed within several days after disease onset. Pleural thickening, interlobular septal thickening may also be noted.

COMPLICATIONS

Complications of COVID-19 virus include pulmonary complications of ARDS and pneumonia. Vascular complications include thromboembolic complications including PE, DVT, and arterial thrombosis (acute stroke, limb ischemia). Cardiac complications include arrhythmias, MI, heart failure, and cardiogenic shock. Infectious complications include septic shock and secondary bacterial or fungal infections. Neurologic complications include encephalopathy, delirium, seizures, ataxia, and motor or sensory deficits. Renal complications include acute kidney injury and rhabdomyolysis.

TREATMENT/MANAGEMENT

The evidence supporting COVID-19 management continues to evolve at a rapid pace. Treatment options are based on severity of respiratory illness and manifestations of system disease.

GENERAL MANAGEMENT

General management includes antipyretics with acetaminophen to alleviate fever; however, nonsteroidal anti-inflammatory drugs (NSAIDs) may be associated with worse outcomes. Aspirin, statin, angiotensin-converting enzyme inhibitors (ACEIs), or angiotensin receptor blockers (ARBs) are recommended if not otherwise contraindicated. If the diagnosis is uncertain, initiate empiric antibiotics for CAP and empiric influenza antiviral treatment.

IMMUNOMODULATORY AGENTS

Immunomodulatory agents include routine use of IV dexamethasone for its anti-inflammatory properties. Other agents that may be used include IL-6 monoclonal antibodies (siltuximab, sarilumab, tocilizumab); antivirals (remdesivir with or without baricitinib [Janus kinase 1 and 2 inhibitor]); tocilizumab (monoclonal antibody against IL-6 receptor); SARS-CoV-2 specific human monoclonal antibodies; and molnupiravir (oral ribonucleoside analog that inhibits SARS-CoV-2 replication).

RESPIRATORY MANAGEMENT

Respiratory management includes initiation of high-flow oxygen for acute hypoxic respiratory failure at 30 to 60 L/min and 21% to 100% FIO_2. For patients with COPD or progressive hypoxia, CPAP may be necessary and, if hypercarbic, will need BiPAP. Mechanical ventilation is common for severe COVID-19 infections. Target ARDS net high PEEP. Institute lung-protective TV to lower respiratory pressures (plateau pressure less than 30 cm H_2O). SpO_2 goals should be 88% to 92%. Early proning is recommended for those who meet ARDS criteria. ECMO could be considered early in severe ARDS with refractory hypoxemia on mechanical ventilation and optimized medical management. Early referral to an ECMO center should be considered.

PREVENTIVE MEASURES

Prevention is key to preventing severe disease. Social distancing (staying 6 ft away from other people), social isolation (staying away from people who are infected), quarantine measures, limited traveling, and working from home can reduce transmission. Screening prior to entry into healthcare facilities including for fever, respiratory symptoms (cough, dyspnea, sore throat), myalgias, and anosmia/hyposmia can help prevent exposure of healthcare providers. Universal masking includes surgical masks for healthcare workers, patients, and visitors; respirator N-95 masks without exhalation valve during medical procedures that generate aerosols; goggles; and face shields to add additional protection for healthcare workers. Respiratory droplet isolation and contact isolation are recommended to prevent in-hospital spread.

AGACNPs should recommend and encourage use of COVID-19 vaccines especially for high-risk patients and family members. Boosters are recommended.

▶ PLEURAL EFFUSION/EMPYEMA

DISEASE OVERVIEW

Pleural effusions are commonly identified in a wide variety of patient conditions, including heart failure, pneumonia, trauma, lung cancer, cirrhosis, and pancreatitis. Pleural effusions can be either transudative or exudative in nature. Use Light's criteria to determine the etiology of the effusion.

CLASSIC PRESENTATION

Patients may have varied symptoms that can range from asymptomatic to dyspnea on exertion (DOE) depending on the patient's ability to expand the thorax. Patients with pleurisy (active pleural inflammation) often complain of sharp, severe, localized pain with breathing or coughing. Constant pain is a classic sign of malignant effusion. Depending on the etiology of effusion, the patient may present with complaints of fever and other systemic symptoms. Physical exam reveals decreased breath sounds and decreased fremitus. Egophony may be present. Pleural rubs are often mistaken for coarse crackles. Fever may be present with empyema.

DIAGNOSTIC CRITERIA

CXR will show blunting of costophrenic angle(s). Upright lateral films can be completed to better identify the volume. When patients are lying supine or recumbent, the fluid will layer posteriorly, thus making quantification difficult. CXR is not the best to differentiate between lung atelectasis/collapse and pleural effusion. Loculated effusions can be seen at the lateral and inferior lung fields as dense convexities that do not layer out in supine or recombinant positions. Bedside ultrasound can be used to identify the presence and quantification of fluid versus atelectasis as well as guide thoracentesis or pigtail catheter placement. CT scans can help differentiate pleural effusion and atelectasis/lobar collapse, quantify volume of pleural effusion, and identify loculations that signify an empyema.

Analysis of fluid should be done in the context of working diagnoses. To determine whether it is transudative or exudative, obtain serum and pleural fluid for protein, and LDH to calculate by Light's criteria (Table 10.10). For ease of use, a phone application or online calculator can calculate the results and aid in diagnosing the etiology. Additional fluid testing can include glucose, cell count differential, cytology, culture, cholesterol/triglycerides, amylase, and culture for *Mycobacterium tuberculosis*.

Table 10.10 Light's Criteria to Differentiate Between Transudate Versus Exudate

Diagnostic	Transudate	Exudate
Pleural to serum protein ratio	Less than 0.5	≥0.5
Pleural to serum LDH	Less than 0.6	≥0.6
Pleural fluid LDH	Less than 2/3 upper limit of normal	≥2/3 upper limit of normal

Main causes	▪ Heart failure
	▪ Hypoalbuminemia
	  ● Cirrhosis
	  ● Nephrotic syndrome
		▪ Malignancy
		▪ Infection
		  ● Pneumonia
		  ● Tuberculosis
		  ● Fungal
		  ● Empyema
		▪ Pancreatitis
		▪ Esophageal rupture
		▪ Chylothorax/hemothorax
		▪ Post-CABG

CABG, coronary artery bypass grafting; LDH, lactate hydrogenase.
Source: Carpenter, D. (2022). *Fast facts for the adult-gerontology acute care nurse practitioner.* Springer Publishing Company.

TREATMENT/MANAGEMENT

Treatment depends on the etiology, and the underlying cause must be treated. Heart failure requires diuresis. Hepatic hydrothorax requires diuresis with Lasix and spironolactone along with treatment of cirrhosis. Small-bore chest tubes or pigtail catheters can be used to drain free-flowing pleural effusions. Temporarily pause chest drainage after ~1,500 mL is drained to prevent re-expansion pulmonary edema. Large-bore chest tubes are needed to drain hemothoraces. Malignant effusions can be treated with thoracentesis, indwelling pleural catheter, or video-assisted thoracoscopy (VAT) with talc pleurodesis. Empyemas require tube thoracostomy to drain combined with antibiotics and may possibly require thoracotomy for decortication.

COMPLICATIONS

Complications of untreated pleural effusions can include a permanently restricted lung from re-expanding. Otherwise, complications of plural effusions are complications of the treatments, specifically thoracentesis and pigtail catheters, including pneumothorax.

▶ ACUTE RESPIRATORY DISTRESS SYNDROME

DISEASE OVERVIEW

ARDS is a clinical syndrome. It includes rapid onset of severe dyspnea, hypoxemia, and diffuse pulmonary infiltrates that progresses to acute respiratory failure. ARDS is caused by diffuse lung injury either by pulmonary or nonpulmonary causes (Table 10.11).

Table 10.11 Risk Factors for ARDS

Direct Lung Injury	Indirect Lung Injury
Aspiration of gastric contents Inhalation injury Near drowning Pneumonia: bacterial, viral, fungal, or opportunistic Pulmonary contusion	Cardiopulmonary bypass Drug overdose Multiple blood transfusions Pancreatitis Reperfusion edema after lung transplant or embolectomy Sepsis Severe trauma: burns, flail chest, head trauma, and multiple bone fractures

ARDS, acute respiratory distress syndrome.

According to the Berlin definition of ARDS, the following criteria must be present to diagnose a patient with ARDS:

- Respiratory symptoms occur within 1 week of known clinical insult or must have new or worsening symptoms during the past week.
- Chest radiography or CT of the chest must show bilateral opacities that are not caused by pleural effusions, lobar collapse, or pulmonary nodules.
- Acute respiratory failure is noncardiac in nature. Fluid overload is not due to cardiac failure. If no risk factors for ARDS are present, an echocardiography is performed to rule out hydrostatic pulmonary edema.
- Presence of moderate to severe oxygenation impairment. The arterial oxygen tension to fraction of inspired oxygen (PaO_2/FIO_2) is used to define the severity of ARDS.
  - Mild ARDS: PaO_2/FIO_2 is greater than 200 mmHg, but ≤300 mmHg on ventilator settings that include PEEP or CPAP ≥5 cm H_2O.
  - Moderate ARDS: PaO_2/FIO_2 is greater than 100 mmHg but ≤200 mmHg on ventilator settings that include PEEP ≥5 cm H_2O.
  - Severe ARDS: PaO_2/FIO_2 is ≤100 mmHg on ventilator settings that include PEEP ≥5 cm H_2O.

PATHOPHYSIOLOGY

ARDS has three phases with clinical and pathological features. The first phase is the exudative phase. The second phase is the proliferative phase, and last, the third phase is the fibrotic phase (Table 10.12).

Table 10.12 Phases of ARDS

Phase	Description
Exudative phase	▪ Occurs after 12–36 hours after insult and lasting up to 7 days ▪ Alveolar-capillary endothelial and type I pneumocytes (alveolar epithelial cells) ▪ Accumulation of protein-rich fluid in interstitial and alveolar spaces (cytokines: interleukins 1 and 8, tumor necrosis factor α, and lipid mediators: leukotriene b4) ▪ Proinflammatory mediator response ▪ Leukocyte infiltration into pulmonary interstitium and alveoli ▪ Aggregation of condensed plasma proteins into airspaces with cellular debris and dysfunctional pulmonary surfactant ▪ Formation of hyaline membrane whorls ▪ Pulmonary vascular injury with vascular obliteration by microthrombi and fibrocellular proliferation ▪ Alveolar edema mainly in dependent areas of lung causing decreased aeration ▪ Atelectasis ▪ Collapse of dependent lung ▪ Decreased lung compliance ▪ Intrapulmonary shunting (hypoxemia, increased work of breathing, dyspnea) ▪ Increased pulmonary dead space causing hypercapnea

(continued)

Table 10.12 Phases of ARDS (*continued*)

Phase	Description

Proliferative phase	■ Occurs during day 7 to day 21
	■ Improvement of disease
	  ● Initiation of lung repair
	  ● Organization of alveolar exudates
	  ● Pulmonary infiltrate shifts from neutrophils to lymphocytes
	  ● Alveolar basement membranes are proliferated by type II pneumocytes
	  ● Type II pneumocytes synthesize into new pulmonary surfactant and differentiate into type I pneumocytes
	■ Progression of disease
	  ● Lung injury
	  ● Pulmonary fibrosis

Fibrotic phase	■ Occurs during 3–4 weeks after pulmonary insult
	■ Alveolar duct and interstitial fibrosis
	■ Disruption of acinar architecture leading to emphysematous-like changes—bullae
	■ Intimal fibroproliferation of pulmonary microcirculation
	  ● Vascular occlusion
	  ● Pulmonary hypertension
	■ Complications
	  ● Pneumothorax
	  ● Increased pulmonary dead space

ARDS, acute respiratory distress syndrome.

CLASSIC PRESENTATION

A 55-year-old male patient presents to the ED with complaints of progressive severe shortness of breath and a productive cough of white to yellow sputum for the past 24 hours. He has a past medical history of HTN for which he takes amlodipine. On presentation, the patient is a well-nourished male sitting up with HOB at 45 degrees and is in acute respiratory distress as he is only able to speak in one-word sentences. Physical examination reveals T 38°C, BP 100/58, HR 115, RR 30, with pulse oximetry 88% on high-flow oxygen at a flow rate of 30 L/min with FIO_2 0.6. Chest has a normal AP diameter and normal contour. No kyphoscoliosis. He has moderate use of accessory muscles. No subcutaneous emphysema is noted; however, he has diffuse crackles throughout. Monitor shows ST, and he has no murmurs, gallops, or rubs. Capillary refill less than 3 seconds. ABG shows pH 7.48, $PaCO_2$ 28, PaO_2 58, Bicarb 22, oxygen saturation 90% on high-flow oxygen at a flow rate of 30 L/min with a FIO_2 0.6. D(A-a). O_2 is elevated at 344 mmHg; BNP less than 100, troponin 0.001; WBC 14, Hgb 12, hematocrit 40. Blood, sputum, and urine cultures are in process. Ultrasound has B-lines with subpleural consolidations, and bronchograms. CXR shows bilateral diffuse alveolar opacities with dependent atelectasis. CT scan of thorax shows widespread patchy airspace opacities that are ground glass in appearance in dependent lung zones.

TREATMENT/MANAGEMENT

Treatment of ARDS is supportive. Early recognition and treatment of underlying condition are essential. Mechanical ventilation is often required and includes lung and diaphragmatic protective measures to decrease mechanical stress of the ventilator and maintain the level of inspiratory diaphragmatic effort that is appropriate for the patient (Table 10.13). Manage dyspnea with sedation and ventilator settings; maintain lighter sedation as appropriate. Conservative fluid management is essential to maintain a dry lung. Proning, paralytics, pulmonary vasodilators, and ECMO are additional therapies used for refractory hypoxemia on mechanical ventilation. Additionally, ongoing management of ICU bundles to prevent complications is essential. Adhere to care bundles, including ventilator, central line, DVT prophylaxis, and stress ulcer prophylaxis. Prompt recognition and treatment of nosocomial infections and focus on liberation from mechanical ventilation improve outcomes.

Table 10.13 Modes of Mechanical Ventilation

Assist Control (Volume or Pressure Control)	Bilevel Ventilation or APRV
■ Low tidal volume 4–8 mL/kg (PBW) with a plateau pressure less than 28 cm H_2O ■ FIO_2: Set to achieve SpO_2 of 88% to 92% and PaO_2 of 55–80 mmHg ■ Rate 20–40 with the goal of avoiding auto-PEEP ■ PEEP: 8–20 cm H_2O to minimize FIO_2 and maximize PaO_2 ■ Patient-ventilator synchrony: avoid triggering, flow, and cycling asynchronies	■ Pressure controlled: time-controlled adaptive ventilation ■ Applies continuous positive airway pressure for prolonged time followed by a release phase of shorter duration ■ FIO_2 and mean airway pressure directly affect oxygenation. P(High) is the pressure to open alveoli which is during most of the respiratory cycle. P(Low) is the release of pressure that allows for elimination of CO_2. T(High) is the amount of time during P(High), and T(Low) is the amount of time during P(Low). Recruits and maintains lung volume and decreases WOB. Limits de-recruitment. Allows spontaneous breathing.
Ongoing Monitoring During Mechanical Ventilation 1. Pulse oximetry, arterial blood gases, calculate PaO_2/FIO_2 ratio 2. Capnography 3. Tidal volume, FIO_2, plateau pressure, PEEP, driving pressure 4. Presence of auto-PEEP 5. Presence of pneumothorax or pneumomediastinum	

APRV, airway pressure release ventilation; PEEP, positive end-expiratory pressure; WOB, work of breathing.

COMPLICATIONS

Complications include refractory hypoxemia leading to end-organ damage, nosocomial infections, DVTs, GI bleeding, delirium, malnutrition, muscle wasting, and deconditioning. They also include alveolar damage from mechanical ventilation, as follows:

■ barotrauma due to excessive airway pressures
■ volutrauma due to overdistention of alveoli from higher TVs
■ atelectrauma due to inspiratory opening and expiratory collapsing causing shearing forces in alveoli
■ biotrauma due to excessive mechanical forces in lung with a resultant release of proinflammatory cytokines

▶ PULMONARY HYPERTENSION

DISEASE OVERVIEW

PH is a heterogeneous disease that is chronic and progressive. PH is defined as an abnormally high mean pulmonary artery pressure greater than 20 mmHg at rest. PH is caused by primary or secondary etiologies that cause remodeling of the pulmonary vasculature leading to increased pulmonary artery pressure and vascular resistance. PH is most commonly due to group II left-sided heart failure or group III lung disease and/or hypoxemia (Table 10.14). PH due to idiopathic pulmonary artery hypertension (PAH) is rare. PH due to CTEPH group IV is 4%. PH is more common in female patients. The functional classifications of PH are described in Table 10.15.

Table 10.14 World Health Organization Classification of Pulmonary Hypertension

Group	Description
Group I	Pulmonary artery hypertension: hereditary, idiopathic, or drug/toxin induced
Group II	Pulmonary hypertension heart disease (left sided)
Group III	Pulmonary hypertension due to lung diseases and/or hypoxia
Group IV	Pulmonary hypertension due to CTEPH and other obstructions in the pulmonary artery
Group V	Pulmonary hypertension due to multifactorial mechanisms

CTEPH, chronic thromboembolic pulmonary hypertension.

Table 10.15 Functional Classification of Pulmonary Hypertension

Class	Description
Class I	▪ Physical activity is unaffected. ▪ Physical activity does not cause fatigue, near-syncopal episodes, dyspnea, or chest pain.
Class II	▪ There are no symptoms at rest. ▪ Physical activities are slightly limited. ▪ Ordinary activities of daily living cause fatigue, dyspnea, and near-syncopal episodes.
Class III	▪ There is no symptomatology at rest. ▪ Minimal physical activity causes fatigue, dyspnea, and near-syncopal episodes.
Class IV	▪ Signs of right-sided heart failure occur during physical activities. ▪ Signs of right-sided heart failure may occur at rest.

The pathophysiology differs between the PH groups (Table 10.16). Group I has progressive vascular remodeling leading to vessel wall changes and lumen narrowing, which restricts blood flow, thus increasing pulmonary vascular resistance (PVR), increasing afterload to right ventricle, increasing right ventricular wall tension, and decreasing right ventricular contractility. In contrast, groups II through V can be due to high postcapillary pressures, vasoconstriction, and remodeling due to hypoxemia, destruction of parenchyma, narrowing or occlusion of arteries due to thromboembolism, compression of proximal vasculature, or hyperdynamic states causing increased circulatory flow.

Table 10.16 Causes and Risk Factors by Group

Group I: Pulmonary Artery Hypertension	Group II: Left Heart Disease	Group III: Chronic Lung Disease or Hypoxia	Group IV: CTEPH Obstruction of Pulmonary Arteries	Group V: Multifactorial
	Venous backpressure from the left heart	Hypoxic vasoconstriction	Obstruction of pulmonary arteries	Multifactorial

▪ Pulmonary veno-occlusive disease/capillary hemangiomatosis
▪ Drug/toxins
  ● Long-standing CCB
  ● Anorexigen
  ● Methamphetamines
  ● Interferons
  ● Bosutinib
  ● Leflunomide
  ● Indirubin
  ● St John's wort
  ● Rapeseed oils
▪ HIV
▪ Connective tissue disease
  ● Scleroderma
  ● RA
  ● SLE
▪ Schistosomiasis
▪ Portal hypertension
▪ CHD
▪ Idiopathic or inheritable mutations
▪ Newborns with persistent PH
	▪ Increased vascular tone and remodeling
	▪ Systolic dysfunction
	▪ Diastolic dysfunction
	▪ Valvular diseases
		▪ Loss of pulmonary capillaries
		▪ Diseases that cause chronic hypoxia
		▪ COPD
		▪ ILD
		▪ OSA
		▪ Other causes of chronic hypoxia
			▪ PE/VTE	▪ Extrinsic compression of pulmonary arteries
				▪ Hematologic disorders
				  ● Chronic hemolytic anemia
				  ● Myeloproliferative disorders
				  ● Splenectomy
				▪ Systemic disorders
				  ● Pulmonary histocytosis
				  ● Lymphangioleiomatosis
				  ● Sarcoidosis
				▪ Metabolic disorders
				  ● Glycogen storage disorders
				  ● Gaucher disease
				  ● Thyroid disorders
				▪ Tumors

CCB, calcium channel blockers; CHD, congenital heart disease; COPD, chronic obstructive pulmonary disease; CTEPH, chronic thrombo-embolic pulmonary hypertension; ILD, interstitial lung disease; OSA, obstructive sleep apnea; PE, pulmonary embolism; PH, pulmonary hypertension; RA, rheumatoid arthritis; SLE, systemic lupus erythematosus; VTE, venous thromboembolism.

Presenting signs and symptoms are often nonspecific. Symptoms may occur on exertion, and in advanced stages, symptoms of PH occur at rest. The principal presenting symptom is usually dyspnea, and hypoxemia may also be present. The most common presenting symptoms are dyspnea, orthopnea, paroxysmal dyspnea, angina, palpitations, fatigue, and peripheral edema. Other symptoms can include paroxysmal nocturnal dyspnea, hemoptysis, hoarseness, hyperventilation, dizziness, presyncope, syncope, dry cough, palpitations, nausea, vomiting, and ascites. Palpation of the precordium may reveal a left parasternal lift, right ventricular heave, downward xiphoid thrust, pulmonary artery tap, or a pulsatile liver. Auscultation findings of the heart may identify an accentuated pulmonary component of S2, pansystolic murmur of tricuspid regurgitation, Carvallo sign (tricuspid regurgitation murmur becomes louder after inspiration due to increased venous return to the right heart), diastolic murmur of pulmonary insufficiency, right ventricular S3, and right-sided S4. Auscultation of the lung may be normal; patient have wheezing or inspiratory crackles. Other signs include signs of right heart failure including jugular vein distention (JVD), hepatomegaly, splenomegaly, hepatojugular reflux, ascites, peripheral edema, along with other signs and symptoms specifically related to the underlying conditions causing PH.

CLASSIC PRESENTATION

A 55-year-old female patient presents to the ED with headache, dizziness, heart palpations, and shortness of breath over the past 6 months that have increased in intensity for the past week. She has a medical history of COPD and HTN for which she takes Symbicort (formoterol and budesonide), hydrochlorothiazide, hydralazine, and amlodipine. The patient is a 20 pack-year cigarette smoker. On presentation, the patient is a well-nourished female sitting up in bed at 45 degrees and is in acute distress. Her vital signs are T 37°C, BP 100/50, HR of 102, RR 30, with a pulse oximetry of 90% on room air. She is positive for tricuspid regurgitation murmur, wheezing throughout all lung fields, and 3+ peripheral edema in lower extremities. ABG shows pH 7.33, PaO_2 55, $PaCO_2$ 58, Bicarb 32, SaO_2 88% on room air. Echocardiogram shows a decrease in right ventricular function, dilated right ventricle, moderate tricuspid regurgitation, and moderate PH. EKG shows sinus tachycardia with a rate of 102, P-pulmonale, and right ventricular hypertrophy. CXR shows hyperinflation of lungs and flattened diaphragm.

DIAGNOSTIC CRITERIA

Transthoracic echocardiogram can be used as a screening tool to estimate pulmonary pressures; however, the gold standard to diagnose PAH and classify the PH group is a right heart catheterization. The WHO definition for PH is a mean pulmonary artery pressure (mPAP) greater than 20 mmHg and Wood units ≥3 (Table 10.17).

Table 10.17 Diagnostic Criteria and Workup by Type of Pulmonary Hypertension

Group I: Pulmonary Artery Hypertension	Group II: Left Heart Disease	Group III: Chronic Lung Disease or Hypoxia	Group IV: CTEPH Obstruction of Pulmonary Arteries	Group V: Multifactorial
mPAP greater than 20 mmHg PCWP less than 15 mmHg Pulmonary vascular resistance ≥3 Wood units TRV Tricuspid annular plane systolic excursion Pulmonary artery dilatation Tricuspid regurgitation (moderate to severe) RV function area change Myocardial performance index	Left heart dysfunction CO reduced mPAP ≥20 mmHg PCWP ≥15 mmHg Left atrial enlargement	Diagnosis of chronic lung disease TRV Tricuspid annular plane systolic excursion Pulmonary artery dilatation Moderate to severe TR RV function area change Myocardial performance index	Presence of occlusion in proximal or distal vasculature by thromboembolism or by other occlusions mPAP ≥20 mmHg PCWP greater than 15 mmHg PVR greater than 3 Wood units or greater than 240 dynes/sec/cm^{-5} Decreased cardiac output	Depends on etiology Extrinsic compression of pulmonary arteries in fibrosing mediastinitis Intrinsic elevations in PVR in sarcoidosis, sickle cell anemia, polycythemia vera, and malignancy

CO, cardiac output; CTEPH, chronic thromboembolic pulmonary hypertension; mPAP, mean pulmonary artery pressure; PCWP, pulmonary capillary wedge pressure; PVR, pulmonary vascular resistance; RV, residual volume; TR, tricuspid regurgitation; TRV, tricuspid regurgitation velocity.

BLOOD WORK

Assess CBC. Chronic hypoxia will increase the HCT and Hgb. Assess BNP. BNP correlates with disease severity in group I PAH and group II due to left systolic heart failure. Initial diagnosis of PAH with a BNP of greater than 150 pg/mL is associated with worse outcomes. A consistent BNP level of greater than 180 pg/mL after treatment is also associated with worse outcomes. Check D-dimer to assess for PE or may need extremity duplex, ventilation-perfusion (VQ) scan, or computed tomography angiography (CTA). Check thyroid stimulating hormone (TSH) and liver function tests (LFTs).

Assess ABGs to monitor for hypoxemia and hypocapnia in PAH. Hypocapnia is an independent marker of mortality in idiopathic PAH.

Specific tests to rule out diseases include HIV to assess for HIV antibodies. Check hepatitis B and C serologies. Obtain antinuclear antibody to assess for connective tissue diseases, including antiphospholipid antibody and lupus anticoagulant.

ELECTROCARDIOGRAM

Assess for right heart strain, right ventricular (RV) hypertrophy, right axis deviation or enlargement in lead II; R wave/S wave ratio greater than one in lead VI; right atrial enlargement, increased P wave amplitude in lead II; and incomplete or complete right bundle branch block (RBB).

VENTILATION-PERFUSION SCAN

Rule out chronic thromboembolic disease or rule out other abnormal shunts in the lungs.

PULMONARY FUNCTION TEST

Assess for obstructive or restrictive pulmonary diseases.

RADIOLOGY

Obtain a baseline CXR, assess for increase in size of proximal pulmonary arteries and narrowing of pulmonary arteries in the medial third of the lung (typically emphysema). A CTA of the chest can assess for pulmonary embolism or other obstructions. CT of the thorax can assess for other diseases of airways, parenchyma, pleura, and mediastinum as well as vascular or cardiac enlargement and extrathoracic organs such as a dilated esophagus or enlarged liver with possible porto-PH.

SIX-MINUTE WALK TEST

The 6-minute walk test can be a predictor of survival in PAH as well as evaluates functional capacity, response to therapy, and monitors for disease progression.

NOCTURNAL OXIMETRY AND SLEEP TESTING

An association exists between OSA and PH, thus warranting evaluation.

TREATMENT/MANAGEMENT

Treatment/management largely depends on the group of PAH being treated (Table 10.18).

Table 10.18 Treatment According to Type of Pulmonary Hypertension

Group I: Pulmonary Artery Hypertension	Group II: Left Heart Disease	Group III: Chronic Lung Disease or Hypoxia	Group IV: CTEPH Obstruction of Pulmonary Arteries	Group V: Multifactorial
First-line therapies (two of three): ■ Macitentan: oral dual ET receptor for subtypes ETA and ETB antagonist; reduces vasoconstriction and decreases proliferation of cells in arteries promoting vasodilation	Manage the underlying heart disease	Manage the underlying lung disease and resolve hypoxia	■ Therapeutic anticoagulation	Manage the underlying disease

(continued)

Table 10.18 Treatment According to Type of Pulmonary Hypertension (*continued*)

Group I: Pulmonary Artery Hypertension	Group II: Left Heart Disease	Group III: Chronic Lung Disease or Hypoxia	Group IV: CTEPH Obstruction of Pulmonary Arteries	Group V: Multifactorial
▪ Tadalafil: oral PDE5 inhibitor; relaxes pulmonary vascular smooth muscle cells and promotes vasodilation of pulmonary vascular bed ▪ Selexipag: oral prostacyclin receptor (IP) agonist that increases vasodilation of arteries, decreases cell proliferation, and inhibits platelet aggregation Other options: ▪ Inhaled treprostinil: a synthetic analog of prostacyclin that causes vasodilation of pulmonary and systemic arterial vascular beds and inhibits platelet aggregation ▪ Calcium channel blockers ▪ Epoprostenol: IV synthetic analog of prostacyclin, causes vasodilation of the pulmonary and systemic vessels and inhibits platelet aggregation ▪ Consider lung transplant for idiopathic pulmonary arterial hypertension for NYHA Functional Class III or IV with rapid progression of disease or refractory to maximal therapy		▪ Oxygen ▪ Inhaled treprostinil, a synthetic analog of prostacyclin that causes vasodilation of pulmonary and systemic arterial vascular beds and inhibits platelet aggregation; used in patients with PH due to ILD	▪ Consider thrombo-endarterectomy for patients with persistent severe symptoms after 3 months of anticoagulation	

ET, endothelin; ILD, interstitial lung disease; NYHA, New York Heart Association; PH, pulmonary hypertension; PDE5, phosphodiesterase type 5.

COMPLICATIONS

Complications of PH include atrial arrhythmias, compression of intrathoracic structures, hemoptysis, cardiac tamponade, and pulmonary artery aneurysm.

▶ THORACIC SURGERY

DISEASE OVERVIEW

Thoracic surgery is performed for several reasons, including traumatic injuries to the chest. Lung cancer and mesothelioma are the most common nontraumatic reasons. Advances in surgical techniques such as minimally invasive VATS and robotic-assisted surgery have enhanced the comfort and healing of patients, with fewer complications. The AGACNP role in guiding patients through this time is varied.

AGACNPs can be involved in the diagnostic workup and preoperative and postoperative care, as well as assist in navigating the patient and family through the healthcare system.

TREATMENT/MANAGEMENT
PREOPERATIVE MANAGEMENT
Perioperative management includes smoking cessation and education on coughing and deep breathing to improve postoperative outcomes. Cardiac workup should include assessment for cardiac viability, including a recent EKG, echocardiogram, and stress testing, or catheterization may be needed. Educate patients on when to stop antiplatelet and anticoagulation preoperatively to prevent intra- and postoperative bleeding.

POSTOPERATIVE CARE
Postoperative care of patients undergoing thoracic surgery includes the management of chest tubes, pain control, volume status, and prevention of complications. Patients who undergo thoracic surgery require close monitoring of their intake and output. "A dry lung is a happy lung"; thus, conservative fluid management is needed. Avoid aggressive volume resuscitation and tolerate mild oliguria. Adequate pain management is critical to ensuring patients can cough and deep breathe. A multimodal pain regimen includes Tylenol, muscle relaxers, epidural or erector spinae plane (ESP), paravertebral, or intrapleural blocks, and opioids. In addition to aggressive pain control, early mobilization prevents postoperative complications of DVTs, atelectasis, and pneumonia.

Chest tubes are a mainstay of postoperative care to evacuate any air, fluid, blood, or purulent material. Bleeding of greater than 200 mL/hr for 2 consecutive hours requires re-exploration. Consider obtaining an HCT on chest tube output to distinguish between bleeding and a lymph leak. Be sure any coagulopathy is corrected.

Chest tubes should be monitored for air leak and to ensure connections are secure. Review chest imaging to ensure the most proximal hole remains inside the pleural space. Palpate the chest wall for subcutaneous emphysema (crepitus). Crepitus may be residual from the initial injury or surgery and should resolve spontaneously. Worsening crepitus signifies an ongoing leak of air from the lung to the pleural space or a chest tube that is not functioning properly from mispositioning or loose connections.

COMPLICATIONS
Complications of thoracic surgery include sequelae of underlying pathology and surgical complications. Patients with underlying pulmonary conditions requiring thoracotomies frequently have atrial arrhythmias, including atrial fibrillation with or without rapid ventricular response. Selective beta-1 blockers are the recommended first-line treatment in the absence of severe COPD or bronchospasm. In this case, diltiazem can be used. Avoid amiodarone in patients with severe lung disease due to the risk of ARDS and pulmonary fibrosis.

Patients with lung cancer are at high risk for PE, and those who develop PE have a decreased survival. Postoperative complications include bleeding, atelectasis, persistent air leak, chylothorax, injury to phrenic or recurrent laryngeal nerve, bronchopleural fistula, pneumonia, empyema, acute respiratory failure, prolonged mechanical ventilation, and death.

▶ SUMMARY

Pulmonary conditions exist in a large percentage of acutely and critically ill patients. AGACNPs must be able to accurately interpret diagnostic tests and distinguish the various diagnoses from each other. Rapid implementation of evidence-based interventions will save lives and prevent complications.

KNOWLEDGE CHECK: CHAPTER 10

1. Which of the following is a major risk factor for the development of acute respiratory distress syndrome (ARDS)?

   A. Cholecystitis
   B. Hyperthyroidism
   C. Massive transfusion
   D. Syncope

2. What diagnostic is the gold standard for diagnosing obstructive sleep apnea (OSA)?

   A. Arterial blood gases (ABGs)
   B. Friedman tongue position (FTP)
   C. Mallampati score
   D. Polysomnography (PSG)

3. What is the most significant risk factor associated with obstructive sleep apnea (OSA)?

   A. Congestive heart failure
   B. Hypothyroid
   C. Obesity
   D. Pulmonary hypertension

4. Pulmonary hypertension is characterized by which of the following?

   A. Mean pulmonary artery pressure (mPAP) greater than 20 mmHg
   B. Pulmonary artery occlusive pressure (PAOP) of 6 mmHg
   C. Pulmonary vascular pressure (PVR) of 80 dynes/sec/cm^{-5}
   D. Cardiac output (CO) of 4 L/min

5. Which of the following diagnostics is recommended for initial screening in patients with suspected pulmonary hypertension?

   A. Pulmonary angiogram
   B. Right-sided heart catheterization
   C. Transthoracic echocardiogram
   D. Ventilation-perfusion lung scan

6. The AGACNP assesses a patient whose vital signs are heart rate (HR) 130, blood pressure (BP) 80/60, respiratory rate (RR) 30, O_2 sat 85%. Two hours ago, the patient had an internal jugular (IJ) central line placement. The patient has distended neck veins and absent breath sounds on the ipsilateral side as the IJ attempt, and the trachea is deviated to the contralateral side. What is the most likely diagnosis?

   A. Septic shock
   B. Simple pneumothorax
   C. Cardiac tamponade
   D. Tension pneumothorax

(See answers next page.)

1. C) Massive transfusion

Risk factors associated with the development of ARDS are direct injury or indirect injury. Direct lung injury is from aspiration of gastric contents, inhalation injuries, near drowning, pneumonia (bacterial, viral, fungal, or opportunistic), and pulmonary contusion. Indirect lung injury is from post cardiopulmonary bypass, drug overdose, multiple blood transfusions, pancreatitis, reperfusion edema after lung transplant or embolectomy, sepsis (most common), and severe trauma (burns, flail chest, head trauma, and multiple bone fractures). Cholecystitis is not a major risk factor for ARDS. If a patient becomes septic due to cholecystitis, then ARDS can develop. Hyperthyroidism is not a risk factor for the development of ARDS. Syncope is not a risk factor for the development of ARDS.

2. D) Polysomnography (PSG)

PSG is the gold standard to diagnose OSA. ABGs assess acid-base balance, oxygenation (PaO_2), ventilation ($PaCO_2$), and compensation. FTP measures obstruction at the oropharyngeal level. Mallampati classification score predicts the difficulty in laryngoscopy and endotracheal intubation.

3. C) Obesity

Body mass index (BMI) greater than 30 kg/m^2 is a significant risk factor for OSA. Congestive heart failure, hypothyroidism, and pulmonary hypertension are medical conditions that are associated with OSA but are not risk factors for OSA.

4. A) Mean pulmonary artery pressure (mPAP) greater than 20 mmHg

The mPAP is high. mPAP is normally 9 to 18 mmHg. The PAOP is within normal range of 6 to 15 mmHg. A PVR of 80 dynes/sec/cm^{-5} is within normal range of 37 to 120 dynes/sec/cm^{-5}. CO is within normal range of 4 to 8 L/min.

5. C) Transthoracic echocardiogram

Transthoracic echocardiogram should be performed to estimate the pulmonary artery pressure and assess ventricular function. Pulmonary angiogram assesses for blood flow to the lungs and to diagnose an obstruction as in a pulmonary embolism. Right heart catheterization is recommended as the confirmatory test to diagnose pulmonary hypertension. Ventilation-perfusion lung scan is performed to identify pulmonary embolism.

6. D) Tension pneumothorax

Classic signs of tension pneumothorax include tracheal deviation away from the pneumothorax, absent breath sounds on the affected side, tachycardia, tachypnea, hypotension, and jugular vein distention (JVD). Cardiac tamponade will have tachycardia, hypotension, JVD, narrow pulse pressure, and muffled heart sounds. This patient has tension physiology; thus, it is not a simple pneumothorax. This patient is in an obstructive shock, not septic shock.

7. The AGACNP assesses a patient with rib fractures whose vital signs are heart rate (HR) 120, blood pressure (BP) 80/60, respiratory rate (RR) 30, O_2 sat 85%. The patient has absent breath sounds on the side of the rib fractures. The trachea is deviated to the contralateral side. What action should the AGACNP take?

   A. Obtain chest x-ray (CXR).
   B. Call interventional radiology (IR) for pigtail catheter placement.
   C. Insert 14-gauge intravenous (IV) in the second intercostal space (ICS) midclavicular line (MCL).
   D. Insert 36-Fr chest tube in the fifth ICS MAL.

8. A patient was admitted with nonspecific complaints of fatigue, breathlessness, and palpitations. She reports progressive shortness of breath over the last 4 to 6 months that is worse with exertion. Vital signs are temperature (T) 37°C, heart rate (HR) 102, blood pressure (BP) 100/50, respiratory rate (RR) 30, O_2 Sat 90% on room air. Arterial blood gases (ABGs) show pH 7.33, $PaCO_2$ 58, PaO_2 55, Bicarb 32, SaO_2 88% on room air. Chest x-ray (CXR) shows clear lungs. transthoracic echocardiogram (TTE) shows pulmonary artery pressure (PAP) 60/30. What is the confirmatory test the AGACNP should order?

   A. Right heart catheterization
   B. Left heart catheterization
   C. CT pulmonary embolism (PE) scan
   D. Ventilation-perfusion (VQ) study

9. Patients who have untreated obstructive sleep apnea (OSA) should be educated that they are at greater risk for:

   A. Hypotension
   B. Septal deviation
   C. Motor vehicle crashes
   D. Mandibular hypoplasia

10. Families of older adult patients with multiple rib fractures should be educated that older adult patients:

    A. Are at greater risk of death
    B. Are more sensitive to pain
    C. Need higher amounts of narcotics
    D. Have greater pulmonary reserves

11. Patients with acute respiratory distress syndrome (ARDS) should:

    A. Be ambulated
    B. Have tidal volume (TV) 4 to 6 mL/kg/ ideal body weight (IBW)
    C. Receive liberal transfusion criteria
    D. Have a Richmond Agitation Sedation Score (RASS) −4

12. A patient in acute respiratory distress syndrome (ARDS) ventilated at 6 mL/kg/ ideal body weight (IBW) has plateau pressures of 35. The AGACNP's next intervention is to:

    A. Decrease tidal volume (TV) to 4 mL/kg/IBW
    B. Increase TV to 8 mL/kg/IBW
    C. Wean positive end-expiratory pressure (PEEP)
    D. Increase sedation

(See answers next page.)

7. **C) Insert 14-gauge intravenous (IV) in the second intercostal space (ICS) midclavicular line (MCL).**

This patient has a tension pneumothorax that requires immediate lifesaving measures. Needle decompression with a 14-gauge IV in the second ICS at the MCL is the initial intervention needed to relieve the tension physiology and restore hemodynamic stability. A chest tube could emergently be inserted but will take longer to set up, and a smaller tube such as a pigtail or 20 French should be used for an isolated pneumothorax. Calling IR for a pigtail would take too long.

8. **A) Right heart catheterization**

This patient has pulmonary hypertension. The confirmatory test is right heart catheterization. The right heart catheterization will be diagnostic of pulmonary hypertension if the mPAP is greater tha 20 mmHg and Wood units ≥ 3.

9. **C) Motor vehicle crashes**

Patients who have OSA are at a greater risk for motor vehicle crashes due to poor quality sleep, resulting in daytime sleepiness. Patients with untreated OSA are at risk for hypertension, not hypotension.

10. **A) Are at greater risk of death**

Older adults, especially frail older adults, have a higher mortality from rib fractures than younger patients. They have less pulmonary reserve. They are less sensitive to pain but more sensitive to narcotics and other sedating medications and should be started on lower doses.

11. **B) Have tidal volume (TV) 4 to 6 mL/kg/ ideal body weight (IBW)**

Patients in ARDS should have protective lung strategies, including low TVs of 4 to 6 mL/kg/IBW. Conservative fluid management and restrictive transfusion criteria are also core management strategies for ARDS. Daily spontaneous awakening trial (SAT) and minimization of sedation are best practices to minimize risk for post-ICU syndrome (PICS) for all critically ill patients. Early mobilization is also recommended to reduce PICS; however, not all patients are able to ambulate.

12. **A) Decrease tidal volume (TV) to 4 mL/kg/IBW**

This patient's lungs are becoming less compliant and thus require additional protective lung measures to prevent barotrauma, by reducing the TV further. PEEP should not be decreased as that will de-recruit alveoli. An increase in sedation can be used to ensure the patient is not fighting the ventilator or coughing or biting on the endotracheal tube (ETT): however, the plateau pressure reflects the alveolar level, not the resistance in the ETT.

13. A female patient who was admitted for a spontaneous intracranial hemorrhage due to uncontrolled hypertension has vomited. The nurse says the patient is awake and coughing, and her O_2 saturations have decreased to 92%. Right lower lung sounds are coarse. The AGACNP should:

    A. Start antibiotics
    B. Encourage pulmonary hygiene
    C. Put head of bed (HOB) to 20 degrees
    D. Intubate the patient

14. The most common immunomodulatory agent used in severe COVID-19 disease is:

    A. Dexamethasone
    B. Remdesivir
    C. Sarilumab
    D. Tocilizumab

15. Which of the following tests is currently considered the gold standard for diagnosing COVID-19?

    A. Real-time (RT) polymerase chain reaction (PCR)
    B. Rapid antigen test
    C. Rapid antibody test
    D. Enzyme-linked immunosorbent assay (ELISA)

16. A 24-year-old female patient with asthma presents with complaints of shortness of breath, chest tightness, wheezing, and nonproductive cough three to four times a week for the past month. This resolves within 30 minutes with the use of her albuterol inhaler and rest. She states that she thought that it would improve but has failed to do so. She denies fever, chills, chest pain, dizziness, syncope, or hemoptysis. Chest x-ray CXR is negative for any acute processes. What would be the next step in management?

    A. Add an inhaled corticosteroid.
    B. Add an inhaled corticosteroid and a long-acting beta-agonist.
    C. Add a long-acting beta-agonist and a systemic corticosteroid.
    D. Add an inhaled corticosteroid and a systemic corticosteroid.

17. A 59-year-old male patient presents with complaints of chest tightness and shortness of breath. He has a medical history of coronary artery disease, hypertension, and hyperlipidemia. Family history is positive for coronary artery disease, hypertension, hyperlipidemia, and asthma. His vital signs are heart rate (HR) 110, blood pressure (BP) 160/86, respiratory rate (RR) 28, SpO_2 96%. On exam, the AGACNP appreciates bilateral expiratory wheezes but no rubs, gallops, or murmurs. Capillary refill time is less than 3 seconds. Which medication should be avoided until asthma has been ruled out?

    A. Nitroglycerin
    B. Morphine
    C. Aspirin
    D. Captopril

(See answers next page.)

13. B) Encourage pulmonary hygiene

The patient has likely aspirated. Antibiotics are not indicated for aspiration pneumonitis. The HOB should be kept minimally at 30 degrees and may need to be up to 45 degrees. The patient is protecting her airway and thus does not need to be intubated.

14. A) Dexamethasone

Dexamethasone is used in patients with COVID-19 due to its anti-inflammatory and immunosuppressant effects. Dexamethasone 6 mg daily is recommended for patients who are on supplemental oxygenation or mechanical ventilation. Dexamethasone improves clinical outcomes and reduces mortality. Remdesivir is an antiviral used to treat patients with severe COVID-19 who are not on mechanical ventilation. Sarilumab is a human monoclonal that binds to interleukin 6 receptors (IL-6R). It is potentially effective in the treatment of lung complications due to COVID-19. Sarilumab is used in conjunction with dexamethasone. Tocilizumab is a human monoclonal antibody against IL-6R. It is used in cytokine release syndrome and severe forms of COVID-19 pneumonia. Tocilizumab is used in patients who are on dexamethasone who are progressing toward high-flow oxygen with elevated inflammatory markers.

15. A) Real-time (RT) polymerase chain reaction (PCR)

RT-PCR assays are the most common nucleic acid amplification tests (NAATs) with high sensitivity and specificity to diagnose current infection. Antigen tests are less sensitive than nucleic acid tests. Serology antibody detection diagnoses previous infection. ELISA test detects antibodies, antigens, proteins, glycoproteins, and hormones. An ultrasensitive ELISA test is an antigen test that is being introduced to diagnose COVID-19.

16. A) Add an inhaled corticosteroid.

Daytime symptoms more than 2 days per week require one step up. This patient was on step one with PRN SABA use only, but now requires step two, which is the addition of an inhaled corticosteroid.

17. C) Aspirin

Aspirin, a COX-1-inhibiting nonsteroidal anti-inflammatory drug (NSAID), can cause severe exacerbation of asthma symptoms from an overproduction of leukotrienes.

18. A 60-year-old male patient presents to the pulmonary clinic for exertional shortness of breath on exertion. The patient reports that he quit smoking cigarettes 3 years ago and that he smoked one pack of cigarettes a day for 40 years. According to the Global Strategy for the Diagnosis, Management, and Prevention of Chronic Obstructive Pulmonary Disease (GOLD), which of the following is found in most adults for a confirmed diagnosis of COPD?

    A. Pre-bronchodilator FEV_1/FVC less than 0.70
    B. Pre-bronchodilator FEV_1/FVC greater than 0.70
    C. Post-bronchodilator FEV_1/FVC less than 0.70
    D. Post-bronchodilator FEV_1/FVC greater than 0.70

19. The AGACNP is seeing a 67-year-old female patient with a medical history of chronic obstructive pulmonary disease (COPD) who has experienced increasing dyspnea, which is now more prominent at rest. She has a slight increase in sputum production for the last 3 days at home. Sputum remains clear to white. The AGACNP notes she is short of breath but able to speak in full sentences. The patient's last hospitalization for COPD was 3 years ago. White blood cell (WBC) 8,800/mm³, Na 142 mmol/L, blood urea nitrogen (BUN) 16 mg/dL, creatinine 0.9 mg/dL. Nasal swab for methicillin-resistant *Staphylococcus aureus* (MRSA) is negative. Based on these findings, what is the best treatment?

    A. Administer supplemental oxygen, albuterol nebulizers, increase long-acting beta-agonist, oral corticosteroids.
    B. Admit to ICU on levofloxacin (Levaquin), piperacillin- tazobactam (Zosyn), ceftriaxone (Rocephin).
    C. Admit to ICU for oxygen, noninvasive ventilation, IV corticosteroids.
    D. Admit to observation, prescribe piperacillin-tazobactam (Zosyn) and vancomycin.

20. Which of the following chronic therapies are shown to improve survival in patients with chronic obstructive pulmonary disease (COPD)? Smoking cessation with:

    A. Correction of hypoxemia with supplemental O_2
    B. All inhaled medications administered via nebulizer
    C. Vaccinations for influenza and pneumonia
    D. Pulmonary rehabilitation

(See answers next page.)

18. **C) Post-bronchodilator FEV$_1$/FVC less than 0.070**

The results of a Pulmonary Function Tests (PFT) confirm a persistent existence of airflow restriction.

19. **A) Administer supplemental oxygen, albuterol nebulizers, increase long-acting beta-agonist, oral corticosteroids.**

For mild acute exacerbation of COPD, antibiotics are not indicated. Supplemental oxygen, short-acting beta-agonists, long-acting beta-agonists, and oral corticosteroids are indicated. Noninvasive ventilation is recommended over intubation. This patient does not warrant admission to the ICU or require antibiotics. Severe acute exacerbation of COPD is defined by at least two of the following: increased dyspnea, increased sputum volume, and increased sputum virulence with respiratory failure for which fluoroquinolone, antipseudomonal penicillin, and third-generation cephalosporin are the treatment of choice for 5 to 7 days.

20. **A) Correction of hypoxemia with supplemental O$_2$**

Smoking cessation with correction of hypoxemia is the only chronic medical therapy shown to improve survival rates of patients with COPD.

KEY BIBLIOGRAPHY

Only key resources appear in the print edition. Access the full bibliography for this chapter on ExamPrepConnect.com.

Carpenter, D. (2022). *Fast facts for the adult-gerontology acute care nurse practitioner*. Springer Publishing Company. https://doi.org/10.1891/9780826152244

Chen, C., Despotovic, V., & Kollef, M. (2016). Critical care. In P. Bhat, A. Dretler, M. Gdowski, R. Ramgopal, & D. Williams (Eds.), *The Washington manual of medical therapeutics* (35th ed., pp. 225–248). Wolters Kluwer

Cloutier, M. M., Baptist, A. P., Blake, K. V., Brooks, E. G., Bryant-Stephens, T., DiMango, E., Dixon, A. E., Elward, K. S., Hartert, T., Krishnan, J. A., Lemanske, R. F., Ouellette, D. R., Pace, W. D., Schatz, M., Skolnik, N. S., Stout, J. W., Teach, S. J., Umscheid, C. A., & Walsh, C.; Expert panel working group of the National Heart, Lung, and Blood institute administered and coordinated National Asthma Education and Prevention Program Coordinating Committee. (2020). 2020 Focused updates to the Asthma Management Guidelines: A report from the National Asthma Education and Prevention Program Coordinating Committee Expert Panel Working Group. *Journal of Allergy Clinical Immunology*, 146(6), 1217–1270. https://doi.org/10.1016/j.jaci.2020.10.003

Hess, D., & Kacmarek, R. (2019). Acute respiratory distress syndrome. In D. R. Hess & R. M. Kacmarek (Eds.), *Essentials of mechanical ventilation* (4th ed., pp. 181–194). McGraw Hill.

Jameson, J., Fauci, A., Kasper, D., Hauser, S., Longo, D., & Loscalzo, J. (2018). *Harrison's principles of internal medicine* (20th ed.). McGraw Hill.

Metlay, J., Waterer, W., Long, A., Anzueto, A., Brozek, J., Crothers, K., Cooley, L., Dean, N., Fine, M., Flanders, S., Griffin, M., Metersky, M., Musher, D., Restrepo, M., Whitney, C., & on behalf of the American Thoracic Society and Infectious Diseases Society of America. (2019). Diagnosis and treatment of adults with community-acquired pneumonia. An official clinical practice guideline of the American Thoracic Society and Infectious Diseases Society of America. *American Journal of Respiratory and Critical Care Medicine*, 200, e45–e67. https://doi.org/10.1164/rccm.201908-1581ST

Gastrointestinal System Review

Mary Anne McCoy and Johnny Isenberger

▶ INTRODUCTION

The AGACNP will encounter patients with ailments linked to the gastrointestinal (GI) system. The GI tract begins at the mouth and extends to the anus. The gut wall has a mucosal layer that is either a barrier to the luminal content or a transfer site for fluid or nutritional exchange. Innervated by the enteric nervous system with principal activity modulated by the parasympathetic nervous system, luminal contents are mechanically propelled through the various regions. The system contains multiple individualized organs, has exocrine and endocrine functions, and plays a principal role in digestion, absorption, and excretion.

▶ IMPAIRED DIGESTION AND ABSORPTION

Digestion of food is the main function of the GI system. Diseases of the stomach, intestine, biliary tree, and pancreas can disrupt the digestion and absorption of nutrients the body needs for normal function and growth. Alteration in the secretion of enzymes, both over- and underproduction, leads to maldigestion syndromes or lack of key vitamin and nutrient absorption for production of red blood cells. Dysregulation of gut secretion, either over- or undersecretion, can cause ulcerations, scarring, or atrophy of specialized mucosal tissue. Inflammation, autoimmune dysfunction, and viral or bacterial infection can cause small-intestinal and colonic diseases that produce fluid loss through impaired absorption or enhanced secretion.

Transit time can be altered, causing challenging problems from achalasia of the esophagus to gastroparesis affecting the stomach.Both the small intestine and the colon can have delayed transit due to enteric nerve or intestinal smooth-muscle injury. Slow-transit constipation is produced by diffusely impaired colonic propulsion. Rapid transits are less common but can be viral, bacterial, or parasitic infections. Irritable bowel syndrome (IBS) can exaggerate small bowel and colonic motor patterns, causing diarrhea, but hyperthyroidism can as well. Mechanical obstructions can occur from adhesions and volvulus, hernias, intussusception, or cancerous growth. Immune dysregulation can occur and be seen in eosinophilic esophagitis, gastroenteritis, ulcerative colitis, and Crohn's disease, whereas impaired gut vascular flow can cause mesenteric ischemia from embolic sources or venous or arterial deficiencies. Dehydration, sepsis, hemorrhage, or decreased cardiac output can be other causes of ischemia.

▶ COMMON MANIFESTATIONS OF GASTROINTESTINAL DISORDERS

ABDOMINAL PAIN

The most frequent complaint in the ED is abdominal pain. Due to the complexity and number of organs in the abdominal cavity and to the frequent overlap of benign and serious conditions, the differential diagnosis process must be thorough in order to arrive at the correct diagnosis. Pain quality can assist with, but not confirm, potential diagnoses. Visceral pain is usually caused by distention of an organ, inflammation, or ischemia, and is usually described as deep, dull, and diffuse, whereas sharp, localized pain is more commonly parietal or peritoneal pain and a result of inflammation. Diffuse abdominal pain should make the clinician consider primary peritonitis versus secondary peritonitis and potential referred pain from the lungs or cardiac cause. The timing of pain onset is a key aspect that must be evaluated within minutes for abrupt onset of pain, which is more closely attributed to perforation, rupture, or infarction or to an organ or spillage of organ contents into the abdominal cavity. With gradual onset of pain within hours, the AGACNP must consider acute inflammation of an organ itself or a cause adjacent or external to the organ (e.g., pancreatitis inflaming the liver). Table 11.1 reviews associated symptoms of abdominal pain.

Table 11.1 Associated Symptoms: Abdominal Pain

Disorder	Clinical Definition	Rome IV Criteria	Associated With
Diarrhea Refer to BSS chart for stool consistency	Frequent defecation, passage of loose or watery stools, fecal urgency, or sense of incomplete evacuation	■ Loose or watery stools, without predominant abdominal pain or bothersome bloating, occurring in more than 25% of stools; BSS 6–7 ■ IBD: Diarrhea is excluded.	■ Diet intolerance ■ Hyperthyroidism ■ Psychological stress, abuse ■ Medications ■ IBS ■ Intestinal parasites ■ Infectious bacteria/viral ■ *Clostridioides difficile* ■ Malnutrition ■ Overconsumption of sugars ■ Inflammatory disease
Constipation Refer to BSS chart for stool consistency	Straining with, or infrequent defecation and hard consistency and volume of can be associated with nonspecific abdominal pain	■ Less than three spontaneous BMs/week ■ Straining greater than 25% of defecation attempts ■ BSS type 1–2 greater than 25% episodes ■ Use of manual maneuvers to support defecation ■ New, or worsening, symptoms of constipation when initiating, changing, or increasing opioid therapy ■ Must also include two of the three criteria previously mentioned ■ IBS-C is excluded	■ Abdominal pain ■ Preceding-> colon motor or passage issues ■ Rectal disorders ■ Diet: fiber or water intake ■ IBS ■ Acute or chronic opioid use
Nausea	■ Stomach queasiness, urge to vomit	■ CNVS ■ Bothersome (i.e., severe enough to impact on usual activities) nausea, occurring at least 1 day per week and/or ≥1 vomiting episodes per week ■ No evidence of organic, systemic, or metabolic diseases with evaluation (including at upper endoscopy)	■ GI bleeding ■ Unexplained iron-deficiency anemia ■ Unintentional weight loss ■ Palpable abdomin ■ GI cancer ■ Influenza ■ Inner ear disorders ■ Dysphagia ■ Food intake or lack of food intake ■ Medications ■ Migraines ■ Pregnancy

(*continued*)

Table 11.1 Associated Symptoms: Abdominal Pain (*continued*)

Disorder	Clinical Definition	Rome IV Criteria	Associated With

Vomiting	Oral eviction of GI contents, due to contractions of the gut and the muscles of the thoracoabdominal wall	1. CVS
		   ● Acute episodic vomiting with a cyclical pattern
		2. CNVS
		   ● Bothersome daily nausea, at least 1 day/week + ≥1 vomiting episode/week
		3. CHS
		   ● Episodic vomiting resembling CVS in terms of onset, duration, and frequency
		   ● Relief of vomiting episodes by sustained cessation of cannabis use
			■ Retching
			■ Influenza
			■ Nausea
			■ CVS: Family history of migraines
			■ CHS: Presentation after prolonged use of cannabis
			■ Food intolerance
			■ Medication side effects

BSS, Bristol stool scale; CHS, cannabinoid hyperemesis syndrome; CNVS, chronic nausea and vomiting syndrome; CVS, cyclic vomiting syndrome; GI, gastrointestinal; IBD, inflammatory bowel disease; IBS, irritable bowel syndrome; IBS-C, IBS with predominantly constipation.

▶ FUNCTIONAL GASTROINTESTINAL DISORDERS

DISEASE OVERVIEW

In recent years, there has been growing recognition that multiple specific pathophysiological processes play a role in functional GI disorders, including imbalance between different types of gut bacteria, increased gut permeability, and altered immune function. The role of inflammation in immune activation with IBS is increased mast cells (causing increased gut pain) along with increased T-cell production. Furthermore, the importance of neural and hormonal interaction between the brain and the gut in producing and modulating the symptoms of the disorders has been recognized. A key difference between IBS and inflammatory bowel disease (IBD) is that abdominal symptoms in IBS are usually relieved with defecation, and patients are usually symptom-free during sleep. There is also an absence of organic abnormalities on colorectal exam. Genetics are thought to be a component as IBS runs in families, with the theory that there is dysfunction in one of the genes that regulates the inflammatory process. In 10% of patients, IBS originates with bacterial, viral, or parasitic infection. Most important to distinguish IBS from IBD is a relative lack of alarm signs or red flag symptoms (Table 11.2), which are associated with several diseases.

Table 11.2 Alarm Signs/Red Flag Symptoms of IBD

Age of Onset	Weight Loss	Diarrhea	Fever and Chills	Nocturnal Symptoms	Hematochezia	Abnormal Labs	Family History
Older than 50 years	Unintentional	Large volume	Recent travel to endemic areas	40%	Positive	Positive	+ IBD + Early colon CA

IBD, inflammatory bowel disease; CA, cancer.

Key associated symptoms include recurrent abdominal pain on average at least 1 day/week in the last 3 months, associated with two or more of the following criteria:

- related to defecation
- associated with a change in frequency of stool
- associated with a change in form (appearance) of stool

Functional GI disorders are also called disorders of gut–brain interaction. See Table 11.3 for further information on types of IBS disorders.

Table 11.3 Types of IBS Disorders[a]

Disorder (IBS Subtypes)	Rome Criteria Definition	Management	Complications
IBS-C	■ Greater tha 25% of stool at BSS 1–2, and less than 25% of stool at BSS 6–7 ■ Patients may report most of their stool is in the constipation form.	■ Laxatives (intermittent) ■ Prokinetics, antidepressants ■ Increase soluble fiber and water consumption	■ Quality of life issues ■ Dependence on medication to induce any stool ■ Bowel obstruction ■ High stool burden complications
IBS-D	■ Greater than 25% of stool at BSS 6–7 Less than 25% at BSS 1–2	■ Maintenance of adequate water consumption ■ Antidiarrheals ■ Anticholinergics, antidepressants (SSRIs; paroxetine [Paxil]) ■ Aldosterone, a serotonin antagonist (5-HT$_3$) ■ Ramosetron, a 5-HT$_3$ receptor agonist	■ Quality of life issues ■ Dependence on medication to control stool consistency ■ Dehydration ■ Incontinence ■ UTI especially older female patients
IBS with mixed bowel habits (IBS-M)	■ 25% of the stool are BSS 1–2 and 25% are BSS 6–7 ■ Patients will complain of mixed constipation and diarrhea, but less "normal"		

[a]Diagnosis should be made with patient off any medication to treat their bowel habits.
BSS, Bristol stool scale; IBS, irritable bowel syndrome; IBS-C, IBS with predominantly constipation; IBS-D, IBS with predominantly diarrhea; SSRIs, selective serotonin reuptake inhibitors; UTI, urinary tract infection.

Table 11.4 Diagnostic Criteria for Dyspepsia and GERD[a]

Clinical Definition	Rome Criteria Definition	Management	Complications
Indigestion	One or more of: ■ Bothersome postprandial fullness ■ Bothersome early satiation ■ Bothersome epigastric pain ■ Bothersome epigastric burning ■ No structural evidence of disorder (including negative endoscopy)	■ Symptom management only if there are no "red flag" symptoms ■ Check serology for *Helicobacter pylori*. If positive, treat appropriately.	■ Older patients on ASA and NSAIDs ■ *H. pylori* infection

(continued)

Table 11.4 Diagnostic Criteria for Dyspepsia and GERD[a] (*continued*)

Clinical Definition	Rome Criteria Definition	Management	Complications
GERD	▪ Non-Rome criteria ▪ Characterized by troublesome symptoms or mucosal lesions due to reflux of gastric contents into the esophagus ▪ Typical GERD syndrome is characterized by heartburn and regurgitation ▪ Adult population (60%) experience, in the United States (two to three times/week)	▪ PPIs mainstay Tx ▪ H₂ blockers ▪ Other medicines ▪ Fundoplication ▪ Bariatric surgery ▪ Endoscopy	▪ Barrett esophagitis ▪ Hemorrhagic episodes ▪ Aspiration pneumonia ▪ Perforation of an esophageal ulcer ▪ May require a Nissen fundoplication if conservative treatment fails

[a]Criteria fulfilled for the last 3 months with symptom onset at least 6 months prior to diagnosis.

ASA, aspirin; GERD, gastroesophageal reflux disease; NSAID, nonsteroidal anti-inflammatory drug; PPI, proton pump inhibitor.

▶ DYSPEPSIA AND GASTROESOPHAGEAL REFLUX DISEASE

DISEASE OVERVIEW

Dyspepsia is described as epigastric burning, gnawing disturbance, bloating, or pain, whereas gastroesophageal reflux disease (GERD) is stomach content backwashing into the esophagus from the stomach due to inappropriate lower esophageal sphincter relaxation. Table 11.4 shows diagnostic criteria.

▶ *CLOSTRIDIOIDES DIFFICILE* INFECTION

DISEASE OVERVIEW

Clostridioides difficile infection is associated with antibiotic use and presents with watery diarrhea (three or more loose stools in 24 hours). Other symptoms are lower abdominal pain and cramping, low-grade fever, nausea, and anorexia. Although *C. difficile* causes relatively benign diarrhea in some cases, with more virulent strains the patient may present with severe life-threatening pseudomembranous colitis, toxic megacolon, sepsis,or septic shock, which has been strongly correlated with high use of fluoroquinolones (Table 11.5).

Table 11.5 Definition, Management, and Complications of *Clostridioides difficile* Infection

Clinical Definition	Management	Complications
CDI is characterized as unexplained new-onset diarrhea (i.e., three or more unformed stools within 24 hours); risks are exposure to antibiotics: + healthcare facility exposure; greater than 65 years; immune suppression	▪ Avoid certain antibiotics in vulnerable patients. (clindamycin; fluoroquinolones) ▪ CDI stool sample for PCR per facility policy ▪ Initiate contact precautions ▪ Vancomycin 125 mg orally four times per day *or* fidaxomicin 200 mg twice daily for 10 days ▪ Flagyl 500 mg orally TID may be given in mild cases	▪ Reoccurrence ▪ Intractable ▪ Toxic megacolon ▪ Death ▪ 9% of patients older than 65 years will die within a month of contracting CDI ▪ *C. difficile* is now the most common cause of HAI in U.S. hospitals

CDI, *Clostridioides difficile* infection; HAI, healthcare-associated infections.

▶ INFLAMMATORY BOWEL DISORDERS

IRRITABLE BOWEL DISEASE
DISEASE OVERVIEW

Irritable bowel disease is thought to occur when there is a dysregulation in the normal relationship between the three key components of the intestines—the intestinal epithelial cells, the microbiota, and the mucosal immune system—which leads to hyperactivation of the immune system associated with the development of IBD. Along with these interrelated factors, genes and specific environmental factors (e.g., smoking, antibiotics, enteropathogens) are influential in a susceptible host, where cumulative interactive disruption of homeostasis culminates in a chronic state of dysregulated inflammation; that is IBD (Tables 11.6–11.8).

Table 11.6 Differentiation of IBDs

Disorder	Pathophysiology/Epidemiology/Incidence
Crohn disease	■ Inflammatory disease that can occur anywhere from the mouth to the anus ■ Symptoms can be vague with appetite loss, abdominal pain, and fever. ■ Fatigue, joint pain, nausea, pain and redness in eyes, red bumps on the skin ■ Typically involves the small and large intestines, in segmental manner with skipped areas—where there is healthy tissue that separates inflamed areas; particular area, 35% incidence each, is terminal ileum and initial ascending colon ■ Can affect all layers, from the mucosa through the adventitia ■ Seen in more industrial, urban areas with higher incidence in North America, Northern Europe, and New Zealand ■ Bimodal incidence ages 15–30 and 40–60 years
Ulcerative colitis	■ Inflammatory disease that is confined to the colon. Symptoms that should warrant an investigation are abdominal pain and blood in the stool. ■ Persistent diarrhea nonresponsive to over-the-counter medications ■ Diarrhea that awakens a person from sleep; an unexplained fever lasting more than 24–48 hours ■ Typically involves the mucosa of the colon only ■ Damage is not patchy but continuous. ■ Usually starts at the rectum and spreads upward into the rest of the colon ■ Commonly flares associated with multiple associated issues (NSAIDs use, stress, missing medications, patient-specific food triggers) ■ Higher incidence in White patients of Jewish descent ■ 20% + family member or relative ■ Age at diagnosis 15–30 years, less frequent at 50–70 years; equally seen in men and women

IBS, inflammatory bowel disease; NSAID, nonsteroidal anti-inflammatory drugs.

Table 11.7 Associated Factors in Crohn Disease and Ulcerative Colitis

Other Disease Features	Crohn Disease	Ulcerative Colitis
Genetic susceptibility	(+++) HLA HLA-DQ2 (90%) or HLA-DQ8 (10%)	(+) Class II HLA
Associated immune disease	No	Yes
ASCA	(+++)	(+)
Antineutrophil cytoplasmic antibodies (p-ANCA)	(+)	(+++)
Long latent period	Yes	No
Osteopenia on diagnosis	Yes	No

(continued)

Table 11.7 Associated Factors in Crohn Disease and Ulcerative Colitis (*continued*)

Other Disease Features	Crohn Disease	Ulcerative Colitis
Smoking	(++) Smokers	Nonsmokers or ex-smokers
Malignancy incidence	Rare	Common
Reoccurrence after surgery	Yes	No (possibly pouchitis)

Note: (+), weakly associated; (++), moderately associated; (+++), strongly associated.
ASCA, anti-*Saccharomyces cerevisiae* antibody; HLA, human leukocyte antigen.

Table 11.8 Diagnostics, Management, and Complications of IBD

Disease	Initial Workup	Management	Complications
Crohn disease	■ CBC; CMP; beta stool sample for C&S and bacterial pathogens ■ *Clostridioides difficile* toxins and leukocyte count ■ Stools for calprotectin and occult blood ■ Two-view chest radiographs ■ CT of the abdomen and pelvis with oral and intravenous contrast ■ CRP or ESR ■ Confirmatory colonoscopy, endoscopy, or capsule endoscopy (required to confirm the diagnosis) ■ Special serology normal ANCA and raised anti-*Saccharomyces cerevisiae* antibodies and (p-ASCA)	The goal is to induce and maintain remission, maintain nutritional status, and decrease risk factors: ■ Sulfasalazine (Azulfidine) a prostaglandin inhibitor, contains 5-ASA and sulfapyridine ■ Mesalamine (5-ASA agent) ■ Corticosteroids ■ Immunosuppressive agents: ● Infliximab (Remicade; a chimeric immunoglobulin G1-kappa monoclonal antibody), is used in refractory Crohn disease for induction and maintenance of remission ● Biologics	Chronic health conditions: ■ Cardiovascular disease ■ Respiratory disease ■ Cancer ■ Arthritis ■ Kidney disease ■ Liver disease ■ Migraine or severe headaches ■ Hip fractures are common among older adults with IBD ■ Bowel obstruction ■ Ulcerations ■ Abscesses ■ Fistulas ■ Cancer is rare unless colon involved ■ *C. difficile* with immunosuppression
UC	UC was part of the differential diagnosis and is included in the prior workup: ■ Abdominal pain more likely LLQ ■ Diarrhea with blood or hematochezia ■ More commonly sigmoidoscopy or colonoscopy for definitive diagnosis ■ (p-ANCA) more strongly associated with UC ■ Smoking classically associated with some relative decrease in symptoms with smokers	The goal is to induce and maintain remission, maintain nutritional status, and decrease risk factors: ■ Sulfasalazine (Azulfidine) ■ Corticosteroid: prednisone, methyl-prednisone, and hydrocortisone ■ Immunosuppressants ■ Azathioprine ■ Possible infliximab ■ Biologics	■ Arthritis ■ Eye inflammation ■ Liver disease (sclerosing cholangitis) ■ Osteoporosis ■ Cancer if have disease more than 8 years, or based on the amount of colon affected and/or poor disease management (5%–32% of patients) ■ Toxic or fulminant colitis ■ Toxic megacolon

5-ASA, 5-aminosalicylic acid; ANCA, antineutrophil cytoplasmic antibody; C&S, culture and sensitivity; CBC, complete blood count; CMP, comprehensive metabolic panel; CRP, C-reactive protein; ESR, erythrocyte sedimentation rate; IBD, inflammatory bowel disease; LLQ, left lower quadrant; UC, ulcerative colitis.

CLASSIC PRESENTATION

A 29-year-old patient presents to the ED with abdominal pain. Pain is diffuse and now located in the right lower quadrant for 3 days. The patient reports associated anorexia, nausea, vomiting, diarrhea, fatigue, weakness, and shortness of breath. The diarrhea is described as Bristol stool scale (BSS)-7, nonbloody, and increased in occurrence to about eight times per day. There is no bowel incontinence or hematochezia. Pertinent positive social history includes smoker, 2.5 pack/years. Pertinent negative social history includes no recent travel history or contact with individuals with similar GI symptoms.

▶ CELIAC DISEASE AND SIMILAR DISORDERS

DISEASE OVERVIEW

Celiac disease (Table 11.9) is characterized by small intestinal enteropathy, systemic symptoms related to malabsorption, and/or immune activation from inappropriate reaction to gliadin (found in gluten) causing autoantibody production to tissue transglutaminase. Early presentations include diarrhea, malodorous stools, abdominal bloating, and poor weight gain. Later presentations are seen with other autoimmune disorders and complications.

Table 11.9 Diagnostics, Management, and Complications of Celiac Disease and Similar Disorders

Disorder	Workup	Management	Complications
Celiac disease	▪ Careful history and risk factor assessment ▪ + Dermatitis herpetiformis ▪ + Family HX ▪ CBC and peripheral smear ▪ ESR and CRP ▪ Antibody testing, IgA-anti-tTG (sensitivity 95%–99%, specificity 95%–97%) ▪ Barium swallow to assess for malabsorption areas ▪ Endoscopic four biopsies from the second half on the duodenum ▪ Marsh classification used to grade villi destruction on biopsies	▪ Electrolyte and fluid replacement in the acute phase ▪ Strict life-long gluten-free diet ▪ Micronutrient supplementation (iron, vitamin B_{12}, folate, zinc, copper, fat-soluble vitamins, vitamin D) ▪ Bone densitometry	▪ Misdiagnosis as IBD ▪ Megaloblastic anemia ▪ Osteoporosis ▪ Coagulopathies ▪ Chronic fatigue ▪ Associated autoimmune diseases such as: type I—DM ▪ Refractory disease with malignant transformation
Brush border disease (tropical sprue)	▪ Travel history is strongly positive for tropical region ▪ CBC; CMP; Beta stool sample for C & S and bacterial pathogens ▪ *Clostridioides difficile* toxins and leukocyte count ▪ Stools occult blood	▪ Supportive care as needed ▪ Tetracycline responsive (may take 3–6 months of treatment) ▪ Folate and vitamin B_{12} if anemic	▪ Malabsorption of vitamins, which causes a megaloblastic anemia ▪ Malabsorption
Nonceliac gliadin sensitivity (gluten intolerance)	▪ Celiac disease–like symptoms but negative immunoassays if done ▪ 10%–15% of Americans estimated to have gliadin intolerance (30% of Northern European descent)	▪ Avoid or reduce gluten foods, more in the form of cereal grains and some legumes ▪ Avoid phenylalanine (in some artificial sweeteners) ▪ CAM therapies: use peppermint oil	▪ Chronic low-grade inflammation ▪ Contributes to cardiovascular disease, cancer, type 2 diabetes, and other conditions

(continued)

Table 11.9 Diagnostics, Management, and Complications of Celiac Disease and Similar Disorders (*continued*)

Disorder	Workup	Management	Complications
Lactase deficiency	◼ Positive lactase breath hydrogen test ◼ Lactose tolerance test	◼ Avoid lactose-containing foods ◼ Supplement with lactase orally before consumption of trigger foods	◼ No significant complications are reported beyond QOL

CAM, complementary and alternative medicine; C&S, culture and sensitivity; CBC, complete blood count; CMP, comprehensive metabolic panel; CRP, C-reactive protein; DM, diabetes mellitus; ESR, erythrocyte sedimentary rate; Hx, history; IBD, inflammatory bowel disease; QOL, quality of life.

The cause of *brush border disease* (tropical sprue) is unknown, but it is assumed that an infectious process is the original initiation of the disease, where there is an injury to the mucosa of the small bowel. This leads to enterocyte damage and bacterial overgrowth, which retards small-intestinal transit. It is seen typically in individuals living in or having visited tropical areas. The disease imitates celiac disease with abdominal distention, diarrhea, and anorexia and can result in inflammation of the intestinal villi.

Lactose intolerance is prevalent in 60% to 70% of the population worldwide. It is an intolerance to lactose due to a deficiency in lactase enzymes to break down lactose. The results are abdominal discomfort, gas, bloating, and diarrhea. Lactose intolerance is most common in South America, Africa, and Asia, and in descendants of people from those regions. Secondary lactose deficiency can be acquired from injury to the small intestine (Crohn disease, celiac disease, brush border disease, bacterial overgrowth, and gastroenteritis).

CLASSIC PRESENTATION: CELIAC DISEASE

A 24-year-old male patient presents to urgent care with a complaint of an off-and-on skin rash that currently is on the patient's elbows and knees. He denies allergies, changes in diet, or environmental triggers. He has tried antihistamine cream without relief and 1% cortisone cream with a slight improvement. Review of systems reveals increased general fatigue, "dry eyes," no cardiovascular or respiratory symptoms, abdominal pain, malodourous diarrhea with blood streaks, abdominal bloating, and anorexia. The patient has been using over-the-counter medication (Lomotil) without much relief. He has seen some improvement in symptoms with cutting down on bread, pasta, and cereal in the diet. He denies genitourinary symptoms. On exam, the "rash" appears to have small, clustered papules and vesicles that are in a somewhat symmetrical pattern on the elbows and knees. Stool smear is positive for guaiac.

▶ PEPTIC ULCER DISEASE

DISEASE OVERVIEW

Gastric and duodenal ulcers (Table 11.10) are included under the umbrella term *peptic ulcer disease* (PUD). The most common symptom of both is epigastric pain, usually described as a gnawing or burning sensation that occurs after eating. Classically, pain ensues shortly after eating in gastric ulcers and 2 to 3 hours afterward with duodenal ulcers. The principal defect is the penetration of the protective superficial "gel" layer of the stomach and duodenum, which is normally impermeable to acid and pepsin. Bicarbonate is also produced by other cells that lie near the mucosa. The other protective agent is prostaglandin type E, which increases both bicarbonate and the mucous layer. Under normal conditions, a healthy balance is maintained. PUD is due to *Helicobacter pylori* infection, drugs (nonsteroidal anti-inflammatory drugs [NSAIDs] in particular), severe physiological stress, hypersecretory states, and genetic factors (blood type O in duodenal ulcer).

Table 11.10 Differentiation Between Gastric and Duodenal Ulcers

Ulcer Type	Management	Complications
Gastric	Incidence male to female 1:1 Age older than 50 years. If PUD is suspected in an acute setting: ■ Obtain: CBC, CMP; Fe studies, LFTs, amylase, and lipase. If critical patient: PT/aPTT/INR; type/screen/crossmatch ■ Urea breath test: detects the activity of bacterial urease ■ Acid suppression to pH greater than 6.0 ■ H$_2$RAs (nonactive bleeding) ■ PPIs (PO or IV depending on severity at presentation of diagnosis) ■ Upper endoscopy for *H. pylori* biopsy and/or treatment (hemostasis) ■ Obtain rapid urea test; histopathology (gold standard) and culture ■ Eliminate NSAIDs (63% of gastric ulcers associated with *H. pylori*) ■ Treat *H. pylori* infections 10–14 days (see Chapter 4)	■ Bowel perforation ■ Gastrocolic fistula ■ GI bleeding ■ Gastric outlet obstruction ■ MALT lymphoma ■ Refractory symptomatic ulcers
Duodenal	■ Male to female incidence; 2–3:1 ■ Age 30–60 years ■ If suspected in an acute setting: ● Obtain labs: CBC, CMP; Fe studies, liver function studies, levels of amylase and lipase. If critical patient PT/aPTT/INR; type and screen/crossmatch based on status ■ Urea breath test: detects the activity of bacterial urease ■ Treat any *H. pylori* infection ■ Smoking cessation if *H. pylori* +	■ Small bowel obstructions ■ Bleeding, perforation, and obstruction

aPTT, activated partial thromboplastic time; CBC, complete blood count; CMP, comprehensive metabolic panel; GI, gastrointestinal; H$_2$RA, H$_2$-receptor antagonist; INR, international normalized ratio; IV, intravenous; LFT, liver function tests; MALT, mucosa-associated lymphoid tissue; NSAIDs, nonsteroidal anti-inflammatory drugs; PPI, proton pump inhibitor; PT, prothrombin time; PUD, peptic ulcer disease.

CLASSIC PRESENTATION: GASTRIC ULCER

A 68-year-old female patient with a past medical history of dyspepsia presents to the ED with epigastric burning and gnawing pain, labeled a 7/10, after ingestion of pizza. The pain started about 30 minutes after eating. The patient has experienced this pain before and usually takes two to three Maalox tablets, after which the pain goes away. She has associated nausea and belching after taking the Maalox. Today she has not gained relief with this same regimen and is worried it could be a heart attack.

CLASSIC PRESENTATION: DUODENAL ULCER

A 32-year-old female patient presents to the ED with epigastric burning and gnawing pain, labeled a 7/10, after eating lunch 3 hours ago. The pain seems to improve when eating but then comes back after a time. This has been occurring on and off for 4 to 6 weeks. The patient noticed a little maroon color to her stool this morning and that it was looser in consistency than usual but not diarrhea.

▶ PANCREATITIS

DISEASE OVERVIEW

Pancreatitis is an acute inflammatory autodigestive process of the pancreas. Classic symptoms are usually an abrupt onset of epigastric abdominal pain, steady, radiating to the back, with guarding. Severity worsens when supine and improves with knee-to-chest positioning or tripod sitting (leaning forward with hands or elbow on knees). The causes are numerous; a mnemonic to remember the causes is "I GET SMASHED" (Table 11.11). Mortality for a patient with acute pancreatitis can be estimated with either the Ranson Criteria or the Bedside Index for Severity in Acute Pancreatitis (BISAP) score (Table 11.12). Two clinical signs associated with pancreatitis are Cullen and Grey Turner signs. The first is subcutaneous periumbilical edema and bruising (also associated with rupture of ectopic pregnancy), and the latter is bruising along the flanks associated with intra-abdominal bleeding.

Table 11.11 Mnemonic for Causes of Pancreatitis

"I GET SMASHED" Differential							
I		**G**		**E**		**T**	
Idiopathic		Gallstones (30%–60% occult)		Ethanol (15%–30%) ESRD		Trauma: blunt or postoperative	
S	**M**	**A**	**S**	**H**		**E**	**D**
Steroids	Mumps	Autoimmune	Scorpion sting	Hypercalcemia Hypertriglyceridemia Hypothermia		ERCP	Drugs: sulfa-based, thiazide and loop diuretics, others

ERCP, endoscopic retrograde cholangiopancreatography; ESRD, end stage renal disease.

Table 11.12 Ranson and BISAP Scores to Predict Mortality in Pancreatitis

Ranson criteria: One of the first prognostic scores. Major limitation: Requires 48 hours of data. One point for each criterion. Not available as prognosticator on admission.	
Criteria first 24 hours (five items)	▪ Age older than 70 years ▪ WBC greater than 18,000 cells/cm ▪ Blood glucose greater than 220 mg/dL ▪ Serum AST greater than 250 IU/L and serum LDH greater than 400 IU/L
Criteria at 48 hours (six items)	▪ Serum calcium less than 8.0 mg/dL ▪ Hematocrit fall greater than 10% ▪ BUN increased by 2 mg/dL or more (despite IV fluid hydration) ▪ Base deficit greater than 5 mEq/L ▪ Sequestration of fluids greater than 4 L
Score interpretation	▪ 0–2 points: mortality 0%–3% ▪ 3–4 points: 15% ▪ 5–6 points: 40% ▪ 7–11: nearly 100%
Bedside Index for Severity in Acute Pancreatitis (BISAP) score: The score identifies five independent criteria in the first 24 hours. One point for each criterion.	
Criteria	▪ B: BUN greater than 25 mg/dL ▪ I: Impaired mental status ▪ S: SIRS ▪ A: Age greater than 60 years ▪ P: Pleural effusions

Note: Ranson and BISAP score ≥3 should be considered for ICU admission.
AST, aspartate aminotransferase; BISAP, Bedside Index for Severity in Acute Pancreatitis; BUN, blood urea nitrogen; IV, intravenous; LDH, lactate dehydrogenase; WBC, white blood count.

CLASSIC PRESENTATION

A 56-year-old male patient comes into the ED with acute epigastric abdominal pain, which radiates to back and is worse when lying supine. He currently is sitting on the side of the stretcher, leaning forward, endorsing 10/10 pain. He is anxious and sweating, feels weak, and states that the pain woke him from sleep. He vomited once without improvement in the pain. Vital signs: heart rate 112 bpm, blood pressure

106/65, respiratory rate 24, temperature 38.3°C. EKG shows no ischemic change. On exam A and O × 4; anxious but cooperative. S1/S2 heart sounds, no murmurs, gallops, or rubs; tachycardic, regular. Bowel sounds clear except for diminished left lower lobe (LLL). Patient refuses to lie supine for abdominal exam. Abdomen confirmed to be distended. Positive for bowel sounds in all quadrants but distant. Guarding epigastric region to light palpation. Noted bruising on left flank (Grey Turner sign).

▶ GALLBLADDER DISEASE

DISEASE OVERVIEW

Gallbladder disease (Table 11.13) affects more than 20 million people in the United States. One million patients are newly diagnosed with gallbladder disease, of which 50% to 70% are asymptomatic at diagnosis. Prevalence rates of cholelithiasis increase with age and are higher in female patients. One of the earliest large-scale ultrasonographic survey studies, known as the NHANES III study, revealed that the overall prevalence of gallbladder disease in men and women was 7.9% and 16.6%, respectively.

Table 11.13 Gallbladder Disorders, Evaluation, Management, and Complications

Disorder	Evaluation	Management	Complications
Asymptomatic cholelithiasis	■ As long as ~10 years before diagnosis ■ Risk factor assessment ■ Pregnancy: progesterone decreases contractility of the GB leading to stasis ■ Obesity ■ Genetics ■ Medications: estrogens, fibrates, somatostatin analogs ■ Stasis of the gallbladder ■ Female sex assigned at birth ■ Metabolic syndrome ■ Rapid weight loss ■ Prolonged fasting ■ Bariatric surgery ■ Crohn disease ■ Ileal resection ■ US is the best test for most GB disorders	■ Avoidance of high-fat meals and eating smaller meals ■ Treatment or control of risk factors if possible	■ Gallbladder inflammation leading to cholecystitis ■ Common bile duct blockage resulting in bile duct infection and jaundice ■ Pancreatic duct blockage can cause pancreatitis ■ Cancer of the gallbladder
Biliary colic	■ Dull and intense visceral pain, RUQ, + Murphy sign; episodic ■ Occurs when a gallstone is being passed and is blocking a bile duct ■ Typically comes and goes in a fairly regular pattern ■ US: may not see stones, but sludge may be present. Single episode usually does not warrant surgery	■ US GB ■ WBC count ■ Liver enzymes ■ Amylase and lipase ■ Surgery not usually urgent ■ Consult general surgery ■ Counsel patient to avoid fatty food and long periods of fasting. ■ Use Tylenol for pain PRN. ■ Actigall may decrease cholesterol production.	■ See earlier ■ May lead to acute cholecystitis

(*continued*)

Table 11.13 Gallbladder Disorders, Evaluation, Management, and Complications (*continued*)

Disorder	Evaluation	Management	Complications
Acute acalculous cholecystitis	■ 20% of patients admitted for biliary tract disease will have acute acalculous cholecystitis. ■ May present with acute RUQ pain but typically presents more insidiously ■ More common in critically ill patients ■ Defined as cholecystitis without a gallstone ■ Critically ill patients are vulnerable due to bile stasis, hypoperfusion, and nonenteric feeding Risk factors: ■ Trauma, burns, sepsis, multi-organ failure ■ Nonbiliary surgery (especially cardiac or aortic surgery) ■ Gallbladder distension ■ Total parenteral nutrition ■ Lack of enteral nutrition ■ Opioids ■ Global hypoperfusion, or heart failure ■ Vascular disease (DM, HTN, atherosclerosis, vasculitis) ■ Check direct and indirect bilirubin levels ■ Check amylase/lipase ■ No symptoms or vague abdominal cramping	■ US GB ■ WBC count ■ Liver enzymes ■ Amylase and lipase ■ May need CT of the abdomen in some complex cases ■ Gallbladder decompression drainage with T-tube placement, usually by IR ■ General surgery consult to monitor ■ If GB perforation has occurred, abscess drainage may be needed with cultures. ■ Usually triple antibiotic coverage with an antifungal is included ■ May need GB removal usually not in the acute phase	■ Acute gallbladder necrosis (50%) and perforation (10%) ■ Perforation will lead to bile peritonitis and contribute to the shock condition ■ Gram-negative sepsis ■ Death (30%–50%) depending on preexisting patient status
Chronic cholecystitis	■ May present as biliary colic ■ GB damaged by repeated acute inflammation, usually due to gallstones, and may become thick-walled, scarred ■ Stone may block the cystic duct ■ The GB usually also contains sludge ■ If scarring is extensive, calcium may be deposited in the walls of the GB; if hardens called porcelain gallbladder	■ Lap or open cholecystectomy ■ Empiric ABX coverage if fever, leukocytosis, and is directed at gram-negative enteric organisms: ■ IV regimens such as ceftriaxone 2 g every 24 hours + metronidazole 500 mg every 8 hours ■ Piperacillin/tazobactam 4 g every 6 hours, or ■ Ticarcillin/clavulanate 4 g every 6 hours	■ Sepsis

(*continued*)

Table 11.3 Gallbladder Disorders, Evaluation, Management, and Complications (*continued*)

Disorder	Evaluation	Management	Complications
Choledocholithiasis with or without cholangitis	■ Primary stones (usually brown pigment stones), form in the bile ducts ■ Secondary stones (usual: cholesterol), form in the GB but migrate to the bile ducts ■ Residual stones, which are missed at the time of cholecystectomy ■ Recurrent stones, which develop in the ducts more than 3 years after surgery	■ An emergent condition ■ Consult GI medicine for ERCP and sphincterotomy ■ Support blood pressure with fluids ■ Antibiotic coverage as earlier	■ Could lead to pancreatitis, hepatitis, or both ■ Common bile duct perforation
Acute cholangitis	■ Charcot triad: fever, RUQ pain, and jaundice ■ Bile duct obstruction allows bacteria to ascend from the duodenum ■ Typically, gram negative: *Escherichia coli, Klebsiella*, or *Enterobacter* ■ Symptoms: abdominal pain, jaundice, fever, or chills (Charcot triad) ■ Abdomen and liver are tender and enlarged (possible abscesses)	■ Treat with antibiotics as earlier and narrow when surgical cultures and sensitivities are resulted	■ Confusion and hypotension, abdominal pain, jaundice, and fever or chills (Reynold pentad) predict about a 50% mortality rate and high morbidity

DM, diabetes mellitus; ERCP, endoscopic retrograde cholangiopancreatography; GB, gallbladder; HTN, hypertension; IR, interventional radiology; PRN, as needed; RUQ, right upper quadrant; US, ultrasound; WBC, white blood count.

▶ OTHER INFECTIOUS GI DISEASES

The AGACNP must be familiar with appendicitis and diverticulitis as well. See Table 11.14 for evaluation, management, and complications.

Table 11.14 Appendicitis and Diverticulitis: Evaluation, Management, and Complications

Disorder	Evaluation	Management	Complications
Appendicitis	■ Common symptoms ■ Abdominal pain (RLQ) ■ Anorexia ■ Nausea and vomiting ■ Pain migration ■ Classic symptom sequence (vague periumbilical pain to anorexia/nausea, unsustained vomiting to migration of pain to RLQ to low-grade fever) ■ Duration of symptoms exceeding 24–36 hours is uncommon in nonperforated appendicitis ■ Other confirmatory peritoneal signs (absence does not exclude appendicitis)	■ Standard for management of nonperforated appendicitis remains appendectomy ■ Periappendiceal abscess ■ Can be treated with antibiotics and/or surgery ■ Also, CT-guided drainage, followed by interval appendectomy 6 weeks to 3 months later	■ Ruptured appendix ■ Sepsis with late presentation and site not walled off ■ Adhesions and potential for SBO in the future

(*continued*)

Table 11.4 Appendicitis and Diverticulitis: Evaluation, Management, and Complications (*continued*)

Disorder	Evaluation	Management	Complications
	▨ Psoas, obturator, or Rovsing sign ▨ Dunphy sign: increased pain with coughing ▨ Patient with hip flexion and knees drawn up for comfort Labs: ▨ Elevated CRP level with leukocytosis and neutrophilia highly sensitive and specific. These missing = no appendicitis		
Diverticulitis	▨ Acute diverticulitis is inflammation due to microperforation of a diverticulum ▨ Pain, tenderness, or sensitivity in the LLQ ▨ Risk factors: low-fiber, high-fat diet with red meats ▨ Obesity and smoking increase the potential for both diverticulitis and diverticular bleeding ▨ Drugs including NSAIDs, steroids, and opiates associated with diverticulitis ▨ Pain can start out mild and increase over several days or come on suddenly ▨ Fever ▨ Nausea and/or vomiting ▨ Chills ▨ Cramps in the lower abdomen ▨ Rectal bleeding, constipation or diarrhea (less common)	Labs and imaging: ▨ WBC, CRP and ESR elevations ▨ Consult colon–rectal or general surgery ▨ Radiological test of choice is CT of the abdomen and pelvis, with water-soluble oral or rectal contrast and IV contrast provided there are no contraindications ▨ Admission criteria: patient cannot tolerate oral intake, excessive vomiting, signs of peritonitis, immune compromised, or at an advanced age should be hospitalized	▨ Abscess formation ▨ Abscesses that are less than 2–3 cm treat conservatively with IV antibiotics ▨ Large abscesses should be drained ▨ Fistula formation ▨ Colovesicular fistula occurs in about 65% of fistulating cases ▨ Peritonitis ▨ Bowel obstruction ▨ Sepsis/septic shock ▨ Bleeding per rectum

CRP, C-reactive protein; ESR, erythrocyte sedimentary rate; IV, intravenous; LLQ, Left lower quadrant; RLQ, right lower quadrant; SBO, small bowel obstruction; WBC, white blood count.

▶ LIVER DISORDERS

DISEASE OVERVIEW

The liver is the largest organ of the body and receives a dual blood supply; about 20% of the blood is from the hepatic artery, and 80% is nutrient-rich blood from the portal vein arising from the stomach, intestines, pancreas, and spleen. Liver inflammation has multiple causes, with viral causes being the most common; other causes include drugs (prescription, nonprescription, and illicit); alcohol, toxins, autoimmune origins, and Wilson disease. The mechanism is either direct toxin-induced or host immune-mediated. Acute hepatitis presents with low-grade fever; jaundice (10 days after the appearance of constitutional symptomatology; it lasts 1–3 months); hepatomegaly (mildly enlarged, soft liver); splenomegaly (in 5%–15%); palmar erythema; and spider nevi (rarely), with or without right upper quadrant and epigastric pain (intermittent, mild to moderate). Aspartate aminotransferase (AST) and alanine aminotransferase (AMT) levels can be 20- to 100-fold above normal levels. Signs of chronic liver disease include hepatomegaly, splenomegaly, muscle wasting, palmar erythema, spider angiomas, and vasculitis (rarely), whereas patients with cirrhosis may have ascites, jaundice, history of variceal bleeding, peripheral edema, gynecomastia, testicular atrophy, hepatic encephalopathy, and abdominal collateral veins (caput medusa).

CLASSIC PRESENTATION: HEPATITIS A

A 21-year-old female patient is seen in the ED with a chief complaint of yellowing of the skin and eyes. These symptoms were preceded by 7 days of progressive fatigue and flu-like symptoms. She admits to having dark urine the last 2 days. She thought she was not drinking enough fluids. She has subjective fevers and nausea. She denies abdominal pain, vomiting, diarrhea, hematuria, or rashes, as well as recent travel and insect or chemical exposures. Her roommate is also ill after returning from a semester abroad.

TREATMENT/MANAGEMENT

See Tables 11.15 and 11.16.

Table 11.15 Liver Disorders: Evaluation, Management, and Complications

Disorder	Cause	Management	Complications
HAV	▪ HAV is an RNA virus that spreads person to person via fecal–oral route. Usually in close contact with contamination of food, water, objects, or sexual contact ▪ Risk factors for HAV: travel to developing areas of the world, exposure to persons with jaundice, and exposure to young children in daycare centers ▪ Clinical features 2- to 6-week incubation with viral shedding 14 days before symptoms ▪ Malaise, diarrhea, jaundice, and RUQ tender	▪ Elevated AST/ALT ▪ LFTs include total and direct bilirubin, albumin, and INR ▪ Once recovered provides immunity to future HAV infections ▪ Contact evaluation and notification as needed in cohorts ▪ Supportive therapy: IV fluids; rest and good nutrition ▪ Vaccines available, in two types: first type—two doses 6 months apart; second type—HAV and HBV combined	▪ Rare complications ▪ Can be fatal in late presentations, immunosuppressed individuals, and coinfections
HBV	▪ Parenteral inoculation or equivalent; direct contact spread ▪ Careful history of sexual activity includes the number of lifetime sexual partners, and for men, a history of having sex with men. Sexual exposure is a common mode of spread of hepatitis B. ▪ Blood transfusion before 1986 (screening for antibody to anti-HBc was introduced, is also a risk factor for hepatitis)	▪ Serologic/virologic studies ▪ HBeAG/anti-HBe ▪ HBV DNA level ▪ Anti-HAV ▪ LFTs with direct bilirubin, albumin, and INR and CBC ▪ Nucleos(t)ide reverse transcriptase inhibitors (tenofovir disoproxil fumarate, tenofovir alafenamide, lamivudine) ▪ Hepatitis B/hepatitis C agents (adefovir dipivoxil, entecavir, telbivudine, Peginterferon alfa-2a, Peginterferon alfa-2b)	▪ Liver inflammation for around 8/10 adults, whereas 2/10 adults will not have symptoms ▪ Acute liver failure can require liver transplantation or lead to death. ▪ Chronic infection can lead to cirrhosis and liver cancer.
HCV	▪ Similar transmission to HBV but poor sexual transmission or vertical transmission ▪ Labs to assess liver function ▪ History of injection drug use ▪ Injection drug use is the single most common risk factor for hepatitis C. ▪ Transfusion with blood or blood products before 1992	▪ Hepatitis C/hepatitis B agents (e.g., adefovir, entecavir, Peginterferon alfa-2a, Peginterferon alfa-2b) DAA tablets Sofosbuvir (Sovaldi) for 8–12 weeks	▪ Cirrhosis ▪ ESLD
HDV	▪ The HDV is unable to replicate on its own and is dependent on the surface antigen of HBV. Coinfection is serious.	▪ Evaluate serum for HBsAg and anti-HDV	▪ High morbidity with HBV superinfections

(continued)

Table 11.15 Liver Disorders: Evaluation, Management, and Complications (*continued*)

Disorder	Cause	Management	Complications
HEV	▪ Hepatitis E is one of the more common causes of jaundice in Asia and Africa but is uncommon in other nations. ▪ Transmission is usually through exposure to fecal-contaminated water. ▪ Occasional cases are associated with eating raw or undercooked pork or game.	Evaluation: ▪ Thorough history, travel, and food consumption evaluation ▪ R/O other forms of hepatitis; serum testing for anti-HEV IgM and HEV RNA	
ALD	▪ Symptoms vary from asymptomatic to fever, jaundice, abdominal pain, and hepatomegaly. ▪ Labs: elevated ALT, AST (2–7× above normal) Usually not greater than 400 IU ▪ AST: ALT: >2 ▪ May see hyperbilirubinemia, hypo-albuminemia, elevated PMNs	▪ Support treatment based on patient presentation ▪ If currently drinker, institute CIWA-AR protocol	Fulminant and subfulminant hepatitis may present with: ▪ Encephalopathy ▪ Somnolence ▪ Disturbances in sleep pattern ▪ Mental confusion ▪ Coma ▪ Ascites ▪ GI bleeding ▪ Coagulopathy

Liver cirrhosis	▪ Chronic liver inflammation leads to scarring and fibrosis
	▪ Multiple causes acute or chronic viral hepatitis C, autoimmune, drug induced, metabolic, alcohol and/or NAFLD
	▪ Evaluation: confirm cause
	▪ CBC, CMP, Pt, INR, liver function tests, liver enzymes
	Imaging:
	▪ US with and without Doppler
	▪ MRI of the abdomen
	▪ Gold standard: Liver bx
	▪ Fibroscan: noninvasive fibrosis staging
	Stages:
	▪ Stage I: asymptomatic
	▪ Stage II: mild portal HTN w/out liver dysfunction
	▪ Stage III: decompensated: see complications
	▪ MELD scores prognosticator of survival next 3 months (range 6–40). Use for transplant assessment referrals to centers at greater than 10
		▪ Cause: viral, autoimmune
		▪ Refer to hepatologist for biopsy and/or antiviral or immunosuppression
		▪ Ascites:
		  ● Dietary sodium restriction
		  ● Diuretics
		  ● Paracentesis
		  ● TIPS procedure
		▪ Variceal hemorrhage
		▪ Stabilize patient: blood products, fluid resuscitation, stat GI medicine, possible esophageal tamponade
		▪ Medications: octreotide: propranolol or nadolol
		▪ SBP: generally gram negative without perforated viscus
		▪ Cultures: PMNs greater than 250 cells/mm
		▪ Treatment: Ceftriaxone or cefotaxime 2 g IV every 4–8 hours
		▪ Orthotopic liver transplantation
			▪ Portal hypertension with development of ascites
			▪ Hepatic encephalitis
			▪ Variceal development and hemorrhage
			▪ Spontaneous bacterial peritonitis
			▪ End-stage liver disease
			▪ May need liver transplantation
			▪ Death

(*continued*)

Table 11.15 Liver Disorders: Evaluation, Management, and Complications (*continued*)

Disorder	Cause	Management	Complications
HE	■ Presents with altered mental status due to impaired clearance of neurotoxins by the liver ■ Cognitive deficits include altered sleep–wake cycles, impaired LOC, inattention, personality alterations ■ Fetor hepaticus refers to the slightly sweet, ammoniacal odor that can develop in patients with liver failure, particularly with portal-venous shunting	■ Removal of neurotoxins especially ammonia through the stool: ● Lactulose: 30–45 mL orally two to four times a day to produce two to three bowel movements/day ● Xifaxan (Rifaximin); dose 550 mg orally twice a day	■ Patients are considered high risk with HE for any other surgery

ALD, Alcoholic liver disease; ALT, alanine transaminase; AST, aspartate aminotransferase; CBC, complete blood count; CMP, comprehensive metabolic panel; DAA, direct-acting antiviral; ESLD, end-stage liver disease; GI, gastrointestinal; HAV, hepatitis A virus; HBV, hepatitis B virus; HCV, hepatitis C virus; HDV, hepatitis D virus; HE, hepatic encephalopathy; HEV, hepatitis E virus; HTN, hypertension; IFN, interferon; INR, international normalized ratio; IV, intravenous; LOC, level of conciousness; MELD, model for end-stage liver disease; NAFLD, nonalcoholic fatty liver disease; RUQ, right upper quadrant; SBP, spontaneous bacterial peritonitis; TIPS, transjugular intrahepatic portosystemic shunt; US, ultrasound.

Table 11.16 Hepatitis B Lab Nomenclature

Lab	Description
HbsAg	*HB surface antigen* Marker of infectivity Presence indicates either acute or chronic infection
Anti-HBs	*Antibody to HB surface antigen* Marker of immunity Presence indicates an immune response to HBV infection, response to vaccination, or presence of passively acquired antibody
Anti-HBc	*Antibody to HB core antigen* Marker of acute chronic, or resolves HBV infection Not a marker of vaccine-induced immunity May be used in prevaccine exposure to HBV infection
IgA anti-HBc	*IgM antibody subclass of anti-HBc* Positivity indicates recent infection with HBV ($\geq$6 months) Presence indicates an acute infection
IgG anti-HBc	*IgG antibody subclass of anti-HBc* Marker of past or current infection with HBV. If it and HbsAg are both positive (in the absence of IgM-anti-HBc), it indicates chronic HBV.
HBeAG	*HB "e" antigen* Marker of a high degree of HBV infectivity; it correlates with a high level of HBV replication. Used in the clinical management of chronic HBV infections
Anti-HBe	*Antibody to HB "e" antigen* may be present in an infected or immune person. In chronic HBV infections, its presence suggests a low viral replication and infectivity.
HBV-DNA	*HBV DNA* is a marker of viral replication; correlates with infectivity; used to monitor chronic HBV infected patients

HBV, hepatitis B virus.

▶ GASTROINTESTINAL BLEEDING

DISEASE OVERVIEW

GI bleeding is generally categorized into two types: upper and lower (Tables 11.17, 11.18, and 11.19). Upper GI bleeding can be further subdivided into variceal and nonvariceal bleeding and typically involves bleeding from the esophagus to the duodenum. Lower GI bleeding encompasses bleeding from the colon and/or rectum.

Table 11.17 Comparison of Upper and Lower GI Bleeding

Bleeding	Upper GI Bleeding	Lower GI Bleeding
Characteristics	▪ Hematemesis and/or melena	▪ Hematochezia
Potential sources	▪ Peptic ulcer disease in a patient with *Helicobacter pylori* infection, NSAIDs, antithrombotic, alcohol use, and smoking ▪ Marginal ulcers in a patient with a GI anastomosis ▪ Varices or portal hypertensive gastropathy in a patient with known liver disease and portal hypertension ▪ Malignancy ▪ Aortoenteric fistula in a patient with a history of aortic aneurysm or an aortic graft ▪ Angiodysplasia in a patient with aortic stenosis, renal disease, or hereditary hemorrhagic telangiectasia	▪ Small bowel ▪ Colon such as ischemia, perforation, infection, malignancy, or diverticulitis ▪ Rectum
	▪ Upper abdominal pain may indicate peptic ulcer disease ▪ Dysphagia and unintentional weight loss may indicate malignancy ▪ Jaundice and ascites would indicate variceal hemorrhage ▪ Emesis, retching, or coughing would indicate Mallory–Weiss tear ▪ Gastroesophageal reflux would indicate esophageal ulcer	▪ Abdominal pain suggests inflammation such as ischemia or perforation ▪ Diarrhea
Physical exam findings	▪ Hematemesis ▪ Tachycardia ▪ Orthostatic hypotension ▪ Narrow pulse pressure	▪ Hematochezia ▪ Tachycardia ▪ Orthostatic hypotension ▪ Narrow pulse pressure
Laboratory findings	▪ Anemia ▪ Elevated blood-urea-nitrogen to creatinine ratio (greater than 30:1)	▪ Anemia ▪ Low MCV
Gold standard	▪ EGD to examine esophagus, stomach, and duodenum	▪ EGD to rule out upper GI bleed ▪ Colonoscopy is the gold standard and requires colon preparation for visualization and is typically done if the patient is hemodynamically stable ▪ Radionuclide imaging must be performed during active bleeding—attempts to localize bleeding site ▪ CT angiography—to localize bleeding site; must be done during active bleeding ▪ Angiography must be done during active bleeding and can be therapeutic

EGD, esophagogastroduodenoscopy; GI, gastrointestinal; MCV, mean corpuscular volume; NSAIDs, nonsteroidal anti-inflammatory drugs.

Table 11.18 General Management: Upper GI Bleeding

	Nonvariceal	Variceal
Resuscitation	For hemodynamic instability: ■ Secure airway ■ Reverse coagulopathy ■ Obtain two large-bore IVs ■ Transfuse blood products in a 1:1:1 ratio of PRBCs, fresh frozen plasma, and platelets For hemodynamically stable: ■ Transfuse PRBCs for Hgb less than 8 g/dL in patient with CAD ■ Transfuse PRBCs for Hgb less than 7 g/dL in lower risk patients	For hemodynamic instability: ■ Secure airway; aspiration is common source of morbidity and mortality ■ Reverse any existing coagulopathy ■ Obtain two large-bore IVs ■ Transfuse blood products in a 1:1:1 ratio of PRBCs, plasma, and platelets For hemodynamically stable: ■ Transfuse PRBCs for Hgb less than 8 g/dL in patient with CAD ■ Transfuse PRBCs for Hgb less than 7 g/dL in lower risk patients
Source control	■ Immediate consultation with gastroenterology for endoscopic evaluation and treatment ■ Consult interventional radiology ■ Large-scale bleeding may require surgical consult; need the source of the bleed localized	■ Immediate consultation with gastroenterology for EGD within 12 hours for endoscopic variceal ligation ■ Balloon tamponade is a temporizing measure until source control ■ If endoscopic variceal ligation fails or the patient is at high risk for rebleeding, TIPS is beneficial.
Pharmacotherapy	■ Protonix 40 mg IV every 12 hours	■ Protonix 40 mg IV every 12 hours ■ Vasopressin infusion *or* ■ Octreotide 50 mcg IV × 1, then 50 mcg/hr ■ Antibiotics for SBP prophylaxis

CAD, coronary artery disease; EGD, esophagogastroduodenoscopy; GI, gastrointestinal; IV, intravenous; PRBC, packed red blood cells; SBP, spontaneous bacterial peritonitis; TIPS, transjugular intrahepatic portosystemic shunt.

Table 11.19 General Management: Lower GI Bleeding

Resuscitation	Same as Upper GI Bleeding
Source control	For hemodynamically stable: ■ Consult gastroenterology for colonoscopy ■ If source identified, then expectant management ■ If source not identified, upper endoscopy or small bowel enteroscopy For hemodynamically unstable: ■ Consult gastroenterology for potential upper endoscopy and colonoscopy ■ If no source of bleeding is identified, consult IR for angiography to localize the source of bleeding and potential embolization ■ Consult surgery if IR unable to obtain source control ■ If no source identified, will need small bowel enteroscopy or capsule study

GI, gastrointestinal; IR, interventional radiology.

CLASSIC PRESENTATION: UPPER GI BLEED

A 56-year-old male patient with a history of coronary artery disease, stent placement 5 months ago, atrial fibrillation on apixaban (Eliquis), diabetes mellitus type 2, and hyperlipidemia presents to the ED with hematemesis for the past 24 hours. Vital signs: temperature 37.0°C, heart rate 134, sinus tachycardia, respiratory rate 30, oxygen saturation 95% on room air. On physical exam, the patient appears anxious and is alert and oriented ×3 without focal weakness. Lung sounds clear to auscultation. S_1/S_2 heart sounds, no murmurs, gallops, or rubs; tachycardic. Upper abdominal pain, guaiac-positive stool, hematemesis.

CLASSIC PRESENTATION: LOWER GI BLEED

A 56-year-old male patient with a history of hypertension, hyperlipidemia, and diabetes mellitus type 2 presents after 1 week of bloody bowel movements. He reports unintentional weight loss of 20 lb over the last 2 months. Temperature 37.0°C, heart rate 122, sinus tachycardia, respiratory rate 20, oxygen saturation 95% on room air. The patient is calm and appropriate, alert and oriented ×3. Lung sounds clear to auscultation. S_1/S_2 heart sounds normal but tachycardic, regular. Mild abdominal pain to palpation, guaiac-positive stool.

COMPLICATIONS

Complications from a GI bleed vary widely and can arise from procedural interventions needed to manage the disease, like endoscopy or colonoscopy. Complications include:

- transfusion reactions
- electrolyte abnormalities
- transfusion-related lung injury (TRALI)
- intubation
- aspiration

▶ ABDOMINOPELVIC TRAUMA

DISEASE OVERVIEW

Abdominopelvic trauma (Table 11.20) may be blunt, penetrating, or blast injury. Blunt injuries are the result of a direct blow that can cause compression and crushing injuries to the abdominopelvic viscera and internal organs, as well as pelvic bones. Shearing injuries are a form of blunt trauma that results when a restraint device, such as a seat belt, is worn inappropriately. Penetrating traumas are commonly caused by stab or gunshot wounds and cause tearing and laceration of abdominopelvic structures. Blast injuries typically occur through penetration of fragments or blunt injuries from projectiles.

Table 11.20 Diagnostic Criteria for Abdominopelvic Trauma

Diagnostic	Clinical Relevance
X-ray	Chest x-ray would evaluate for hemothorax and pneumothorax, and in the case of penetrating trauma, evaluate the trajectory of the missile.
	Abdominopelvic x-ray (KUB) would evaluate for the presence of foreign bodies and pelvic fractures.
FAST	*Indications:* abnormal vital signs in a patient with blunt abdominal trauma or penetrating injury without indications for immediate abdominal surgery
	Advantages: can be performed rapidly at the bedside, noninvasive, and can inform regarding the need for surgery
	Disadvantages: can be difficult in patients with a large body habitus and is operator-dependent; will miss injuries of the diaphragm, pancreas, bowel, and retroperitoneal space; bowel gas or subcutaneous air will hinder images for proper assessment
	Positive findings: include finding free fluid (anechoic material) in Morrison pouch, peri-splenic area, or above the bladder
DPL	*Indications:* done in hemodynamically unstable patients with blunt injury or penetrating injury without indications for immediate abdominal surgery
	Advantages: can be completed rapidly at the bedside to determine fecal spillage and the need for immediate surgical intervention
	Disadvantages: invasive procedure with a high risk of complications and would limit interpretation from CT scans and/or FAST
	Positive findings: the presence of blood or fecal contents with lavage

(continued)

Table 11.20 Diagnostic Criteria for Abdominopelvic Trauma (*continued*)

Diagnostic	Clinical Relevance
CT scan	*Indications:* done in hemodynamically stable patients with blunt or penetrating injuries; will also be done in patients with trauma and no immediate need for surgery
	Advantages: noninvasive, repeatable, and will deliver the clearest visualization of the retroperitoneal space, bones, soft tissue, and extraluminal space
	Disadvantages: higher cost that requires patient transport and may not be immediately available; could miss injuries of the diaphragm, pancreas, and bowel; also exposes the patient to IV contrast and radiation
	Positive findings: extraluminal air, bloody ascites, and bowel perforation with fecal contamination seen on a positive CT scan

DPL, diagnostic peritoneal lavage; FAST, focused assessment with sonography for trauma; IV, intravenous; KUB, kidney, ureter, and bladder.

CLASSIC PRESENTATION

A 23-year-old male patient arrives to the ED after a stab wound to the right lower quadrant. There is evisceration of omentum and bowel. Temperature 34.5°C, heart rate 154, respiratory rate 35, blood pressure 88/66, oxygen saturation 90% on room air. The patient is anxious and in obvious pain. Lungs are clear to auscultation. S_1/S_2 heart sounds, tachycardic, regular. Abdomen is distended, tender, obvious eviscerated bowel and omentum. Extremities are cold; weak and thready pulse. A Foley catheter is placed and has minimal dark amber urine.

TREATMENT/MANAGEMENT

See Table 11.21.

Table 11.21 Treatment/Management for Abdominopelvic Trauma

Injury Type	Specific to Treatment/Management
Penetrating injuries	*Indications for laparotomy* Hemodynamic instability Bowel evisceration Gunshot wound with transperitoneal trajectory Peritonitis
	Nonoperative management Nonoperative management can be considered in patients who are hemodynamically stable and without peritonitis or bowel evisceration. Specifically, these patients have anterior abdominal wounds or flank and back injuries. These patients can be evaluated with a CT scan, serial physical exams, serial FAST exams, DPL, or diagnostic laparoscopy.
Liver, spleen, and kidney	*Hemodynamic instability* Ensure airway and ventilation/oxygenation. Massive transfusion protocol may be needed. Consult IR for angioembolization. If unable to embolize, then laparotomy for damage control surgery. In the case of a splenic injury, a total splenectomy may be necessary. These patients require vaccination prior to discharge.
	Hemodynamically stable Ensure adequate airway and ventilation/oxygenation. Serial physical exam Serial FAST exam Serial hematocrit and hemoglobin measurements

(*continued*)

Table 11.21 Treatment/Management for Abdominopelvic Trauma (*continued*)

Injury Type	Specific to Treatment/Management
Pancreatic injuries	*Determine the classification*
	Low grade (I–II): ERCP or MRCP If ductal injury, will need surgical diversion If no ductal injury, nonoperative management and/or simple drainage
	High grade (III–V): Needs surgical intervention for diversion
Diaphragm injuries	Can be missed on initial chest x-ray High suspicion in patients with penetrating injury May require surgical management depending on severity
Duodenal injuries	Suspect in patients with a direct frontal impact Requires surgical management
Hollow viscus injuries	Suspect in patients with a "seat belt" sign or chance fracture on x-ray Requires evaluation by surgery with possible surgical intervention
Pelvic injuries	Consult orthopedics Ensure adequate airway and ventilation/oxygenation Massive transfusion protocol for hemorrhagic shock Apply a pelvic binder If intraperitoneal blood, then laparotomy required If there is no intraperitoneal blood, then angioembolization or preperitoneal packing Requires placement of an external fixation device

DPL, diagnostic peritoneal lavage; ERCP, endoscopic retrograde cholangiopancreatography; FAST, focused assessment with sonography for trauma; MRCP, magnetic resonance cholangiopancreatography.

COMPLICATIONS
See Table 11.22.

Table 11.22 Complications of Abdominopelvic Trauma

Complication	Specifics Related to the Complication
Resuscitative complications	Airway: trauma, malposition of endotracheal or chest tubes Ventilation: barotrauma, ARDS, ventilator-associated pneumonia Transfusion: transfusion reactions, TRALI, transmission of infection, electrolyte abnormalities, coagulopathy Central line–related complications Abdominal compartment syndrome Fluid overload
Injury-related complications	Bleeding Infection Fistula formation Prolonged mechanical ventilation Prolonged "open" abdomen Biliary leak with biloma Hepatic artery or splenic artery pseudoaneurysm Urinary leak

ARDS, acute respiratory distress syndrome; TRALI, transfusion-related lung injury.

▶ BOWEL PERFORATION

DISEASE OVERVIEW

Bowel perforation is the result of full-thickness injury of the bowel resulting in the release of GI contents into the perineum, causing peritonitis. Several etiologies exist and include trauma, ischemia (due to bowel obstruction or vascular obstruction), neoplasm (as the result of instrumentation during surgery or endoscopy), IBDs, connective tissue disorders, and PUD.

CLINICAL MANIFESTATIONS

Acute abdominal or chest pain, fever, shortness of breath, subcutaneous emphysema.

CLASSIC PRESENTATION

A 56-year-old female patient presents with a 3-day history of abdominal pain. She states that it started in the left lower quadrant but now has progressed to the entire abdomen. She has not had a bowel movement in 5 days. Temperature 39.4°C, heart rate 134, respiratory rate 42, oxygen saturation 93% on room air. She appears anxious and is in obvious pain. Clear lung fields, diminished over left lower lobe. S_1/S_2 heart sounds, tachycardic, regular rhythm. Abdomen is distended, tympanitic with diffuse tenderness to palpation. Extremities are cold with capillary refill time greater than 3 seconds. Urine is dark with minimal output.

DIAGNOSTIC CRITERIA

To make the diagnosis of bowel perforation, an upright chest x-ray can be obtained to detect free air under the diaphragm, and ultrasound is also useful for its ability to detect pneumoperitoneum or pneumomediastinum. However, both of these methods will not determine the site of the perforation. Abdominal CT scan can be the most useful to detect any amount of free air and determine the location and even the possible cause of the perforation.

TREATMENT/MANAGEMENT

See Table 11.23.

Table 11.23 Treatment/Management of Bowel Perforation

Treatment/ Management	Specifics
Resuscitation	Volume resuscitation Vasopressors Lactate, cap refill, central venous oxygen saturation are end points of resuscitation
Antibiotics	*Low-risk community-acquired (perforated appendix)* Low risk for antibiotic resistance or treatment failure Coverage against streptococci, anaerobes, and *Enterobacter* Cephalosporin or fluoroquinolone plus metronidazole Piperacillin–tazobactam as a single agent
	High-risk community-acquired (severely ill or high risk for antibiotic resistance) Need coverage against *Pseudomonas* and resistant *Enterobacter* Antifungal coverage for upper GI perforation Piperacillin–tazobactam Cefepime or ceftazidime with metronidazole Antifungal agents: fluconazole, micafungin, caspofungin ESBL risk: add carbapenem such as imipenem or meropenem Aztreonam may be used for allergy to carbapenems or beta-lactams Vancomycin for known MRSA colonization
	Healthcare-associated (resistance is high) Meropenem, or imipenem, or piperacillin–tazobactam Cefepime or ceftazidime plus metronidazole and vancomycin

(continued)

Table 11.23 Treatment/Management of Bowel Perforation (*continued*)

Treatment/ Management	Specifics
Source control	Need surgical consultation Initially with damage control surgery and "open" abdomen to prevent abdominal compartment syndrome Avoid/correct hypothermia
Nutrition	Enteral nutrition as soon as possible Parenteral nutrition may be necessary if malnourished or NPO for greater than 7 days
Ostomy care	Consult wound ostomy nurse Ensure adequate patient education for ostomy care Assess skin integrity frequently for signs of breakdown

ESBL, extended spectrum beta-lactamase; MRSA, methicillin-resistant staphylococcus aureus.

COMPLICATIONS

Complications can be short term, such as volume overload and pulmonary edema. Longer-term complications include antibiotic resistance, *C. difficile* infection, malnutrition, fistula formation, bleeding, and hypovolemia.

▶ ACUTE LIVER FAILURE

DISEASE OVERVIEW

Acute liver failure is rare. It is defined as liver dysfunction in a patient with encephalopathy and an international normalized ratio (INR) of ≥1.5 in a patient without preexisting liver dysfunction and with an illness of less than 26 weeks' duration. Patients may have jaundice, encephalopathy, confusion, asterixis, and abdominal pain.

CLASSIC PRESENTATION

A 19-year-old female patient is brought to the ED after being found unconscious. She was noted to have an empty acetaminophen bottle next to her. Temperature 35.4°C, heart rate 150, respiratory rate 42, oxygen saturation 83% on room air. She is comatose with jaundice. She is decorticate posturing to stimulus, pupils are 5 mm and reactive to light, and there is no corneal reflex. She has a gag reflex and a cough. Rhonchi are noted over right lung fields. The patient is tachycardic. Abdomen is flat, without evidence of ascites. Extremities are warm with palpable pulses. A Foley catheter is placed with dark urine and minimal output.

DIAGNOSTIC CRITERIA

The patient presenting with acute liver failure can have a wide range of physical exam findings, including fever, jaundice, abdominal pain, bleeding or bruising, and ascites. Alterations in laboratory data can induced elevated AST/alanine transaminase (ALT) and INR. To make the diagnosis of acute liver failure, the patient will have an INR greater than 1.5.

TREATMENT/MANAGEMENT

Acute liver failure is treated/managed based on the etiology (Table 11.24).

Table 11.24 Treatment and Management of Acute Liver Failure

Treatment/Management	Specifics
Initial labs to determine etiology	PT/INR Chemistries Hepatic function panel Arterial blood gas Arterial lactate Complete blood count Blood type and screen Acetaminophen level Comprehensive toxicology screen Viral hepatitis serologies: anti-HAV IgM, HBsAg, anti-HBc IgM, anti-HEV, anti-HCV, HCV RNA, HSV$_1$ IgM, VZV Ceruloplasmin level Consider serum and urinary copper levels Pregnancy test (as applicable) Ammonia Consider autoimmune markers: ANA, ASMA, immunoglobulin levels HIV-1, HIV-2 Amylase and lipase
Treat specific etiology	*Acetaminophen toxicity:* ■ Activated charcoal if ingested within 4 hours ■ Start NAC infusion *For all nonacetaminophen ALF* ■ NAC infusion *Mushroom toxicity* ■ NAC infusion and penicillin G ■ List for transplant *Drug-induced liver injury* ■ Get detailed history of ingestion ■ NAC infusion *Viral hepatitis* Hepatitis A and E are supportive ■ Hepatitis B: nucleotide analogues ■ Hepatitis C: antiviral treatment ■ Varicella or herpes simplex virus: acyclovir *Wilson disease* ■ Liver biopsy to confirm ■ List for transplantation
	HELLP syndrome ■ Prompt delivery of the fetus ■ Supportive care ■ List for transplantation if liver dysfunction does not resolve *Acute ischemia* ■ Treatment of shock ■ Supportive care *Budd–Chiari* ■ List for transplantation *Malignancy* ■ Liver biopsy for diagnosis ■ Supportive care *Indeterminate* ■ Liver biopsy

(*continued*)

Table 11.24 Treatment and Management of Acute Liver Failure (*continued*)

Treatment/Management	Specifics
Treat encephalopathy and cerebral edema	*Grade I/II encephalopathy* ■ Lactulose and/or rifaximin ■ Obtain head CT to rule out other etiologies *Grade III/IV encephalopathy (in addition to Grade I/II tx)* ■ Airway protection ■ Place ICP monitor ■ Keep head of bed elevated greater than 30 degrees ■ Avoid fever ■ Target sodium level of 145–155 ■ Sedate to target RASS-3 ■ Hyperosmotic therapy for elevated ICP ■ Treat seizures if present ■ Induced hypothermia, pentobarbital, or indomethacin for refractory ICP elevation
Coagulopathy	■ Correct INR with FFP for active bleeding or procedures ■ Platelets only for active bleeding or procedures ■ Consider TEG for targeted coagulopathy treatment ■ H_2 or proton pump inhibitor for stress ulcer prophylaxis
Hemodynamic support	■ Volume replacement with crystalloid infusion ■ Vasopressor support with norepinephrine
Renal failure	■ Renal replacement therapy if indications exist
Metabolic support	■ Early enteral nutrition ■ Glycemic control

ALF, acute liver failure; ANA, antinuclear antibodies; ASMA, anti-smooth muscle antibodies; FFP, fresh frozen plasma; HAV, hepatitis A virus; HCV, hepatitis C virus; HEV, hepatitis E virus; ICP, intracranial pressure; INR, international normalized ratio; NAC, *N*-acetylcysteine; TEG, thromboelastogram; VZV, varicella zoster virus.

COMPLICATIONS

Patients with acute liver failure are at high risk for seizures, brain herniation, and death. Bleeding is common. Infections such as ventilator-associated pneumonia, central line–associated infections, catheter-associated urinary tract infection, infectious diarrhea, and peritonitis can occur. As with all ICU patients, depending on the severity, patients can experience malnutrition, delirium, and ICU-acquired weakness; multi-organ dysfunction syndrome, risks associated with blood transfusion, and post–intensive care syndrome can all occur.

▶ HEPATORENAL SYNDROME

DISEASE OVERVIEW

Hepatorenal syndrome (HRS) is the most common complication in patients with cirrhosis. It is subdivided into two types: (a) HRS–acute kidney injury (AKI), previously known as type 1 HRS, which is the acute form; and (b) HRS–non-AKI, previously known as type 2 HRS, which is the chronic form. HRS–AKI is defined as renal dysfunction in the presence of cirrhosis with ascites, in a patient without shock or parenchymal renal disease and not currently receiving nephrotoxic agents. An increase in serum creatinine of greater than two to three times the baseline without improvement with volume expansion with albumin is seen. HRS–non-AKI is a slow progression of renal dysfunction in the setting of cirrhosis with ascites. Prognostically, HRS–AKI carries a higher mortality, and without treatment, median survival is days to weeks.

CLASSIC PRESENTATION

A 45-year-old female patient with a history of alcoholic cirrhosis presents to the hospital with abdominal pain and is found to have spontaneous bacterial peritonitis. She is now hospital day 3 and is noted to have creatinine of 3.54 (baseline 1.2) and oliguria. Temperature 35.4°C, heart rate 100, respiratory rate 12, oxygen saturation 93% on room air. The patient is anxious and jaundiced and is currently alert but oriented only ×1. Bilateral rales are noted in the bilateral lower lung fields. She has generalized abdominal pain and ascites with fluid present. Lower extremities show 3+ pitting edema. Urine is scant and dark. Laboratory data reveal sodium 125, potassium 5.6, chloride 96, CO_2 15, blood urea nitrogen 109, creatinine 3.54, and calcium 6.6.

DIAGNOSTIC CRITERIA

Patients presenting with HRS can have findings of jaundice, ascites, hypotension, and oliguria or anuria. Laboratory findings of hyponatremia, elevated serum creatinine, and hepatic function are consistent with HRS. The gold standard for diagnosis includes the presence of the following: (a) cirrhosis with ascites, (b) serum creatinine greater than two to three times baseline, (c) absence of shock, (d) no improvement after withdrawal of diuretics and volume expansion with albumin, (e) absence of renal parenchymal disease, and (f) absence of nephrotoxic **agents.**

TREATMENT/MANAGEMENT

Treatment includes albumin administration (1.5 g/kg at day 1 and 1 g/kg at day 3), plus a vasoconstrictor, which includes vasopressin or norepinephrine or midodrine and octreotide. Ongoing monitoring will identify the need for renal replacement therapy; signs include worsening acidosis, hyperkalemia, fluid overload, or uremic complications such as bleeding, encephalopathy, or pericarditis. Consult the transplant team for liver and/or simultaneous liver and kidney transplant. If transplant services are not available, consider transferring the patient to a transplant center.

COMPLICATIONS

HRS–AKI without treatment portends a poor prognosis. Severe acidosis, severe electrolyte disturbances, fluid overload leading to poor oxygenation, and uremic complications are common. Dialysis line-associated complications include vessel injury, thrombus, lung injury, and infection. Dialysis-related complications include disequilibrium syndrome, dehydration, and electrolyte disturbances.

KNOWLEDGE CHECK: CHAPTER 11

1. A 26-year-old female patient is involved in a motor vehicle crash and is intubated at the scene for a Glasgow Coma Scale score of 5. Upon arrival at the ED, she is noted to have a heart rate of 154 beats/min and a blood pressure of 92/60 mmHg. Her capillary refill is greater than 3 seconds. A focused assessment with sonography for trauma (FAST) reveals hypoechoic material in Morrison pouch. What is the *most* appropriate next intervention?

   A. Admit to the ICU.
   B. Check hematocrit.
   C. Obtain a CT scan.
   D. Initiate damage control surgery.

2. A 78-year-old male patient is brought to the ED after suffering a fall at home. Upon arrival, he is noted to have a heart rate of 135 beats/min and a blood pressure of 84/67 mmHg. He has bruises throughout his lower abdomen and into his testicles. Imaging reveals a grossly displaced pelvic fracture. Which is the *most* appropriate immediate intervention?

   A. Apply a pelvic binder.
   B. Obtain a CT scan.
   C. Check an arterial blood gas.
   D. Give two units of packed red blood cells.

3. An 18-year-old male patient was involved in an altercation resulting in multiple stab wounds to his right lower quadrant and right upper quadrant. He is hemodynamically stable but has severe pain with palpation of his abdomen. Which of the following statements is true?

   A. The patient should be admitted for serial abdominal exams.
   B. Peritonitis is an indication for exploratory surgery.
   C. The patient does not need surgery because there is no bowel evisceration.
   D. He should be treated nonoperatively given his hemodynamic stability.

4. An 18-year-old female patient is brought to the ED after being found unresponsive beside an empty acetaminophen bottle. What should be administered to this patient?

   A. Fresh frozen plasma
   B. Penicillin G
   C. Nucleotide analogues
   D. *N*-acetylcysteine

5. A 42-year-old male patient is admitted to the ICU for altered mental status. He was admitted to the general wards for acute liver failure 3 days ago. Upon arrival to the ICU, he is unresponsive and is intubated. What is the most appropriate next intervention?

   A. Obtain a noncontrast head CT.
   B. Start sedation with midazolam.
   C. Start valproic acid 15 mL/kg intravenous (IV) × 1.
   D. Give fresh frozen plasma.

(See answers next page.)

1. D) Initiate damage control surgery.

The patient has evidence of hemorrhagic shock and free fluid in the abdomen, presumably around the liver. Damage control surgery would provide source control. Admitting the patient to the ICU, obtaining a hematocrit, and obtaining a CT scan would delay appropriate intervention in treating the primary problem.

2. A) Apply a pelvic binder.

The patient has evidence of shock due to a pelvic fracture. Immediate treatment and source control would be to apply a pelvic binder. A CT scan will be obtained once the patient is stable enough. Giving two units of blood would not provide source control and would not be enough product. Checking an arterial blood gas would not resolve the primary cause of the patient's shock.

3. B) Peritonitis is an indication for exploratory surgery.

Peritonitis is an indication for exploratory surgery following penetrating injury. Nonoperative treatment or serial abdominal exams would delay the necessary surgery.

4. D) *N*-acetylcysteine

N-acetylcysteine is given as a therapy for suspected acetaminophen toxicity. Penicillin G would be given for mushroom toxicity. Nucleotide analogues are given for suspected hepatitis B. Fresh frozen plasma would offer no benefit for this patient.

5. A) Obtain a noncontrast head CT.

The patient is exhibiting grade 4 encephalopathy and is at risk for cerebral edema, which may be revealed on a noncontrast head CT. Sedation with midazolam may be necessary but would inhibit essential neurological examinations. Valproic acid would be given if the concern was for seizures. Fresh frozen plasma would offer no benefit.

6. A 45-year-old male patient with a history significant for hypertension presents to the ED with a fever, shortness of breath, and abdominal pain that is diffuse but improves when sitting up with knees flexed. On exam, he is tachycardic and has abdominal guarding. The abdomen is distended and diffusely tender to palpation. Labs are notable for a white blood cell count of 15,000 and a lactate of 5.4. A chest x-ray is obtained, which reveals free air under the right hemidiaphragm. Initial management of this patient should include:

   A. STAT surgical consult, intravenous (IV) antibiotics, and IV fluids
   B. H_2 blockers and bowel prep
   C. Right upper quadrant ultrasound, IV antibiotics, and IV fluids
   D. Nasogastric tube placement, admission to the ICU, and frequent observation

7. A 64-year-old male patient with a history of colon cancer presents to the ED with diffuse abdominal tenderness, fever, and tachycardia. The AGACNP is concerned about a possible bowel perforation. Which of the following diagnostic modalities has the greatest sensitivity for bowel perforations?

   A. Chest x-ray
   B. Abdominal x-ray
   C. CT scan
   D. Ultrasound

8. A 65-year-old female patient is admitted to the ICU after damage control surgery for a sigmoid colonic perforation. She was at home and suffered from constipation for 5 days leading to a stercoral ulcer and subsequent perforation. The AGACNP should order which of the following antibiotic regimens?

   A. Clindamycin and vancomycin
   B. Metronidazole
   C. Levofloxacin and vancomycin
   D. Ceftriaxone and metronidazole

9. A 72-year-old male patient with a history of hypertension and hyperlipidemia presents to the ED after vomiting bright red blood. He reports that he has had nausea and vomiting for several days, but the emesis has been bilious up until today. The AGACNP suspects that the patient may have an upper gastrointestinal (GI) bleed due to which of the following?

   A. Malignancy
   B. Mallory–Weiss tear
   C. Esophageal varices
   D. Peptic ulcer disease

10. A 73-year-old male patient presents to the ED after vomiting approximately 5 cups of bright red blood. On exam, heart rate is 126 beats/min, blood pressure is 92/46 mmHg, and capillary refill time is 5 seconds. Initial management of this patient should include:

    A. Admission to the ICU, placement of a triple lumen central catheter, administration of 2 L of intravenous (IV) fluids
    B. Placement of a nasogastric tube and Foley catheter for strict intake/output monitoring
    C. Gastroenterology consult for endoscopy, transfused packed red blood cells (PRBCs), administration of proton pump inhibitor (PPI)
    D. Abdominal CT scan, administration of empiric antibiotics, administration of IV fluids

(*See answers next page.*)

6. **A) STAT surgical consult, intravenous (IV) antibiotics, and IV fluids**

The patient has signs of a bowel perforation and requires surgery and sepsis management with fluids and antibiotics. Bowel prep should not be given to this patient. A right upper quadrant ultrasound would not be useful. The patient will need a nasogastric tube as well as admission to the ICU, but surgery should not be delayed.

7. **C) CT scan**

CT scan is the most useful modality and not only can detect small amounts of free air but also can provide information on the location of the perforation.

8. **D) Ceftriaxone and metronidazole**

This patient has a low-risk community-acquired bowel perforation. The most appropriate antibiotic regimen would be a cephalosporin and metronidazole to cover against streptococci, anaerobes, and *Enterobacter*. Clindamycin and vancomycin, metronidazole, and levofloxacin and vancomycin are incomplete regimens and would not cover what is required.

9. **B) Mallory–Weiss tear**

Mallory–Weiss tears often occur in patients with a history of significant nausea and vomiting. Malignancy often presents with a reported unintentional weight loss. Esophageal varices would occur in a patient with cirrhosis and portal hypertension. Peptic ulcer disease could be possible, but it is often associated with upper abdominal pain, which this patient has not reported.

10. **C) Gastroenterology consult for endoscopy, transfused packed red blood cells (PRBCs), administration of proton pump inhibitor (PPI)**

The patient is experiencing an upper gastrointestinal (GI) bleed. Therapy would consist of source control via endoscopy, blood transfusion, and administration of a PPI. He may need admission to the ICU, but placement of a triple lumen central line is unnecessary and inappropriate for multiple blood transfusions. Placement of a nasogastric tube may be necessary but should not take priority. Abdominal CT and antibiotics would offer no benefit.

11. A 45-year-old female patient with a history of alcoholic cirrhosis is in the ICU for management of hepatic encephalopathy, which has improved with lactulose and rifaximin. She is on a 2-L nasal cannula and is on a restricted diet. However, this morning she is noted to be vomiting copious amounts of bright red blood. The AGACNP understands that which of the following is a *priority* for this patient?

   A. Immediate intubation to secure airway
   B. Administration of a proton pump inhibitor
   C. Administration of blood products
   D. Starting an octreotide infusion

12. > A 56-year-old male patient with a history of cirrhosis due to nonalcoholic fatty liver disease is admitted to the ICU after vomiting bright red blood at home. He has a history of hepatic encephalopathy and ascites. TheAGACNP understands that management of this patient would include:

   A. Paracentesis
   B. Bowel prep for colonoscopy
   C. Right upper quadrant ultrasound
   D. Empiric antibiotics

13. A 63-year-old female patient is admitted with a lower gastrointestinal (GI) bleed. She is hemodynamically stable, and her abdominal exam is benign, but she continues to have melanotic stools. The AGACNP should prepare the patient for which of the following?

   A. CT scan of the abdomen and pelvis
   B. Ultrasound of the abdomen
   C. Upper endoscopy
   D. Colonoscopy

14. A 65-year-old male patient with a history of cirrhosis due to alcohol use disorder is admitted to the hospital with fever, abdominal pain, and jaundice. Paracentesis labs are concerning for spontaneous bacterial peritonitis, and the patient is placed on ceftriaxone 1 g intravenous (IV) daily. On hospital day 3, the AGACNP notes that his creatinine has doubled, and he is oliguric. Which one of the following should be started?

   A. Hemodialysis
   B. Furosemide
   C. Albumin
   D. Lactated Ringer solution

15. A 43-year-old female patient with cirrhosis is admitted to the ICU for sepsis and is noted to have a worsening acute kidney injury due to hepatorenal syndrome. Which one of the following is an indication for renal replacement therapy?

   A. Creatinine of 4.6
   B. Blood urea nitrogen of 100
   C. Oxygen saturation of 85% on 100% FIO_2
   D. Sodium of 124

(See answers next page.)

11. A) Immediate intubation to secure airway

Patients with a variceal hemorrhage have a difficult airway and are at risk for aspiration, which is the leading cause of morbidity and mortality in this patient population. Proton pump inhibitors, blood products, and octreotide infusion are also necessary; however, securing the airway is the priority.

12. D) Empiric antibiotics

Patients with variceal hemorrhage and ascites should be given empiric antibiotics to prevent spontaneous bacterial peritonitis.

13. D) Colonoscopy

The patient with a lower gastrointestinal (GI) bleed who is hemodynamically stable will undergo a colonoscopy to localize the bleed and to offer treatment. CT scan, abdominal ultrasound, or upper endoscopy would not treat the underlying issue.

14. C) Albumin

The patient is in hepatorenal syndrome and should be treated with volume expansion with albumin. He may need hemodialysis but currently does not have an indication for urgent hemodialysis. Furosemide will deplete the patient of necessary volume. Lactated Ringer solution will not expand volume as effectively as albumin.

15. C) Oxygen saturation of 85% on 100% FIO_2

The indications for renal replacement therapy include acidosis, hyperkalemia, poor oxygenation, and complications of uremia.

16. The AGACNP is caring for a 78-year-old patient in the ICU with previous medical history of congestive heart failure (CHF). The patient was in a recent motor vehicle collision with subsequent cardiac
arrest from hemorrhagic shock and is intubated and on two vasopressor therapies: Levophed and
vasopressin. Lab data reveal a worsening aspartate aminotransferase (AST)/alanine transaminase
(ALT) elevation, so the AGACNP orders an abdominal ultrasound. The ultrasound reveals peri-
cholecystic fluid and gallbladder distention with associated sludge. The patient is febrile, despite
antimicrobial therapy with meropenem, and has normal renal function. The AGACNP obtains a stat
CT of the abdomen and pelvis with contrast and finds an abscess to the gallbladder area without
obstructing stones. The *best* treatment would be to:

   A. Add Flagyl to the patient's antibiotic regimen
   B. Consult interventional radiology for a percutaneous cholecystostomy tube
   C. Consult general surgery for an emergency cholecystectomy
   D. Initiate trickle enteric feeding to decompress the gallbladder

17. A 75-year-old female patient is seen in urgent care for respiratory distress. She has a history of rheumatoid arthritis (RA) and gastroesophageal reflux disease (GERD) and is a moderate social drinker.
She also has a 20 pack-year smoking history. She is postmenopausal and has a surgical history of
total hip replacement 4 years ago. Her review of systems is negative except for generalized joint
stiffness, right knee pain, and heartburn and belching. She is on Ultram for management of her RA
and omeprazole for her GERD, which she feels is not helping anymore. She has had two episodes
of community-acquired pneumonia in the past 18 months that her primary care doctor said were
precipitated by her occasional aspiration R/T her GERD. Her exam is positive for substernal chest
pain and wheezing, but there are no clinical exam findings for pneumonia. An aerosol bronchodila-
tor treatment relieves the bronchospasms, and her chest x-ray is normal. The AGACNP feels a gastrointestinal (GI) medicine referral is appropriate for further evaluation of her GERD regimen. What
is the AGACNP's *next* step in the treatment for complications of GERD?

   A. Upper GI series (barium swallow)
   B. 24-hr pH esophageal and pharyngeal pH monitoring
   C. Flexible endoscopy
   D. Nissen fundoplication

18. The AGACNP knows that treatment for patients with *Helicobacter pylori* (*H. pylori*) infection should
aim to achieve high eradication rates in the setting of ever-increasing antibiotic resistance. Therefore,
the evidence-based, first-line treatment for a patient with prior exposure to a macrolide antibiotic is:

   A. A proton pump inhibitor (PPI), clarithromycin, and amoxicillin or metronidazole for 14 days
   B. Bismuth quadruple therapy (PPI, bismuth, tetracycline, and a nitroimidazole for 10–14 days)
   C. A PPI and clarithromycin, tetracycline, and a nitroimidazole for 10 to 14 days
   D. Sequential therapy consisting of a PPI and amoxicillin for 5 days followed by clarithromycin
   and nitroimidazole for an additional 5 days

19. Acute appendicitis (AA) is the most common abdominal emergency. Diagnosing AA is often ham-
pered by diagnostic uncertainty and the need for risk stratification. Which of the following diagnostic studies or clinical criteria is the *most* accurate in the process of AA diagnosis?

   A. Low-grade fever, nausea, and vomiting
   B. An Alvarado score of greater than 8
   C. CT imaging of the abdomen
   D. Abdominal ultrasound

(See answers next page.)

16. B) Consult interventional radiology for a percutaneous cholecystostomy tube

Given this patient's critical condition, the percutaneous cholecystectomy tube is the appropriate conservative management as the patient will have very poor outcomes if taken to the operating room. Nasogastric tube (NGT) to low wall suction (LWS), gentle intravenous hydration given the history of CHF, pain medications, antiemetics, and antimicrobial therapy are all most appropriate at this time, until the patient is more stable for surgical intervention. The patient is on appropriate antimicrobial therapy with guidelines recommending second-or third-generation cephalosporins or carbapenems, or Flagyl with a fluoroquinolone like ciprofloxacin. Early cholecystectomy is the gold standard for the management for certain patient populations. However, the surgical management of older adult and critically ill patients is thought to be associated with poor outcomes with high rates of morbidity and mortality. Current guidelines, including the Tokyo guidelines, recommend gallbladder drainage by percutaneous cholecystostomy tube placements in this patient population of those who are critically ill. The patient should remain NPO. Trickle feeding may be an option to prevent gallbladder distension.

17. D) Nissen fundoplication

The classic hallmark symptoms of GERD are substernal burning or warmth that is aggravated by the supine position and ingestion of large meals. The Nissen fundoplication is a surgical treatment for GERD and would be needed to prevent the patient's aspiration pneumonia and improve her quality of life (QOL) as she ages. Most diagnoses and treatment can be started with acid reduction and lifestyle alterations. This patient can still benefit from counseling for the latter. However, some patients with known GERD require more involved treatment. Diagnostic tests may include a barium swallow, pH monitoring, and often a flexible endoscopy.

18. B) Bismuth quadruple therapy (PPI, bismuth, tetracycline, and a nitroimidazole for 10–14 days)

In the United States and Canada, the incidence of *Helicobacter pylori* infection is generally lower than for people born outside these countries. The first-line treatment for patients with *H. pylori* with no previous history of macrolide exposure, who reside in areas where clarithromycin resistance among *H. pylori* isolates is known to be low (less than 15%) can be clarithromycin triple therapy (PPI, clarithromycin, and amoxicillin or metronidazole for 14 days). However, resistance patterns may not be known, or patients may have had macrolide antibiotic exposure in the past, so *most* patients will be better served by first-line treatment with the addition of bismuth quadruple therapy (PPI, bismuth, tetracycline, and a nitroimidazole for 10 to 14 days) or concomitant therapy consisting of a PPI, clarithromycin, amoxicillin, and metronidazole for 10 to 14 days or sequential therapy: PPI and amoxicillin 5 to 7 days, followed by PPI and clarithromycin plus nitroimidazole for 5 to 7 days.

19. C) CT imaging of the abdomen

CT is the most accurate mode of imaging in suspected appendicitis; however, radiation is a concern. Ultrasound is beneficial while decreasing the need for CT in some situations. Laboratory markers and clinical signs have very limited diagnostic utility on their own but show promise when used in combination with diagnostics such as the Alvarado score. Low-grade fever, nausea, and vomiting are too generalized to be diagnostic for appendicitis, alone.

20. A 35-year-old male patient with a history of Crohn disease since age 20 years has been recently managed on azathioprine. He presents to the clinic this morning with complaints of malodorous diarrhea, left lower quadrant (LLQ) abdominal pain, weakness, and malaise. The AGACNP orders stool culture for *Clostridioides difficile* and what other test?

A. Stool for occult blood and a complete blood count (CBC)

B. Enzyme-linked immunosorbent assay (ELISA) for cytomegalovirus

C. Barium enema to evaluate for fistula

D. CT with oral and intravenous (IV) contrast

(*See answers next page.*)

20. B) Enzyme-linked immunosorbent assay (ELISA) for cytomegalovirus

Patients with inflammatory bowel disease (IBD) may be more prone to infectious complications based on their underlying inflammatory disease and variations in their microbiome. Immunosuppressant medications commonly used to treat patients with Crohn disease play a role in predisposing these patients to acquiring these infections. The most common infections of the gastrointestinal (GI) tract in patients with IBD are *C. difficile* infections and cytomegalovirus.

KEY BIBLIOGRAPHY

Only key resources appear in the print edition. Access the full bibliography for this chapter on ExamPrepConnect.com.

Hart, P. A., Conwell, D. L., & Krishma, S. G. (2021). Acute and chronic pancreatitis. In J. Loscalzo, A. S. Fauci, D. L. Kasper, S. L. Houser, D. L. Longo, & J. L. Jameson (Eds.), *Harrison's principle of internal medicine* (21st ed.). McGraw Hill.

Hart, P. A., Conwell, D. L., & Krishma, S. G. (2021). Nausea, vomiting and Indigestion. In J. Loscalzo, A. S. Fauci, D. L. Kasper, S. L. Houser, D. L. Longo, & J. L. Jameson (Eds.), *Harrison's principle of internal medicine* (21st ed., chap. 45). McGraw Hill.

Lee, W. M., Stravitz, R. T., & Larson, A. M. (2012). Introduction to the revised American Association for the Study of Liver Diseases position paper on acute liver failure 2011. *Hepatology, 55*(3), 965–967. https://doi.org/10.1002/hep.25551

Polson, J., & Lee, W. M. (2005). AASLD position paper: The management of acute liver failure. *Hepatology, 41*(5), 1179–1197. https://doi.org/10.1002/hep.20703

Strate, L. L., & Gralnek, I. M. (2016). ACG clinical guideline: Management of patients with acute lower gastrointestinal bleeding. *American Journal of Gastroenterology, 111*(5), 755. https://doi.org/10.1038/ajg.2016.155

Renal, Genitourinary, and Reproductive System Review

Alexander Menard and Danielle Hebert

▶ INTRODUCTION

The AGACNP must be prepared to diagnosis, treat, and manage patients presenting with acute and acute-on-chronic conditions of the renal, genitourinary, and reproductive systems. Kidney disease, also known as chronic kidney disease (CKD), causes more deaths than breast cancer or prostate cancer. It is the underrecognized public health crisis. Kidney disease affects approximately 37 million people in the United States, and one in three adults are at risk for kidney disease. The AGACNP will care for patients with conditions that range from sexually transmitted infections (STIs) to acute kidney injury (AKI) to genitourinary trauma and many ailments in between.

▶ ACUTE KIDNEY INJURY

DISEASE OVERVIEW

AKI is defined by the deterioration of kidney filtration and excretory abilities over a short period of time, hours to 1 week. Altered filtration and/or excretion results in retention of nitrogen waste products normally cleared by the kidney. This alteration also negatively impacts the kidney's ability to maintain effective circulating volume, the excretion of nitrogenous wastes and metabolic toxins, acceptable electrolyte levels, and the acid-base levels within the plasma. AKI is not a simple disease but rather a result of many compounding factors. There are varying phenotypes of AKI that can range from asymptomatic and/or transient changes to significant expressions that can result in death (Tables 12.1 and 12.2).

Table 12.1 Types of Acute Kidney Injury

Prerenal	Any cause of reduced blood flow to the kidney
Intrarenal	Glomerular or tubular injury
Post-renal	Obstruction of outflow from kidney

Table 12.2 Causes of Acute Kidney Injury

Prerenal	▪ Hypovolemia ▪ Decreased cardiac output ▪ Decreased renal perfusion due to medications
Intrinsic	▪ Acute tubular necrosis ▪ Toxins (drugs or heavy metals) ▪ Glomerular disease (glomerulonephritis, lupus, vasculitis) ▪ Vascular disease (atherosclerosis, aortic aneurysms, thromboses) ▪ Microvascular disease (embolic, heparin-induced thrombocytopenia, disseminated intravascular coagulation, thrombotic thrombocytopenic purpura, hemolytic uremic syndrome, HELLP syndrome) ▪ Macrovascular disease (renal artery occlusion) ▪ Interstitial disease (allergic reaction to drugs, autoimmune disease)

(continued)

Table 12.2 Causes of Acute Kidney Injury (*continued*)

Post-renal	▪ Prostatic hypertrophy (benign or malignant) ▪ Cervical cancer ▪ Obstruction (renal calculi, urate crystals) ▪ Pelvic mass ▪ Intraluminal bladder mass (clot, tumor) ▪ Neurogenic bladder ▪ Ureteral strictures

CLASSIC PRESENTATION

The AGACNP is caring for a 72-year-old patient with a past medical history of hypertension and diabetes. The patient reports increased shortness of breath and decreased enteral/nutritional intake over the last 2 to 3 days. A diagnosis of community-acquired pneumonia is made. On hospital day 4, the patient is noted to have minimal urine output that is dark yellow and a creatine that has doubled from baseline.

DIAGNOSTIC CRITERIA

A thorough history and physical exam will provide significant clues as to the underlying cause of AKI. AKI is often an acute process that is a result of another pathology. Examples include AKI due to dehydration from excessive vomiting or diarrhea or use of nephrotoxic agents, or other disease states that can decrease renal blood flow such as heart failure, sepsis, hypotension, and all shock states (Table 12.3).

Table 12.3 Diagnostic Criteria of Acute Kidney Injury

	RIFLE	AKIN	KIDGO
Diagnostic criteria	See staging criteria	Increase in serum creatinine of ≥0.3 mg/dL or ≥50% within 48 hours OR Urine output of less than 0.5 mL/kg/hr for 6–12 hours	Increase in serum creatinine of ≥0.3 mg/dL within 48 hours or ≥50% within 7 days OR Urine output of less than 0.5 mL/kg/hr for 6–12 hours
Staging Criteria			
Risk (RIFLE) or Stage 1 (AKIN/KDIGO)	Increase in serum creatinine to 1.5 times baseline OR Urine output of less than 0.5 mL/kg/hr for 6–12 hours	Increase in serum creatinine of ≥0.3 mg/dL or to 150%–200% baseline OR Urine output of less than 0.5 mL/kg/hr for 6–12 hours	Increase in serum creatinine of ≥0.3 mg/dL or 1.5 to 1.9 times baseline OR Urine output of less than 0.5 mL/kg/hr for 6–12 hours
Injury (RIFLE) or Stage 2 (AKIN/KDIGO)	Increase in serum creatinine of to two times baseline OR Urine output of less than 0.5 mL/kg/hr for 12–24 hours	Increase in serum creatinine to 200%–300% baseline OR Urine output of less than 0.5 mL/kg/hr for 12–24 hours	Increase in serum creatinine to 2.0–2.9 times baseline OR Urine output of less than 0.5 mL/kg/hr for 12–24 hours

(*continued*)

Table 12.3 Diagnostic Criteria of Acute Kidney Injury (*continued*)

	RIFLE	AKIN	KIDGO
Failure (RIFLE) or Stage 3 (AKIN/KDIGO)	Increase in serum creatinine to three times baseline OR Increase in serum creatinine by greater than 0.5 mg/dL to greater than 4.0 mg/dL OR Urine output of less than 0.3 mL/kg/hr for greater than 24 hours or anuria for greater than 12 hours OR Initiation of kidney replacement therapy	Increase in serum creatinine to greater than 300% baseline OR Increase in serum creatinine by greater than 0.5 mg/dL to ≥4.0 mg/dL OR Urine output of less than 0.3 mL/kg/hr for greater than 24 hours or anuria for greater than 12 hours OR Initiation of kidney replacement therapy	Increase in serum creatinine to ≥3.0 times baseline OR Increase in serum creatinine of ≥0.3 mg/dL to ≥4.0 mg/dL OR Urine output of less than 0.3 mL/kg/hr for ≥24 hours or anuria for ≥ 12 hours OR Initiation of kidney replacement therapy
Loss (RIFLE)	Need for kidney replacement therapy for greater than 4 weeks		
End stage (RIFLE)	Need for kidney replacement therapy for greater than 3 months		

AKIN, Acute Kidney Injury Network; KDIGO, Kidney Disease Improving Global Outcomes; RIFLE, Risk, Injury, Failure, Loss of kidney function, End-stage renal disease.

Laboratory data (Table 12.4) needed for the evaluation of AKI include:

- comprehensive metabolic panel, including evaluation of blood urea nitrogen (BUN) to creatinine ratio
- urinalysis with urine specific gravity
- microscopic evaluation for urine sediment examination to assess for muddy brown casts
- urine sodium, BUN, and creatinine to calculate the fractional excretion of sodium (FeNa) and fractional excretion of urea (FeUrea)

Table 12.4 Laboratory Findings by Type of Acute Kidney Injury

Acute Kidney Injury Type	Associated Labs
Prerenal	FeNa less than 1% FeUrea less than 20%–30% Urine sodium less than 20 mEq/L
Intrarenal	FeNa greater than 1% FeUrea greater than 40%–70% UA with microscopy results: muddy casts, oxalate crystals, eosinophils
Post-renal	Variable; location of the obstruction must be identified

TREATMENT/MANAGEMENT

- Identify and treat the underlying cause of the AKI.
- Discontinue nephrotoxic drugs.
- Optimize hemodynamics (goal is mean arterial pressure greater than 60–65).
- Correct fluid and electrolyte abnormalities.
- Initiate renal replacement therapy (think "vowels" for indications for dialysis: *A*cidosis, *E*lectrolytes, *I*ngestions, *O*verload, *U*remia).

COMPLICATIONS

See Table 12.5.

Table 12.5 Complications of Acute Kidney Injury

■ Uremia	■ Hyperphosphatemia
■ Hypervolemia or hypovolemia	■ Hypocalcemia
■ Hyponatremia	■ Bleeding
■ Hyperkalemia	■ Infections
■ Acidosis	■ Cardiac complications (arrhythmias, pericarditis,
■ Malnutrition	pericardial effusion)

▶ RHABDOMYOLYSIS

DISEASE OVERVIEW

Rhabdomyolysis is a clinical syndrome resulting from skeletal muscle breakdown. Skeletal muscle breakdown can result from trauma, particularly crush injuries; medications; toxins; infections; hypothermia; hyperthermia; and extreme exercise.

CLASSIC PRESENTATION

The AGACNP is caring for a 34-year-old patient who suffered a crush injury while working at an automotive shop. The patient presented with a significant right lower extremity deformity. On admission, the patient was noted to have dark "cola-colored" urine and labs significant for creatinine 1.5× baseline and creatine kinase of 19,000 U/L with a repeat 6 hours later of 23,000 U/L.

DIAGNOSTIC CRITERIA

Rhabdomyolysis is suspected based on clinical presentation and history and confirmed with a creatine kinase that is 5× that of the upper limit of normal.

TREATMENT/MANAGEMENT

The mainstay of therapy is volume expansion with intravenous (IV) fluids to flush out the kidneys. Address or resolve the underlying cause and manage complications. There is no clear evidence for the use of sodium bicarbonate for urinary alkalinization.

COMPLICATIONS

- AKI
- Disseminated intravascular coagulation
- Hypoalbuminemia
- Electrolyte disturbances

▶ CHRONIC KIDNEY DISEASE

DISEASE OVERVIEW
CKD includes a spectrum of changes associated with abnormalities of kidney function or structure that has been present for 3 or more months with a gradual decline of the glomerular filtration rate (GFR):

- *systemic disease:* diabetes, autoimmune, infection (HIV, SARS-CoV-2), toxic therapy exposure (chemotherapies), hypertension
- *genetics:* age, sex, family history (polycystic kidney disease)
- *childhood/adolescent risks:* increased body mass index (BMI), kidney disease, premature birth, persistent microscopic hematuria, increased blood pressure
- *adulthood risks:* preeclampsia, AKI, kidney donation
- *lifestyle:* physical activity, smoking, diet
- *nephrotoxic medications:* nonsteroidal anti-inflammatory drugs (NSAIDs), antimicrobials, chemotherapy agents, cyclooxygenase-2 (COX-2) inhibitors, proton pump inhibitors, antiretroviral agents, lithium, and phosphate-containing bowel laxatives
- estimated that at least 6% of adults in the United States have CKD in stages 1 and 2, with 4.5% estimated to have stages 3 and 4
- *most frequent cause:* diabetic nephropathy due to diabetes mellitus (DM) type 2
- stages classified according to cause, GFR category, and albuminuria (nephron injury) category (Table 12.6)
- patients in stages 1 and 2 usually without symptoms, noted incidentally on lab work
- patients in stages 3 and 4 may have anemia; fatigue; decreased appetite with malnutrition; changes in lab values for calcium, phosphorus, vitamin $1,25(OH)_2 D_3$, and parathyroid hormone; and changes in electrolytes

Table 12.6 Stages of CKD

CKD Stage According to GFR	Kidney Function	GFR Result
G1	Normal or high	≥90
G2	Mildly decreased	60–89
G3a	Mildly to moderately decreased	45–59
G3b	Moderately to severely decreased	30–44
G4	Severely decreased	15–29
G5	Kidney failure	Less than 15
CKD Albuminuria Categorization	**Albumin Amounts/Kidney Function**	**Albumin Result**
A1	Normal to mildly increased	Less than 30 mg/g or less than 3 mg/mmol
A2	Moderately increased	30–300 mg/g or 3–30 mg/mmol
A3	Severely increased	Greater than 300 mg/g or greater than 30 mg/mmol

CKD, chronic kidney disease; GFR, glomerular filtration rate.

CLASSIC PRESENTATION
The AGACNP is caring for a 58-year-old male patient with a medical history of hypertension, hyperlipidemia, and DM type 2 and notes a gradual decline in his eGFR. Initial results were 75 about 5 years ago and now are 59. His last office visit was 9 months ago. His blood pressure reading was 149/94,

HbA1C was 8.2, low-density lipoprotein (LDL) was 132, and high-density lipoprotein (HDL) was 24. He is currently taking lisinopril 10 mg/hydrochlorothiazide 25 mg daily, atorvastatin 20 mg daily, metformin 1,000 mg twice daily, and dulaglutide (Trulicity) 1.5 mg weekly.

DIAGNOSTIC CRITERIA

One of the following is present for more than 3 months, indicating kidney damage: albuminuria, urine sediment, abnormal electrolytes secondary to a tubular disorder, abnormal histology, abnormal structure, or history of kidney transplant; *or* GFR reading less than 60 mL/min/1.73 m²:

- *Determine contributing cause:* complete full history and physical exam (medications, family history, environmental or social factors, labs, and appropriate imaging)
- *Blood pressure:* Check for target organ damage due to hypertension, edema, or polyneuropathy.
- *Labs:* serum and urine protein electrophoresis for patients older than 35 years of age and unexplained CKD (evaluating for multiple myeloma); autoimmune or infectious disease if glomerulonephritis is present (lupus, hepatitis B and C, HIV); serum creatinine; estimated serum GFR (eGFR); calcium; phosphorus; vitamin D; parathyroid hormone (PTH); complete blood count (CBC); iron; vitamin B$_{12}$; folate
- *Imaging:* renal ultrasound
- Albuminuria is measured by the urinary albumin-to-creatinine ratio (UACR) using one or more samples obtained from first morning urination. Persistent UACR greater than 2.5 mg/mmol (male patient) or greater than 3.5 mg/mmol (female patient) is an early detector of primary kidney disease and systemic microvascular disease.
- Kidney failure risk (KFR) equation can be used to determine patient risk to progress to stage 5 kidney disease: uses age, sex, geographical region, GFR, and UACR.
- CKD stage 2 or 3 is stable without proteinuria: monitor with lab work.
- Nephrology referral indicated if stable labs worsen, albuminuria develops, or blood pressure cannot be controlled.

TREATMENT/MANAGEMENT

See Table 12.7.

Table 12.7 Treatments for Chronic Kidney Disease by Etiology

Potential Cause	Treatment
Extracellular fluid volume expansion (edema) due to sodium retention secondary to decreased sodium excretion	■ Dietary salt restriction ■ Consider furosemide, bumetanide, or torsemide ● May need higher doses due to resistance ■ Consider addition of metolazone if lack of response in edema
Hyperkalemia due to dietary potassium intake, hemolysis, or medications	■ Dietary potassium restriction ■ Use potassium-sparing medications cautiously: RAS inhibitors, spironolactone, amiloride, eplerenone, triamterene

Hypertension	■ Good blood pressure control:
	  ● Less than 130/80 if DM or proteinuria greater than 1 g/24 hr
	■ Angiotensin-converting enzyme or angiotensin receptor blocker to slow decline of kidney function
	  ● Discontinue use if GFR continues to decline

DM, diabetes mellitus; GFR, glomerular filtration rate; RAS, renin angiotenin system.

COMPLICATIONS

- Metabolic acidosis due to decreased urine acid secretion
- *Bone manifestations:* increased bone turnover due to elevated PTH levels, osteomalacia, and low bone turnover due to normal to low PTH level. This can present with bone pain, fractures, or calcinosis.

- Increased cardiovascular mortality with CKD and hyperphosphatemia
- Increased morbidity and mortality due to cardiovascular disease in any stage of CKD. It is important to identify and treat cardiovascular risk factors early in diagnosis.
- Anemia of CKD presents as normocytic, normochromic; it is noted in stage 3 and present by stage 4.
- Abnormal hemostasis due to prolonged bleeding time; aggregation and adhesiveness of platelets is abnormal; platelet factor III has decreased activity; impaired consumption of prothrombin. May see increased bruising and bleeding.
- *Neuromuscular:* changes in memory and concentration, musculature, peripheral neuropathy
- Pruritis

Clinical Pearls

- It is normal for GFR to gradually decline by 1 mL/min/y/1.73 m² due to normal aging process (e.g., by 70 mL/min/1.73 m² by age 70 years).
- Avoid use of nephrotoxic drugs or other potential causes of AKI.
- Dose-adjust medications according to CKD stage or switch to alternative treatment regimen.

▶ CONTRAST-INDUCED NEPHROPATHY

DISEASE OVERVIEW
Contrast-induced nephropathy (CIN) is a common cause of AKI in hospitalized patients. It is most often observed within 72 hours of iodinated contrast exposure (can be up to 1 week) with an associated rise in serum creatinine of 0.5 mg/dL or a 25% increase from baseline.

CLASSIC PRESENTATION
A 60-year-old patient with a past medical history of hypertension and CKD presents after a motor vehicle crash. The initial workup includes a CT scan of the chest, abdomen, and pelvis with IV contrast. On hospital day 2, the patient is noted to have a doubling of baseline serum creatinine.

DIAGNOSTIC CRITERIA
CIN is an increase in the plasma creatinine level of at least 0.5 mg/dL (44 mcmol/L) or at least a 25% increase from the baseline level within 2 to 5 days after exposure to contrast material.

The Kidney Disease Improving Global Outcomes (KDIGO) working group proposed the term "contrast-induced acute kidney injury" and suggested a definition based on a plasma creatinine level that has increased by a factor of 1.5 times or more over the baseline value within 7 days after exposure to contrast medium; a plasma creatinine level that has increased by at least 0.3 mg/dL (26.5 mcmol/L) over the baseline value within 48 hours after exposure to contrast medium; or a urinary volume of less than 0.5 mL/kg of body weight per hour that persists for at least 6 hours after exposure.

TREATMENT/MANAGEMENT
Prevention is key as there is no definitive treatment for CIN. Prevention techniques include minimizing use of contrast by evaluating whether the test is absolutely necessary and using the lowest necessary total dose of low osmolality or iso-osmolality contrast medium. If contrast study or intervention is needed, use intravascular volume expansion with IV crystalloids as prophylaxis. There is no role for bicarbonate infusion or acetylcysteine (Mucomyst). Renal replacement therapy should be initiated only in the setting of CIN for clinical indications for renal replacement therapy (acidosis, hypervolemia, electrolyte abnormalities, ingestions, uremia).

COMPLICATIONS
Complications include acceleration/worsening of underlying CKD and increased morbidity and mortality.

▶ FLUID AND ELECTROLYTE IMBALANCES

DISEASE OVERVIEW

Acute, acute-on-chronic, and chronic illnesses are often associated with a variety of fluid and electrolyte imbalances. Elevations and deficiencies in electrolytes and intravascular volume status play roles in clinical conditions and complications that warrant AGACNP attention, aggressive interventions, and frequent reassessment.

CLASSIC PRESENTATION: FLUID AND ELECTROLYTE IMBALANCE

The AGACNP is caring for an adult patient who presents with nausea and diarrhea for 3 days. The patient reports palpitations and lower leg cramping. On exam, the patient appears dehydrated and has a basic metabolic panel notable for a potassium of 2.2 mEq/L.

DIAGNOSTIC CRITERIA

The AGACNP must know normal ranges as well as clinical symptoms (Tables 12.8 and 12.9).

Table 12.8 Normal Ranges for Electrolytes

Electrolyte	Normal Range
Sodium	135–145 mEq/L
Potassium	3.5–5.5 mEq/L
Chloride	95–105 mEq/L
Calcium	Total = 8.6–10.2 mg/dL Ionized = 1.12–1.3 mmol/L
Magnesium	1.5–2.4 mg/dL
Phosphorus	2.5–4.5 mg/dL

Table 12.9 Clinical Findings of Electrolyte Abnormalities

Electrolyte	Hypo- Findings	Hyper- Findings
Sodium	Less than 135 mEq/L: Neurologic deficits ■ Confusion ■ Agitation ■ Disorientation ■ Forgetfulness ■ Dizziness ■ Seizures ■ Coma Fatigue Headache Anorexia Nausea and vomiting	Greater than 145 mEq/L: Variable depending on cause, acuity Neurologic abnormalities ■ Irritability ■ Coma ■ Polyuria ■ Nausea and vomiting ■ Generalized muscle weakness
Potassium	Less than 3.5 mEq/L: Palpitations Arrhythmia Nausea and Vomiting Constipation Muscle weakness Muscle cramping Postural hypotension Paralysis (severe)	Greater than 5.5 mEq/L: Malaise Weakness Nausea, vomiting, diarrhea Muscle twitching Hyperreflexia Paresthesia
Chloride	Weakness/fatigue	Metabolic acidosis

(continued)

Table 12.9 Clinical Findings of Electrolyte Abnormalities (*continued*)

Electrolyte	Hypo- Findings	Hyper- Findings
Calcium	Total ≤8.6 mg/dL Ionized ≤1.12 mmol/L Perioral numbness Tetany (severe) Seizures (severe) Prolonged QT interval Paresthesia	Total ≥10.2 mg/dL Ionized ≥1.3 mmol/L Fatigue Anorexia Confusion Nausea, vomiting, constipation
Magnesium	Less than 1.5 mg/dL Hyperreflexia Carpopedal spasm Tetany Seizures EKG changes: torsades de pointes (severe)	Greater than 2.4 mg/dL Loss of deep tendon reflex Nausea and vomiting Hypotension Bradycardia Increased PR and QRS intervals
Phosphorus	Less than 2.5 mg/dL Muscle weakness Diaphragmatic weakness Irritability Paresthesia Hemolysis and platelet dysfunction	Greater than 4.5 mg/dL See hypocalcemia section (due to calcium phosphate precipitation)

DETERMINING VOLUME STATUS

There are three main categories for volume status: hypervolemic, euvolemic, and hypovolemic. Determining a patient's intravascular volume status requires an astute diagnostician to interpret a wide range of clinical and diagnostic information. Options to evaluate volume status and/or fluid responsiveness include:

- vital signs (heart rate, respiratory rate, blood pressure)
- point-of-care ultrasound to evaluate cardiac function and inferior cava variability
- pulse pressure variation
- esophageal Doppler monitor readings
- passive leg raises
- pulmonary artery catheter data
- imaging (including but not limited to chest radiograph, CT scan)
- physical exam findings (edema, adventitious breath sounds, skin turgor, jugular venous distension, hepatojugular reflex, capillary refill, skin color and temperature, skin tenting, dry mucous membranes)
- weight (trend)
- intake and output data
- laboratory data including but not limited to comprehensive metabolic panel, CBC, and lactic acid

TREATMENT/MANAGEMENT

The mainstay of treatment for all fluid and electrolyte imbalances is to address the underlying cause. Use caution in replacing electrolytes in AKI or CKD (Table 12.10).

Table 12.10 Treatment of Electrolyte Abnormalities

Electrolyte Disturbance	Treatment
Hypokalemia	Replete potassium, PO/NGT or IV
Hyperkalemia	Stop/reduce supplemental potassium Administer IV calcium gluconate or chloride Administer regular insulin and dextrose IV Administer Kayexalate or patiromir Hemodialysis or CRRT

(*continued*)

Table 12.10 Treatment of Electrolyte Abnormalities (*continued*)

Electrolyte Disturbance	Treatment
Hypomagnesemia	Replete magnesium PO or IV
Hypermagnesemia	Stop/reduce supplemental magnesium Hemodialysis
Hypocalcemia	Replete calcium IV
Hypercalcemia	Stop/reduce supplemental calcium Calcium-binding agents Hemodialysis
Hypophosphatemia	Replace phosphorus IV or PO/NGT
Hyperphosphatemia	Stop/reduce supplemental phosphorus Phosphate binders (e.g., sevelamer, Phos Lo, Renagel) Hemodialysis or CRRT
Hyponatremia	Depends on cause but may include: ■ Fluid restriction ■ Hypertonic saline (1.5% or 3% IV infusion or PO via salt tablets or dietary) ■ Vaptans (tolvaptan, lixivaptan, and satavaptan)
Hypernatremia	Stop/reduce supplemental sodium Fluid resuscitation Reduce diuresis

CRRT, continuous renal replacement therapy; IV, intravenous; NGT, nasogastric tube; PO, by mouth.

COMPLICATIONS

Complications of fluid and electrolyte abnormalities vary depending on the electrolyte and the severity of the abnormality, as well as patient-specific factors.

■ Hypovolemia can cause organ hypoperfusion leading to kidney failure, liver failure, heart failure, brain damage, and potentially death.
■ Hypervolemia can cause ileus, increased permeability of bacterial translocation, impaired liver function, myocardial edema, arrythmia, pulmonary edema, kidney injury, and potentially death.
■ Electrolyte abnormalities (see Table 12.9) can cause arrythmias, fatigue, lethargy, nausea, vomiting, hemolysis, constipation, tetany, seizures, and potentially death.

▶ URINARY TRACT INFECTION

DISEASE OVERVIEW

Urinary tract infection (UTI) is an umbrella term for symptomatic disease that includes acute cystitis, asymptomatic bacteriuria, prostatitis, and pyelonephritis. In patients younger than 50 years, UTI occurs primarily in women. After age 50 years, UTI occurs in male and female patients equally due to obstruction secondary to prostatic hypertrophy.

■ *Uncomplicated UTI* (infection located in the bladder):
  ● *Presentation:* urinary urgency, dysuria, urinary frequency, hematuria, suprapubic discomfort, hesitancy
  ● *Risk factors in premenopausal women:* frequent sexual intercourse, diaphragm and spermicide use, or UTI history
  ● *Risk factors in postmenopausal women:* DM, frequent sexual intercourse, urinary incontinence
  ● *Risk factors in men:* anatomic or functional abnormality, being uncircumcised
  ● *U.S. pathogens: Escherichia coli* (75%–90%); *Staphylococcus saprophyticus* (5%–15%); *Klebsiella, Proteus, Enterococcus, Citrobacter* species (5%–10%)

- *Complicated UTI* (infection located beyond the bladder, seen with symptoms suggestive of systemic illness and/or fever):
  - *Presentation:*
    - ❑ *Mild:* low-grade fever, costovertebral-angle pain (CVAT)
    - ❑ *Severe:* high fever, flank pain, nausea, vomiting, rigors
  - *U.S. pathogens: E. coli, Pseudomonas aeruginosa, Klebsiella, Proteus, Citrobacter, Acinetobacter, Morganella.* Can see gram-positive bacteria (enterococci, *S. aureus,* yeast)
- *Recurrent UTI* (complicated or uncomplicated presentation):
  - *Recurrence within 2 weeks of infection:* considered to be reinfection
  - *May have clustering:* multiple recurrences following initial infection
  - *Risk factors in premenopausal women:* spermicide use, frequent sexual intercourse
  - *Risk factors in postmenopausal women:* previous history of UTI when premenopausal, anatomic factors affecting emptying of the bladder (urinary incontinence, cystoceles, or residual urine)
- *Pyelonephritis* (infection located in the renal parenchyma of the kidneys):
  - *Risk factors for women:* diabetes, frequent sexual intercourse, new sexual partner, history of UTI in preceding 12 months, urinary incontinence, or maternal history of UTI
- *Catheter-associated bacteriuria* (CAUTI; presents with or without symptoms):
  - *U.S. pathogens: E. coli, P. aeruginosa, Klebsiella, Proteus, Citrobacter, Acinetobacter, Morganella.* Can see gram-positive bacteria (enterococci, *S. aureus,* yeast)
- *Asymptomatic bacteriuria* (presence of bacteria in urinary tract without symptoms, found incidentally on urine testing): more frequently seen in older men and women (40%–50%) and may not require treatment:
  - In pregnancy, screening and treatment are indicated to prevent preterm delivery secondary to pyelonephritis.
- *Prostatitis* (prostate gland demonstrates infectious or noninfectious abnormalities):
  - *Presentation:*
    - ❑ *Acute bacterial:* urinary frequency, dysuria, pain (pelvic or perineal), fever, chills, bladder outlet obstruction symptoms
    - ❑ *Chronic bacterial:* cystitis episodes that are recurrent, may have pelvic or perineal pain

CLASSIC PRESENTATION

A healthy female patient who is sexually active with a new partner presents with complaints of urinary frequency, urinary urgency, hematuria, and suprapubic pressure and/or discomfort. She denies fever or chills. Her urine dip is positive for nitrites and blood.

DIAGNOSTIC CRITERIA

A detailed history can provide the diagnosis. In these instances, with a healthy, nonpregnant patient, laboratory testing with urine dip or culture is not indicated unless concern for resistance is present.

- 50% probability of acute cystitis or pyelonephritis if one presenting symptom (hematuria, back pain, dysuria, frequency) and no complicating factors
- 90% probability of recurrent UTI if risk factors present and no complicating factors or vaginal discharge
- Urine dipstick
  - There is a probability of UTI (50%–80%) when positive for nitrites or leukocyte esterase on urine dipstick AND one UTI symptom is present.
  - Nitrite levels may be normal due to increased fluid intake and frequent urination.
  - Test is confirmatory for uncomplicated cystitis and a high pretest probability.
  - Negative results require exploration for other symptom causes and urine culture.
  - For pregnancy, a negative result is not sensitive enough to rule out bacteriuria.
- Urine culture
  - This confirms the diagnosis if bacteria are detected.
  - In women, symptoms of cystitis and colony count threshold $\geq 10^2$ bacteria/mL is 95% sensitive and 85% specific than threshold $\geq 10^5$/mL.
  - In men, it is strongly recommended to complete urine culture when UTI symptoms are present to document the presence of bacteria. Consider infection with colony count threshold $\geq 10^3$.

TREATMENT/MANAGEMENT

See Table 12.11.

Table 12.11 Treatment/Management for Urinary Tract Infections

Infection	Treatment/Medication

Acute uncomplicated cystitis in women	■ First line:
	  ● Nitrofurantoin 100 mg twice daily × 5 days
	  ● Trimethoprim-sulfamethoxazole 1 DS tablet twice daily × 3 days
	■ Alternative regimens:
	  ● Fosfomycin 3 gram single-dose sachet
	  ● Ciprofloxacin 250 mg twice daily × 3 days
	  ● Ciprofloxacin ER 500 mg once daily × 3 days
	  ● Levofloxacin 250 mg once daily × 3 days
	  ● Amoxicillin-clavulanate 875/125 mg twice daily × 5–7 days
	  ● Cephalexin 500 mg twice daily × 5–7 days
	  ● Cefdinir 300 mg twice daily × 3–7 days
	■ In pregnancy patients:
	  ● Amoxicillin 500 mg orally every 8 hours × 7 days
	  ● Amoxicillin 875 mg orally every 12 hours × 7 days
	  ● Nitrofurantoin (DO NOT USE IN THIRD TRIMESTER OF PREGNANCY) 100 mg twice daily × 5–7 days

Acute cystitis in men	■ First-line:
	  ● Nitrofurantoin 100 mg twice daily × 7 days
	  ● Trimethoprim-sulfamethoxazole-DS 1 tablet twice daily × 7 days
	  ● Ciprofloxacin 500 mg twice daily × 7 days
	  ● Ciprofloxacin ER 1,000 mg once daily × 7 days
	  ● Levofloxacin 750 mg once daily × 7 days
	■ Alternative regimens:
	  ● Fosfomycin 3-g single-dose sachet orally every other day × 1–3 days
	  ● Amoxicillin-clavulanate 875/125 mg twice daily × 7 days
	  ● Cephalexin 500 mg four times daily × 7 days
	  ● Cefdinir 300 mg twice daily × 7 days

Asymptomatic bacteriuria	■ Patients who are not pregnant: no treatment indicated
	■ Pregnant patients (asymptomatic group B streptococcus):
	  ● Amoxicillin 500 mg orally every 8 hours × 4–7 days
	  ● Amoxicillin 875 mg orally every 12 hours × 4–7 days

Complicated UTI or catheter-associated UTI	■ Ciprofloxacin 500 mg orally twice daily ■ Ciprofloxacin ER 1,000 mg orally once daily × 7–14 days ■ Ciprofloxacin 400 mg IV every 12 hours ■ Levofloxacin 750 mg orally or IV every 24 hours ■ Nitrofurantoin 100 mg orally twice daily ■ Trimethoprim-sulfamethoxazole-DS 1 tablet orally twice daily

Pyelonephritis	■ Empiric therapy for low-risk bacteria resistance:
	  ● Ciprofloxacin 500 mg orally twice daily × 5–7 days
	  ● Ciprofloxacin ER 1,000 mg orally once daily × 5–7 days
	  ● Ciprofloxacin 400 mg IV every 12 hours × 5–7 days
	  ● Levofloxacin 750 mg orally once daily × 5–7 days
	  ● Levofloxacin 750 mg IV once daily × 5–7 days
	  ● Ceftriaxone 1 g IV daily × 10 days
	■ Alternative regimen empiric therapy for low-risk bacteria resistance:
	  ● Ertapenem 1 g IV every 24 hours
	  ● Gentamicin 5 mg/kg IV every 24 hours
	■ Empiric therapy for high-risk bacteria resistance:
	  ● Ertapenem 1 g IV every 24 hours

(continued)

Table 12.11 Treatment/Management for Urinary Tract Infections (*continued*)

Infection	Treatment/Medication
	▪ Alternative regimen empiric therapy for high-risk bacteria resistance:
	● Piperacillin-tazobactam 3.375 gm IV every 6 hours
	● Cefepime 2 g IV every 12 hours
	● Ceftazidime-avibactam 2.5 gm IV every 8 hours
	● Plazomicin 15 mg/kg IV every 24 hours

IV, intravenous.

COMPLICATIONS
Untreated UTI can lead to pyelonephritis.

▶ UROGENITAL/RENAL TRAUMA

DISEASE OVERVIEW
The kidneys are the most commonly injured genitourinary organs and are particularly susceptible to deceleration injuries. Fractured ribs and flank ecchymosis are findings suggestive of renal trauma.

CLASSIC PRESENTATION
A 74-year-old patient presents after a fall from standing 24 hours previously. The patient presents due to flank ecchymoses and chest wall pain and hematuria.

DIAGNOSTIC CRITERIA
Diagnostic imaging with IV contrast–enhanced CT of the abdomen and pelvis should be obtained on patients with a mechanism of injury or exam findings concerning for renal injury (Table 12.12).

Table 12.12 Diagnostic Testing of Genitourinary Trauma

Trauma	Diagnostics
Renal	CT of the abdomen and pelvis with IV contrast
Ureteral	CT of the abdomen and pelvis with IV contrast with delayed post contrast phase, urogram *or* direct inspection of ureters if patient taken emergently to the operating room for a laparotomy
Bladder	Retrograde cystography
Urethral	Retrograde urethrography
Genital	Clinical suspicion, ultrasound, surgical exploration

MECHANISM OF INJURY OR EXAM FINDINGS CONCERNING FOR RENAL INJURY
▪ Injury related to rapid deceleration
▪ Significant blow or force to the flank with ecchymosis
▪ Lower rib fractures
▪ Penetrating injury to the abdomen, flank, or lower chest
▪ Pelvic fractures

TREATMENT/MANAGEMENT
Treatment of urogenital injuries is specific to the injury itself (Table 12.13). Treatment specific to renal injuries has largely shifted to noninvasive management strategies when appropriate. For the hemodynamically unstable patient, despite appropriate resuscitation, the surgical team must perform immediate intervention (surgery or angioembolization).

Table 12.13 Treatment/Management of Genitourinary Trauma

Trauma	Treatment
Renal	▪ Noninvasive when appropriate ▪ Surgical or angioembolization
Ureteral	▪ Stable and underwent laparotomy surgical repair of laceration ▪ Unstable patients can be managed with temporary urinary drainage follow by delayed definitive management ▪ Stenting for ureteral contusions or resection with primary repair
Bladder	▪ Surgical repair ▪ Catheter drainage
Urethral	▪ Surgical repair ▪ Catheter drainage
Genital	▪ Surgical repair

COMPLICATIONS

Renal trauma can result in a wide range of complications (Table 12.14).

Table 12.14 Complications of Genitourinary Trauma

Complications	
▪ Reduced glomerular filtration rate ▪ Renal failure ▪ Urinary tract infection or pyelonephritis ▪ Urine leak/fistula ▪ Urinoma ▪ Abscess ▪ False aneurysm	▪ Arteriovenous fistula ▪ Vascular thrombus ▪ Persistent bleeding ▪ Incomplete repair ▪ Infarct or parenchymal loss ▪ Renal dysfunction

▶ SEXUALLY TRANSMITTED INFECTIONS

DISEASE OVERVIEW

Adolescents and young adults in the United States have the highest rates of STIs. Higher risk is associated with early initiation of sexual activity, habitation in a detention facility, being a transgender youth, substance misuse, mental health disorder, being a youth with a disability, sex trafficking, or being a young male having sex with males. In transgender patients, evaluate for symptoms of STI and screen according to patient's anatomy, sexual practices, and guidelines.

SEXUALLY TRANSMITTED INFECTION SCREENING

▪ Annual screening of all sexually active women ≤25 years of age and older women at increased risk (partner with STI, partner with multiple partners, new partner, more than one partner, inconsistent condom use when not in monogamous relationship, previous or coexisting STIs, exchanging sex for money or drugs) is recommended.
▪ Self-collected samples (collected by the patient) have been found to have high specificity and sensitivity when compared with clinician-collected samples.
▪ In pregnancy, screen if patient ≤25 years of age or high risk (multiple sex partners, new partner with or without STI, partner with additional sex partners, or obtaining money and/or drugs in exchange for sex). Rescreen 3 months following treatment.
▪ Screen anyone for both chlamydia and gonorrhea whose sexual partner was positive for *Neisseria gonorrhoeae* within the previous 60 days.
▪ Syphilis screening in pregnancy: Screen at first prenatal visit and again in the third trimester. Perform test at 28 weeks' gestation if patient is high risk (drug abuse, STI during pregnancy, high rate of syphilis in community, multiple sex partners or new partners, partner with an STI).
▪ See Tables 12.15 to 12.22 for screening and treatment of STIs.

Table 12.15 STI Symptoms, Diagnostics, Treatment, and Complications

STI	Signs and Symptom	Diagnostic Test	Treatment	Complications
Chlamydia	▪ Women may present with a mucopurulent vaginal discharge, cervical inflammation, and/or pelvic pain. ▪ Men may present with *urethritis*: purulent discharge, dysuria, frequency, urgency. ▪ MSM may present with symptoms of *prostatitis* (discharge, rectal bleeding, pain on defection, or pain during anal sex).	▪ NAAT is most sensitive for endocervical specimens. ● Vaginal swab collection is preferred for females. First-catch urine sample can be used but may detect 10% fewer infections. ● Urethral swab or first-catch urine are equivalent in detection infections for male patients. ● Oropharyngeal or rectal sample collection: Aptima Combo 2 Assay or Xpert CT/NG	See Table 12.16.	
Gonorrhea	▪ Women are commonly asymptomatic or may have purulent vaginal discharge, dysuria, urinary frequency, and inflammation, burning or itch of the vulva, vagina, cervix, or urethra (similar to PID). ▪ Men: *urethritis*: frequency, urgency, difficulty initiating urine stream, urethral discharge; *epididymitis*: pelvic discomfort, testicular pain, red or swollen scrotum; *proctitis*: rectal pain, diarrhea, rectal bleeding	▪ The recommended test is NAAT for both women and men. ● Vaginal swab is preferred for women. ● First-catch urine sampling is recommended for men. ● Oropharyngeal or rectal samples can be tested with NAAT and POC NAATs. ▪ Culture testing requires endocervical or urethral swab sampling.	See Table 12.17.	
HSV	▪ HSV may be asymptomatic and without lesions (commonly seen with HSV-1). ▪ Patients often have multiple, painful, vesicular genital lesions and/or ulcerations. ▪ Lesions may also look similar to those associated with syphilis and chancroid.	▪ Culture antigen testing or PCR for genital herpes is preferred test. ▪ PCR assay for HSV DNA is considered to be more sensitive. ▪ Conduct serologic testing for type-specific herpes simplex virus antibody.	See Table 12.18.	Disseminated infection can manifest as hepatitis, pneumonitis, or CNS changes (meningoencephalitis). Hospitalization is required.

(continued)

Table 12.15 STI Symptoms, Diagnostics, Treatment, and Complications (*continued*)

STI	Signs and Symptom	Diagnostic Test	Treatment	Complications
	▨ With first infection, patient may also have fever, headache, and malaise. ▨ After initial infection, the virus remains dormant and can present as recurring genital lesions. ▨ Infection remains transmissible in the absence of genital lesions.	▨ Provide counseling and education when HSV-2 antibody is present—this is indicative of an anogenital infection. ▨ HSV-1 antibody can be difficult to interpret as it may be due to an oral herpes lesion from childhood.		
Syphilis	See Tables 12.19 and 12.20.	▨ Serologic screening, dark-field microscopy, or PCR to detect *Treponema pallidum* DNA using sampling from lesion exudate or tissue is considered definitive method to diagnose early syphilis. ▨ Dark-field microscopy is required for all suspected primary lesions. Repeat serologic testing every week × 6 weeks. ▨ Nontreponemal tests with VDRL or RPR are nonspecific and may result in false positives. In the presence of symptoms, further testing is needed. ▨ A presumptive diagnosis requires two lab serologic tests: nontreponemal test: VDRL or RPR test, and a treponemal test (TP-PA) assay, various EIAs, CIAs and immunoblots, or rapid treponemal assays.	See Tables 12.19 and 12.20.	If not treated may progress into tertiary syphilis that presents as destructive lesions on skin, bone, cardiovascular system (aortic aneurysm), and the nervous system (meningitis).
Bacterial vaginosis (BV)	▨ BV presents with milky, homogenous vaginal discharge with fishy odor.	▨ Amsel criteria: must have three of the following four criteria: ● Homogenous vaginal discharge ● Positive "whiff test": presence of fishy odor when potassium hydroxide added to vaginal secretions	See Table 12.21.	Without pregnancy: cellulitis of the vaginal cuff following hysterectomy, infection following abortion, and PID Pregnancy: increased risk of preterm labor and delivery

(*continued*)

Table 12.15 STI Symptoms, Diagnostics, Treatment, and Complications (*continued*)

STI	Signs and Symptom	Diagnostic Test	Treatment	Complications
		• Presence of clue cells in vaginal secretions on saline wet mount microscopy • Vaginal pH more than 4.5 ▪ Nugent score: • Presence of large gram-positive rods (*Lactobacillus* morphotypes, scored 0–4) • Presence of small gram-variable rods (*Gardnerella vaginalis* morphotypes, scored 0–4) • Presence of curved gram-variable rods (*Mobiluncus* spp. morphotypes, scored 0–2) • Diagnosis of BV seen with score of 7–10 • DNA probe-test for presence of *Gardnerella*		
PID	▪ Classifications: • Acute (≤30 days) • Chronic (more than 30 days) ▪ Subclinical: no symptoms ▪ Mild: dyspareunia, dysuria or GI symptoms ▪ Moderate symptoms: pelvic pain aggravated by intercourse, UTI symptoms, vaginal discharge, or intermittent post-intercourse cervical bleeding ▪ Severe symptoms: fever, chills, nausea, vomiting and purulent vaginal discharge	▪ No confirmatory test for PID; diagnosis based on clinical presentation ▪ Imaging: transvaginal ultrasound or MRI: fallopian tubes may appear thickened and fluid filled; may see free fluid in the pelvis ▪ Laparoscopy: for severe cases confirms diagnosis and can visualize salpingitis ▪ Presumptive diagnosis: sexually active women and those at risk for STIs presenting with pelvic or lower abdominal pain; no other cause can be identified; and at least one: cervical motion tenderness, or uterine tenderness or adnexal tenderness	See Table 12.22.	If untreated, PID can result in infertility, chronic pelvic pain, or ectopic pregnancy. Tubo-ovarian abscess (~30% of women will develop). Symptoms include abnormal vaginal bleeding, pelvic or abdominal pain, fever, vaginal discharge and nausea.

BV, bacterial vaginosis; CIA, chemiluminescence immunoassay; CNS, central nervous system; EIA, enzyme immunoassay; GI, gastrointestinal; HSV, herpes simplex virus; MSM, men who have sex with men; NAAT, nucleic acid amplification test; PCR, polymerase chain reaction; PID, pelvic inflammatory disease; POC, point of care; RPR, rapid plasma reagin; STI, sexually transmitted infection; TP-PA, *T. pallidum* particle agglutiniation.

Table 12.16 Treatments for Chlamydia Infections

Recommended regimen	▦ Azithromycin 1 g orally in a single dose OR ▦ Doxycycline 100 mg orally two times daily × 7 days PLUS ▦ Ceftriaxone 250 mg IM in a single dose OR ▦ Cefixime 400 mg orally in a single dose (covers for *Neisseria gonorrhea* infection) ● CDC recommends testing men and women 3 months after treatment for possible repeat infection
Alternative regimen	▦ Erythromycin base 500 mg orally four times daily × 7 days ▦ Erythromycin ethyl succinate 800 mg orally four times daily × 7 days ▦ Levofloxacin 500 mg orally once daily × 7 days ▦ Ofloxacin 300 mg orally twice daily × 7 days
In pregnancy	▦ Azithromycin 1 g orally single dose ▦ Amoxicillin 500 mg orally three times daily × 7 days ▦ Perform NAAT as test of cure 4 weeks and retest 3 months after treatment
Partner therapy	▦ If allowed by law and/or regulations, should be offered to any sexual partners 60 days prior to diagnosis. Include patient education with treatment.
Considerations/counseling	▦ Advise patients to abstain from intercourse for 7 days after single-dose therapy or completion of 7-day regimen with resolution of symptoms. Refrain from intercourse until all partners are treated.

CDC, Centers for Disease Control and Prevention; IM, intramuscular; NAAT, nucleic acid amplification test.

Table 12.17 Treatment Options for Gonorrhea

Uncomplicated infection of cervix, urethra, or rectum	▦ Ceftriaxone 500 mg IM single dose if weight less than 150 kg; 1 g ceftriaxone if weight greater than 150 ▦ Treat for chlamydia if not excluded: doxycycline 100 mg orally two times daily × 7 days ▦ If ceftriaxone not available: cefixime 800 mg orally single dose and treat for chlamydia if not excluded with doxycycline 100 mg two times daily × 7 days
Uncomplicated (pharynx)	▦ Ceftriaxone 500 mg IM single dose if weight less than 150 kg, ceftriaxone 1 gm if weight greater than 150 kg
Cephalosporin allergy	▦ Gentamicin 240 mg IM single dose *PLUS* azithromycin 2 g orally single dose
In pregnancy	▦ Ceftriaxone 500 mg single IM dose plus treat for chlamydia if not excluded: azithromycin 1 g orally single dose or amoxicillin 500 mg orally three times daily × 7 days. Consult Infectious Disease if cephalosporin allergy is present.
Partner therapy	▦ If allowed by law and/or regulation, should be offered to any sexual partners 60 days prior to diagnosis. Include patient education with treatment.
Follow-up	▦ Uncomplicated pharynx infection: CDC recommends to complete test of cure with culture or NAAT 14 days after treatment (risk of possible false-positive result if done prior to 14 days). If NAAT is positive, complete culture before providing retreatment and complete antimicrobial susceptibility testing. ▦ Uncomplicated infection of cervix, urethra, or rectum: CDC recommends to test men and women 3 months after treatment for possible repeat infection. ▦ If suspected treatment failure, perform culture (Thayer–Martin or chocolate agar) and antimicrobial susceptibility testing.
Considerations/counseling	▦ Advise patients to abstain from intercourse for 7 days after single-dose therapy or completion of 7-day regimen with resolution of symptoms. Refrain from intercourse until all partners have been treated.

CDC, Centers for Disease Control and Prevention; IM, intramuscular; NAAT, nucleic acid amplification test.

Table 12.18 Treatment of Herpes Simplex Virus

First infection	▪ Acyclovir 400 mg orally three times daily × 7–10 days* ▪ Acyclovir 200 mg orally five times daily × 7–10 days* ▪ Famciclovir 250 mg orally three times daily × 7–10 days* ▪ Valacyclovir 1 g orally two times daily × 7–10 days* *Continue treatment longer than 10 days if lesions are still present.
Suppressive therapy	▪ Acyclovir 400 mg orally two times daily ▪ Famciclovir 250 mg orally two times daily ▪ Valacyclovir 500 mg orally one time daily (may be less effective if patient has more than 10 episodes/year) ▪ Valacyclovir 1 g orally once daily
Episodic therapy	▪ Acyclovir 400 mg orally three times daily × 5 days ▪ Acyclovir 800 mg orally two times daily × 5 days ▪ Acyclovir 800 mg orally three times daily × 2 days ▪ Famciclovir 125 mg orally two times daily × 5 days ▪ Famciclovir 500 mg orally once, followed by 250 mg two times daily × 2 days ▪ Famciclovir 1 g orally twice daily × 1 day ▪ Valacyclovir 500 mg orally twice daily × 3 days ▪ Valacyclovir 1 g orally once daily × 5 days
Suppressive therapy in pregnancy	▪ Acyclovir 400 mg orally three times daily ▪ Valacyclovir 500 mg orally two times daily ▪ Consider suppression therapy (if not already in place) at 36 weeks to prevent neonatal transmission.
HIV + suppressive therapy	▪ Acyclovir 400–800 mg orally two to three times daily ▪ Famciclovir 500 mg orally two times daily ▪ Valacyclovir 500 mg orally two times daily
HIV + episodic therapy	▪ Acyclovir 400 mg orally three times daily × 5–10 days ▪ Famciclovir 500 mg orally two times daily × 5–10 days ▪ Valacyclovir 1 gm orally two times daily × 5–10 days

Table 12.19 Stages of Syphilis

Primary syphilis (10–90 days after disease is contracted)	▪ Usually presents as a single painless ulcer or chancre or multiple atypical or painful lesions on anus, labia, vulva, vagina, cervix, nipples, and lips. ▪ Patients may have rubbery, painless lymphadenopathy in affected region followed by generalized lymphadenopathy during infection weeks 3–6. ▪ Dark-field microscopic findings will be present. ▪ Positive serologic testing is seen in 70% of primary syphilis cases.
Secondary syphilis (14–180 days after primary lesion develops)	▪ May present with papulosquamous rash on palms and soles, condyloma latum (white patches in moist lesions, considered infectious), and lymphadenopathy. Lesions may be scattered over the trunk of the body as macular, maculopapular, papular, or pustular. ▪ Dark-field microscopic findings will be positive with samples from moist lesions. ▪ Serologic testing will be positive.
Tertiary syphilis (≥4–20 years after primary lesion)	▪ This may present with cardiac involvement, gummatous lesions, and general paresis. ▪ Lesions may be present in cardiac, neurological, ophthalmic, and auditory systems.
Latent syphilis infections (may develop after secondary syphilis, may last lifetime)	▪ Clinical symptoms and lesions may be absent, but 25% may relapse in the first year with symptoms of secondary syphilis. ▪ Patients are infectious for first 1–2 years of latency period. ▪ It is usually detected by serologic testing that shows previous infection.

Table 12.20 Treatment of Syphilis

Preferred (primary, secondary, and early latent syphilis less than 1 year in duration)	◾ Penicillin G preferred for all stages: ● Benzathine penicillin G 2.4 million units IM single dose
Latent syphilis* (or unknown duration of infection)	◾ Benzathine penicillin G 7.2 million units in 3 doses of 2.4 million units IM spread over course of 3 weeks (1-week intervals) *Refer to Infectious Disease for treatment and monitoring
PCN allergy (without pregnancy)	◾ Doxycycline 100 mg orally two times daily × 14 days ◾ Tetracycline 500 mg orally four times daily × 14 days
In pregnancy*	◾ Parenteral penicillin G is only therapy with documented efficacy for syphilis in pregnancy. Those with penicillin allergy require desensitization and treatment with penicillin. *Refer to Infectious Disease for treatment and monitoring as there is risk of treatment failure, and second treatment may be indicated
HIV-positive patient	◾ Benzathine penicillin G 2.4 million units IM in a single dose

Partner therapy	◾ If allowed by law and/or regulations should be offered to any sexual partners 90 days prior to diagnosis. Include patient education with treatment.
	◾ Partners should be evaluated clinically and serologically, treatment if indicated:
	  ● If contact with a person who has diagnosis of primary, secondary, or early latent syphilis less than 90 days before diagnosis—treat presumptively even if serological testing is negative.
	  ● If contact was more than 90 days before diagnosis, treat presumptively for early syphilis if serologic test results not immediately available and follow-up is uncertain. If serologic tests are negative, no treatment is indicated. If positive, treat according to clinical and serologic evaluation and syphilis stage.
	  ● Check local health department requirements for treatment of partners when duration of syphilis is unknown.

Follow-up	◾ Repeat clinical and serologic evaluation at 6 and 12 months following treatment.

IM, intramuscular; PCN, penicillin.

Table 12.21 Treatment of Bacterial Vaginosis

Patients who are not pregnant	◾ Metronidazole 500 mg orally two times daily × 7 days ◾ Metronidazole gel 0.75%, one full applicator (5 g) intravaginally, once daily × 5 days ◾ Clindamycin cream 2%, one full applicator (5 g) intravaginally at bedtime × 7 days Alternative regimen: ◾ Clindamycin 300 mg orally two times daily × 7 days ◾ Clindamycin ovules 100 mg intravaginally once at bedtime × 3 days ◾ Tinidazole 2 gm orally once daily × 2 days ◾ Tinidazole 1 gm orally once daily × 5 days
Pregnant patients	◾ Metronidazole 250 mg orally three times daily × 7 days ◾ Clindamycin 300 mg orally two times daily × 7 days

Table 12.22 Treatment of Pelvic Inflammatory Disease

Recommended outpatient treatment option 1	◾ Ceftriaxone 250 mg IM single dose (or alternative parenteral third-generation cephalosporin) PLUS ◾ Doxycycline 100 mg orally twice daily × 14 days, WITH OR WITHOUT ◾ Metronidazole 500 mg twice daily × 14 days

(continued)

Table 12.22 Treatment of Pelvic Inflammatory Disease (*continued*)

Recommended outpatient treatment option 2	▪ Cefoxitin 2 g IM single dose and probenecid 1 g orally single dose administered concurrently PLUS ▪ Doxycycline 100 mg twice daily × 14 days OR ▪ Metronidazole 500 mg orally twice daily × 14 days
Alternative outpatient treatment regimens:	▪ Ceftriaxone 250 mg IM single dose PLUS ▪ Azithromycin 1 g orally once per week × 2 weeks OR ▪ Azithromycin 500 mg IV daily × 1–2 doses followed by azithromycin 250 mg orally daily × 12–14 days *Consider addition of metronidazole for all alternative regimens
Alternative outpatient quinolone treatment regimen for cephalosporin	▪ Levofloxacin 500 mg orally once daily × 14 days OR ▪ Ofloxacin 400 mg twice daily × 14 days OR ▪ Moxifloxacin 400 mg orally once daily × 14 days *Quinolones are not recommended due to building resistance by *Neisseria gonorrhoeae* but can be used if cephalosporins not feasible and there is low community prevalence and patient risk is low for gonorrhea
Recommended inpatient treatment option 1	▪ Cefotetan 2 g IV every 12 hours OR ▪ Cefoxitin 2 g IV every 6 hours PLUS ▪ Doxycycline 100 mg orally or IV every 12 hours
Recommended inpatient treatment option 1	▪ Clindamycin 900 mg IV every 8 hours PLUS ▪ Gentamicin loading dose IV or IM (2 mg/kg body weight) then maintenance dose (1.5 mg/kg) every 8 hours
Alternative inpatient treatment regimen	▪ Ampicillin/sulbactam 3 g IV every 6 hours PLUS ▪ Doxycycline 100 mg orally or IV every 12 hours *Oral doxycycline preferred to avoid discomfort associated with IV infusion .
In pregnancy	▪ Hospitalize patient and avoid use of doxycycline

IM, intramuscular; IV, intravenous.

▶ SUMMARY

This renal, genitourinary, and reproductive system review contains a tremendous amount of content. It is a broad overview to prepare for board certification as an AGACNP. The AGACNP will be expected to be knowledgeable about this content.

● KNOWLEDGE CHECK: CHAPTER 13

1. Which of the following glomerular filtration rate (GFR) result is associated with chronic kidney disease (CKD) stage G2?

   A. 45 to 59 mL/min/1.73 m^2
   B. 60 to 89 mL/min/1.73 m^2
   C. <30 mg/g
   D. 30 to 300 mg/g

2. A 52-year-old male patient is noted to have sediment in two different urinalyses over a 3-month time frame. He has a past medical history (PMH) of hypertension, which is controlled with lisinopril 5 mg daily. His electrolytes are normal, and his estimated serum glomerular filtration rate (eGFR) is 59. Which imaging would the AGACNP order first?

   A. MRI abdomen with contrast
   B. Abdominal ultrasound
   C. CT scan abdomen without contrast
   D. Renal ultrasound

3. A 76-year-old female patient with a history of hypertension, diabetes mellitus type 2, hyperlipidemia, and chronic kidney disease stage G2 has recently completed labs for her 3-month follow-up appointment. There is a noted drop in her glomerular filtration rate (GFR) from 63 to 57. Her vital signs are stable, and her recent A$_{1c}$ is 7.6. After completing a medication reconciliation, the AGACNP advises the patient to stop which of the following medications:

   A. Atorvastatin 20 mg
   B. Diltiazem 180 mg
   C. Celecoxib 200 mg
   D. Famotidine 10 mg

4. Which of the following is the most frequently reported bacterial infectious disease in the United States?

   A. Herpes simplex
   B. Gonorrhea
   C. Chlamydia
   D. Syphilis

5. Risk factors for sexually transmitted infections among adolescents and young adults include all of the following *except:*

   A. Living in a detention facility
   B. Mental health disorders
   C. Substance misuse
   D. Later initiation of sexual activity

6. Which of the following is the most common bacterial cause for urinary tract infections?

   A. *Escherichia coli*
   B. *Staphylococcus saprophyticus*
   C. *Klebsiella* species
   D. *Citrobacter* species

(See answers next page.)

1. B) 60 to 89 mg/min/1.73 m²

GFR results between 45 and 59 mg/min/1.73 m² correlate to chronic kidney disease (CKD) stage G3a. Measurement results of less than 30 or 30 to 300 mg/g are associated with categorization of CKD albuminuria, listed as A1, A2, or A3.

2. D) Renal ultrasound

A renal ultrasound will provide information regarding kidney size and determine if there is a kidney stone or blockage as well as the presence of a cyst(s) or mass. This is the safest first-step test to obtain while limiting the patient's exposure to radiation and contrast at a time when kidney function is decreased. A CT scan without contrast would be indicated if there was concern for infection, pyelonephritis, a kidney stone not seen on ultrasound, or renal artery stenosis.

3. C) Celecoxib 200 mg

Nonsteroidal anti-inflammatory agents and cyclooxygenase-2 (COX2) inhibitors are known to be nephrotoxic medications and should be stopped when there is a noted deterioration of the GFR.

4. C) Chlamydia

Chlamydia infection is the most frequently reported bacterial infectious disease in the United States, with the highest prevalence among women age 25 years and younger.

5. D) Later initiation of sexual activity

Higher risk for sexually transmitted infections among adolescents and young adults is associated with early initiation of sexual activity, habitation in a detention facility, being a transgender youth, substance misuse, mental health disorders, being a youth with a disability, sex trafficking, and being a young male having sex with males.

6. A) *Escherichia coli*

Escherichia coli accounts for 75% to 90% of urinary tract infections in the United States, followed by *Staphylococcus saprophyticus* (5%–15%), *Klebsiella*, and *Citrobacter* species (5%–10%).

7. A 22-year-old female patient is reporting 2 days of fever up to 100.4°F, left back pain, nausea, and dysuria. Which of the following is the most likely diagnosis?

    A. Bacterial vaginosis
    B. Uncomplicated urinary tract infection (UTI)
    C. Pyelonephritis
    D. Chlamydia

8. A 52-year-old male patient who is in a monogamous relationship with a male partner is reporting dysuria, urinary frequency and urgency, greenish penile discharge, and rectal discomfort. Which of the following tests is the most likely diagnosis?

    A. Complicated urinary tract infection (UTI)
    B. Syphilis
    C. Gonorrhea
    D. Epididymitis

9. A 22-year-old female patient is being seen for her annual exam and requires testing for chlamydia. Which of the following is the preferred testing method for female patients?

    A. Dark-field microscopy
    B. Serologic testing
    C. First-catch urine sample
    D. Vaginal swab

10. A 28-year-old-female patient who received an injection of penicillin for early syphilis 6 hours ago is presenting at urgent care with new onset fever, headache, and myalgia. Which of the following is the probable cause for this presentation of symptoms?

    A. Worsening of syphilis infection
    B. Jarish–Herxheimer reaction
    C. Incorrect diagnosis of syphilis
    D. Presence of co-infection

11. A 56-year-old female patient presents with a history of urinary frequency and urgency for 3 days. She has an allergy to penicillin. Her urinalysis is positive for nitrites and blood. Which of the following antibiotics would the AGACNP select?

    A. Ciprofloxacin ER 500 mg twice daily for 5 days
    B. Trimethoprim-sulfamethoxazole 1 DS tablet twice daily for 7 days
    C. Amoxicillin-clavulanate 875/125 mg twice daily for 5 days
    D. Nitrofurantoin 100 mg tablet twice daily for 5 days

12. The AGACNP is caring for a 38-year-old male patient who has transferred to the office. He presents today with concern of painful vesicular lesions located on the penis, lower pelvic region, and scrotum for the past week. He reports he is heterosexual and has not been sexually active for the past year. He reports he has had the rash twice over the past year and has had successful treatment with a pill when the rash is present. Which of the following treatments will the AGACNP prescribe?

    A. Benzathine penicillin G 2.4 million units intramuscular (IM) single dose
    B. Ceftriaxone 500 mg IM single dose
    C. Levofloxacin 250 mg once daily for 3 days
    D. Acyclovir 400 mg orally three times a day for 5 days

(See answers next page.)

7. C) Pyelonephritis

Symptoms of pyelonephritis include fever, flank pain, nausea, vomiting, and rigors. Bacterial vaginosis usually presents with a milky vaginal discharge that has a fishy odor; an uncomplicated UTI will present with dysuria, urinary urgency, and hesitancy. Chlamydia will present with a mucopurulent vaginal discharge and possibly pelvic discomfort.

8. C) Gonorrhea

Gonorrhea infection in males will present with symptoms like a UTI (dysuria, frequency, urgency) and purulent penile discharge. Men who have anal sex with men may experience rectal pain that may indicate an anal gonorrhea infection. Syphilis will present with either a painless ulcer or chancre or atypical or painful lesions in the anus or pelvic region with rubbery lymphadenopathy in the affected region. Epididymitis will present with symptoms of pain in the pelvic region, a red or swollen scrotum, and testicular pain.

9. D) Vaginal swab

Vaginal swab is the preferred testing modality for female patients when screening for chlamydia, whereas first-catch urine sample is the preferred testing modality for male patients. Dark-field microscopy would be used to test for syphilis, and there are no recommendations for use of serologic testing to screen for chlamydia.

10. B) Jarish–Herxheimer Reaction

Approximately 50% to 75% of patients with early syphilis will develop this reaction within 4 to 12 hours of receiving a penicillin injection. It will usually resolve on its own within 24 hours.

11. D) Nitrofurantoin 100 mg tablet twice daily for 5 days

Nitrofurantoin 100 mg twice daily for 5 days is the recommended first-line treatment for an uncomplicated urinary tract infection in an adult female patient. Ciprofloxacin ER is an extended-release tablet that would be dosed once daily, and the recommended time frame is 3 days. Trimethoprim-sulfamethoxazole is recommended as a first-line treatment for a total of 3 days. Amoxicillin-clavulanate would be contraindicated due to the patient's penicillin allergy.

12. D) Acyclovir 400 mg orally three times a day for 5 days

The patient is displaying vesicular lesions that have a history of recurrence that respond to episodic treatment, which is consistent with herpes simplex virus. The dosing and length of treatment of acyclovir are appropriate for an episodic treatment. Benzathine penicillin G would be indicated for a syphilis infection, which would present with painful or painless ulcer(s) or lesions during the primary syphilis stage and as papulosquamous rash on the palms and soles or maculopapular on the trunk as part of the secondary syphilis stage (14–180 days after primary lesion develops). Ceftriaxone would be indicated for a possible gonorrheal infection, which presents with symptoms of urinary frequency and urgency and purulent urethral discharge. The dose and time frame of levofloxacin is indicated for a female patient presenting with uncomplicated urinary tract infection.

13. A 39-year-old female patient has a homogenous, white milky vaginal discharge for 3 days. On exam, she has a positive "whiff test" and clue cells in the vaginal secretion. Her last menstrual period was 2 weeks ago. Which of the following treatments would the AGACNP order?

A. Metronidazole 500 mg orally twice daily for 7 days
B. Over-the-counter (OTC) vaginal douching once per week for 2 weeks
C. Doxycycline 100 mg twice daily for 14 days
D. No treatment as it is normal to have a vaginal discharge mid-cycle

14. A 24-year-old male patient has an oozing, painless ulceration on the penile shaft for the past 7 days and noticed some lymph node swelling in his left and right groin. Which of the following tests would the AGACNP order?

A. Rapid plasma reagin (RPR) test
B. Urinalysis and reflex to culture and sensitivity
C. Polymerase chain reaction (PCR) test for *Treponema pallidum*
D. Nucleic acid amplification test (NAAT)

15. The AGACNP is caring for a patient who was involved in a motor vehicle crash with a crush injury to their left lower extremity. On hospital day 1, they are noted to have dark-colored urine and a doubling of their creatinine. What is the next best thing for the AGACNP to order?

A. Creatine kinase STAT
B. 1 L crystalloid bolus STAT
C. Consult with nephrology for renal replacement therapy
D. Mannitol 50 g intravenously (IV) STAT

16. The AGACNP is caring for a male middle-aged patient with a past medical history of end-stage renal failure (ESRD). He was admitted to the hospital 3 days ago secondary to a community-acquired pneumonia. This morning's labs reveal a potassium level of 6.8 mmol/L. After receiving this information, a 12-lead electrocardiogram (EKG) was ordered, and it revealed diffuse peaked T waves not present on the patient's admission EKG. What will the AGACNP order next?

A. 10 units of regular insulin IV and 50 mL of 50% of dextrose intravenous (IV) STAT
B. Nephrology consult
C. Albuterol 10 mg nebulized STAT
D. 150 mEq sodium bicarbonate infusion at 50 mL/hr

17. An older adult patient presents from home with report of a fall 48 hours ago. The patient fell in the bathroom, striking their right flank. The patient now presents with flank ecchymosis and pain and gross hematuria. What is the AGACNP most concerned about?

A. Traumatic brain injury
B. Urinary tract injury
C. Rib fractures
D. Delirium

18. The AGACNP is caring for a patient on hospital day 3 after presenting with hypoxia and having a computed tomography angiogram (CTA) to evaluate for a pulmonary embolism. The CTA was negative. The AGACNP notes that the patient has had a rapid doubling of their creatinine on today's labs. What is the AGACNP most concerned about?

A. Contrast-induced nephropathy
B. Acute pulmonary embolism
C. Kidney stones
D. Medication-induced acute kidney injury

(See answers next page.)

13. A) Metronidazole 500 mg orally twice daily for 7 days

This patient has three of the four Amsel criteria for bacterial vaginosis, and metronidazole would be a recommended first-line treatment for the patient. Vaginal douching would be contraindicated because bacterial vaginosis is due to a decrease of *Lactobacillus* in the vaginal flora, and douching could further decrease the *Lactobacillus*. Doxycycline 100 mg twice daily for 2 weeks would be indicated treatment for pelvic inflammatory disease, which would present with a purulent vaginal discharge and pelvic or abdominal pain. While it is normal to have a vaginal discharge at the time of ovulation, or mid-cycle of menses, the discharge is usually sticky and clear, not milky white.

14. C) Polymerase chain reaction (PCR) test for *Treponema pallidum*

Syphilis can present as a painful or painless lesion, with bilateral lymphadenopathy. PCR testing of discharge directly from the lesion is considered the definitive method to diagnose early syphilis. RPR testing is nonspecific and can result in false-positive results. It would be better to perform the PCR testing on the lesion discharge. Urinalysis with reflex to culture and sensitivity would be indicated if the patient had urinary symptoms consistent with urethritis. NAAT is indicated for testing vaginal or penile discharge for chlamydia or gonorrhea.

15. A) Creatine kinase STAT

The patient has other potential reasons for the dark urine and acute kidney injury. To confirm the diagnosis of rhabdomyolysis, a creatine kinase level greater than 1,000 U/L or at least five times the upper limit of normal is needed. Prompt crystalloid resuscitation is the mainstay of therapy for rhabdomyolysis.

16. A) 10 units of regular insulin IV and 50 mL of 50% of dextrose intravenous (IV) STAT

The patient requires an immediate intervention to reduce the serum potassium level due to hyperkalemia with associated EKG changes. The best option for a patient with ESRD would be insulin and dextrose IV administration. While albuterol can reduce potassium, in 20% of ESRD this method is not effective and thus should not be administered as solitary therapy.

17. B) Urinary tract injury

The patient is presenting with reported abdominal/chest trauma with associated ecchymoses on the side of the trauma with gross hematuria. Renal and genitourinary injury must be suspected.

18. A) Contrast-induced nephropathy

The patient had a greater than 1.5 times baseline increase in creatine within 7 days of contrast exposure. Kidney stones can cause acute increase in serum creatinine, but there is nothing in this case to suggest such a diagnosis. The patient was ruled out for a pulmonary embolism on admission, and no information is provided to suspect worsening hypoxia or hypotension. While medications can cause increases in serum creatinine, there is no mention of the patient taking medication.

19. A patient with a past medical history of end-stage renal disease presents from their dialysis appointment with altered mental status. Transport reports that the patient did not receive dialysis today, and the family reports that the patient missed an appointment earlier this week. The patient is noted to have peaked T waves and a wide QRS complex across all leads on the electrocardiogram (EKG). What does the AGACNP suspect is causing these EKG changes?

    A. Hypokalemia
    B. Hyperkalemia
    C. Hypercalcemia
    D. Hypermagnesemia

20. A patient with a past medical history of end-stage renal disease presents from their dialysis appointment with altered mental status and hypotension. Transport reports that the patient did not receive dialysis today, and the family reports that the patient missed an appointment earlier this week. The patient is noted to have peaked T waves across all leads and a serum potassium of 7.2 What is the next best order the AGACNP can place?

    A. Lasix (furosemide) 20 mg intravenously (IV) STAT
    B. Nephrology consult for emergent dialysis
    C. Kayexalate (sodium polystyrene) 15 g PO STAT
    D. Low-potassium diet

(See answers next page.)

19. B) Hyperkalemia

The patient has presented with hyperkalemia based on the EKG findings and known history of end-stage renal disease with recent missed dialysis sessions. The other electrolyte abnormalities can increase chances of arrythmia, but the pattern of diffuse peaked T waves and widening QRS is concerning for hyperkalemia.

20. B) Nephrology consult for emergent dialysis

The patient has presented with symptomatic hyperkalemia based on the electrocardiogram findings, serum potassium, and known history of end-stage renal disease with recent missed dialysis sessions. The patient is symptomatic given the alteration in mental status and hypotension. The patient requires emergent dialysis to correct the hyperkalemia. Lasix is unlikely to work with end-stage renal disease, PO Kayexalate will not work quickly enough, and the patient has an altered mental status. Diet restrictions do not help in the acute phase of symptomatic hyperkalemia.

KEY BIBLIOGRAPHY

Only key resources appear in the print edition. Access the full bibliography for this chapter on ExamPrepConnect.com.

Bargman, J. M., & Skorecki, K. (2022). Chronic kidney disease. In J. Loscalzo, A. Fauci, D. Kasper, S. Hauser, D. Longo, & J. L. Jameson (Eds.), *Harrison's principles of internal medicine* (21st ed.). McGraw Hill Education

Kidney Disease Improving Global Outcome. (2016). *KDIGO guidelines*. https://kdigo.org/guidelines/

Lam, A. Q., & Seifter, J. L. (2017). Assessment and management of patients with renal disease. In S. C. McKean, J. J. Ross, D. D. Dressler, & D. B. Scheurer (Eds.), *Principles and practice of hospital medicine* (2nd ed.). McGraw-Hill Education.

Mehran, R., Dangas, G. D., & Weisbord, S. D. (2019). Contrast-associated acute kidney injury. *New England Journal of Medicine*, *380*(22), 2146–2155. https://doi.org/10.1056/NEJMra1805256

Waikar, S. S., & Bonventre, J. V. (2022). Acute kidney injury. In J. Loscalzo, A. Fauci, D. Kasper, S. Hauser, D. Longo, & J. L. Jameson (Eds.), *Harrison's principles of internal medicine* (21st ed.). McGraw Hill Education.

Hematology, Oncology, and Immunology Review

Jean Boucher and Kimberly J. Langer

▶ INTRODUCTION

Hematology, oncology, and immunology is a broad and scoping topic that the AGACNP must be well versed in to be a safe entry-level practitioner. These conditions can be either acute or chronic and can range from mild anemia to life-threatening conditions and complications. Failure to diagnose oncologic crises can lead to death. Thus, the AGACNP must be astute in diagnosing these life-threatening conditions.

▶ ANEMIA

DISEASE OVERVIEW

Anemia is defined as a lowering of the hemoglobin (Hgb) blood level. The hematocrit (HCT) and/or red blood cells (RBCs) are also reduced, but Hgb measurement is considered to be a more accurate test for determining anemia (Table 13.1).

Causes of anemia include three major categories: bone marrow failure, hemorrhage, and shortened RBC survival (Table 13.2). Additional workup for anemia should be based on clinical signs and symptoms.

Table 13.1 Glossary of Anemia-Related Tests

Test	Results	
Hemoglobin (Hgb)	WHO: For men, Hgb less than 13 For women, Hgb less than 12	NCI: Mild: 10–11 Moderate: 8–10 Severe: less than 8 Life-threatening: less than 6.5
Reticulocyte (retic) count Normal corrected retic count: 0.5%–2.5% Corrected retic count: Reticulocyte count × HCT count Normal HCT count	Measures immature RBCs in bone marrow response as either: low production versus destruction or blood loss: ■ *Low* (RBC production problem—marrow dysfunction or lack of EPO stimulus) ■ *High* (RBC destruction from hemolysis, prosthetic heart valve, spherocytosis, drugs, or blood loss problem)	
RDW Normal: approximately 13.5%	Measures homogeneity of the red cell population ■ Elevated in iron, folate, and vitamin B_{12} deficiency ■ RDW is normal with thalassemia	
Ferritin	Measures iron (Fe) storage	
Transferrin	Measures plasma iron (Fe) transport	
Iron	Measure plasma iron levels (normal range 60–150 mcg/dL)	
TIBC Reflects transferrin saturation by iron, 33%	A combined measure of serum-free iron and iron bound to transferrin reflects iron storage	

(continued)

Table 13.1 Glossary of Anemia-Related Tests (*continued*)

Test	Results
Folate or folic acid	Measures vitamin B$_9$ required for normal growth including production of RBCs, WBCs, and platelets Drugs that decrease folate: alcohol, amino-salicylic acid, birth control pills, estrogens, tetracyclines, ampicillin, chloramphenicol, erythromycin, methotrexate, penicillin, aminopterin, phenobarbital, phenytoin, drugs to treat malaria
Vitamin B$_{12}$	Significant in the synthesis of DNA and red blood cells. not produced by human body. Vitamin B$_{12}$ is stored in liver. Vitamin B$_{12}$ deficiency can be due to: ■ Poor nutrition ■ Atrophic gastritis ■ Pernicious anemia, hard for body to absorb vitamin B$_{12}$ ■ Conditions that affect small intestines: Crohn disease, celiac disease, bacterial growth, or parasites ■ Alcohol ■ Immune system disorder: Graves disease or lupus ■ Certain medications: PPIs, H$_2$ blockers, metformin
Iron studies: serum iron, TIBC, ferritin level	Iron studies: ■ Falsely elevated when taking iron or when vitamin B$_{12}$ or folate deficient ■ Falsely low during erythropoiesis (placed on vitamin B$_{12}$ or folate)
ESR: 0–22 mm/hr for men 0–29 mm/hr for women	Measures inflammation, infection, or injury May increase or decrease (sickle cell) with anemia Note: elevates with infection, pregnancy, malignancies, collagen vascular diseases, rheumatic heart disease, and other chronic disease states (e.g., HIV)
Lactate dehydrogenase Bilirubin Haptoglobin	Elevated with hemolytic anemias

EPO, erythropoietin; ESR, erythrocyte sedimentation rate; H$_2$ blockers, histamine H$_2$ receptor antagonist; HCT, hematocrit; Hgb, hemoglobin; NCI, National Cancer Institute; PPIs, proton pump inhibitors; RBC, red blood cell; RDW, red cell distribution width; TIBC, total iron-binding capacity; WHO, World Health Organization.

Table 13.2 Major Causes of Anemia

Bone Marrow Failure (Can Be Microcytic, Normocytic, Macrocytic)	Hemorrhage (Usually Normocytic)	Shortened RBC Survival
■ Low RBC dysfunction ■ Low WBC, low platelets ■ Lack of EPO stimulus (renal disease) ■ Low reticulocyte count ■ RBC destruction/hemolysis ■ Reticulocyte count low due to certain drugs with induced bone marrow suppression ■ Calcium channel blockers, theophylline, angiotensin-converting enzyme inhibitors, angiotensin-receptor blockers, beta-adrenergic blockers *Acquired disorders:* ■ Aplastic anemia, paroxysmal nocturnal hemoglobinuria ■ Leukemias, diseases such as cancer with bone marrow infiltration *Inherited disorder:* Fanconi anemia, dyskeratosis congenital	■ Loss of RBCs can be seen ■ Increased reticulocytes *Acute loss:* abrupt drop in RBCs *Causes:* arterial damage, aneurysm bleed, gastrointestinal bleeding, surgery, trauma, menstruation, pregnancy, postpartum bleeding. Hematology and oncology malignancies may also cause acute hemorrhage. Classification of hemorrhagic shock: Class I (less than 15% blood loss) Class II (15%–30% blood loss) Class III (30%–40% blood loss) Class IV (40% blood loss)	■ Inability of kidneys to secrete EPO such as with CKD ■ Hemolysis: intracorpuscular (within RBC defect) versus extracorpuscular (external to the RBC) RBC destruction (e.g., malaria) ■ Excessive RBC loss from bacterial, parasitic, viral infections ■ Insufficient RBCs: Nutrition-related causes of vitamin B$_{12}$, folic acid, and/or iron deficiency

CKD, chronic kidney disease; EPO, erythropoietin; RBC, red blood cell; WBC, white blood count.

DIAGNOSTIC CRITERIA
SYMPTOMS

- *General:* fatigue, exercise intolerance
- *Central nervous system (CNS):* dizziness, headache (H/A), irritability, insomnia, difficulty concentrating
- *Cardiovascular (C/V):* tachycardia, palpitations; systolic ejection murmur, S_3 when severe
- *Pulmonary:* dyspnea on exertion, shortness of breath at rest
- *Gastrointestinal (GI)/genitourinary (GU):* anorexia, indigestion, menstrual problems, impotence
- *Skin:* pallor, hypersensitivity to cold, creases lighter in color in hands
- *Associated symptoms:* koilonychia (spoon nails: iron deficiency); jaundice (hemolytic or megaloblastic anemias); leg ulcers (sickle cell and hemolytic anemias); bone deformities (thalassemia major and severe congenital hemolytic anemias); spontaneous bruising and excess infections indicating thrombocytopenia, neutropenia, and possible bone marrow failure; retinal hemorrhages (rare and found in severe anemia)
- *Acute bleeding signs:* flank ecchymosis (Grey Turner sign) suggesting retroperitoneal hemorrhage; umbilical ecchymosis (Cullen sign) suggestive of intraperitoneal or retroperitoneal bleeding

DIAGNOSTIC WORKUP

The initial steps to evaluate anemia include obtaining a complete blood count (CBC) with differential including peripheral blood smear (PBS) to help determine type of anemia and reticulocyte count.

- *PBS with RBC indices:* the most important element to obtain. Evaluate the PBS for appearance; normal RBCs are flexible, concave disks, whereas abnormally shaped RBCs are elliptocytes, spherocytes, schistocytes, or sickle cells.
- *Reticulocyte count:* normal 0.5% to 2.5%; reflects bone marrow response to make RBCs. It is an important value to determine bone marrow failure:
  - Low = underproduction/bone marrow dysfunction or lack of erythropoietin (EPO)
  - High = destruction or blood loss

LABORATORY ASSESSMENT

- *RBC:* indices include mean corpuscular volume (MCV), mean corpuscular Hgb (MCH), MCH concentration (MCHC), and red cell distribution width (RDW)
- Hgb less than 13 g/dL, HCT less than 40% for male patients; Hgb less than 12 g/dL and HCT less than 36% for female patients
  - RBC size and Hgb content via MCV, MCH, and MCHC
- *RDW:* measures size and volume of RBC
- *MCV:* microcytic, normocytic, or macrocytic reflecting RBC production
- *Other associated labs:* lactate dehydrogenase (LDH), blood urea nitrogen (BUN)/creatinine, EPO level, vitamin B_{12}, folate, iron, ferritin, transferrin level

ANEMIA CLASSIFICATIONS

Microcytic anemia is classified as an MCV less than 80; normocytic anemia has an MCV of 80 to 100, and macrocytic anemia has an MCV greater than 100 (Tables 13.3 and 13.4).

Table 13.3 Microcytic/Normocytic Anemia Causes

Iron Deficiency (Can Be Normocytic)	Acute Bleed, Splenomegaly	Sideroblastic Anemia, Lead Poisoning, Thalassemia
Causes: GI bleed Menstruation for premenopausal patients Decreased iron intake or lack of absorption (e.g., celiac disease) Other causes: TB, blood donation, pregnancy, coagulopathies	*Diagnostic findings:* ▪ MCV less than 80 ▪ High reticulocyte count ▪ High LDH, bilirubin: evaluate for hemolysis ▪ Low EPO production: kidney damage or disease, thyroid metabolism, hyperviscosity	*Diagnostic findings:* ▪ MCV less than 80 Check medication history, INH, ETOH; inflammatory or chronic disease to *sideroblastic anemia*, check bone marrow biopsy for ringed sideroblasts or iron granules

(continued)

Table 13.3 Microcytic/Normocytic Anemia Causes (*continued*)

Iron Deficiency (Can Be Normocytic)	Acute Bleed, Splenomegaly	Sideroblastic Anemia, Lead Poisoning, Thalassemia
Medications: antacids, H$_2$ blockers, proton pump inhibitors, tetracyclines *Diagnostic findings:* ■ Low reticulocyte count; MCV less than 80 (not common) or MCV normocytic ■ Low RBC, iron, transferrin ■ Decreased ferritin (happens first) ■ Increased TIBC	*Anemia of chronic disease* (can be normocytic): Hgb less than 10 g/dL ■ Low retic count, iron, RBC, transferrin, and low TIBC ■ Increased ferritin ■ Check diet, UGI, barium enema, hemoccult to rule out GI bleed; if negative, then colonoscopy to rule out cancer	*Thalassemia minor:* Low MCV, increased RBC; PBS with target cells, basophilic stripping; osmotic fragility, *check Hgb electrophoresis* to evaluate for beta-thalassemia versus alpha-thalassemia ■ Normal TIBC ■ Increased iron, transferrin, ferritin *Lead poisoning:* ■ Hypochromic, red cell stippling, MCV lower ■ Heme synthesis disorder ■ Can mimic a form of porphyria ■ Check for mild hemolysis, can be normocytic, blood cell stippling on smear, sideroblastic rings, blood/urine lead levels ■ May see porphyria precursors in blood tests

EPO, erythropoietin; ETOH, ethyl alcohol; GI, gastrointestinal; INH, Isoniazid; LDH, lactate dehydrogenase; MCV, mean corpuscular volume; PBS, peripheral blood smear; RBC, red blood cell; TB, tuberculosis; TIBC, total iron-binding capacity; UGI, upper gastrointestinal.

Table 13.4 Macrocytic Anemias Subtypes

Megaloblastic (MCV greater than 100, low retic count)	*Vitamin B$_{12}$ deficiency:* Causes: dietary restrictions (vegetarians), impaired absorption (gastrectomy, bariatric surgery), Crohn disease, Zollinger–Ellison syndrome Medications (protein pump inhibitors, antacids, H$_2$ receptor antagonists, metformin) Diagnostic findings: ■ Marked decreased serum B$_{12}$ ■ Increased serum iron, LDH ■ Normal or increased serum folic acid (folate) ■ Methylmalonic acid and homocysteine may be elevated ■ Diagnosis: Schilling test *Pernicious anemia:* Causes: lack of intrinsic factor with inability to absorb vitamin B$_{12}$ Found in with bowel surgery, bacterial overgrowth Diagnostic findings: ■ Schilling test *Folate deficiency:* Causes/risks: ETOH, sprue, poor diet, hemodialysis, TPN, older age, premature infants, pregnancy, Crohn disease. Medications (methotrexate, trimethoprim, phenytoin) Diagnostic findings: ■ Assess for hypothyroidism: check thyroid function tests ■ Confirmatory test: homocysteine ■ Primary marrow disorders: bone marrow biopsy to evaluate for myelodysplastic syndrome, aplastic anemia ■ Peripheral blood smear: revealing big think red cells
Non-megaloblastic (MCV greater than 100, low retic count)	Causes: medications, hypothyroidism, liver disease, alcohol Vitamin B$_{12}$, folate, and hypothyroidism can be normocytic Evaluate for mixed deficiency state: iron and vitamin B$_{12}$ deficiency

ETOH, ethyl alcohol; LDH, lactate dehydrogenase; MCV, mean corpuscular volume; TPN, total parenteral nutrition.

MICROCYTIC ANEMIA

Pathogenesis includes iron metabolism disorders due to:

- heme synthesis defect, including iron deficiency
- anemia of chronic disorders
- globin synthesis defects such as alpha- and beta-thalassemias, hemoglobin E syndromes (AE, EE, E-beta-thalassemia), hemoglobin C syndromes, and unstable Hgb disease
- sideroblastic anemias (e.g., hereditary sideroblastic anemia: X-linked or autosomal)
- acquired: refractory anemia with ringed sideroblasts, sickle cell disease
- malignancies: myeloproliferative disorders, reversible acquired sideroblastic anemia (alcoholism)

Classic Presentation: Microcytic/Normocytic Anemia

A 72-year-old patient presents with complaints of fatigue, dyspnea on exertion, and anorexia. The patient also endorses the feeling of a racing heartbeat, and family have commented that the patient's complexion appears paler than normal. CBC reveals Hgb 8.8, HCT 28%.

MACROCYTIC ANEMIAS

MCV greater than 100; macrocytic anemia can further be delineated into megaloblastic and non-megaloblastic.

Classic Presentation: Macrocytic Anemia

A 74-year-old patient presents with loss of appetite, fatigue, and reports of poor concentration. Blood work reveals RBC 2.9, reticulocyte count low, transferrin low, RDW 15% (high), ferritin 10 (low), B_{12} 250 (normal), folate 200 (normal), iron 28 (low), LDH 148, total iron-binding capacity (TIBC) 455 (high), creatinine 1.2, EPO level normal.

TREATMENT/MANAGEMENT: TRANSFUSION CRITERIA

The patient's underlying condition guides transfusion criteria (Table 13.5). Acute coronary syndrome (e.g., elevated troponins, active chest pain) requires a Hgb greater than 8.0 g/dL. Hemodynamically unstable patients (e.g., tachycardic, hypotensive, vasopressor use) can benefit by an Hgb level 7.0 to 8.0 g/dL, whereas most hemodynamically stable patients are safe to transfuse below 7.0 g/dL. For patients with active hemorrhage, see Chapter 19 for mass transfusion protocol. Patients with end-stage liver disease (ESLD) can have significantly elevated international normalized ratio (INR) and very low platelet counts and typically need transfusions only for planned procedures or active bleeding.

Table 13.5 Transfusion Criteria

Product	Transfusion Guidelines
Red blood cells	■ Active bleeding, symptomatic (tachycardia, hypotension, vasopressor use) or hemorrhage regardless of Hgb ■ Active ACS: Hgb less than 8.0 g/dL ■ All others: Hgb less than 7.0 g/dL
Plasma	■ Intracranial bleeding: INR greater than 1.5 ■ Active bleeding: INR greater than 1.5 ■ ESLD: only for active bleeding regardless of INR level
Platelets	■ Active bleeding, planned surgery/procedures less than 50,000 ■ Less than 10,000 given risk for spontaneous hemorrhage
Cryoprecipitate	■ Fibrinogen less than 150 mg/dL

ACS, acute coronary syndrome; ESLD, end-stage liver disease; Hgb, hemoglobin; INR, international normalized ratio.

▶ HEMOCHROMATOSIS

DISEASE OVERVIEW

Iron-overload autosomal recessive disorder in White patients involves the mutated *HFE* C282Y variant gene or can be acquired from frequent blood transfusions. The condition can cause liver failure, diabetes, heart disease, and thyroid disease.

CLASSIC PRESENTATION

A 68-year-old male patient with a past medical history of hypertension, diabetes mellitus, and chronic kidney disease (CKD) stage IIIa is admitted to the hospital service with pneumonia. On admission, his vital signs are stable. Laboratory studies include a CBC revealing white blood cells (WBCs) 8.2, Hgb 16.6, platelets 235,000, HCT 49%, and ferritin level on 1,000 ng/mL. Basic metabolic panel (BMP) shows Na 136, K 4.1, Cl 101, BUN 18, creatine 1.6, glucose 106. Creatine clearance (CrCl) is 52 mL/min/BSA.

SYMPTOMS

Symptoms of hemochromatosis include jaundice, lethargy, and abnormal heart rhythm with hepatitis and diabetes.

DIAGNOSTIC CRITERIA

Assess for elevated iron, transferrin, and ferritin levels and perform liver biopsy to confirm.

TREATMENT/MANAGEMENT

Patients with hemochromatosis require lifelong phlebotomy based on iron saturation. Proton pump inhibitors increase iron absorption and may decrease need for phlebotomy. Patients should avoid vitamin C and uncooked seafood, and obtain genetic consultation.

▶ ERYTHROCYTOSIS

DISEASE OVERVIEW

Erythrocytosis is a disorder of excessive RBCs (increased HCT). Erythrocytosis is categorized as either primary or secondary based on etiologies.

PRIMARY CAUSE

Polycythemia rubra vera caused by abnormal cell production in bone marrow is a myeloproliferative disorder. Approximately 95% have a Janus kinase 2 gene (*JAK2*) mutation as the cause for excessive production. A small percentage may develop myelofibrosis or acute leukemia.

SECONDARY CAUSES

Secondary causes include dehydration, burns, vomiting, anabolic steroids, chronic obstructive pulmonary disease (COPD), high altitudes, carbon monoxide poisoning, and tumors. Check to see if the patient is on diuretics.

DIAGNOSTIC CRITERIA
SYMPTOMS

Symptoms include headache, lightheadedness, weakness, shortness of breath, fatigue, night sweats, nose bleeds, and pruritus after bathing.

LABORATORY

- *CBC:* HCT elevated greater than 53% in male patients, 51% in female patients, + splenomegaly (primary and secondary). Monitor platelets and iron level, which may decrease.
- *Goal:* Keep HCT 42% to 47% for both primary and secondary hemochromatosis.
- *Primary cause:* Check EPO level (decreased).
- *Secondary cause:* Check HCT as earlier and EPO level (increased).
- *Secondary cause:* Evaluate smoking history and COPD history, exposure to high altitudes for prolonged periods of time, history of cardiovascular disease, severe obesity, tumor, renal disease (EPO level high); plasma volume decrease (dehydration).

TREATMENT/MANAGEMENT

Consult hematology for considerations: phlebotomy, hydroxyurea (antineoplastic), targeted therapies of *JAK2* gene kinase pathway.

COMPLICATIONS

Patients are at risk for blood clots from excessive RBCs. First presenting symptoms may be fingertip necrosis; face, hand, and foot flushing; and risk for thrombocythemia.

▶ SICKLE CELL ANEMIA

DISEASE OVERVIEW

Sickle cell disease is more common in those who have ancestors from sub-Saharan Africa, Spanish-speaking regions in the Western hemisphere, Saudi Arabia, India, or Mediterranean countries.

CLASSIC PRESENTATION

A Black patient presents to the ED with severe joint pains, dyspnea on exertion, and headache. The pain is unrelenting even after attempts to manage at home with short-acting morphine 15 to 30 mg orally every 4 hours.

DIAGNOSTIC CRITERIA

Symptoms of sickle cell disease vary between patients. Symptoms can include fatigue, headache, dizziness, joint pain, chest pain, shortness of breath, hand and foot swelling, jaundice, and leg skin ulcerations. Patients who become dehydrated or hypoxic are at increased risk for pain crisis, clots, joint necrosis, infection, and renal impairment. A PBS will show sickled erythrocytes; an Hgb electrophoresis reveals HBS.

TREATMENT/MANAGEMENT

Treatment includes maintaining hydration, pain control, and monitoring for infection, vaso-occlusive crisis, stroke, kidney or eye damage, and anemia crisis.

COMPLICATIONS

Sickle cell crisis describes several acute conditions such as vaso-occlusive crisis (acute painful crisis), aplastic crisis, splenic sequestration crisis, hyperhemolytic crisis, hepatic crisis, acute chest syndrome, and dactylitis. Other acute complications include pulmonary nodular amyloidosis, meningitis, sepsis, stroke, avascular necrosis, and venous thromboembolism (VTE). Patients can present with any of these conditions, and treatment is based on it. Early detection and rapid initiation of appropriate treatment for most of these conditions are extremely important to prevent mortality. If a patient has severe bone pain, concerns for avascular necrosis and acute osteomyelitis are suggested. If the patient has an aplastic crisis, it is treated with supportive care and simple transfusions.

▶ HEMOLYTIC ANEMIAS

DISEASE OVERVIEW

Hemolytic anemias (Table 13.6) are disorders in which RBCs are destroyed faster than they can be made.

Table 13.6 Causes of Hemolytic Anemia

Type	Etiology
Congenital	Hereditary spherocytosis; hereditary elliptocytosis
Acquired	Spurr cell anemia (cirrhosis); paroxysmal nocturnal hemoglobinuria
Drug-induced	Piperacillin, ceftriaxone, diclofenac, methyldopa, quinine, primaquine, sulfa drugs, nitrofurantoin
Clinical conditions	DIC, TTP, HUS, hypersplenism
Enzyme defects	G6PD deficiency: Check level; PBS shows bite or blister cells; PK deficiency
Hgb defects	Sickle cell; Heinz body

DIC, disseminated intravascular coagulation; HUS, hepatic uremic syndrome; PK, pyruvate kinase; TTP, thrombotic thrombocytopenia purpura.

DIAGNOSTIC CRITERIA

Check a peripheral smear for RBC parasites to evaluate for malaria and babesiosis and Coombs test to check for two types: immune-mediated (autoimmune hemolytic anemia) and microangiopathic hemolysis.

▶ PANCYTOPENIAS

DISEASE OVERVIEW

Pancytopenia is defined as low levels of WBCs (neutropenia), RBCs (anemia), and platelets (thrombocytopenia). Pancytopenia can occur for a number of reasons, including bone marrow failure/suppression (e.g., autoimmune diseases, aplastic anemia, myelodysplasia, drugs, and leukemias), nutritional (e.g., vitamin B_{12} or folate deficiency), or destruction (e.g., infection, lymphomas) from infiltration/replacement (e.g., infection, leukemias, multiple myeloma, and metastatic cancer), or inherited/congenital.

DIAGNOSTIC CRITERIA

Check CBC with differential and comprehensive metabolic panel (CMP) to assess renal and hepatic function. Uric acid will be elevated, calcium will be low, and phosphorous will be elevated. Bone marrow biopsy will be done by the hematologist. Lumbar puncture is needed for patients with WBC greater than 50,000.

▶ APLASTIC ANEMIA

DISEASE OVERVIEW

Aplastic anemia is a disease involving pancytopenia and hypocellular marrow. WBC, RBCs, and platelets are dangerously low. It is idiopathic or drug/chemical induced and requires transfusion support.

SYMPTOMS

Symptoms include fever, fatigue, dizziness, or fever, skin rash of small purplish spots, petechiae, bruising, gum or nose bleeding, shortness of breath, tachycardia, and infections.

DIAGNOSTIC CRITERIA

Workup includes bone marrow biopsy that reveals severe hypocellularity with a high risk for morbidity due to infection or bleeding. Check for hypersplenism (pancytopenia).

TREATMENT/MANAGEMENT

Treatment of aplastic anemia includes blood transfusions, immunosuppressive drugs, and allogeneic bone marrow transplant (BMT).

▶ MYELODYSPLASTIC SYNDROMES

DISEASE OVERVIEW

Syndromes include clonal hematopoiesis, cytopenias (anemia, neutropenia, and/or thrombocytopenia), and abnormal cellular maturation.

CLASSIC PRESENTATION

A 68-year-old male patient who is a Vietnam veteran reports history of exposure to Agent Orange. Physical exam reveals cracked lips, cheilosis, severe fatigue, dehydration, abnormal bruising. Hgb 15 g/dL; HCT 45%; platelet count 30; absolute reticulocyte count 89,000; MCV 78; and absolute neutrophil count (ANC) 0.5.

▶ THROMBOCYTOPENIA

DISEASE OVERVIEW

Thrombocytopenia is defined as a decrease in platelet count. The AGACNP should perform a full history and physical exam to help determine the cause. Thrombocytopenia includes production decrease, abnormal distribution, autoimmune disease, or increased destruction. In this section, categories of causes of thrombocytopenia are discussed.

INFECTION-INDUCED THROMBOCYTOPENIA

Infection-induced thrombocytopenia is a decline in platelet counts associated specifically with viral and bacterial infections. Thrombocytopenia may or may not be associated with disseminated intravascular coagulation (DIC), which is typically seen in those with more severe systemic infections in critically ill patients.

CLASSIC PRESENTATION

A 32-year-old female patient presented with 5-day history of lethargy, shortness of breath on exertion, bruising with petechiae to her extremities, and gum bleeding. She has history of recurrent urinary tract infections and has been treated recently with ciprofloxacin twice in the past 6 months. Labs show Hgb 11, RBCs 4.3, with a critical value platelet count of 15,000. Prothrombin time (PT), partial PT (PTT), and D-dimer are normal. Urinalysis is normal.

DIAGNOSTIC CRITERIA

History and physical exam should explicitly assess for infectious processes and workup including assessment for infection or reactivation of viral processes. Test for cytomegalovirus (CMV), Epstein-Barr virus, and gram-negative/-positive infections, which can be associated with thrombocytopenia due to their ability to affect both platelet production and platelet consumption.

TREATMENT/MANAGEMENT

Treatment should focus on treating the underlying infection and transfuse as the clinical condition warrants.

DRUG-INDUCED THROMBOCYTOPENIA

Many medications, including chemotherapy agents, can cause a decline in platelet counts. For example, within a week after receiving myelosuppressive chemotherapy, there can be a notable decline in platelet count (Table 13.7).

Table 13.7 Drugs That Can Cause or Have a High Probability to Cause Thrombocytopenia

Acetaminophen	Diazepam	Piperacillin
Amiodarone	Eptifibatide	Quinine
Amlodipine	Furosemide	Quinidine
Ampicillin	Haloperidol	Ranitidine
Carbamazepine	Heparin	Rosiglitazone
Ceftriaxone	Ibuprofen	Roxifiban
Cephamandole	Lorazepam	Sulfsoxazole
Ciprofloxacin	Mirtazapine	Suramin
Diazepam	Naproxen	Tirofiban
Eptifibatide	Oxaliplatin	Tranilast
Furosemide	Penicillin	Trimethoprim/Sulfamethoxazole
Gold	Phenytoin	Vancomycin

TREATMENT/MANAGEMENT

If a patient has notable thrombocytopenia after starting one of these medications, stop the agent, if possible.

▶ IMMUNE-MEDIATED THROMBOCYTOPENIC PURPURA OR IDIOPATHIC THROMBOCYTOPENIC PURPURA

DISEASE OVERVIEW

This is an immune-mediated disorder with destruction of platelets, with inhibition of platelet release causing thrombocytopenia.

DIAGNOSTIC CRITERIA

Idiopathic thrombocytopenic purpura (ITP) can present with bleeding of the mucosa, low platelet counts with a normal peripheral smear, and ecchymosis and/or petechiae; rarely, retinal hemorrhage or wet purpura can occur. Workup for ITP includes CBC and peripheral smear (which may show large platelets); secondary testing to look for other causes of ITP includes testing for HIV, hepatitis C, and other infections. A bone marrow biopsy can be reserved for patients who may show signs/symptoms of other disease processes in addition to ITP.

TREATMENT/MANAGEMENT

In patients without significant bleeding or severe thrombocytopenia, ITP can be managed in the outpatient setting and can include steroid therapy such as prednisone (1 mg/kg) with subsequent taper, pending the result to therapy. Administration of intravenous (IV) gamma globulin can be added as a secondary treatment option in a total dose of 1 to 2 g/kg total given over 1 to 5 days. Note that severe thrombocytopenia (platelets <less than 5,000/mcL) may warrant admission.

- *Refractory ITP:* Rituximab, a CD20 antibody, has been shown to provide long-lasting remission in about 30% of patients.
- *Relapse:* Splenectomy could be considered for those who relapse with ITP after treatment with steroids, but only after all other treatment options have been exhausted.

▶ THROMBOSIS

Thrombosis can occur due to coagulopathies, venous thrombosis embolism, and thrombophilia (Table 13.8).

Table 13.8 Causes of Thrombosis

Cause	As a Result of/Example
Endothelial damage	Shock states Hypoxia ARDS Cardiopulmonary arrest MI Cancer Obstetrics
Factor X activation	Pancreatitis Venom Liver disease

ARDS, acute respiratory distress syndrome; MI, myocardial infarction.

▶ DISSEMINATED INTRAVASCULAR COAGULATION

DISEASE OVERVIEW

Diffuse coagulation occurs simultaneously as fibrinolysis, which causes bleeding. Decreases in circulating platelets occur due to consumption in clots. Circulation of plasmin occurs, which degrades fibrin and increases fibrin degradation products (FDPs). Inhibition of platelets results in bleeding and activation of the complement and kinin systems. Finally, major organs develop thromboemboli, causing multisystem organ failure and death. Endothelial damage is a result of sepsis, hypoxia, acute respiratory distress syndrome (ARDS), cardiopulmonary arrest, release of thrombotic ITP due to trauma, myocardial infarction, cancer, obstetrics, and factor X activation resulting from pancreatitis, venom, liver disease, and miscellaneous hematologic conditions, anaphylaxis, pulmonary embolus, and necrotizing enterocolitis.

DIAGNOSTIC CRITERIA
SYMPTOMS

Symptoms include hypotension, shortness of breath, chest pain, hypoxia, acidosis, proteinuria, gangrene, renal failure, shock, bleeding, tachycardia, petechiae, and purpura; edema with increased permeability, dilation, fluid, and plasma protein shift.

LABORATORY

Laboratory tests include a positive D-dimer with other laboratory tests: CBC, PT, PTT, FDP, protein C and protein S, bleeding time, factor assay, and fibrinogen.

TREATMENT/MANAGEMENT

Treatment should focus on treating the underlying cause of the DIC. Second, restoration of hemostasis should be accomplished with transfusions if bleeding (fresh frozen plasma, platelets, and packed RBCs and cryoprecipitate). Additionally, organ function should be maintained with fluid resuscitation vasopressors. Heparin should be considered cautiously for extensive fibrin deposition or thrombosis without evidence of substantial hemorrhage.

▶ HYPERCOAGULABLE STATES

VENOUS THROMBOEMBOLISM

Includes deep vein thrombosis (DVT) and pulmonary embolism (PE; see Chapter 10). Thrombophilia disorders can result in DVT or PE, such as:

▪ antithrombin III deficiency: can be caused by *SERPINC1* gene mutation
▪ protein C deficiency (type I: inadequate amount, type II: defective molecules)
▪ protein S deficiency (free and bound): type I: inadequate amount; type II: defective molecules; type III: low amount of free only
▪ factor V Leiden: most common hereditary blood coagulation disorder in the United States. Increased risk of venous thrombosis (three- to eight-fold) occurs for heterozygous individuals (one damaged gene inherited). The risk increases substantially more (30- to 140-fold) for homozygous (two damaged genes inherited) individuals, increasing their risk for DVT, PE, stroke, and transient ischemic attacks.

▶ HEPARIN-INDUCED THROMBOCYTOPENIA

DISEASE OVERVIEW

Heparin-induced thrombocytopenia (HIT) is most common in surgical or trauma patients with greater than 5 days' use of heparin resulting in an antibody reaction. Patients may develop venous or arterial VTE that can result in loss of digits or limbs, necrosis of skin at injection sites, organ failure, and death. Diagnosis should be based on a pretest probability with the 4T model (Table 13.9) followed by HIT antibody testing when indicated.

Table 13.9 4T Model to Diagnose HIT

4T's	Points
Thrombocytopenia	▪ 2 – platelet count fall ≥50%, and platelet nadir greater than 20×10^9/L ▪ 1 – platelet count fall 30%–50%, and platelet nadir greater than 10×10^9/L ▪ 0 – platelet count fall less than 300%, and platelet nadir less than 10×10^9/L
Timing (of platelet decrease)	▪ 2 – clear onset between 5 and 10 days or platelet fall ≤1 day (prior heparin exposure within 30 days) ▪ 1 – consistent with fall days 5–10 but not clear; onset after 10 days, or fall ≤1 day (prior heparin exposure 30–100 days ago) ▪ 0 – platelet count fall less than 4 days without recent exposure
Thrombosis	▪ 2 – new thrombosis (confirmed); skin necrosis; acute systemic reaction after IV unfractionated heparin bolus ▪ 1 – progressive or recurrent thrombosis; nonnecrotizing (erythematous skin lesions; suspected thrombosis (not proven) ▪ 0 – none

(continued)

Table 13.9 4T Model to Diagnose HIT (*continued*)

4T's	Points
Other (causes for thrombocytopenia)	■ 2 – no apparent cause for thrombocytopenia ■ 1 – possible other causes for thrombocytopenia ■ 0 – definite other causes for thrombocytopenia
Interpretation: Score 0–3: low pretest probability; 4–5: intermediate pretest probability; 6–8: high pretest probability for HIT.	

HIT, heparin-induced thrombocytopenia; IV, intravenous.

TREATMENT/MANAGEMENT

If HIT is suspected, stop all heparin products (unfractionated heparin and enoxaparin) and change to nonheparin anticoagulation such as lepirudin, argatroban, danaparoid, bivalirudin, or fondaparinux.

▶ COAGULOPATHY

- Hemophilia is an inherited bleeding disorder involving factor VIII (hemophilia A or classic hemophilia) or factor IX (hemophilia B or Christmas hemophilia), where spontaneous bleeding can occur in the mouth, gums, nose, joints, skin regions, urine/stool, or head. Treatment is prevention. If patient is bleeding, transfuse missing clotting factor.
- Von Willebrand disease is an inherited autosomal dominant trait with risk of bleeding. Check bleeding time, PT/PTT, von Willebrand factor, factor VIII activity, and fibrinogen. Can be acquired due to other diseases.

▶ HEMATOLOGIC AND SOLID TUMORS

SOLID TUMOR OVERVIEW

In 2022, 1.9 million new cases of cancer were diagnosed, with lung cancer as the leading cause of death in men and women (21%), followed by prostate (11%) and colorectal (9%) cancers for men, and breast (15%) and colorectal (8%) cancers for women. Prostate cancer is the most common cancer among men (27%), followed by lung (12%) and colorectal (8%) cancers. Among women, breast (31%), lung (13%), and colorectal (8%) cancers are the most common.

CANCER CLASSIFICATION

- *Epithelial tissue:* adeno or squamous cell
- *Connective tissue:* bone (osteo), chondro (cartilage), lipo (fat), rhabdo (skeletal muscle), leiomyo (smooth muscle) sarcomas
- *Hematologic cell origin:* lymphocytes (B- or T-cell lymphomas), myeloid or lymphocytic leukemias, plasma proteins (multiple myeloma)
- *Location:* ductal, infiltrating, or inflammatory breast cancer

Staging describes the TNM system:

- *Tumor:* size and local extent
- *Node:* lymph node number
- *Metastases:* sites of spread to other tissues (bone, brain, liver, and lung)

Grading is a classification of stage of cancer and ranges from 1 to 4 or A to D or well to poor differentiation and is achieved via biopsy (histology) and cytology.

DIAGNOSTIC CRITERIA

SYMPTOMS

Patients may have unintentional weight loss (cachexia), bloating, fatigue, pain, fever, diaphoresis, shortness of breath, anemia, leukopenia, thrombocytopenia, constipation, urine retention, or frequency.

WORKUP
- Screening tests: x-rays of chest and kidney–ureter–bladder, CT scan, ultrasound, and MRI
- Lab tests such as CBC/differential, chemistry panel, serum immunoglobulins (Ig), and urinalysis
- Tumor-specific antigen markers such as CEA, CA-125, PSA, AFPRO, and HCG
- Biopsy/cytology
- PET, bone scan bronchoscopy, upper/lower endoscopy or colonoscopy, endoscopic retrograde cholangiopancreatography

TREATMENT/MANAGEMENT
Treatment is based on the type of cancer, extent of spread, and whether the intent is cure, control, or palliative. Treatment can include chemotherapy, radiation, surgery, immunotherapy with CAR-T cells, monoclonal antibodies, or targeted therapies such as vascular endothelial growth factors, epidermal growth factor receptors, multi-kinase, and/or mammalian target of rapamycin (mTOR) inhibitors.

CHEMOTHERAPY
Chemotherapy affects both cancer cells and normal cells. Risks include immunosuppression predisposing to infection and/or bleeding and anemia. Side effects requiring symptom management include pain, nausea/vomiting, anorexia, cachexia, mucositis, esophagitis, gum bleeding, thrush, fatigue, loss of concentration, changes in appearance/body image, alopecia, gastroesophageal reflux disease, diarrhea or constipation, cystitis, hematuria, and electrolyte imbalances.

RADIATION THERAPY
Radiation therapy can include external beam, brachytherapy, and implanted seeds. Side effects include risk for immunosuppression, anorexia, fatigue, skin changes, cachexia, and effects on certain organs depending on site: oropharynx (mucositis, dysphagia, dry mouth); esophagus (esophagitis, fungal infection); bladder (cystitis, hematuria); bowel (diarrhea/colitis); and lung (pneumonitis, dyspnea).

SURGERY
Resection of tumor for cure or palliation is done in conjunction with chemotherapy or radiation. Implantation of devices such as ports and hepatic pumps can be used to administer chemotherapy. Side effects and complications include bleeding, infection, wound dehiscence, edema, anorexia, and mucositis.

IMMUNOTHERAPY
Immunotherapies are targeted to stimulate the immune system. Immunotherapies are available to treat non–small-cell lung cancer, bladder cancer, melanoma, renal cell carcinoma, Hodgkin lymphoma, and squamous cell carcinoma of the head and neck. B cells are lymphocytes that stimulate plasma cells to produce antibodies (immunoglobin (Ig) G, IgA, IgM, IgE, IgD; humoral immunity). T cells are lymphocytes that recognize antigens and attack them (cell-mediated immunity). Types of immunotherapies include the following:

- Interferon and interleukin are used to treat melanoma and renal cancers; they can cause severe flu-like symptoms.
- Monoclonal antibodies can be used (e.g., Rituximab is used with lymphomas).
- Immune checkpoint inhibitors are drugs that block checkpoint proteins such as CTLA-4, PD-1, or PD-L1, preventing them from binding with their partner proteins.
- CAR-T cell therapy involves T cells treated with chimeric antigen receptor (CAR) proteins that are given back to patients to attack cancer cells.
  - Side effects include monitoring for cytokine release syndrome (CRS), in which a large number of cytokines is released into the blood, causing systemic inflammatory response. Signs and symptoms of CRS mimic sepsis and septic shock: fatigue, fever, nausea, headache, tachycardia, hypotension, and shortness of breath. Other side effects are rash, pruritus, diarrhea (colitis), hepatitis, endocrinopathies, loss of appetite, neurotoxicity, pancreatitis, pneumonitis, and hematologic toxicity.

▶ HEMATOLOGIC OVERVIEW

LEUKEMIA

Leukemia is a type of blood cancer in which there is rapid production of abnormal WBCs that are unable to fight infection. Overproduction of these cells causes crowding in the bone marrow, leading to a decrease in platelet and Hgb production. Leukemia can also be found in extramedullary tissues with poorly differentiated cells of the hematopoietic stem cell system. Leukemias can be differentiated as acute or chronic, myeloid or lymphoid. Commonly, there are four types of leukemia: acute myeloid leukemia, acute lymphoid leukemia, chronic myeloid leukemia, and chronic lymphoid leukemia.

CLASSIC PRESENTATION

A patient presents due to increased bruising, bleeding of the gums, and ongoing upper respiratory symptoms unrelieved by antibiotic therapy. Routine blood work with a CBC reveals WBC 65, Hgb 6.5, and platelets 19,000. Chemistries are normal.

SYMPTOMS

Patients can present with a multitude of symptoms or can be completely asymptomatic. Symptoms can include fatigue, anorexia, weight loss, abnormal bleeding, cough, lymphadenopathy, or headache. On physical exam, patients may present with fever, bleeding, splenomegaly, hepatomegaly, and/or lymphadenopathy.

DIAGNOSTIC CRITERIA

Diagnostic tests include CBC with differential, CMP, peripheral smear, and lactate dehydrogenase. Pending the extent of the WBC, patients may undergo a bone marrow biopsy with aspirate, which is reviewed by a pathologist to confirm the diagnosis; cytogenetic testing and molecular testing can also be performed to determine if there are molecular markers. Patients with concern or confirmed leukemia will be referred to Hematology. Leukapheresis may be warranted to reduce the WBC burden.

TREATMENT/MANAGEMENT

Treatment varies depending on the confirmed diagnosis, extent of disease, and patient condition. Common pathways for treatment of leukemia include induction chemotherapy followed by maintenance chemotherapy. Most types of leukemia warrant BMT as the best chance for ongoing remission.

▶ LYMPHOMA OVERVIEW

Lymphomas are a type of cancer of the lymphatic system and can include the lymph nodes, spleen, thymus gland, and bone marrow. There are many different types of lymphoma. The two most common classes are non-Hodgkin lymphoma (NHL) and Hodgkin lymphoma. NHL affects mature B, T, and natural killer (NK) cells. Hodgkin lymphoma has the distinct presence of Reed–Sternberg cells and has different biologic characteristics than NHL. The subclasses associated with NHL are more associated with relapse and/or higher mortality rate. Each type of lymphoma has its own subset of characteristics; thus, a thorough workup with general and specialized testing is warranted.

CLASSIC PRESENTATION

A 41-year-old male patient is admitted for vague symptoms, including a 15-lb weight loss in the past 4 months, significant pruritis, and night sweats with fever. On physical exam, cervical and axillary lymphadenopathy are present bilaterally. Routine blood work, including CBC and CMP, is unremarkable.

SYMPTOMS

Patients may be asymptomatic, and the disease is found during a routine workup. It is prudent to obtain a complete history and physical exam to determine the onset of symptoms to determine the severity or how aggressive the disease is. Some patients may develop what is referred to as "B symptoms" associated with lymphoma, which consist of fever, night sweats, and unexplained weight loss. On physical exam, patients may have rash or areas of erythema/lesions due to scratching from pruritis and may appear fatigued. Weight loss and lymphadenopathy may be present, more so in the cervical nodes, axillary nodes, inguinal nodes, and submandibular nodes, although all lymph nodes should be assessed.

DIAGNOSTIC CRITERIA

CBC, CMP, serum protein electrophoresis, lactate dehydrogenase, bone marrow biopsy, PET/CT or basic CT scan, and possible cerebral spinal fluid analysis may be used. A basic CT scan may be ordered initially; a PET/CT scan helps determine the level of aggressiveness of the disease.

TREATMENT/MANAGEMENT

Treatment includes chemotherapy, which can be targeted based on the specific type of disease. Based on response to the chemotherapy, some patients may proceed to a stem cell transplant for the best chance at ongoing remission. If the disease is refractory to the chemotherapy, alternative chemotherapy regimens would need to be considered. Allogeneic stem cell transplant and CAR-T therapy are additional lines of therapy that can be considered as well.

▶ MULTIPLE MYELOMA OVERVIEW

Multiple myeloma is a malignancy of the plasma cells for which the cause is unknown. Multiple myeloma is a plasma cell proliferative disorder that can lead to a multitude of organ dysfunctions including bone pain or fracture, acute renal failure, anemia, hypercalcemia, thrombosis (or abnormal clotting), hyperviscosity, and possibly infection. The cause of multiple myeloma is unknown, although literature has shown an increase in frequency in those exposed to radiation, farmers, workers exposed to petroleum products, and woodworkers. Multiple myeloma is further defined or staged based on the criteria in Table 13.10.

Table 13.10 CRAB Criteria

	Symptom	Diagnostic Criteria	Management
C	Hypercalcemia	Corrected serum calcium greater than 11.5 mg/dL	Hydration and IV bisphosphonates; may require steroids and calcitonin
R	Renal insufficiency	Serum creatinine greater than 2 mg/dL	Correct hypercalcemia and possible dehydration; avoid nephrotoxic medications
A	Anemia	Hgb less than 10 g/dL or greater than 2 g/dL below the lower limit of normal range	Correct iron, folate, and vitamin B_{12} deficiency, if present; use erythropoietic agents, if symptomatic
B	Bone disease	Severe osteopenia, lytic lesions, pathologic fractures, and/or pain	Monitor; use of bisphosphonates for the prevention of skeletal-related injuries

CRAB, criteria used in the diagnosis of multiple myeloma; IV, intravenous.

A complete history and physical are crucial because many patients may be asymptomatic, or their presenting symptoms will be ongoing bone pain that is unrelieved by traditional measures including physical therapy and can lead to fractures.

CLASSIC PRESENTATION

A patient presents for a routine blood donation. Upon review of Hgb, the patient is found to be anemic with an Hgb of 8.5 g/dL. Vitamin B_{12}, ferritin, and folate levels are all within range. Later, while moving furniture, the patient feels a "pop" in the back when bending over, resulting in ongoing back pain. The patient subsequently presents due to this back pain. During that time, imaging is done that confirms multiple lytic lesions throughout.

DIAGNOSTIC CRITERIA

Diagnostic criteria include anemia, including pallor, fatigue, and shortness of breath. On physical exam, the patient may have tender bony areas and/or masses that are palpable. Persons with bone pain may present with fractures. Workup should include imaging starting with a chest x-ray that subsequently will lead to MRI for more sensitive results; PET/CT can assess for bone damage and extramedullary disease.

Routine blood work consists of CBC, CMP, M-protein, Ig levels (IgG, IgA, and IgM), 24-urine protein for protein electrophoresis and immunofixation, serum-free light chain and ratio, bone marrow biopsy,

LDH, serum monoclonal protein, serum protein electrophoresis, and fixation. A skeletal x-ray survey may also be done to assess for bone lesions.

TREATMENT/MANAGEMENT

Treatment varies if the disease is caught in the early stages, where it may be diagnosed as smoldering myeloma or monoclonal gammopathy of undetermined significance. Patients may be observed until the disease progresses. Active multiple myeloma will start with induction chemotherapy followed by maintenance chemotherapy. Many of these patients will go on to undergo autologous stem cell transplant(s) and possibly CAR-T therapy. There is no cure for myeloma, and the goal is to stabilize the disease at the lowest disease burden possible, although depending on the staging, myeloma can progress quickly, which warrants changes in therapy. Even after stem cell transplant and/or CAR-T therapy, most patients will require ongoing maintenance therapy.

▶ ONCOLOGY-RELATED PROCEDURES

BONE MARROW BIOPSY

Bone marrow aspiration and biopsies are used for diagnosis and monitoring of more common hematologic or blood-related cancers. Conditions to be evaluated for include anemias, hemochromatosis, lymphomas, leukemias, multiple myelomas, and infection. Samples are often procured from the iliac crest. Two samples that can be obtained are (a) bone marrow aspirate, which allows for a quick review of the cells, gives a description of the quantity of the cells, and provides materials for more detailed testing including molecular and flow studies, but bone marrow aspirate does not represent all cells in the bone marrow; and (b) core biopsy, which analyzes all cells and stromal cells in the bone marrow and requires a longer processing time.

CATHETER VENOUS ACCESS

Most patients with oncologic or hematologic malignancies require either an implanted port or a peripherally inserted central catheter (PICC) line for chemotherapy, blood product administration, laboratory draws, medications, and/or nutrition.

OMMAYA RESERVOIR

A more specific type of port, the Ommaya reservoir, is commonly used for patients who require ongoing access to the intrathecal space for aspiration of cerebral spinal fluid and the administration of medications, including intrathecal chemotherapy for treatment of intracranial neoplasms or hematological cancers such as leukemias. An Ommaya reservoir is a small cerebral ventricular access device inserted under the scalp, typically in the frontal area with access to cerebral spinal fluid. The device consists of an intraventricular catheter where the distal end is surgically positioned into the ipsilateral anterior horn with the proximal end connected to the reservoir.

▶ PROCEDURES FOR CANCER CELL–RELATED FLUID ACCUMULATION

THORACENTESIS

A malignant pleural effusion is fluid with cancer cells occurring in the pleural space between the lung and the chest wall. Malignant pleural effusions occur most commonly in breast and lung cancers and is also seen in lymphomas and gastrointestinal cancers. Symptoms of malignant pleural effusions include dyspnea, cough, chest pain, fever, and fatigue. Confirmation of malignant pleural effusion is by cytology and Light criteria (see Chapter 10). Management may include chemotherapy, immunotherapy/and or radiation, thoracentesis, pleurodesis, or indwelling pleural catheter.

PARACENTESIS

Malignant ascites is fluid in the peritoneum from cancer lining the organs or primary organ tumors caused by cancer cells related to liver, colon, ovarian, and pancreatic cancers. Symptoms of malignant ascites include swelling, tightness, distension, fullness with eating, fever, pain, shortness of breath, and possible infection. Treatment includes paracentesis for diagnosis and/or management. Paracentesis for diagnostics would include checking cytology for cancer cells, WBCs, blood, and bacteria. Consider diuretics for management of large volume of ascites.

LUMBAR PUNCTURE

Lumbar punctures sample cerebral spinal fluid to evaluate for blood cancer cells,; most commonly lymphomas, but may also be used to inject chemotherapy for treatment. Monitor for headaches, infection, bleeding, and numbness of the legs and lower spine.

BONE MARROW TRANSPLANT

Hematopoietic stem cell transplantation (HSCT) was harvested from peripheral blood stem cells (PBSCs) or bone marrow aspiration (more rapid engraftment rate compared with bone marrow). PBSCs can come from the patient themselves (autologous SCT) or from someone who is donating cells (allogenic SCT). Prior to collection, the patient receives medications to stimulate production of PBSCs. Once the cells are collected, they are frozen until ready for transplant.

Allogeneic BMT: Human leukocyte antigen (HLA) typing is done to identify a donor who is HLA matched. This can be a family member, an unrelated matched donor, or mismatched family donors (haploidentical).

Autologous BMT: An autologous BMT is collected from the patient and reinfused after purification methods. Patients are then prepared for the BMT by having high-dose chemotherapy/and or total body irradiation before receiving the infusion of stem cells. The process of engraftment occurs when infused transplanted hematopoietic stem cells produce mature progeny in the peripheral circulation.

COMPLICATIONS OF BONE MARROW TRANSPLANT

Acute complications of BMT occur in the first 90 days and include myelosuppression with neutropenia, anemia, thrombocytopenia, sinusoidal obstruction syndrome or vaso-occlusive disease, mucositis, acute graft versus host disease (GVHD), gram-positive/gram-negative infections (*Pseudomonas, Klebsiella pneumonia* [PNA], *Haemophilus influenzae*) that can lead to sepsis/septic shock, herpes simplex virus (HSV), CMV, *Candida*, and *Aspergillus*. Chronic complications include chronic GVHD, infection with encapsulated bacteria and varicella-zoster virus (VZV), *Pseudomonas, Klebsiella*, and *H.influenzae*.

Graft Versus Host Disease

GVHD is almost always in allogenic transplants and is very rare in autologous. Acute GVHD happens right after ANC starts to rise, within days to 2 weeks after transplant. Signs of acute GVHD include diarrhea (most common) and skin rash. Biopsy diagnoses GVHD and is done during colonoscopy or skin biopsy of rash. Liver GVHD is less common, and rarely is GVHD seen within the eyes. Chronic GVHD would occur more than 100 days after transplant and most commonly occurs when immunosuppression is stopped or decreased.

Neutropenia After Bone Marrow Transplant

Neutropenia is defined as an ANC less than 1,000. Treatment includes levofloxacin orally or intravenously until ANC is greater than 1,000.

Bone Marrow Transplant Prophylaxis

Patients who receive a BMT require prophylaxis to prevent *Pneumocystis jiroveci* pneumonia (PJP; formerly referred to as *Pneumocystis carinii* pneumonia), fungal infections, and viral infections. PJP prophylaxis post BMT includes trimethoprim–sulfamethoxazole (TMP-SMX) given 2 days per week until off immunosuppression. Antifungal infection prophylaxis includes fluconazole recommended for 1 month following transplant. Voriconazole is commonly used in patients with a high-risk profile of developing severe forms of antifungal infection or drug-resistant fungal infections. HSV and VZV prophylaxis includes acyclovir continued for 1 month for the prevention of HSV and for 1 year for prevention of VZV. CMV prophylaxis is recommended only in patients who test positive for CMV by polymerase chain reaction and is treated with ganciclovir.

▶ONCOLOGIC EMERGENCIES

Oncologic emergencies include neutropenic fever, tumor lysis syndrome (TLS), neoplastic cardiac tamponade, superior vena cava syndrome, spinal cord compression, hypercalcemia, and syndrome of inappropriate antidiuretic hormone (SIADH). An overview is provided; symptoms, diagnostics and treatment are shown in Table 13.11.

Table 13.11 Oncologic Emergencies, Symptoms, Diagnostics, and Treatments

Emergency	Symptoms	Diagnostics	Treatment
Neutropenic fevers	Fatigue, fever chills, diaphoresis, rigors, confusion, dehydration, mucositis, cough/sputum, pain, vomiting, diarrhea, urinary burning/discomfort, and skin rash	Seek source of infection: ■ Chest x-ray ■ Blood cultures ■ Urinalysis ■ Consider LP ■ Wound culture ■ RVP Check lactate Consider procalcitonin level	Assess and treat the etiology of the sepsis/septic shock: ■ Culture, IVF bolus 30 mL/kg; pressors as needed ■ Broad-spectrum antibiotics with *Pseudomonas* coverage (e.g., cefepime, Zosyn) ■ Anaerobic coverage (metronidazole or Zosyn) ■ MRSA coverage with vancomycin ■ Daptomycin or linezolid for VRE ■ For patients with ANC less than 1.0 or if beta-D-glucan or galactomannan are elevated, need antifungal coverage (e.g., posaconazole, isavuconazonium) ■ Patients with febrile neutropenia may decompensate quickly, a low threshold to transfer to the ICU
Tumor lysis syndrome	Nausea with or without vomiting; lack of appetite and fatigue; dark urine, reduced urine output, or flank pain; numbness, seizures, or hallucinations; muscle cramps and spasms, and heart palpitations	Hyperkalemia Hyperuricemia Hyperphosphatemia Hypocalcemia AKI Elevated uric acid level Elevated LDH	Treatment aimed at preserving renal function: ■ Allopurinol 300 mg/mg^2/day prior to starting chemotherapy to prevent uric acid–mediated nephropathy ■ IV volume hydration with NS or 0.45% NS ■ Rasburicase ■ Hold chemotherapy ■ Dialysis
Neoplastic cardiac tamponade	Muffled heart sounds, JVD, narrow pulse pressure, hypotension, tachycardia	Transthoracic echocardiogram	■ Pericardiocentesis ■ Pericardial window
SVC syndrome	Symptoms include facial, neck, and arm swelling; dilated neck veins; and may have shortness of breath	■ CT scan of chest with IV contrast	■ Emergent treatment of the underlying etiology
Spinal cord compression	Depends on the area of cord compressed: ■ Weakness ■ Bowel/bladder incontinence ■ Paresthesia ■ Paralysis	MRI of the spine for best visualization of the soft tissues	■ Steroids such as Decadron ■ Hospital admission ■ Consult Oncology (medical, radiation, surgical)

(*continued*)

Table 13.11 Oncologic Emergencies, Symptoms, Diagnostics, and Treatments (*continued*)

Emergency	Symptoms	Diagnostics	Treatment
Hypercalcemia	Patients with hypercalcemia may be immobilized, dehydrated, and have renal insufficiency. Chvostek sign Trousseau sign	▪ BMP shows hypercalcemia ▪ Ionized calcium level to confirm or ▪ Calculate a corrected serum calcium level	▪ IV bisphosphonate ▪ IV hydration with or without diuretics ▪ Serial monitoring of calcium level
SIADH	Muscle weakness, cramps, loss of appetite, irritability, restlessness, nausea/vomiting, confusion, hallucinations, seizures, coma	▪ Hyponatremia ▪ Low serum osmolality (less than 275 mOsm/L) ▪ High urine osmolality (greater than 100 mOsm/L) ▪ High urine sodium	▪ Fluid restriction (1.5 L/24 hr) ▪ Critical care monitoring ▪ Treat cancer

ANC, absolute neutrophil count; AKI, acute kidney injury; BMP, basic metabolic profile; IV, intravenous; IVF, intravenous fluid; JVD, jugular venous distention; LDH, lactate dehydrogenase; LP, lumbar puncture; MRSA, methicillin-resistant *Staphylococcus aureus*; NS, normal saline; RVP, respiratory viral panel; VRE, vancomycin-resistant enterococcus.

NEUTROPENIC FEVER

Neutropenic fever, commonly known as febrile neutropenia, is a serious complication related to chemotherapy treatments. Patients with neutropenia are more susceptible to infections and may need to defer or stop chemotherapy treatments for infectious workup. Neutropenia typically occurs about 7 to 12 days after receiving cytotoxic chemotherapy agents. The degree and duration of neutropenia vary by the type and dose of cytotoxic chemotherapy.

- *Neutropenia* is defined as a reduction in the ANC of less than 500 cells/mcL and can be confirmed on the CBC with differential.
- *Neutropenic fever* is defined as a patient who is neutropenic and has a temperature of 101°F in a single reading or an oral temperature of 100.4°F in two consecutive readings over a 2-hour period.

TUMOR LYSIS SYNDROME

TLS can occur with induction chemotherapy, secondary to tumor burden. Cytotoxic chemotherapy agents cause the rapidly dividing cancer cells to lyse, releasing the contents of their internal environment. The release of the internal contents is too much for the renal system to excrete. Those who develop TLS are at risk of developing acute kidney injury. TLS is more commonly associated with cancers such as Burkitt lymphoma and acute lymphoblastic leukemia but can present in those cancers with rapid proliferation including other lymphomas and leukemias. TLS is rarely noted in solid tumors except small-cell lung cancers. Common electrolyte abnormalities related to TLS include hyperkalemia, hyperuricemia, hyperphosphatemia, and hypocalcemia, due to the release of the intracellular contents of the destructed cancer cells.

NEOPLASTIC CARDIAC TAMPONADE

Neoplastic cardiac tamponade is excess fluid accumulation due to malignancy in the pericardial sac, which impedes normal contraction and ejection capacity. Capillary permeability induces fluid extravasation from leukemia, cytosine arabinoside, and cytokines such as interleukin-2 and tumor necrosis factor. Severe venous congestion can occur from cardiomyopathy, pulmonary tumors, or infection. Hemorrhage from severe thrombocytopenia can also be a cause. Malignancies from breast, lung, lymphoma, head and neck cancer, and leukemia can place a person at risk for this emergency.

SUPERIOR VENA CAVA SYNDROME

Superior vena cava syndrome is the compression of the superior vena cava resulting in reduced venous blood return to the heart (low cardiac output). Edema of the upper torso and arms can form due to impeding blood return. Internal or external superior vena cava obstruction results in low cardiac output.

Extrinsic compression occurs from tumors, lymph node enlargement, radiation scarring, or direct tumor involvement such as from bronchogenic, lymphoma, metastatic breast cancer (most common), head and neck cancers, melanoma, and renal cell cancers. Intraluminal thrombosis can occur from indwelling venous catheters. Hypercoagulability can occur (e.g., mucin-producing tumors seen with adenocarcinomas, procoagulants from myelocytic leukemia, and hyperviscosity from myeloma and lymphomas).

SPINAL CORD COMPRESSION

Spinal cord compromise occurs from compression or compromised blood flow to the spinal cord or cauda equina. Direct compression results from tumor (e.g., lung, prostate, breast, kidney cancer), lymph node growth, or hematogenous spread. Vascular supply can be compromised or pathologic fracture or vertebral collapse by lymphomas, myeloma, and neuroblastoma can occur.

HYPERCALCEMIA

Hypercalcemia is caused by bone demineralization due to tumor in bone (breast, lung, head and neck, or renal cancer) or increased levels of parathyroid hormone or osteoclast-activating factors (myeloma, lymphoma, or leukemia).

SYNDROME OF INAPPROPRIATE ANTIDIURETIC HORMONE

Risk factors for SIADH include small-cell lung cancer (80% of cases) and head and neck, pancreas, prostate, brain, lymphatic, or duodenal cancer. (See Chapter 15 for more on SIADH.)

▶ SUMMARY

The acute care of adult patients with hematological and oncological malignancies requires an understanding of classifications, causes, diagnostic workup, and management. Consultation with hematology and oncology specialists should be considered for newly diagnosed malignancies, treatments, and management of complications.

KNOWLEDGE CHECK: CHAPTER 13

1. A 72-year-old female patient presents to urgent care after complaining of fatigue, dyspnea on exertion, and anorexia with a noted hemoglobin (Hgb) 8.8, hematocrit (HCT) 28%. The most important blood test to first order for this patient to evaluate for anemia is:

   A. Complete blood count (CBC), electrolyte panel, blood urea nitrogen (BUN), and creatinine
   B. CBC/differential, peripheral blood smear
   C. CBC, red cell distribution width (RDW), erythrocyte sedimentation rate (ESR), total iron-binding capacity (TIBC)
   D. CBC, erythropoietin (EPO) level, albumin, IgG, IgA

2. A 72-year-old patient's bloodwork reveals red blood cells (RBCs) 2.9, reticulocyte count low, transferrin low, red cell distribution width (RDW) 15% (high), ferritin 10 (low), B_{12} 250 (normal), folate 200 (normal), iron 28 (low), lactate dehydrogenase (LDH) 148, total iron-binding capacity (TIBC) 455 (high), creatinine 1.2, erythropoietin (EPO) level normal, indicating:

   A. Pernicious anemia
   B. Iron-deficiency anemia
   C. Hemolytic anemia
   D. Thalassemia

3. A 68-year-old male patient with a past medical history of hypertension, diabetes mellitus, and chronic kidney disease (CKD) stage IIIa is admitted to the hospitalist service with pneumonia. On admission, his vital signs are stable. His laboratory studies include a complete blood count (CBC) revealing white blood count (WBC) 8.2, hemoglobin (Hgb) 9.6, platelets 235,000, and hematocrit (HCT) 27.5%. His basic metabolic panel (BMP) shows Na 136, K 4.1, Cl 101, blood urea nitrogen (BUN) 18, Cr 1.6, glucose 106. CrCl is 52 mL/min/BSA. There are no previous laboratory studies for comparison. The next *best* step for the AGACNP is to:

   A. Order vitamin B_{12} and folate levels
   B. Order ferritin and folate levels
   C. Reassess labs the next morning
   D. Order vitamin B_{12}, folate, and ferritin levels

4. An adult female patient presents in sickle cell crisis with severe joint pains, dyspnea on exertion, and headache after trying to manage at home with short-acting morphine, 15 to 30 mg orally every 4 hours. The *most important* immediate intervention, which may also reduce hospital length of stay, would be to administer:

   A. Hydration intravenously
   B. Oxygen supplementation
   C. Blood transfusions
   D. Parental opioids

5. A 20-year-old male patient presents with jaundice and scleral icterus with anemia, with hemoglobin (Hgb) 9.5, hematocrit (HCT) 27.5, and splenomegaly. He does not have any recent trauma. Family history reveals that his mother has spherocytosis. Further findings that most likely indicate the cause of hemolytic anemia include:

   A. Elevated lactate dehydrogenase (LDH), haptoglobin, and indirect bilirubin
   B. Increased blood-urea-nitrogen (BUN), creatinine, and total bilirubin
   C. Low reticulocyte count, transferrin, and iron
   D. Elevated erythrocyte sedimentation rate (ESR), C-reactive protein, and mean corpuscular volume (MCV)

(See answers next page.)

1. B) CBC/differential, peripheral blood smear

Peripheral blood smear is the gold standard for assessing size, shape, and appearance of red blood cells, white blood count, and platelets to test for anemia and related disease.

2. B) Iron-deficiency anemia

Iron deficiency is associated with low RBCs, low reticulocyte count (low RBC production), high TIBC, low transferrin saturation level (serum iron/TIBC), and low ferritin (low iron stores). LDH is normal, indicating no RBC destruction related to hemolysis. Low B_{12} is associated with pernicious anemia. Thalassemia has normal iron levels.

3. D) Order vitamin B_{12}, folate, and ferritin levels

CKD is an underlying cause of anemia—more specifically, anemia of chronic disease. Given that there are no previous laboratory studies to compare, it would be prudent to ensure the proper underlying cause of the anemia. This would lead the AGACNP to check the various sources of anemia, including checking ferritin, folate, and vitamin B_{12} levels to ensure that no other causes of anemia, other than CKD, are present.

4. D) Parental opioids

A person with sickle cell crisis needs immediate parental opioids to stabilize pain due to many disease-related factors, including vaso-occlusive disease that causes this pain.

5. A) Elevated lactate dehydrogenase (LDH), haptoglobin, and indirect bilirubin

The findings associated with hemolytic anemia include elevated LDH, haptoglobin, and indirect bilirubin. The patient may have inherited spherocytosis, which can cause hemolytic anemia.

6. A 32-year-old female patient presents to the hospital with a 5-day history of lethargy, shortness of breath on exertion, and bruising with petechiae to her extremities and bleeding gums. She has history of recurrent urinary tract infections and has been treated recently with ciprofloxacin twice in the past 6 months. Labs show hemoglobin (Hgb) 11, red blood cells (RBCs) 4.3, with a platelet count of 15,000. Prothrombin time (PT)/partial prothrombin time (PTT), and D-dimer are normal. Urinalysis is normal. The most likely cause of thrombocytopenia is:

   A. Disseminated intravascular coagulation (DIC)
   B. Drug-induced thrombocytopenia
   C. Infection-induced cytopenia
   D. Immune thrombocytopenic purpura

7. A 24-year-old patient presents to the hospital with increased symptoms of shortness of breath, oxygen desaturation, chest pain, abdominal swelling, gastrointestinal (GI) bleeding, and leg swelling. The patient was recently diagnosed with gastric lymphoma. The AGACNP suspects disseminated intravascular coagulation (DIC) based on which confirmatory blood test?

   A. Prothrombin time (PT)/partial prothrombin time (PTT)
   B. Platelet count
   C. Fibrinogen
   D. D-dimer

8. A patient presents due to increased bruising, bleeding of the gums, and ongoing upper respiratory symptoms unrelieved by antibiotic therapy. Labs reveal white blood count (WBC) 65, hemoglobin (Hgb) 6.5, and platelets 19,000. Based on the laboratory findings, the *next best step* for the AGACNP would be to:

   A. Obtain a bone marrow biopsy and peripheral smear
   B. Initiate chemotherapy
   C. Initiate an infectious workup including blood cultures
   D. Start intravenous antibiotics

9. A 41-year-old male patient is admitted for a 15-lb weight loss in the past 4 months, significant pruritis, and night sweats with fever. On physical exam, cervical and axillary lymphadenopathy are present bilaterally. Routine bloodwork including complete blood count (CBC) and comprehensive metabolic panel (CMP) is unremarkable. The AGACNP's *next best step* is to:

   A. Obtain a chest/pelvis CT scan and bone marrow biopsy
   B. Order a chest x-ray
   C. Repeat routine blood work including CBC, basic metabolic panel (BMP), Mg, and Phos
   D. Refer to dermatology

10. A patient presents for a routine blood donation. Upon review of hemoglobin (Hgb), the patient is found to be anemic with an Hgb of 8.5 g/dL. Vitamin B_{12}, ferritin, and folate levels are all within range. Later, while moving furniture, the patient feels a "pop" in the back when bending over, resulting in ongoing back pain. The patient subsequently presents due to this back pain. During that time, imaging is done that confirms multiple lytic lesions throughout. The AGACNP should also check:

    A. Chemistries including creatinine
    B. Liver function studies
    C. Urinalysis
    D. B-natriuretic peptide

(See answers next page.)

6. B) Drug-induced thrombocytopenia

Drugs such as ciprofloxacin can cause new-onset drug-induced thrombocytopenia. There is no evidence of infection, and normal D-dimer indicates no DIC. Workup for immune thrombocytopenic purpura is indicated if treatment for drug-induced thrombocytopenia does not resolve it.

7. D) D-dimer

D-dimer is the gold standard test to evaluate for DIC.

8. A) Obtain a bone marrow biopsy and peripheral smear

High WBC with low Hgb and low platelets indicate bone marrow problems. Peripheral blood smear is important to look at appearance, shape, and size to evaluate, and bone marrow biopsy evaluates bone marrow suppression, bone marrow failure, infection, inflammation, leukemia, platelet dysfunction, cancer, or an immune system disorder.

9. A) Obtain a chest/pelvis CT scan and bone marrow biopsy

Signs and symptoms are concerning for "B symptoms" associated with lymphoma. Repeating blood-work and chest x-ray will not be beneficial at this time based on previous bloodwork. Also, enlarged lymph nodes are not always seen on chest x-ray. Dermatology consult would not be beneficial because the patient has pruritis but lacks rash. Thus, a bone marrow biopsy and a chest/pelvis CT scan will be prudent to check for bone marrow involvement and to determine the extent of the lymphadenopathy.

10. A) Chemistries including creatinine

This case is concerning for multiple myeloma given the anemia and the imaging showing lytic lesions. With multiple myeloma, the free light chains have the potential to cause subsequent kidney damage in the form of acute renal failure. Urinalysis could be helpful but would not help to determine if acute renal failure is present. Liver function studies and B-natriuretic peptide would not be helpful in this case.

11. The use of the patient's own bone marrow cells for transplant occurs during which type of transplantation?

    A. Autologous
    B. Allogeneic
    C. Unrelated donor
    D. Cord blood

12. A 48-year-old male patient who had an allogeneic bone marrow transplant (BMT) for lymphoma presents with fever, gastroenteritis symptoms of diarrhea and abdominal pain, a new prominent skin rash on his extremities, and fatigue. Exam reveals normal heart and lung sounds, no organo-megaly, and no peripheral edema. The AGACNP suspects:

    A. Viral infection
    B. Graft versus host disease
    C. Venous occlusive disease
    D. Lymphoma relapse

13. A 22-year-old female college student had an autologous bone marrow transplant (BMT) 3 years ago for leukemia and now presents with flu-like symptoms and abdominal discomfort. The AGACNP knows that:

    A. There is no risk for leukemia relapse
    B. Immune system reconstitution has taken place
    C. Delayed effects of BMT can occur at any time
    D. Infertility should always be assumed for patients with BMT

14. A 68-year-old male patient was diagnosed with acute lymphoblastic leukemia approximately 6 months ago. In the past 3 days, he completed his second cycle of chemotherapy. He presents with a fever of 102.1°F. Complete blood count (CBC) shows white blood count (WBC) 0.2 with absolute neutrophil count (ANC) 0, hemoglobin (Hgb) 9.4, and platelets 85,000. Chemistries are all within normal range. Blood cultures are pending, and lactate is 0.7. The patient is hemodynamically stable. He is started on intravenous (IV) antibiotics and admitted for further care. The AGACNP's *next best step* is to:

    A. Await culture results and continue IV antibiotics
    B. Stop IV antibiotics once fever resolves
    C. Transfer the patient to the ICU
    D. Change to oral antibiotics

15. A 55-year-old male patient is diagnosed with acute lymphoblastic leukemia. At diagnosis, complete blood count (CBC) shows white blood count (WBC) 75, hemoglobin (Hgb) 7.8, and platelets 35,000. Chemistries are within normal range except for a creatinine of 1.3. Prior to starting chemotherapy, the AGACNP should consider what additional intervention to perform due to concern for tumor lysis syndrome?

    A. No additional interventions are needed
    B. Start IV rasburicase
    C. Start IV hydration, diuretics, and allopurinol
    D. Start IV methylprednisolone

(See answers next page.)

11. A) Autologous
An autologous bone marrow transplant (BMT) involves harvesting, treating, and transplanting back a patient's own bone marrow cells.

12. B) Graft versus host disease
The patient is presenting with symptoms of graft versus host disease, which can occur after an allogeneic BMT.

13. C) Delayed effects of BMT can occur at any time
Patients are at persistent risk of complications at any time after BMT.

14. A) Await culture results and continue IV antibiotics
In the setting of neutropenic fever, it is essential to rule out the source of infection. If the patient is hemodynamically stable, the patient has the ability to remain on the medicine floor depending on institutional guidelines; thus, this patient does not warrant transfer to the ICU. IV antibiotics are not stopped until neutrophil recovery occurs, and the route would not change. Thus, awaiting blood cultures and continuing IV antibiotics is the best choice.

15. C) Start IV hydration, diuretics, and allopurinol
The patient has a significantly elevated WBC and is thus at risk for tumor lysis syndrome upon the initiation of chemotherapy. With the destruction of the cancer cells, there is risk of the development of hyperkalemia, hyperphosphatemia, hypocalcemia, and hyperuricemia. To prevent these laboratory abnormalities, laboratory studies must be checked at least twice daily or more. Pharmacological interventions include aggressive IV hydration to prevent renal failure, diuretics to assist with elimination of electrolytes from cell rupture, and initiation of allopurinol, which inhibits urate production. IV rasburicase is used as a secondary measure if IV hydration, diuretics, and allopurinol prove unsuccessful. IV methylprednisolone would not be warranted.

● KEY BIBLIOGRAPHY

Only key resources appear in the print edition. Access the full bibliography for this chapter on ExamPrepConnect.com.

Bayer, V., Amaya, B., Baniewicz, D., Callahan, C., Marsh, L., & McCoy, A. S. (2017). Cancer immunotherapy: An evidence-based overview and implications for practice. *Clinical Journal of Oncology Nursing, 21*(2), 13–21. https://doi.org/10.1188/17.CJON.S2.13-21

Gupta, A., & Moore, J. A. (2018). Tumor lysis syndrome. *JAMA Oncology, 4*(6), 895. https://doi.org/10.1001/jamaoncol.2018.0613

Holcomb, S. S. (2005). Recognizing and managing anemia. *The Nurse Practitioner, 30*(12), 16–33. https://doi.org/10.1097/00006205-200512000-00004

Khaddour, K., Hana, C. K., & Mewawalla, P. (2022, April 30). Hematopoietic stem cell transplantation. [Updated]. In *StatPearls* [Internet]. StatPearls.

Swerdlow, S. H., Campo, E., Harris, N. L., Jaffe, E. S., Pileri, S. A., Stein, H., & Thiele, J. (Eds.). (2017). *WHO Classification of Tumours of Haematopoietic and Lymphoid Tissues* (rev. 4th ed.). International Agency for Research on Cancer (IARC).

Infectious Disease Review

Stefanie La Manna

▶ INTRODUCTION

AGACNP students are commonly challenged in choosing antibiotics to treat infectious etiologies. Some infectious processes are reviewed within the specific body system chapters in this book. This chapter encompasses a select review of infectious etiologies and their treatments (see Chapter 4 for a detailed review of antibiotics to supplement exam study).

▶ HEALTHCARE-ASSOCIATED INFECTIONS

Healthcare-associated infections (HAIs) are nosocomially acquired infections that were not present or incubating upon admission to a hospital or within the first 48 hours of admission. HAIs include *catheter-associated urinary tract infections* (CAUTIs), *central line–associated bloodstream infections* (CLABSIs), *surgical site infections* (SSIs), hospital- and ventilator-acquired pneumonia (HAP and VAP), and *Clostridioides difficile* infections (CDIs). HAIs in the United States cost hospitals at least $28.4 billion annually. Mortality related to HAIs is substantial. For example, the overall mortality attributed to just HAP is 30% to 50%. AGACNPs must implement preventive measures to increase survivability and reduce healthcare costs.

CATHETER-ASSOCIATED URINARY TRACT INFECTIONS
DISEASE OVERVIEW
CAUTIs are the most common HAIs and affect 900,000 inpatients in the United States annually. Approximately 25% of inpatients have urethral catheters inserted during their hospital stay. *Escherichia coli* and other gram-negative bacteria, *Pseudomonas aeruginosa*, and gram-positive bacteria such as staphylococci, enterococci, and yeast are the most common organisms that are isolated. All patients with indwelling catheters are at risk for CAUTI and pose one of the greatest concerns for multidrug-resistant organisms (MDROs).

CLASSIC PRESENTATION
Fever is the most common symptom. Localizing symptoms may include flank pain, suprapubic discomfort, or costovertebral angle (CVA) tenderness. Patients with spinal cord injury may have atypical and nonspecific symptoms that include spasticity, malaise, lethargy, and autonomic dysreflexia. Pyuria is a common finding in catheterized patients.

DIAGNOSTIC CRITERIA
The diagnosis of CAUTI is made by finding bacteriuria in a catheterized patient who has signs and symptoms that are consistent with urinary tract infection (UTI). The UTI is diagnosed in a patient with a catheter that has been present for 48 hours or was removed within 48 hours. Signs and symptoms of CAUTI can be nonspecific, and a fair amount of clinical judgment is required. Urinalysis and culture should be obtained by removing the indwelling catheter and obtaining a midstream specimen. If ongoing catheterization is needed, then the catheter should be replaced prior to collecting a urine sample for culture, as this will avoid culturing bacteria present in the biofilm as opposed to the bladder. In the setting of condom catheters, it is difficult to distinguish true infection from skin and mucosal contamination.

Therefore, a clean-catch midstream specimen should be obtained, or urine should be collected from a freshly applied condom catheter after cleaning the glans.

TREATMENT/MANAGEMENT

Removal of the infected catheter is the cornerstone of CAUTI treatment. If medically necessary, a new catheter can be inserted after starting antibiotic treatment. Treatment will depend on the offending organism and the clinical presentation. Antibiotic selection for both acute and complicated UTIs poses risk factors for resistant infection. The approach to empiric antimicrobial therapy for patients with CAUTI depends in part on the presentation, the patient's clinical history of recurrent UTIs and the associated organisms, and whether there are features that suggest an infection has extended past the bladder.

COMPLICATIONS

The important complications of CAUTI include sepsis, bacteremia, and association of the upper urinary tract. Approximately 20% of healthcare-associated bacteremia arise from the urinary tract, and the mortality associated with this condition is about 10%.

CLOSTRIDIOIDES DIFFICILE INFECTIONS
DISEASE OVERVIEW

C. difficile is a spore-forming gram-positive obligate anaerobe. CDI should be suspected in any patient who has diarrhea and association with antibiotic exposure. It is the most common hospital-acquired (nosocomial) infection and is the most frequent cause of morbidity and mortality in the older adult population. The most important modifiable risk factor is exposure to antimicrobial agents. CDI results in acute inflammation of the colonic mucosa. Disease results from spore germination, overgrowth, and toxin production. Pathogenic strains produce toxins A and B or B alone. Patients have profuse watery or green mucoid, foul-smelling diarrhea with cramping abdominal pain that usually begins 4 to 10 days after starting antibiotic therapy with a range of 24 hours to 8 weeks. Patients may develop toxic megacolon, perforation, and peritonitis.

CLASSIC PRESENTATION

A patient was admitted 5 days ago with pneumonia. They now have profuse watery or green mucoid, foul-smelling diarrhea with cramping abdominal pain. They report having six episodes of diarrhea in the last 24 hours. Leukocytosis that was improving is now worsening and is currently 28,000.

DIAGNOSTIC CRITERIA

Testing should be carried out only in patients with new-onset greater or equal to three unformed stools in 24 hours. Multistep testing of stool is recommended. Detection of *C. difficile* glutamate dehydrogenase antigen using enzyme immunoassay (EIA) or detection of *C. difficile* nucleic acid using nucleic acid amplification testing is usually the first step. This must be followed by an EIA detecting toxins A and B or toxin B. Endoscopy may be useful, but pseudomembranous colitis is seen in only about half of patients.

TREATMENT/MANAGEMENT

If able, stop the offending antibiotics. The treatment regimen is specific to an episode of CDI occurrence (Table 14.1).

Table 14.1 CDI Treatment by Episode of CDI Occurrence

Treatment Options for Patients With an Initial Occurrence of CDI
▪ Fidaxomicin 200 mg orally twice daily for 10 days OR ▪ Vancomycin 125 mg orally four times daily for 10 days OR ▪ Metronidazole 500 mg every 8 hours for 10–14 days
Treatment Options for Patients With an Initial Occurrence of CDI

▪ Fidaxomicin
  ● 200 mg PO BID for 10 days OR
  ● 200 mg PO BID for 5 days, followed by once every other day for 20 days

Table 14.1 CDI Treatment by Episode of CDI Occurrence (*continued*)

Treatment Options for Patients With an Initial Occurrence of CDI

■ Vancomycin in a tapered and pulsed regimen, for example:
  ● 125 mg PO QID for 10–14 days, then
  ● 125 mg PO BID for 7 days, then
  ● 125 mg PO once daily for 7 days, then
  ● 125 mg PO every 2–3 days for 2–8 weeks
■ Consider adjunctive treatment with bezlotoxumab 10 mg/kg IV once during antibiotic course

Treatment Options for Second and Subsequent Recurrences of CDI

■ Fidaxomicin
  ● 200 mg PO BID for 10 days, OR
  ● 200 mg PO BID for 5 days, followed by once every other day for 20 days OR
■ Vancomycin in a tapered and pulsed regimen as above OR
■ Vancomycin 125 mg PO QID for 10 days followed by rifaximin 400 mg TID for 20 days
■ Consider fecal microbiota transplantation
■ Consider adjunctive treatment with bezlotoxumab 10 mg/kg IV once during antibiotic course

Treatment Options for Fulminant CDI
■ Vancomycin 500 mg four times daily by mouth or by nasogastric tube ■ If ileus, add rectal instillation of vancomycin and metronidazole 500 mg IV every 8 hours

BID, twice daily; CDI, *Clostridioides difficile* infection; PO, orally; QID, four times daily; TID, three times daily.

COMPLICATIONS

Patients may develop peritonitis, perforation, sepsis, toxic megacolon, septic shock, and death.

CENTRAL LINE–ASSOCIATED BLOODSTREAM INFECTIONS
DISEASE OVERVIEW

A CLABSI is a laboratory-confirmed bloodstream infection that meets at least one of the following criteria:

■ The patient has a recognized bacterial or fungal pathogen cultured from one or more blood cultures, and the pathogen is not related to an infection at another site.

■ The patient has a common commensal organism such as coagulase-negative *Staphylococcus* in two or more blood cultures collected on different days or from different sites that are not related to an infection at another site and that occur in the setting of one of the following signs or symptoms: fever (greater than 38.0°C), chills, or hypotension.

If a patient has positive blood cultures with a gram-positive organism such as *Staphylococcus*, obtain an echocardiogram to ensure no vegetations are noted on the heart valves. Gram-positive organisms tend to seed in heart valves.

CLASSIC PRESENTATION

A patient is admitted for septic shock due to diverticulitis and has a central venous catheter placed for vasopressors that have since been weaned off as the patient recovered. The patient is ready for transfer to the floor and develops a new fever and is more somnolent, tachycardic, and hypotensive. The nurse reports erythema and purulence at the peripherally inserted central catheter (PICC) line site.

DIAGNOSTIC CRITERIA

The diagnosis should be suspected in patients with fever, chills, or hypotension in the setting of a catheter placed at least 48 hours prior to the development of symptoms. Physical examination findings include erythema, pain, swelling, or purulence at the central line insertion site. Blood cultures are positive for an organism commonly associated with catheter-related bloodstream infection (coagulase-negative staphylococci, *Staphylococcus aureus*, enterococci, *Candida* species, and other common commensals).

WBC count, C-reactive protein, and procalcitonin are not useful as specific indicators to diagnose CLABSI.

TREATMENT/MANAGEMENT

Start with empirical antibiotic treatment that will cover gram-positive and gram-negative bacteria and anaerobes. Once sensitivities are known, streamline antibiotics to the appropriate organism and antibiotic.

COMPLICATIONS

Complications include septic thrombophlebitis, infective endocarditis, metastatic musculoskeletal infection, and death.

HOSPITAL-ACQUIRED PNEUMONIA AND VENTILATOR-ACQUIRED PNEUMONIA

HAP and VAP are more likely to be caused by resistant pathogens and therefore are treated differently from community-acquired pneumonia. HAP is the most common hospital-acquired infection.

- HAP develops more than 48 hours after admission to a hospital or within 48 hours after discharge.
- VAP is any pneumonia that develops more than 48 hours after endotracheal intubation or within 48 hours after extubation.

The most common organisms causing HAP and VAP are drug-resistant pathogens including methicillin-resistant *Staphylococcus aureus* (MRSA), *E. coli*, *Klebsiella*, *Serratia*, *Stenotrophomonas*, *Burkholderia*, *Pseudomonas*, and *Acinetobacter*. However, community organisms such as *Streptococcus pneumoniae* and *Haemophilus* are not uncommon. Viruses, atypical bacteria, and fungal pathogens rarely cause nosocomial pneumonia, but these pathogens should be kept in the differential diagnosis in immunocompromised hosts, in patients who do not respond to therapy or very ill, and during influenza season.

CLASSIC PRESENTATION

Patients will frequently present with productive tachypnea, cough, fever, dyspnea, and pleuritic chest pain. Additionally, new or progressive infiltrates on chest x-ray, fever, hypothermia, purulent sputum or increase in sputum production, leukocytosis, and hypoxia or increased oxygen requirements are common findings.

DIAGNOSTIC CRITERIA

The goal of diagnostic testing is twofold:

1. Confirm pneumonia as the diagnosis.
2. Isolate the organism to narrow the antibiotic spectrum. Bronchoscopy may be needed in patients unable to provide an adequate sputum sample and strongly considered when the diagnosis is in question.

Other Laboratories

Consider obtaining urine pneumococcal antigen, urine legionella antigen, multi-organism polymerase chain reaction (PCR), nasopharyngeal swab, and urine histoplasmosis antigen to assess for other organisms.

Imaging

Chest x-ray is required to differentiate between tracheobronchitis and pneumonia. CT scan of the chest is to be considered if the diagnosis is in question.

TREATMENT/MANAGEMENT

Empiric treatment of HAP and VAP in adults with normal kidney function can encompass many antibiotic options (Table 14.2). Renal dosing of antibiotics is critical to avoid acute kidney injury (AKI). Consult with a pharmacist is suggested to ensure appropriate renal dosing.

Table 14.2 HAP and VAP Treatment

Category	Other Factors	Empiric Therapy
HAP	Low risk of MRSA	Piperacillin-tazobactam 4.5 g IV q6h OR Cefepime 2 g IV q8h OR Levofloxacin 750 mg IV q24h OR Imipenem 500 mg IV q6h
	Risk of MRSA	ADD: Vancomycin 15 mg/kg IV q12h
	Septic shock or IVDU in the prior 90 days	ADD a second antipseudomonal agent (Avoid 2 beta-lactams) such as Aztreonam 2 g IV q8h OR Amikacin 15 mg/kg IV daily
VAP	Gram-positive antibiotic with MRSA activity Beta-lactam with gram-negative antibiotic with antipseudomonal activity	Vancomycin 15 mg/kg IV q8–12h OR Linezolid 600 mg IV q12h
	Beta-lactam with gram-negative antibiotic with antipseudomonal activity	Piperacillin-tazobactam 4.5 g IV q6h OR Cefepime 2 g IV q8h OR Imipenem 500 mg IV q6h
	Non-beta-lactam with gram-negative antibiotic with antipseudomonal activity	Aztreonam 2 g IV q8h OR Amikacin 15 mg/kg IV daily OR Levofloxacin 750 mg IV q24h

HAP, hospital-acquired pneumonia; IV, intravenous; IVDU, intravenous drug use; MRSA, methicillin-resistant *Staphylococcus aureus*; VAP, ventilator-acquired pneumonia.

COMPLICATIONS
Complications of HAP and VAP include, sepsis, septic shock, complicated parapneumonic effusion, empyema, and death.

SURGICAL SITE INFECTIONS
DISEASE OVERVIEW
SSI is the most common HAI following surgery. There is significant morbidity and mortality, and most patients require transfer to the ICU, are readmitted to the hospital, and have prolonged hospital admissions. Approximately 2% to 4% of patients will develop an SSI in the United States, placing an economic burden on healthcare.

The Centers for Disease Control and Prevention (CDC) define SSI as an infection related to a surgical procedure that occurs near the surgical site within 30 days after surgery or up to 90 days after surgery when an implant is involved. Incisional SSIs are divided into those involving only skin and subcutaneous tissues (superficial incisional SSI) and those involving deeper tissues of the incisions, to include organ space infections that include abscess, anastomotic leak for intra-abdominal operations, and implant-associated infections.

The CDC describes three types of SSIs: superficial incisional, deep incisional, and organ/space. Superficial incisional presents with peri-incisional pain or tenderness, localized peri-incisional swelling, erythema, and warmth. Deep incisional also has fevers and localized pain. Organ/space SSI commonly presents with nausea and vomiting, abdominal pain or tenderness, fever (greater than 38°C), and hypotension. Elevated transaminases and jaundice can be present depending on the source and severity of infection.

CLASSIC PRESENTATION
A 50-year-old man presents 8 days after a colonic resection for colon cancer. He complains of fevers, chills, and abdominal pain that started 2 days ago and is getting progressively worse. His incision is red but does not have purulent drainage. He is tachycardic to 110, respiratory rate (RR) 20, blood pressure (BP) 100/52. He reports nausea and vomits while the AGACNP is examining him.

DIAGNOSTIC CRITERIA

Superficial SSI can be fully evaluated through direct observation of the wound. In the presence of signs and symptoms of systemic infection, ultrasound can identify the presence of fluid in subcutaneous tissues. In the presence of deep or organ space, CT or MRI provides a more detailed assessment of the underlying soft tissue and organ space. In the setting of prior gastrointestinal resection with the probability of an underlying anastomotic leak or intra-abdominal infection, oral contrast aids in diagnosis.

TREATMENT/MANAGEMENT

General Management

Wound exploration and debridement is the mainstay of treatment of superficial incisional infections. Open the wound and drain any infected fluid and culture. Debride of any necrotic tissue. Cultures and sensitivities should guide antimicrobial therapy.

Organ/Space Surgical Site Infection

Patients with organ/space SSI have higher morbidity and mortality. Antibiotics are warranted. Conservative management with antibiotics is used for smaller collections. CT and ultrasound are used to guide the placement of percutaneous drains into larger abscess collections, if possible. In some cases, it is difficult to differentiate an abscess from an anastomotic leak. Surgical exploration may be warranted.

Antimicrobial

Antimicrobial therapy is determined by the extent of the infection, systemic signs and symptoms of infection, and patient comorbidities. Antibiotics are not always necessary to treat superficial SSI. Antibiotics are required in the setting of surrounding cellulitis or in the presence of systemic signs and symptoms of infection. Antibiotics are nearly always required to treat deep and organ/space SSIs. Antibiotics are initiated under the following conditions:

- Cellulitis is associated with intact but indurated surgical incisions even in the absence of wound drainage or subcutaneous fluid collection.
- Persistent or worsening cellulitis is in the surrounding skin after wound opening.
- Subcutaneous or deeper tissue has persistent inflammation after debridement or drainage.
- Implanted material such as mesh, vascular grafts, and orthopedic hardware is present within the infected area.
- Systemic signs of infection exist (fever, tachycardia, tachypnea, hypotension, leukocytosis).
- Septic shock is present.

COMPLICATIONS

Complications of SSI include sepsis, septic shock, and sequelae of septic shock including AKI, loss of limbs, acute respiratory failure, and death.

▶ COMMON MULTIDRUG-RESISTANT ORGANISMS

The occurrence of *multidrug-resistant organisms* (MDROs) is rising, with ~3 million antibiotic-resistant infections in the United States each year resulting in ~35,000 deaths. IV antibiotic use within the previous 90 days is the principal factor causing MDROs. The severity of resistance is increasing, and a classification system of different levels of drug resistance has come into existence (Table 14.3). This section reviews a few MDROs that AGACNPs commonly see in practice, including methicillin-resistant *Staphylococcus*, vancomycin-resistant enterococcus, extended-spectrum beta-lactamases, carbapenem resistance, *Pseudomonas*, and *Candida auris*.

Table 14.3 Classifications of Resistance

MDR	XDR	PDR
Isolate is not susceptible to at least one agent in three or more antimicrobial categories	Isolate is not susceptible to at least one agent in in all but two or fewer antimicrobial categories	Not susceptible to any agents in any antimicrobial categories

MDR, multidrug resistant; PDR, pan drug resistant; XDR, extensively drug resistant.
Source: Carpenter, D. (2022). *Fast facts for the adult-gerontology acute care nurse practitioner.* Springer Publishing Company.

METHICILLIN-RESISTANT *STAPHYLOCOCCUS AUREUS*

Prevention and control of methicillin-resistant *S. aureus* (MRSA) infection are among the most important challenges of infection prevention. Optimal use of antimicrobial agents such as choice of drug, dose, route, and duration may help to reduce the prevalence of resistant *S. aureus*, including MRSA, and may reduce the risk of MRSA colonization. Measures to help reduce the transmission of MRSA include:

- regularly washing hands with soap and water or an alcohol-based hand gel
- maintaining good general hygiene with regular bathing, particularly after activities with skin-to-skin contact; keeping fingernails cut short and clean
- using a proper over-the-counter detergent or disinfectant that specifies *S. aureus* on the product label to clean equipment and environmental surfaces that multiple people touch with bare skin

Counseling for patients or caregivers of patients with MRSA skin and soft tissue infections (SSTIs) includes:

- Keep draining wounds covered with clean, dry bandages.
- Wash hands with soap and water or an alcohol-based hand gel immediately after touching infected skin or items that directly touch a draining wound.
- Avoid reusing or sharing items that directly contacted a draining wound, including bathtubs, towels, clothing, bedding, bar soap, razors, and athletic equipment.
- Wash linens at least weekly, and wash towels and washcloths after each use.
- Wash and thoroughly dry clothing that comes in contact with wound drainage after each use.

Decolonization regimens suggested by the Infectious Disease Society of America are as follows:

- mupirocin ointment applied to the anterior nares twice daily for 5 to 10 days OR
- mupirocin ointment applied to the anterior nares twice daily for 5 days twice per month for 6 months
- chlorhexidine applied with the hands or a clean washcloth and rinsed off once daily for 5 to 14 days OR
- chlorhexidine applied with the hands or a clean washcloth and rinsed off once daily for 5 to 14 days

With these recommendations and education prevention, MRSA transmission can be decreased.

VANCOMYCIN-RESISTANT ENTEROCOCCUS

Vancomycin-resistant enterococci (VRE) is a common yet difficult-to-treat cause of hospital-acquired infections. Transmission can occur by direct contact with hands of healthcare workers and indirectly from environmental surfaces.

The risk factors for VRE colonization and infection include previous antimicrobial therapy and patient characteristics such as immunosuppression, colonization pressure, exposure to contaminated surfaces, and residence in long-term facilities. Colonization pressure is an infection-control metric defined as the proportion of patients who are colonized in a geographic area in the hospital during a specific period of time.

Good hand hygiene (handwashing, not use of alcohol-based products) is considered an essential measure in reducing the spread of the pathogen. Patients who are colonized with VRE have ~8% rate of developing a VRE infection in hospital or after discharge, and the rate is higher in those who are severely ill or immunocompromised. VRE colonization can spread to other patients. Contact precautions are recommended to be followed for patients with VRE infection or colonization.

EXTENDED-SPECTRUM BETA-LACTAM

Extended-spectrum beta-lactamases (ESBLs) are enzymes that give resistance to most beta-lactam antibiotics, which include penicillin, cephalosporins, and monobactam aztreonam. Infections that result in ESBL are often associated with poor outcomes. Carbapenems are the best antimicrobial agent to treat ESBL. ESBLs have been found exclusively in gram-negative organisms, primarily *Klebsiella pneumoniae*, *Klebsiella oxytoca*, *Escherichia coli*, *Acinetobacter*, *Burkholderia*, *Citrobacter*, *Enterobacter*, *Morganella*, *Proteus*,

Pseudomonas, Salmonella, Serratia, and *Shigella* spp. The most common organism that ESBL is found in is *E. coli.* The most common reservoir for ESBL Enterobacteriaceae is in the gastrointestinal (GI) tract.

TREATMENT/MANAGEMENT

The preferred treatment options that produce the best outcomes are meropenem, ertapenem (although it does not cover pseudomonas), and imipenem. As a result, the spread of ESBL-producing organisms within hospitals can be slowed using barrier protection and restriction of later-generation cephalosporins.

CARBAPENEM-RESISTANT ENTEROCOCCUS

The CDC identified carbapenem-resistant Enterobacteriaceae (CRE) as an urgent public health threat and ESBL-producing Enterobacteriaceae as a serious public health threat. CRE can spread across many regions when a person is infected or colonized or is transferred between healthcare facilities without infection-control measures in place. Healthcare facilities can prevent CRE spread by implementing best practices in infection control and antimicrobial stewardship. Additional risk factors that have been associated with infection or colonization with carbapenemase-producing organisms are trauma, diabetes, malignancy, organ transplantation, mechanical ventilation, indwelling urinary or venous catheters, overall poor functional status or severe illness, and residence in a long-term facility.

When a carbapenemase-producing isolate is identified, clinicians should ask for additional antibiotic susceptibility testing, such as:

- ceftazidime–avibactam, meropenem–vaborbactam, and/or imipenem–cilastatin–relebactam
- cefiderocol
- ceftolozane–tazobactam (particularly for *P. aeruginosa*)
- aminoglycosides (particularly plazomicin, if available)
- colistin or polymyxin B
- aztreonam
- tigecycline and eravacycline (if available)
- fosfomycin (particularly for urinary tract isolates)

For CRE infections, a consultation with infectious disease is warranted. If an outbreak occurs, then empiric therapy against carbapenemase-producing bacteria should be considered for patients with serious infections until culture and susceptibility data become known.

PSEUDOMONAS AERUGINOSA

P. aeruginosa is a gram-negative aerobic bacillus. This organism is important to know as it is often antibiotic-resistant and can cause severe hospital-acquired infections associated with high mortality rates, specifically in immunocompromised hosts. Monotherapy is generally adequate, but combination therapy (double coverage) is indicated in certain high-risk patients and in severe infections.

Risk factors for infection with resistant *P. aeruginosa* include an ICU stay, bedridden status, presence of invasive devices, prior use of broad-spectrum cephalosporins, aminoglycosides, carbapenems, fluoroquinolones, diabetes mellitus, and surgery. Antimicrobial resistance among *P. aeruginosa* is associated with increased length of hospitalization and increased mortality. Prior use of a carbapenem, to include ertapenem, that does not have antipseudomonal activity results in an increased rate of morbidity and mortality.

The use of combination therapy may increase the probability that an active agent is used for potentially resistant organisms and may result in better outcomes. Combination antibiotics that are used for MDROs are as follows:

- novel beta-lactam–beta-lactamase inhibitor combinations: ceftolozane–tazobactam OR ceftazidime–avibactam
- novel cephalosporin: cefiderocol
- novel carbapenem–beta-lactamase combination: imipenem–cilastatin–relebactam
- polymyxins: polymyxin B and colistin

CANDIDA AURIS

Candida auris can develop resistance quickly and is considered an MDRO to several antifungal classes. It should be considered that the target for initial treatment is with echinocandin such as micafungin. Based on susceptibility breakpoints recognized for other *Candida* species, most *C. auris* isolates have been highly resistant to fluconazole. Voriconazole resistance has been variable (3%–73%), whereas posaconazole, itraconazole, and isavuconazole have displayed better activity. Resistance to amphotericin B has been reported in 13% to 35% of isolates. Patients diagnosed with resistant *C. auris* should be immediately placed on contact precautions; consult the infectious disease team.

▶ TUBERCULOSIS

DISEASE OVERVIEW

Tuberculosis (TB) is now the most common infectious cause of death worldwide. Approximately one third of the world's population is infected with latent TB. In poorly controlled HIV and otherwise impaired immune systems, the annual progression rate from latent to active TB is 10%. Only a small fraction of immunocompetent patients with latent TB progress to active TB. The lifetime risk of progression is 10%. TB is spread by aerosolized droplets from patients with active pulmonary disease. Patients at high risk of TB exposure include immigrants from high-prevalence countries, homeless people, IV drug users, migrant farm workers, and prisoners. If infected, risk of progression to active TB includes HIV/AIDS patients, alcoholic patients, immunocompromised patients, diabetic patients, and patients who have received antitumor necrosis factor agents.

CLASSIC PRESENTATION

Patients with latent TB are often asymptomatic, whereas, in active pulmonary TB, patients frequently present with nonproductive cough of 3 weeks or more in duration, fevers, chills, night sweats, and weight loss. Hemoptysis may also occur. Physical examination findings are often nonspecific in TB (Table 14.4).

Table 14.4 Comparison of Latent and Active TB

	Latent TB	Active TB Disease
Classic presentation	Asymptomatic, but can still spread the bacteria	Symptoms include: ■ Cough for longer than 3 weeks ■ Hemoptysis ■ Chest pain ■ Fever, chills, night sweats ■ Weight loss
Diagnostic criteria	■ + TB test ■ Nucleic acid amplification ■ Chest x-ray ■ Early morning sputum cultures ■ HIV serology in all patients with unknown status ■ CT scan may be helpful	■ + TB test ■ Nucleic acid amplification ■ Early morning sputum culture ■ Chest x-ray ■ HIV serology in all patients with unknown status ■ CT scan may be helpful
Treatment	Treatment is necessary, rifapentine in combination with INH	■ Isolation until three negative cultures (approximately 2–4 weeks) ■ Initial empiric treatment: INH, rifampin, pyrazinamide and with ethambutol or streptomycin ■ Directly observed therapy is recommended.
Complications	May develop active TB disease if left untreated	■ Relapse of the disease ■ Aspergiloma ■ Bronchiectasis ■ Broncholithiasis ■ Fibrothorax ■ Possible carcinoma

TB, tuberculosis; INH, Isoniazid.

DIAGNOSTIC CRITERIA

Sputum via natural cough, induction, or bronchoscopy is the gold standard to diagnose pulmonary TB.

Samples should ideally be cultured in both solid and liquid mycobacterial cultures. A nucleic acid amplification test should be performed on all patients if available. Active pulmonary TB is made with laboratory findings of acid-fast organisms in sputum and/or positive nucleic acid amplification test for *Mycobacterium tuberculosis* complex, plus culture growing of *M. tuberculosis*.

Culture-negative pulmonary TB is diagnosed with active TB symptoms, no alternative diagnosis, and improvement on TB therapy. TB skin testing cannot be used to rule out active TB infections. Latent TB is diagnosed with a positive purified protein derivative (PPD) or interferon-gamma release assay. Interferon-gamma release assay is preferred in patients who had the bacille Calmette-Guerin vaccine.

Respiratory isolation can be removed after three consecutive negative acid-fast bacillus sputum smears collected 8 to 24 hours apart with at least one specimen obtained in the early morning and alternate diagnosis.

TREATMENT/MANAGEMENT

Consult infectious disease specialists to assist with drug prescribing. Commonly, four drug regimens are required to prevent multidrug-resistant TB. The most common antibiotics are a combination of rifampin, isoniazid INH, pyrazinamide, and ethambutol, also referred to as RIPE.

COMPLICATIONS

Complications of TB include hemoptysis, pleurisy, pleural effusion, empyema, pneumothorax, aspergilloma, endobronchitis, bronchiectasis, laryngitis, cor pulmonale, enteritis, miliary TB, and HIV-related opportunistic infections.

▶ HUMAN IMMUNODEFICIENCY VIRUS

DISEASE OVERVIEW

Acute HIV infection may present with influenza-like symptoms or nonspecific symptoms. If there is no suspicion of HIV, then the diagnosis can be missed; therefore, a good history and physical are warranted to make the proper diagnosis. Risk factors include unprotected sexual intercourse, especially receptive anal intercourse; mucosal contact with infected blood; a large number of sexual partners; prior or current sexually transmitted infections (specifically, gonorrhea and chlamydia infections, syphilis, and genital herpes); sharing of IV drug paraphernalia; receipt of blood products prior to 1985 (in the United States); needlestick injuries; and maternal–child HIV infection.

Symptoms vary, but in general, fever, fatigue, and myalgias are the most common symptoms. Additional symptoms include adenopathy, pharyngeal edema, recurrent vaginal or oral thrush, generalized rash, nausea, vomiting, diarrhea, and anorexia with a weight loss averaging 5 kg.

CLASSIC PRESENTATION

A 28-year-old male patient presents with complaints of fever, chills, nausea, and diarrhea. He reports having no appetite for several days. Exam reveals cervical adenopathy and white plaques of the tongue and oral pharynx. Rapid strep test is negative. The AGACNP notes that the patient's arms have what appear to be needle tracks.

DIAGNOSTIC CRITERIA

In early HIV infection, in CD4 T cells, the viral RNA level is typically very high (e.g., greater than 100,000 copies/mL), and the CD4 cell count can drop transiently. The AGACNP should order complete blood count (CBC) with differential and CD4/CD8 count, P24 antigen, HIV 1 and 2 with viral load, comprehensive metabolic panel (CMP), rapid plasma reagin (RPR), herpes simplex virus (HSV), and hepatitis panel including hepatitis A, hepatitis B surface antigen and antibody, hepatitis B core, and hepatitis C.

TREATMENT/MANAGEMENT

Unless an AGACNP specifically works for an infectious disease team, they are not likely to be expected to initiate therapies for HIV. Thus, for patients who are newly diagnosed, consult infectious disease specialists, who are well versed in the ever-changing drug regimens and drug resistance patterns. For patients already diagnosed and on antiretroviral therapies, continue therapy while hospitalized unless the patient is critically ill or does not have a functioning GI tract; then, hold the oral antiretrovirals during this critical illness.

COMPLICATIONS

Oral and esophageal candidiasis is the opportunistic infection most often seen. Other opportunistic infections include cytomegalovirus infection, *Pneumocystis jirovecii* pneumonia, and prolonged, severe cryptosporidiosis.

▶ SUMMARY

AGACNPs treat infectious processes on a daily basis. Early recognition, accurate diagnosis, and precise treatments will save lives and improve outcomes for these patients. Prevention of HAIs is paramount to AGACNP practice. Ensuring catheters are removed as early as possible, minimizing patient time on ventilators, and antibiotic stewardship are key to preventing the most severe HAIs.

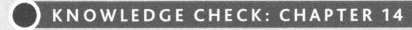

KNOWLEDGE CHECK: CHAPTER 14

1. The most common clinical presentation of catheter-associated urinary tract infection is:

   A. Fever
   B. Malaise
   C. Spasticity
   D. Frequency

2. The AGACNP understands that the cornerstone for catheter-associated urinary tract infection (CAUTI) treatment is:

   A. Amoxicillin
   B. Zosyn
   C. Beta-lactams
   D. Removal of infected catheter

3. A patient is reluctant to have her Foley catheter removed as she has limited mobility to get out of bed. The AGACNP educates her that removal is needed to prevent a catheter-associated urinary tract infection (CAUTI), which can cause:

   A. Sepsis
   B. Chills
   C. Frequency
   D. Dysuria

4. A patient presents with abdominal cramping and six episodes of watery, green diarrhea that has a foul smell. The patient had a 7-day course of levaquin that completed 2 days ago. The AGACNP's most likely diagnosis is:

   A. Rotavirus
   B. *Shigella*
   C. *Escherichia coli*
   D. *Clostridioides difficile* colitis

5. The AGACNP is caring for a patient with *Clostridioides difficile* colitis. The patient complains of increasing abdominal distention, increased abdominal pain. Vital signs: temperature 38.0°C, heart rate (HR) 110, respiratory rate (RR) 20, O_2 Sat 93%. The AGACNP is most concerned the patient is developing:

   A. Toxic megacolon
   B. Hypotension
   C. Murphy sign
   D. Rosving sign

6. The AGACNP understands that hospital-acquired pneumonia (HAP) and ventilator-acquired pneumonia (VAP) are treated differently from community-acquired pneumonia (CAP) because:

   A. VAP and HAP are most likely to be caused by resistant pathogens
   B. CAP is most likely to be caused by resistant pathogens
   C. VAP and HAP are most likely caused by nonresistant pathogens
   D. CAP is more common and more easily spread to hospitalized patients

(See answers next page.)

1. A) Fever

Fever is the most common sign of a catheter-associated urinary tract infection. Malaise, spasticity, and frequency are atypical symptoms found in patients with spinal cord injury.

2. D) Removal of infected catheter

Removal of the infected catheter is the cornerstone of treatment in CAUTI. Amoxicillin, Zosyn, and beta-lactams are not the cornerstone for CAUTI treatment and will build up antibiotic resistance if unnecessarily used.

3. A) Sepsis

Bacteremia, sepsis, and septic shock are severe complications of CAUTI that can lead to significant morbidity and mortality. Frequency, chills, and dysuria are common symptoms of urinary tract infection and CAUTI but are not complications.

4. D) *Clostridioides difficile* colitis

Based on the classic symptoms of profuse watery and green diarrhea that is foul smelling and recently completed course of antibiotics, the most likely diagnosis is *C. difficile* colitis.

5. A) Toxic megacolon

Toxic megacolon, sepsis, and perforation are all complications associated with a high mortality rate. Leukocytosis and hypotension are signs of sepsis. Murphy sign is a clinical finding associated with cholecystitis. Rosving sign is a clinical sign associated with acute appendicitis.

6. A) VAP and HAP are most likely to be caused by resistant pathogens

VAP and HAP are most likely caused by resistant pathogens including methicillin-resistant *Staphylococcus aureus* (MRSA), *Escherichia coli*, *Klebsiella*, *Serratia*, *Stenotrophomonas*, *Burkholderia*, *Pseudomonas*, and *Acinetobacter*. However, community organisms such as *Streptococcus pneumoniae* and *Haemophilus* are not uncommon. CAP is less likely to be caused by resistant pathogens.

7. The AGACNP is caring for a patient admitted with acute respiratory failure due to pneumonia treated with 3 days of ceftriaxone and azithromycin. The patient now has worsening hypoxia and a new infiltrate on chest radiograph. The AGACNP suspects the patient now has:

   A. Community-acquired pneumonia (CAP)
   B. Ventilator-associated pneumonia (VAP)
   C. Hospital-acquired pneumonia (HAP)
   D. Adult respiratory distress syndrome (ARDS)

8. The AGACNP is caring for a patient admitted with acute respiratory failure due to pneumonia treated with 3 days of ceftriaxone and azithromycin. The patient now has worsening hypoxia and a new infiltrate on chest radiograph. The AGACNP should prescribe:

   A. Ceftriaxone and azithromycin
   B. Moxifloxacin and azithromycin
   C. Doxycycline and vancomycin
   D. Cefepime and vancomycin

9. A patient had a Cesarean section 10 days ago and presents with symptoms of peri-incisional pain, tenderness, localized swelling, and erythema to the mid-abdomen. The AGACNP diagnoses the patient with:

   A. Surgical site infection–superficial incision
   B. Surgical site infection–deep incisional
   C. Surgical site infection–organ/space
   D. Cellulitis

10. An adult presents with fever, shaking, chills, and malaise. They deny cough, shortness of breath, nausea, vomiting, and urinary symptoms. Past medical history is significant for hypertension, hyperlipidemia, diabetes mellitus, and sick sinus syndrome for which they had a permanent pacemaker implanted 6 months ago. Upon inspection, the AGACNP notes dark areas on the tip of one finger and under two toenails. Auscultation reveals a murmur. The AGACNP expects which of the following is the causative organism?

    A. *Streptococcus*
    B. *Enterococcus*
    C. *Staphylococcus*
    D. *Corynebacterium*

11. A patient visiting from Africa presents with a persistent fever, cough, and 20-lb weight loss over 2 months. Chest x-ray shows right upper lobe infiltrate with an air–fluid level. CT scan is pending. The AGACNP's first step is to:

    A. Consult infectious disease
    B. Prescribe isoniazid, rifampin, pyrazinamide
    C. Obtain tuberculin skin testing and HIV testing
    D. Place in negative-pressure isolation room

(See answers next page.)

7. C) Hospital-acquired pneumonia

The patient presented with CAP and failed to improve and now has new worsening symptoms and new radiographic evidence of infection more than 48 hours after admission, qualifying the patient for a HAP diagnosis. The patient is not on a ventilator, so VAP is not likely.

8. D) Cefepime and vancomycin

The patient presented with community-acquired pneumonia (CAP) and failed to improve and now has new worsening symptoms and new radiographic evidence of infection more than 48 hours after admission, qualifying the patient for a hospital-acquired pneumonia diagnosis. The patient requires broad-spectrum antibiotics covering gram positives and gram negatives including pseudomonas. Ceftriaxone, azithromycin, moxifloxacin, and doxycycline are all for CAP coverage.

9. A) Surgical site infection–superficial incision

Classic symptoms of the superficial incision are peri-incisional pain or tenderness, localized peri-incisional swelling, peri-incisional erythema or heat, and deep incisional classic symptoms including fever (greater than 38°C) and localized pain. Organ/space includes intra-abdominal infection. While this case presents similarly to cellulitis, in this case the surgical site infection is a more accurate diagnosis.

10. C) *Staphylococcus*

This patient likely has endocarditis related to the cardiovascular implantable electronic device, which can occur up to 12 months after implantation. *Staphylococcus aureus* is the most common organism. Streptococcus is associated with recent upper respiratory infections, whereas enterococcus species originate from the gastrointestinal tract. Corynebacterium is an unusual organism to cause endocarditis.

11. D) Place in negative-pressure isolation room

The highest priority is prompt recognition and detection of cases and prevention of further transmission. The infectious disease team will be consulted, but not before the patient is placed into isolation and appropriate precautions are implemented. African countries have high prevalence of HIV-associated tuberculosis (TB), and HIV testing is indicated along with culture and sensitivity to confirm mycobacterium TB. Multidrug resistances are common; thus, obtaining sensitivities is important but not the highest priority. Treatment of active TB typically begins with four agents due to the high prevalence of multidrug-resistant organisms.

12. A patient admitted with septic shock related to community-acquired pneumonia received the sepsis bundle, including central line placement, fluid resuscitation, vasopressor therapy, and broad-spectrum antibiotics. The patient has weaned off pressors and completed a 7-day course of antibiotics. On hospital day 8, the patient spiked a new fever to 103.3°F (39.6°C), heart rate (HR) 120, respiratory rate (RR) 24, blood pressure (BP) 86/40. Chest x-ray (CXR) shows improved right lower lobe infiltrate, urinalysis shows 1+ hetones, 1+ glucose, 2 white blood count (WBC), no leukocytes or nitrates. Upon exam, the patient is warm and flushed, lungs are clear, abdomen is soft, nontender, nondistended. The most likely cause of this new fever is:

   A. Catheter-related urinary tract infection
   B. *Clostridium difficile*
   C. Catheter-related bloodstream infection
   D. Hospital-acquired pneumonia

13. A frail elderly male patient is admitted after a fall, sustaining right rib fractures, 6 to 10. He is admitted to the ICU for pain control and pulmonary toileting. On hospital day 4, he develops a fever and increased oxygen requirements and requires bilevel positive airway pressure. Repeat complete blood count (CBC) shows a rising white count to 16.5 with a bandemia, up from 11 yesterday. Chest x-ray shows worsening atelectasis with new air bronchograms in the right lower and middle lung fields. The AGACNP diagnoses this as:

   A. Worsening atelectasis
   B. Community-acquired pneumonia (CAP)
   C. Hospital-acquired pneumonia (HAP)
   D. Ventilator-associated pneumonia (VAP)

14. An adult female patient is admitted for severe community-acquired pneumonia. She is dehydrated and receives 2 L lactated Ringer over the first 24 hours. She is on day 3 of ceftriaxone and azithromycin. She is requiring less oxygen. Her blood urea nitrogen (BUN) to creatinine ratio and white blood count (WBC) normalized on hospital day 2. She had three loose stools yesterday and today and is now complaining of abdominal pain. Her WBC is back up to 18,000 mc/L. The AGACNP suspects:

   A. Gastroenteritis
   B. Side effects from antibiotics
   C. Treatment failure of pneumonia
   D. *Clostridioides difficile* infection

15. A culture of a patient in the ICU has just resulted as *Candida auris*. What is the first intervention the AGACNP should take?

   A. Start fluconazole
   B. Start Zosyn and vancomycin
   C. Place patient on contact precautions
   D. Place patient on airborne precautions

(See answers next page.)

12. C) Catheter-related bloodstream infection

Catheter-related bloodstream infection is the most likely cause of this patient's change of condition. The patient has a new episode of sepsis. CXR is improving, urinalysis is negative for infection, and abdominal exam is benign, thus lowering the possibility of catheter-related urinary tract infection, *Clostridium difficile* infection, and hospital-acquired pneumonia.

13. C) Hospital-acquired pneumonia (HAP)

HAP is defined as pneumonia that is not incubating at the time of hospital admission and occurs 48 hours or more after admission. VAP is defined as a pneumonia occurring more than 48 hours after endotracheal intubation. While this patient may have atelectasis, the presence of leukocytosis, bandemia, and air bronchograms are indicative of consolidation or an inflammatory process that is associated with pneumonia. CAP is defined as pneumonia that incubates within 48 hours of admission. The concept of healthcare-associated pneumonia has been removed from HAP and VAP guidelines.

14. D) *Clostridioides difficile* infection

This patient likely has *C. difficile*. Manifestations of *C. difficile* infection include more than three loose stools per day, abdominal pain, and leukocytosis greater than 15,000 mc/L, although patients can have a dynamic ileus, causing no stool. Side effects of antibiotics can cause diarrhea or loose stools; they would not cause a recurrent leukocytosis. Treatment failure of the pneumonia would not demonstrate improved oxygenation. Gastroenteritis is a less likely diagnosis in the inpatient setting.

15. C) Place patient on contact precautions

Candida auris is highly drug resistant. Stopping the spread of this deadly organism is the highest priority. *C. auris* is not airborne and thus does not need airborne precautions. *C. auris* is resistant to fluconazole and requires infectious disease consultation for appropriate antifungal coverage. *C. auris* is a fungal organism, thus Zosyn and vancomycin are not indicated.

KEY BIBLIOGRAPHY

Only key resources appear in the print edition. Access the full bibliography for this chapter on ExamPrepConnect.com.

Centers for Disease Control and Infection. (2021). *Healthcare associated infections (HAIs)*. https://www.cdc.gov/hai/

Johnson, S., Lavergne, V., Skinner, A. M., Gonzales-Luna, A. J., Garey, K. W., Kelly, C. P., & Wilcox, M. H. (2021). Clinical practice guideline by the Infectious Diseases Society of America (IDSA) and Society for Healthcare Epidemiology of America (SHEA): 2021 focused update guidelines on management of *Clostridioides difficile* infection in adults. *Clinical Infectious Diseases, 73*(5), e1029–e1044. https://doi.org/10.1093/cid/ciab549

Kalil, A. C., Metersky, M. L., Klompas, M., Muscedere, J., Sweeney, D. A., Palmer, L. B., Napolitano, L. M., O'Grady, N. P., Bartlett, J. G., Carratalà, J., El Solh, A. A., Ewig, S., Fey, P. D., File, T. M., Restrepo, M. I., Roberts, J. A., Waterer, G. W., Cruse, P., Knight, S. L., & Brozek, J. L. (2016). Management of adults with hospital-acquired and ventilator-associated pneumonia: 2016 clinical practice guidelines by the Infectious Diseases Society of America and the American Thoracic Society. *Clinical Infectious Diseases, 63*(5), e61–e111. https://doi.org/10.1093/cid/ciw353

Kirmani, N., Durkin, M. J., & Liang, S. Y. (2020). *Infectious diseases subspeciality consult*. Washington School of Medicine.

McDonald, L. C., Gerding, D. N., Johnson, S., Bakken, J. S., Carroll, K. C., Coffin, S. E., Dubberke, E. R., Garey, K. W., Gould, C. V., Kelly, C., Loo, V., Sammons, J. S., Sandora, T. J., & Wilcox, M. H. (2018). Clinical practice guidelines for *Clostridium difficile* infection in adults and children: 2017 update by the Infectious Diseases Society of America (IDSA) and Society for Healthcare Epidemiology of America (SHEA). *Clinical Infectious Diseases, 66*(7), e1–e48. https://doi.org/10.1093/cid/cix1085

Rizzo, K., Horwich-Scholefield, S., & Epson, E. (2019). Carbapenem and cephalosporin resistance among Enterobacteriaceae in healthcare associated infections, California, USA. *Emerging Infectious Disease, 25*(7), 1389–1393. https://doi.org/10.3201/eid2507.181938

Endocrine System Review

Al-Zada Aguilar and Helen Miley

▶ INTRODUCTION

The endocrine system is composed of hormone-secreting organs responsible for regulating bodily functions and homeostatic mechanisms. Endocrine gland dysfunction often results in multi-organ dysfunction, resulting in multisystem nonspecific clinical manifestations. A stepwise approach while adhering to overarching and disease-specific diagnostic and treatment principles will improve diagnostic testing accuracy and multimodal management strategies.

▶ DIABETES MELLITUS AND HYPERGLYCEMIA

DISEASE OVERVIEW

The most well-known disorder of dysglycemia, diabetes mellitus (DM) is categorized into types 1 and 2 (Table 15.1). Type 1 DM (DM1) is an autoimmune disorder resulting in pancreatic beta-cell destruction that leads to an absolute insulin deficiency. Type 2 DM (DM2) is the result of inadequate endogenous insulin production and increased insulin resistance leading to impaired glycemic control.

Table 15.1 Characteristics of DM Subtypes

Characteristics	DM1	DM2
Incidence	~10%	~90%
Pathophysiology	Insulin deficiency and ketone production; beta-cells cease insulin production	Excess hepatic gluconeogenesis; beta-cell dysfunction; increased insulin resistance (in muscle cells)
Risk factors	■ High-risk ethnic group (Caucasian) ■ Concomitant autoimmune disease ■ Viral beta-cell destruction (e.g., cytomegalovirus, rubella, adenovirus)	■ High-risk group (African Americans, Hispanic Americans, Native Americans) ■ Concomitant metabolic syndrome ■ Gestational
Age	Younger than 40 years	Older than 40 years
Insulin levels	Diminished	Variable
Autoantibodies	+/−	−
Complications	Microvascular	Macrovascular
Oral agent response	No	Yes

DM, diabetes mellitus; DM1, type 1 diabetes mellitus; DM2, type 2 diabetes mellitus.

CLASSIC PRESENTATION: DIABETES MELLITUS

A 22-year-old male patient with no previous medical history presents to the emergency department (ED) with lethargy, hypotension, and "increased urination." Family history is significant for DM. On physical exam, the patient is lethargic but oriented ×3. He reports "partying" 72 hours previously and drinking "a lot" of alcohol. Vital signs: blood pressure (BP) 80/40, heart rate (HR) 130, respiratory rate (RR) 32, normothermic. Fingerstick blood sugar is 450 mg/dL. Initial workup: pH 7.2, HCO_3 5, glucose

452 mg/dL, lactate 7, blood urea nitrogen (BUN) 35, creatinine 1.8. The patient is started on lactated Ringer solution and insulin infusion protocol. An endocrinologist is consulted given concern for diabetic ketoacidosis (DKA). A positive autoantibody test confirms a diagnosis of DM1.

DIAGNOSTIC CRITERIA
CLINICAL MANIFESTATIONS
Nonspecific findings include fatigue, weakness, weight loss, and paresthesia. Classic findings include the three Ps: polyuria, polydipsia, and polyphagia.

DIAGNOSTIC TESTING
Glycosylated hemoglobin (HgbA$_{1c}$; 5.5%–6.4%) is the gold standard. Adjunct diagnostic tests include fasting plasma glucose and 2-hour post-oral glucose tolerance test. A patient is considered to have DM if HgbA$_{1c}$ is ≥6.5% with a fasting plasma glucose greater than 125 mg/dL on two separate occasions and/or plasma glucose is greater than 200 mg/dL on a 2-hour post-oral glucose tolerance test.

TREATMENT/MANAGEMENT
Optimal inpatient glycemic control (140–180 mg/dL) requires (a) glucose monitoring 4×/day; (b) dietary adherence under nutritionist guidance; and (c) an individualized insulin-centered regimen (Table 15.2).

Table 15.2 Insulin Characteristics: Onset, Peak, and Duration

Insulin Types	Example	Onset	Peak	Duration
Rapid acting	Humalog, Novolog	10–30 mins	30–90 mins	3–5 hours
Short acting	Regular	30–60 mins	2–6 hours	5–8 hours
Intermediate acting	NPH	2–4 hours	6–8 hours	12–15 hours
Long acting	Levemir, Lantus	1–2 hours	4–6 hours	24 hours

NPH, neutral protamine hagedron.

Insulin infusion is the ideal option for optimal glycemic control; however, due to resource limitations, a subcutaneous insulin regimen with basal insulin (50% total daily dose [TDD]) plus a rapid- (or short-) acting insulin analog (50% TDD) is a reasonable alternative (Table 15.3).

Table 15.3 Optimizing Inpatient Glycemic Control

Conditions	Subtype	Recommendations
NPO status (preprocedural or preoperative)	DM1	Do *not* hold insulin or at risk for going into DKA! Half dose long-acting insulin. Use dextrose infusion to prevent hypoglycemia.
	DM2	Stop rapid-/short-acting insulin. Half dose long-acting insulin. Hold metformin (contrast exposure: risk for type B lactic acidosis). Hold thiazolidinediones (if cardiac and/or hepatic issues).
Diet (is eating)	DM2	Use basal *plus* rapid-acting insulin (add and/or adjust). Add adjunct sliding scale. Hold PO anti-hyperglycemic agents.
Insulin-dependent DM (IDDM)	DM1 or DM2	Use long-acting *plus* rapid-acting with meals. Add adjunct sliding scale.
	DM1	Do *not* hold insulin or at risk for going into DKA if held! Use dextrose infusion to prevent hypoglycemia.
Insulin pumps	DM1	*Continue:* if alert, reliable; adequate glycemic control *Hold:* if HHS and/or DKA; switch to insulin infusion; consult endocrinologist

DKA, diabetic ketoacidosis; DM1, type 1 diabetes mellitus; DM2, type 2 diabetes mellitus; HHS, hyperosmolar hyperglycemic syndrome; NPO, nothing by mouth; PO, oral.

There may be conditions that result in more difficult-to-control hyperglycemia. Morning (7 a.m.) hyperglycemia can be divided into two subsets: Somogyi effect and dawn phenomenon (Table 15.4).

Table 15.4 Morning (7 a.m.) Hyperglycemia: Somogyi Effect Versus Dawn Phenomenon

	Somogyi Effect	Dawn Phenomenon
Etiology	Excess basal insulin → 3 a.m. Hypoglycemia → counterregulatory Hormones → increased a.m. glucose	Spiking growth hormone → decreased night Insulin sensitivity → increased a.m. glucose
3 a.m. glucose check	Low	High
Management	▪ Decrease basal insulin dose ▪ Give basal insulin earlier ▪ Switch to shorter-acting basal insulin with decreased dose	▪ Increase basal insulin dose

COMPLICATIONS

Microvascular complications include retinopathy, nephropathy, and the most common, peripheral and autonomic neuropathy. Macrovascular complications include atherosclerotic cardiovascular disease (ASCVD), such as myocardial infarction (MI), cerebral vascular accident, or peripheral arterial disease. Additional complications include immune dysfunction, which can lead to frequent bacterial, fungal, and viral infections as well as impaired wound healing.

▶ HYPERGLYCEMIC EMERGENCIES

DIABETIC KETOACIDOSIS AND HYPEROSMOLAR HYPERGLYCEMIC SYNDROME
DISEASE OVERVIEW

Poorly controlled DM results not only in long-term multisystem microvascular and macrovascular issues but in acute life-threatening hyperglycemic emergencies. DKA occurs because of insulin deficiency (absolute more than relative) causing hyperglycemia and ketone accumulation that leads to high anion gap metabolic acidosis (HAGMA). On the other hand, hyperosmolar hyperglycemic syndrome (HHS) occurs because of insulin deficiency (relative more than absolute) leading to severe hyperglycemia with dehydration and electrolyte imbalances (Table 15.5).

Table 15.5 DKA Versus HHS

Characteristics	DKA	HHS
Risk factors	Usually DM1	Usually DM2, older patient, impaired water access
Signs and symptoms	Kussmaul respirations, "fruity" breath	CNS symptoms (confusion → coma), severe dehydration (e.g., prerenal azotemia)
Serum glucose	Greater than 250 mg/dL	Greater than 600 mg/dL
pH	Less than 7.30	Greater than 7.30
Serum HCO_3	Less than 15 mEq/L	Greater than 15 mEq/L
Anion gap	Greater than 12	Variable
Serum osmolarity	Less than 320 mOsm/kg	Greater than 320 mOsm/kg
Ketones	Positive in serum and/or urine	Trace or small

CNS, central nervous system; DKA, diabetic ketoacidosis; DM1, type 1 diabetes mellitus; DM2, type 2 diabetes mellitus; HHS, hyperosmolar hyperglycemic syndrome.

CLASSIC PRESENTATION: HYPEROSMOLAR HYPERGLYCEMIC SYNDROME

A 50-year-old patient with obesity with no previous medical history presents to the ED after being found at home on the floor. The patient is lethargic and protecting the airway; it is unclear how long they have been this way. Initial vital signs: BP 80/60, HR 140, RR 32, temperature (T) 98°F. Initial workup: pH 7.25, glucose 1309 mg/dL, Na^+ 140 mEq/L, K^+ 5.0 mmol/L, BUN 65 mg/dL, creatinine 4.0, osmolarity 403 mOsm/kg, lactate 5.0, creatine phosphokinase 21,000. Urinalysis is negative for ketones but concerning for a urinary tract infection (UTI). The patient is aggressively hydrated, started on insulin infusion protocol, and given antibiotics. A diagnosis of HHS complicated by rhabdomyolysis with severe acute renal failure and UTI is made.

DIAGNOSTIC CRITERIA

Hyperglycemic emergencies present with the three Ps as well as nonspecific symptoms (e.g., nausea, vomiting, abdominal pain, weakness, malaise). Hyperglycemia with an HAGMA is *not always* DKA; the AGACNP must evaluate for other causes of HAGMA.

TREATMENT/MANAGEMENT

Treatment of hyperglycemic crises (Table 15.6) has significant overlap, but there are also distinct differences when managing DKA versus HHS. When addressing hyperglycemic crises, it is pivotal to address the underlying triggers (Table 15.7).

Table 15.6 Treatment of Hyperglycemic Crises

Management	Description
Replenish free water deficit; restore hemodynamics	Administer isotonic fluids (watch Na^+, HCO_3^-, glucose)
Normalize glucose	Start with insulin bolus (0.15 unit/kg) then infusion (0.1 unit/kg/hr) Transition to SQ long-acting (e.g., Lantus) *plus* rapid-acting (e.g., Novolog) once anion gap closes (in DKA) or serum osmolarity less than 320 mOsm/kg (in HHS)
Address electrolyte and acid-base disorders	Replete K^+ and phosphate (PO_4) Metabolic acidosis: $NaHCO_3$ supplement only if pH less than 6.90, refractory decreased BP, and/or increased K^+-associated arrhythmias
Identify and treat triggers	See Table 15.7.
Treatment endpoints	DKA: Improve glucose (150–200 mg/dL); close anion gap
	HHS: Improve glucose (200–300 mg/dL) and serum osmolarity (less than 320 mOsm/kg)

BP, blood pressure; DKA, diabetic ketoacidosis; HHS, hyperosmolar hyperglycemic syndrome; SQ, subcutaneous.

Table 15.7 Triggers of Hyperglycemic Emergencies ("Is" Mnemonic)

Trigger	Description
Infraction (noncompliance; 25%)	Medication (e.g., missed insulin) and/or diet
Infection (40%)	Pneumonia, UTI, gastroenteritis, skin/soft tissue
Infarction	Myocardial infarction
Inflammation	Pancreatitis
Illness (severe acute)	Pulmonary embolism, trauma, intra-abdominal
Iatrogenic	Corticosteroids, SGLT-2 inhibitors; surgery
Infant (pregnancy)	Gestational DM
Illicit (drugs)	Cocaine, excessive alcohol intake
Idiopathic (unknown)	

DM, diabetes mellitus; UTI, urinary tract infection.

COMPLICATIONS

Common complications are electrolyte/acid-base abnormalities. Less common ones are cerebral or pulmonary edema, venous thromboembolism, and rhabdomyolysis (in HHS).

HYPOGLYCEMIA
DISEASE OVERVIEW

Hypoglycemia is a syndrome of low plasma glucose levels, most commonly a complication of diabetic agents (e.g., oral antihyperglycemic agents, insulin) and malnutrition, especially in those with underlying DM. Non-DM–associated conditions (e.g., sepsis, end-stage renal disease, cirrhosis, advanced heart failure, adrenal insufficiency [AI], systemic lupus erythematosus, insulinoma, nesidioblastosis) that cause hypoglycemia are rare. Medications associated with hypoglycemia include quinolones, pentamidine, quinine, and beta-blockers.

CLASSIC PRESENTATION

A 68-year-old patient with previous history of hypothyroidism and DM2 who is taking glipizide presents with confusion and lethargy. Workup includes negative CT scan of the head, normal thyroid-stimulating hormone (TSH), vitamin B_{12}, folate, ammonia, and noninfectious urinalysis. The patient is found to have a blood sugar of 48 mg/dL and is given parenteral 50% dextrose (D50) with transient improvement in mental status. However, the patient has recurrent hypoglycemia with confusion and lethargy.

CLINICAL MANIFESTATIONS

- Surge in autonomic activity (glucose less than 60 mg/dL): anxiety, hunger, nausea, palpitations, paresthesia, diaphoresis, and tremulousness
- Central nervous system (CNS) symptoms (glucose less than 50 mg/dL): blurred or double vision, confusion, difficulty speaking, and headache to seizures or coma. *Stroke must be ruled out.*

DIAGNOSTIC CRITERIA

- Plasma glucose less than 60 mg/dL along with clinical findings that improve post dextrose administration
- Additional workup includes plasma C-peptide, insulin, and proinsulin levels.

TREATMENT/MANAGEMENT

If patient is conscious, 15 g carbohydrates can be administered orally two times, but if the hypoglycemia is persistent, parenteral dextrose should be administered. If the patient is unconscious, one ampule of D50 with consideration for continuous parenteral dextrose can be administered. Glucose should be checked at least 15 to 20 minutes after each intervention to evaluate for efficacy. The underlying cause should also be investigated.

COMPLICATIONS

Complications include seizures, dysrhythmias, and even cardiac arrest.

▶ ADRENAL INSUFFICIENCY

DISEASE OVERVIEW

AI is an endocrine disorder characterized by destruction or dysfunction of the hypothalamic–pituitary–adrenal axis leading to absolute or relative glucocorticoid (GC) and mineralocorticoid deficiency. AI is classified based on area of dysfunction: primary AI (PAI; adrenal) or secondary AI (SAI; pituitary and/or hypothalamus). Addison disease is the most common cause of PAI. Other less common causes include infections (e.g., HIV, cytomegalovirus, tuberculosis) and adrenal disorders (e.g., hemorrhage, hyperplasia, metastases). The most common cause of SAI is exogenous GC use. Less common causes include opioids, immune checkpoint inhibitors, etomidate, anticonvulsants, and anticoagulants.

CLASSIC PRESENTATION

A 45-year-old patient with no previous medical history presents to the ED with a 3-day history of fevers, myalgias, and malaise. The patient reports a 13-month history of unintentional 30-lb weight loss, intermittent abdominal discomfort, lethargy, and skin darkening. Vital signs: BP 80/40, HR 120. Body mass index is 18. Workup: Na$^+$ 128 mEq/L, K$^+$ 5.2, creatinine 1.7, HbA1C 6.4, normal thyroid function tests. Morning cortisol 5 mcg/dL with adrenocorticotropic hormone (ACTH) 120 pg/mL and ACTH-stimulated cortisol 8 mcg/dL.

DIAGNOSTIC CRITERIA

Common manifestations (e.g., fatigue, dizziness, weight loss) are nonspecific and therefore lead to misdiagnoses and/or diagnostic delays (Tables 15.8 and 15.9).

Table 15.8 Clinical Manifestations of AI

Findings	Description
General	■ Hyponatremia ■ Fever ■ Neuropsychiatric (e.g., depression, impaired memory, delirium) ■ Reproductive dysfunction (e.g., reduced libido, axillary/pubic hair, amenorrhea in female patients)
PAI	Due to mineralocorticoid deficiency: ■ Postural hypotension, GI (e.g., abdominal pain, diarrhea), salt craving, hyperkalemia Due to ACTH stimulation → increased melanocyte-stimulating hormone: ■ Hyperpigmentation
SAI	Due to ACTH suppression → decreased melanocyte-stimulating hormone: ■ Hypopigmentation

ACTH, adrenocorticotropic hormone; AI, adrenal insufficiency; GI, gastrointestinal; PAI, primary adrenal insufficiency; SAI, secondary adrenal insufficiency.

Table 15.9 Diagnostic Criteria for AI

Steps	Description/Results
1. Check morning cortisol level (before 9 a.m.)	Cortisol less than 5 mcg/dL = likely AI Cortisol 5–14 mcg/dL = check ACTH or cosyntropin stimulation test Cortisol greater than 14 mcg/dL = less likely AI
2. Cosyntropin or ACTH stimulation test (before 9 a.m.; if cortisol 5–14 mcg/dL)	***Gold standard confirmatory test*** 250 mcg synthetic ACTH, check cortisol 30 and 60 minutes after ACTH given: Cortisol less than 16 mcg/dL at 30 minutes, less than 18 mcg/dL at 60 minutes = likely AI Cortisol greater than 18 mcg/dL at 30 or 60 minutes = less likely AI
3. ACTH levels (once AI confirmed)	ACTH greater than 100 pg/mL = PAI ACTH less than 10 pg/mL = SAI
4a. PAI workup (once PAI confirmed)	Aldosterone (low/normal), renin (high) = PAI Rule out autoimmune disorders: check autoantibodies (e.g., 21-hyroxylase), CT adrenal glands Rule out genetic conditions in male patients: check very long–chain fatty acids
4b. SAI workup (once SAI confirmed)	Rule out pituitary gland issues: thyroxine, ADH, MRI

ACTH, adrenocorticotropic hormone; ADH, antidiuretic hormone; AI, adrenal insufficiency; PAI, primary adrenal insufficiency; SAI, secondary adrenal insufficiency.

TREATMENT/MANAGEMENT

■ Hydrocortisone (15–25 mg/d) is considered first-line GC replacement in those with AI; those with SAI (15–20 mg/d) require less than those with PAI (20–25 mg/d).

■ Dexamethasone and prednisolone are alternatives; however, they are less preferred for long-term use due to increased risk for metabolic syndrome and iatrogenic Cushing syndrome.

■ PAI also requires mineralocorticoid replacement (i.e., fludrocortisone 0.05–0.25 mg/dL).

■ Patients with AI should be familiar with "sick day rules"—GC dosing recommendations during inter-current illness (e.g., infection, gastrointestinal losses) and/or stressors (e.g., exercise, procedures, surgery, trauma) to prevent adrenal crisis (Table 15.10).

Table 15.10 The 5S's of Acute AI (Adrenal Crisis) Management

Treatment Strategy	Description
Salt replacement	Aggressive resuscitation with isotonic fluids (3–6 L/d) Monitor volume status, urinary excretion, Na^+ levels Encourage Na^+ consumption, especially in suspected PAI
Sugar replacement	Add dextrose in continuous infusion given high risk for hypoglycemia (e.g., from infection, nausea, vomiting)
Steroid replacement	Parenteral hydrocortisone 100 mg then total 200 mg/24 hour (infusion more than bolus) Taper within 24–72 hours post-recovery (*if prolonged exogenous steroid use previously, will require gradual taper*)
Supportive care	ABCDEs (airway, breathing, circulation, disability, exposure) Continuous monitoring, treat comorbidities, and address electrolyte, fluid, and nutritional imbalances
Seek and treat precipitants	Address triggers of the crisis (expect improvement in 24 hours; if not, evaluate alternative causes)

AI, adrenal insufficiency; HCT, hydrocortisone; PAI, primary adrenal insufficiency.

COMPLICATIONS

The most life-threatening AI complication is adrenal crisis, which results in refractory shock due to inadequate cortisol production. The most common trigger is sepsis—specifically, gastroenteritis. Other triggers include surgeries, injuries, life stressors, extreme temperatures, medication noncompliance, and failure to observe sick day rules. If untreated, it can lead to death. Other complications from long-term GC use include metabolic syndrome, bone metabolism dysfunction (e.g., osteoporosis, fracture), neuropsychiatric disorders, decreased quality of life, and death.

▶ PRIMARY ALDOSTERONISM/HYPERALDOSTERONISM

Primary aldosteronism (PA) is the most common potentially treatable cause of endocrine-associated secondary hypertension (HTN). PA occurs due to autonomous aldosterone hypersecretion from one or both adrenal glands, despite hypokalemia and intravascular volume expansion.

CLINICAL MANIFESTATIONS

PA's classic triad is HTN, hypokalemia, and (hypochloremic) metabolic alkalosis.

CLASSIC PRESENTATION: PRIMARY ALDOSTERONISM

A 60-year-old patient presents with a 30-year history of HTN, obstructive sleep apnea on continuous positive airway pressure (CPAP), and HTN nephropathy (chronic kidney disease, Stage 3b) with proteinuria. Since the HTN diagnosis, the patient has never had adequate BP control. They have had frequent hospitalizations with HTN with severe hypokalemia. The patient is compliant with their multidrug BP regimen. Despite this, the BP remains uncontrolled (160/90 mmHg). Secondary HTN workup is negative except for low renin (plasma renin activity [PRA] 0.5 ng/mL/h), elevated aldosterone (PAC 16 ng/dL), and elevated ARR (35 ng/dL per ng/mL/h), suggestive of PA.

DIAGNOSTIC CRITERIA

Diagnosis of PA involves three phases: (a) screening, (b) confirmatory testing, and (c) subtype classification or lateralization testing (Table 15.11).

Table 15.11 Screening Indications, Screening, and Confirmatory Tests for PA

Screening Indications	
Sustained HTN greater than 150/100 mmHg (measured on 3 different days)	
HTN: severe or resistant (greater than 130/80 or greater than 140/90 to three antihypertensive drugs; including a diuretic) or controlled (less than 140/90 mm Hg) requiring four or more antihypertensive drugs	
HTN with family history of early-onset HTN or CVA (less than 40 years old)	
Hypertensive first-degree relatives of patients with PA	
HTN with hypokalemia (spontaneous or diuretic-induced, including on low-dose thiazide diuretics), adrenal incidentaloma, and/or OSA	
Screening Tests	**PA**
PAC (1–14 ng/dL)	PAC greater than 15 ng/dL
PRA (greater than 1 ng/mL/hr) or DRC (greater than 10 pg/mL)	PRA less than 1 ng/mL/hr *or* DRC less than 10 pg/mL
PAC/PRA ratio or ARR (less than 30 ng/dL per ng/mL/hr)	ARR greater than 30 ng/dL per ng/mL/hr
Confirmatory Tests	
1. Oral salt loading with urinary aldosterone 2. Saline infusion with PAC 3. Fludrocortisone suppression with PAC 4. Captopril challenge with PAC and renin activity	

ARR, aldosterone–renin ratio; CVA, cerebrovascular accident; DRC, direct renin concentration; HTN, hypertension; OSA, obstructive sleep apnea; PA, primary aldosteronism; PAC, plasma aldosterone concentration; PRA, plasma renin activity.

Subtype classification or lateralization testing involves adrenal imaging and adrenal vein sampling (AVS). The purpose of adrenal imaging includes (a) differentiation between unilateral and bilateral disease, (b) ruling out adrenocortical carcinoma, and (c) providing mapping for proceduralists. Selective AVS is the gold standard (greater than 95% diagnostic accuracy) for PA subtyping or localizing causes of PA.

TREATMENT/MANAGEMENT
- Laparoscopic unilateral adrenalectomy: gold standard treatment for unilateral PA
- Mineralocorticoid antagonists (spironolactone 25–400 mg/d or eplerenone 25–400 mg/d): for patients unable or unwilling to have surgery with unilateral PA or for patients with bilateral PA

COMPLICATIONS
Patients with PA have higher rates of adverse cardiovascular (e.g., ASCVD, MI, congestive heart failure, arrhythmias), cerebrovascular (e.g., stroke), and renal-associated (e.g., chronic kidney disease) morbidity and mortality compared with age- and sex-matched patients with essential HTN or independent of BP control.

▶ PHEOCHROMOCYTOMA

DISEASE OVERVIEW
Pheochromocytoma (Table 15.12) is caused by excess catecholamine release (norepinephrine and epinephrine) from an adrenal medullary tumor. Triggers include intravenous (IV) contrast dye, anesthesia, trauma, surgery, and medications (e.g., monoamine oxidase inhibitors [MAOIs], selective serotonin reuptake inhibitors [SSRIs], stimulants, decongestants, corticosteroids).

Table 15.12 Clinical Manifestations of Pheochromocytoma

Clinical Manifestations	Incidence (%)
Hypertension (paroxysmal or sustained; *hypertensive crisis = hallmark*)	80
Clinical triad: palpitations, severe headache, (profuse) diaphoresis	~60
Nonspecific spells (e.g., sense of impending doom, visual disturbances, paresthesia, nausea, tachypnea, angina)	~60
Multisystem crisis: severe hyper- or hypotension, ARDS with cardiac, liver, and/or renal dysfunction or failure	rare

ARDS, acute respiratory distress syndrome.

CLASSIC PRESENTATION

A 28-year-old patient with no previous medical history presents to the ED with acute onset of headache, chest pain, and panic attack. Vital signs: BP 190/110, HR 140 and regular, RR 38, afebrile. Physical exam: S_3 gallop, jugular vein distention, and coarse crackles. Lab tests are unrevealing. Nitroglycerin drip is started; the patient has minimal response and so is switched to a nicardipine drip, with better response. Secondary HTN workup is unrevealing except for plasma metanephrines greater than 3× upper limit of normal (ULN) and 24-hour urine metanephrines greater than 135 mcg/g creatinine. He undergoes a CT abdomen, confirming an adrenal tumor.

DIAGNOSTIC CRITERIA

- Plasma metanephrines greater than 3× ULN (97% sensitivity)
- Confirmatory testing with 24-hour urine metanephrines (97% sensitivity)
- Additional adjunct testing: serum chromogranin A, plasma catecholamines, and clonidine suppression test
- Imaging: CT or MRI of adrenal gland (greater than 90% sensitivity and specificity) in detecting adrenal pheochromocytoma (greater than 0.5 cm); nuclear imaging with 1 to 123 iodine meta-iodobenzylguanide (MIBG) or gallium-68 should be considered

TREATMENT/MANAGEMENT

Treatment of choice is a surgical resection of the catecholamine-releasing tumor. Medical management involves BP optimization (less than 140/90 mm Hg supine) with use of alpha-blockers such as doxazosin or phenoxybenzamine (selective more than nonselective to minimize risk of hypotension) as first-line, and Dihydropyridine Calcium Channel Blockers (DH-CCBs; e.g., amlodipine) as adjuncts. Beta-blockers (e.g., labetalol, metoprolol, esmolol) are helpful with arrhythmia control; their use is limited given (a) increased risk for unopposed alpha-stimulation leading to worsening HTN, (b) interference with biochemical testing, and (c) decreased tumor uptake of radioisotopes. Therefore, BP needs to be adequately controlled with alpha-blockers and/or DH-CCBs prior to initiating beta-blockers.

COMPLICATIONS

Complications include hypertensive emergency or shock (paroxysm), multisystem crisis, or pheochromocytomatosis, a surgical complication in which metastatic cells seed the peritoneum, leading to recurrent intra-abdominal tumors.

▶ SYNDROME OF INAPPROPRIATE ANTIDIURETIC HORMONE

DISEASE OVERVIEW

Syndrome of inappropriate antidiuretic hormone (SIADH) is a disorder of persistent vasopressin (i.e., ADH) secretion without osmotic or hemodynamic stimulus characterized by euvolemic hyponatremia (Table 15.13) and impaired urinary dilution without renal disease. Causes of SIADH include drugs (e.g., antiepileptics, vasopressin analogs, SSRIs, tricyclic antidepressants, venlafaxine, ecstasy); CNS disorders (e.g., brain tumor, infections, stroke); malignancy (e.g., small cell lung, gastrointestinal, head and neck, hematologic malignancy); pneumonia (bacterial or viral); and uncontrolled postsurgical or procedural pain and/or nausea.

Table 15.13 Clinical Manifestations of Hyponatremia

Onset	Severity	Signs and Symptoms
Chronic (greater than 48 hours or unclear duration)	Mild to moderate	Minimally symptomatic: headache, fatigue, nausea
	Moderate to severe	Headache, fatigue, nausea, vomiting, confusion, muscle weakness, cognitive impairment and decline, gait instability, falls, Ca^{2+} stones
Acute (less than 48 hours)	Mild to moderate	Nausea, vomiting, headache
	Severe	Vomiting, confusion, hallucinations, seizures, respiratory arrest, coma (Glasgow Coma Scale score ≤8), signs and symptoms of increased intracranial pressure (e.g., decerebrate posturing), death

CLASSIC PRESENTATION

A 55-year-old patient with previous medical history of DM2, HTN, chronic tobacco use (100+ pack-years), and depression on venlafaxine presents with 3-week history of progressive fatigue and dizziness. Initial BP is 80/50. The patient has no neurologic focal deficits. The patient's spouse died 4 months ago, and since then, that patient has had decreased oral intake with an unintentional 20-lb weight loss. Initial workup: Na^+ 115 mEq/L, urine Na^+ 80 mmol/L, urine osmolality 600 mOsm/kg. The patient is given 2 L of IV 0.9 normal saline and has improved BP (130/80) and Na^+ (118 mEq/L). The patient's hyponatremia is thought to be hypovolemic from poor oral intake and SIADH from the venlafaxine. Stopping the venlafaxine and restricting free water intake do not resolve this issue. Given the tobacco use, the patient undergoes a CT chest showing a 4-cm left upper lobe mass, confirming a lung malignancy–induced SIADH.

DIAGNOSTIC CRITERIA

As a type of euvolemic hyponatremia with impaired urinary dilution, SIADH must be differentiated from other forms of hyponatremia (isotonic [or pseudo-hyponatremia], hypotonic, hypertonic; Table 15.14).

Table 15.14 Criteria for SIADH

Main Criteria	Supportive Criteria
Hyponatremia (≤134 mEq/L)	Hypouricemia (uric acid less than 4 mg/dL)
Low serum osmolality (less than 275 mOsm/kg)	Fractional excretion of Na^+ (FeNa) greater than 1%
Urine osmolality greater than 100 mOsm/kg (concentrated urine)	Fractional excretion of urea (FeUrea) greater than 55%
Urine Na^+ greater than 40 mmol/L	Fractional excretion of uric acid (FeUA) greater than 10%
Urine greater than serum osmolality	Worsened hyponatremia with IV 0.9 NS
Clinical euvolemia (no edema)	Decreased BUN less than 10 mg/dL
Normal thyroid and adrenal function	

(continued)

Table 15.14 Criteria for SIADH (*continued*)

Main Criteria	Supportive Criteria
Absence of advanced kidney disease, heart failure, and cirrhosis	Inappropriate vasopressin, copeptin despite hypotonicity and/or euvolemia

BUN, blood urea nitrogen; NS, normal saline; SIADH, syndrome of inappropriate antidiuretic hormone.

TREATMENT/MANAGEMENT

Inpatient management of hyponatremia should be based on (a) presence or absence and severity of symptoms, (b) chronicity and risk for osmotic demyelination syndrome, and (c) determination of and addressing of the underlying cause. If clinical manifestations are mild to moderate, initial treatment includes fluid restriction and increasing solute load with use of NaCl or urea tabs. If these interventions are not successful in improving Na$^+$, then vaptans such as IV conivaptan (20 mg bolus, then 20- to 40-mg infusion/24 hours) and oral tolvaptan (7.5–60 mg/d) are reasonable alternatives. If clinical manifestations are severe, rapid correction with 3% NaCl (bolus or continuous infusion) may be warranted (increased Na$^+$ ≤ 4–6 mEq until symptoms resolve; ≤8 mEq/24 hours or ≤18 mEq/48 hours).

COMPLICATIONS

Cerebral osmotic dysregulation or rapid overcorrection of Na$^+$ (i.e., osmotic demyelination syndrome; greater than 10 mEq/24 hours) leading to cerebral edema is a potential complication.

▶ DIABETES INSIPIDUS

DISEASE OVERVIEW

Diabetes insipidus (DI) is a form of polyuria–polydipsia syndrome characterized by hypotonic polyuria (excessive urination greater than 50 mL/kg/24 hours and urine osmolality less than 300 mOsm/kg) and polydipsia (excessive drinking greater than 3 L/day). Acquired forms are much more common (~90%) than hereditary (or familial) forms of DI (less than 10%). DI subtypes include central, nephrogenic, dipsogenic (or primary polydipsia), and gestational (Table 15.15).

Table 15.15 Differentiating Polyuria–Polydipsia Syndromes

	Primary Polydipsia (Dipsogenic DI)	Central DI	Nephrogenic DI	Gestational DI
Defect	Abnormally low thirst threshold with excessive thirst	Deficiency in AVP synthesis or secretion from pituitary gland	Decreased renal response to antidiuretic effect of arginine vasopressin	Increased placental vasopressinase levels
Causes	Psychosis intermittent hyponatremia–polydipsia syndrome, compulsive water drinking	Trauma, malignancy, vascular, granulomatous, infectious, inflammatory, autoimmune, drug or toxin, idiopathic, genetic	Drug (e.g., lithium, demeclocycline), hypercalcemia, hypokalemia, infiltrative, vascular, mechanical	Pregnancy, especially with complications (e.g., HELLP, preeclampsia)

AVP, arginine vasopressin DI, diabetes insipidus.

CLASSIC PRESENTATION

A 40-year-old 70-kg male patient with previous history of depression controlled by sertraline (Zoloft) initially presents to the primary care provider for headache, increased polyuria (15 times per day), and thirst (prompting him to drink 5 L of water per day). His headache has been worsening despite use of over-the-counter medications. A 24-hour urine collection confirms 4 L urine/24 hours. Further workup shows HbA1C 5.5, serum osmolality 300 mOsm/kg, serum Na$^+$ 148 mEq/L, urine osmolality 200 mOsm/kg, urine specific gravity 1.003 (normal is 1.005–1.030):

- *intact thirst mechanism:* polyuria (greater than 50 mL/kg in a 24-hour period), polydipsia, increased thirst
- *inadequate compensation for polyuria:* dehydration, hypotension, neurologic dysfunction (mild: cognitive dysfunction, irritability; severe: seizure, lethargy, coma, focal neurologic deficits)

DIAGNOSTIC CRITERIA

Diagnosis involves (a) obtaining history of present illness and history, (b) evaluating for polyuria, (c) checking for plasma and urine osmolality, (d) checking plasma Na$^+$, and (e) water deprivation testing (Table 15.16).

Table 15.16 Differentiating Polyuria–Polydipsia Syndromes Based on Biochemical Testing

	Primary Polydipsia	Central DI	Nephrogenic DI	Gestational DI
Sodium	Low	High	High	Normal/high normal
Serum osmolality	Low/normal	High	High	High
Urine osmolality	Normal	Low	Low	Low
Urine osmolality	Normal	High	Low	Water deprivation test recommended

DI, diabetes insipidus.

TREATMENT

See Table 15.17.

Table 15.17 Treatment of DI

Steps	Description	
1. Correct water deficits	Acute: Correct Na$^+$ $\leq$1 mEq/h Chronic: Correct Na$^+$ $\leq$0.5 mEq/h Use enteral and/or parenteral hypotonic fluids (e.g., 0.45 NaCl greater than D5W)	
2. Treat underlying condition	Central DI	DDAVP (intranasal greater than oral; parenteral if decreased consciousness)
	Nephrogenic DI	Lithium-induced: diuretics (amiloride, HCTZ, acetazolamide) Electrolyte-induced: normalize Ca^{2+} and/or K$^+$ Adjunct: low Na$^+$ diet, NSAIDs *Watch for renal dysfunction!*
	Dipsogenic DI	Cognitive behavioral intervention Clozapine
	Gestational DI	DDAVP (intranasal greater than oral; parenteral if decreased consciousness)

D5W, detrose 5% in water; DDAVP, desmopressin; DI, diabetes insipidus; HCTZ, hydrochlorothiazide.

COMPLICATIONS

Severe and rapid dehydration leading to hyperosmolality, hypernatremia, renal dysfunction, hypovolemic shock, and, potentially, death. Hyponatremia with risk for osmotic demyelination syndrome during Na$^+$ correction is another major complication in patients with chronic central DI on long-term desmopressin.

▶ THYROID DISORDERS

THYROIDITIS

Thyroiditis is a group of inflammatory thyroid disorders that may cause hypo- or hyperthyroidism. Types include autoimmune (or Hashimoto), painful subacute, infectious (suppurative), painless postpartum/sporadic subacute, and Reidel (Table 15.18).

Table 15.18 Comparison of Thyroiditis

Type	Etiology	Clinical Findings	Diagnostic Findings	Treatment
Autoimmune	Dietary, iodine, autoimmune disorder, occupational, exposure, smoking	Chronic fatigue, Sjogren syndrome, myasthenia gravis symptoms, depression	Increase TSH, increased anti-thyroglobulin Ab, increased anti-thyroperoxidase Ab, no detectable antithyroid Ab US = diffuse heterogenous, decreased echogenicity	See treatment for hypothyroidism or hyperthyroidism
Painful subacute	Viral URI, younger woman	Fevers, pain Hallmark sign: tender thyroid gland with painful dysphagia	Increased ESR, decreased antithyroid Ab US = normal/decreased vascularity, radioiodine update = very low	ASA (drug of choice) ± steroids, treat transient hyperthyroidism → hypothyroidism
Infectious	Immunocompromised, nonviral	Fevers, pain	Increased ESR, increased WBC US = normal/decreased vascularity, swelling, abscess formation, FNA with gram stain and culture	Antimicrobials ± drainage
Painless postpartum/ sporadic subacute	DM1, pregnancy, family history of Hashimoto thyroiditis	No palpable goiter	US = normal/decreased vascularity	Treat transient hyperthyroidism (1–6 months) → hypothyroidism (4–8 months)
Reidel	Autoimmune thyroiditis; middle-aged or older female patient	Enlarged asymmetric, hard, fixed, with dysphagia, pain due to compression of esophagus and/or trachea	Increased ESR, increased anti-thyroglobulin Ab, increased anti-thyroperoxidase Ab, RAI uptake low, biopsy with fibrin + eosinophilic infiltrates	Tamoxifen, steroids, rituximab if refractory to tamoxifen and/or steroids

DM1, type 1 diabetes mellitus; ESR, erythrocyte sedimentation rate; ESR, erythrocyte sedimentation rate; FNA, fine needle aspiration; RAI, radioactive iodine; TSH, thyroid-stimulating hormone; URI, upper respiratory infection; US, ultrasound; WBC, white blood count.

Thyroiditis can often cause hypothyroidism or hyperthyroidism. Autoimmune thyroiditis is the most common cause of hypothyroidism; Graves disease is the most common cause of hyperthyroidism (Table 15.19).

Table 15.19 Body System–Based Clinical Manifestations in Hypothyroidism and Hyperthyroidism

Body System	Hypothyroidism	Hyperthyroidism
Neuropsychiatric	Lethargy, fatigue, weakness Delirium, psychosis Depression, flat affect Paresthesias Memory impairment Slow deep tendon reflexes	Hyperactivity Delirium/hyper-delirium Insomnia
HEENT	Puffy face and eyelids	Eyelid lag and retraction Ophthalmopathy*
Cardiopulmonary	Exertional dyspnea Decreased HR, increased BP Pericardial effusion (rare) Pleural effusion (late) Peripheral edema	Increased HR (palpitations, A-fib) Widened pulse pressure High-output heart failure
Gastrointestinal	Constipation	Loose stools/diarrhea
Metabolic	Hypothermia/cold intolerance Weight gain	Fevers/heat intolerance/sweating Weight loss
Musculoskeletal/integumentary	Arthralgias or myalgias Hair thinning, brittle nails Skin pallor	Muscle weakness or cramps Osteoporosis Symmetric flaccid paralysis Pretibial myxedema (i.e., Graves dermopathy)* Thyroid acropachy*
Miscellaneous	Menorrhagia	

*More common in smokers.
BP, blood pressure; HEENT, head, eyes, ears, nose, throat; HR, heart rate.

HYPOTHYROIDISM AND HYPERTHYROIDISM

Classic Presentation: Hypothyroidism

A 70-year-old patient with obesity with unknown previous medical history is found unresponsive in their home after a welfare check by the police. A friend saw the patient the day before and stated that they had exertional dyspnea. The patient's Glasgow Coma Scale (GCS) score is 4, and the patient is subsequently intubated for airway protection. Initial vital signs before intubation: T 90°F, BP 80/40, RR 10, SpO_2 80% on room air. Exam: absent deep tendon reflexes; only withdraws to pain. The patient is given IV fluid boluses, cultured, and started on antibiotics. Initial workup: Na^+ 125, BUN 70, creatinine 2.6, HCO_3 8, K^+ 5.4, glucose 136, lactate 5.0, white blood cells 20. Follow-up workup: negative CT head and urine drug screen, high thyroid stimulating hormone (TSH), low free T_4/T_3 (FT_4/FT_3). Plasma free metanephrines normal. Cortisol level is 10.

Diagnostic Testing

Diagnosis of hypo- and hyperthyroidism involves checking TSH, FT_4, and radioactive iodine thyroid scan (Table 15.20).

Table 15.20 Differentiating Thyroid Disorders Based on Biochemical Testing

Thyroid Disorder Subtypes	Diagnostic Findings
Primary hypothyroidism (thyroid dysfunction)	Increased TSH, decreased T_4
Secondary hypothyroidism (pituitary dysfunction)	Decreased TSH, decreased T_4
Tertiary hypothyroidism (hypothalamic dysfunction)	Decreased TRH, decreased TSH, decreased T_4

(continued)

Table 15.20 Differentiating Thyroid Disorders Based on Biochemical Testing (*continued*)

Thyroid Disorder Subtypes	Diagnostic Findings
Thyroiditis, ectopic thyroid hormone	Decreased TSH, increased T_4, low uptake RAI scan
Graves disease, toxic goiter or adenoma	Decreased TSH, increased T_4, high uptake RAI scan

RAI, radioactive iodine; TRH, thyrotropin-releasing hormone; TSH, thyroid stimulating hormone.

Treatment
See Table 15.21.

Table 15.21 Treatment/Management of Hypothyroidism and Hyperthyroidism

Treatment	Hypothyroidism	Hyperthyroidism
General ***First-line treatment	***Levothyroxine (LT4): check TSH 4–6 weeks Start lower dose in stable CAD and/or age older than 60 years: increased risk of angina, ACS, arrhythmia, or clinical hyperthyroidism	***Propranolol ***Thiourea drugs (methimazole greater than PTU) [watch for cytopenias] Lithium Radioactive iodine therapy Thyroid surgery
For severe cases	**Myxedema Coma**	**Thyrotoxic crisis ("Thyroid storm")**
	Levothyroxine IV *Hypothermia:* do not warm quickly (decreased BP) *Decreased Na⁺: avoid* hypotonic solutions, use 0.9% or 3% NaCl *Decreased glucose:* use fluids with dextrose *Volume overload:* diuretics (loop greater than thiazide given decreased Na⁺) *Hypercapnic respiratory failure:* monitor use of sedatives/opioids (decreased metabolism with prolonged effects) → respiratory support *AI:* hydrocortisone IV	Beta-blockers Thiourea agents Iodine preparations (e.g., sodium iodine, Lugol solution) *AI:* hydrocortisone IV (inhibit T4 → T3 conversion, improve adrenal axis dysfunction) *Hyperthermia:* acetaminophen, *avoid* NSAIDs and ASA (interfere with T_4 and thyroid-binding globulin → worsen hypermetabolism)

AI, adrenal insufficiency; ASA, acetylsalicylic acid (aspirin); IV, intravenous; NSAID, nonsteroidal anti-inflammatory drug; PTU, propylthiouracil

Complications
Hypothyroidism-related complications include sepsis (e.g., bacterial pneumonia), ASCVD, HTN, and in its most life-threatening and severe form, myxedema coma. Hyperthyroidism-related complications include tachyarrhythmias, orbitopathy, angina, Graves dermopathy, severe thyroid acropachy, and in its most life-threatening and severe form, thyrotoxic crisis or "thyroid storm."

▶ SUMMARY

Patients who are admitted for management of acute illness or exacerbation of chronic illnesses may have endocrine conditions that are preexisting or the primary reason for admission. AGACNPs must be knowledgeable about managing diabetic and endocrine-related conditions to improve patient outcomes. Restarting or continuing home diabetic medications in the acute care setting should be a priority when it is medically safe to do so. It is critical to master the transition between IV and subcutaneous or oral agents. Identifying and treating symptoms of complications related to these conditions and their associated treatments is essential to prevent untoward events or death.

KNOWLEDGE CHECK: CHAPTER 15

1. A 70-year-old male patient with a previous medical history of bacterial pneumonia 2 weeks ago presents with generalized weakness. He is otherwise asymptomatic. Lab work shows: Na^+ 118 mEq/L, serum osmolarity of 270 mOsm/kg, and urine osmolality of 170 Osm/kg. How should this patient be treated?

   A. Begin 3% normal saline and increase the Na level by 2 mEq/L per hour
   B. Begin normal saline and increase the Na level by 15 mEq/L over the next 24 hours
   C. Initiate 1-L daily fluid restriction and salt tabs (1 g NaCl twice per day)
   D. Do nothing and monitor because the patient is asymptomatic

2. A 25-year-old 7-day postpartum female patient presents with a fever of 104°F, diaphoresis, agitation, and diarrhea. Thyroid storm is suspected. Which agent should be *avoided* in this patient?

   A. Acetylsalicylic acid (ASA)
   B. Propranolol
   C. Acetaminophen
   D. Propylthiouracil (PTU)

3. A 70-year-old male patient with previous medical history of coronary artery disease (CAD) presents with a 3-month history of unintentional weight gain, fatigue, memory impairment, and severe constipation. Workup reveals a high thyroid-stimulating hormone and low FT_4. The AGACNP begins low-dose levothyroxine because they are concerned about which potential complication from initiating treatment?

   A. Hypercapnic respiratory failure
   B. Volume overload
   C. Angina
   D. Hyponatremia

4. The AGACNP is caring for a 40-year-old female patient with previous medical history of type 1 diabetes mellitus (DM1) admitted for *Escherichia coli* urinary tract infection now complicated by difficult-to-control glucose levels. It has been difficult to manage this patient's glucose over the past 48 hours, with periods of hyperglycemia and hypoglycemia occurring. The AGACNP reviews the chart and notes the following blood sugars:

   Day 1: 7 a.m. (380), 11 a.m. (300), 6 p.m. (289), 11 p.m. (300)

   Day 2: 3 a.m. (40), 7 a.m. (344), 11 a.m. (285), 6 p.m. (290), 11 p.m. (300)

   Insulin regimen: Lantus 30 units nightly, Lispro 8 units 3×/day before meals, Lispro sliding scale before meals and nightly. Based on these findings, the AGACNP decides to:

   A. Increase Lantus to 35 units nightly
   B. Discontinue Lantus
   C. Increase Lantus to 40 units nightly
   D. Administer Lantus 30 units earlier in the evening

(See answers next page.)

1. C) Initiate 1-L daily fluid restriction and salt tabs (1g NaCl twice per day)

This patient has syndrome of inappropriate antidiuretic hormone (SIADH) with euvolemic hyponatremia, a complication of the bacterial pneumonia. If there were severe central nervous system symptoms, 3% NaCl should be started in order to increase Na^+ $\leq$4 to 6 mEq over 4 hours until symptoms resolve. The goal is Na^+ $\leq$ 8 mEq/24 hours or $\leq$18 mEq/48 hours. 0.9% NaCl may worsen hyponatremia in SIADH, so this is not an ideal choice of fluids. Monitoring is appropriate; however, the patient is still symptomatic, although mild. Additionally, because symptoms are chronic (more than 48 hours), Na^+ should be corrected slowly. In those with mild chronic symptoms, initial treatment should include fluid restriction and increasing solute load with NaCl or urea tablets.

2. A) Acetylsalicylic acid (ASA)

In thyroid storm, ASA or other NSAIDs should be avoided because they interfere with T_4 and thyroid-binding globulin, which worsens hypermetabolism in this syndrome. Propranolol and PTU are the mainstay of management. Acetaminophen is a safe option for addressing hyperthermia in this patient.

3. C) Angina

When initiating levothyroxine, caution should be taken with patients who are older than 60 years and/or have stable CAD given increased risk for cardiac manifestations such as angina, acute coronary syndrome (ACS), arrhythmias, and clinical hyperthyroidism. Hypercapnic respiratory failure, volume overload, and hyponatremia are complications that may occur in untreated and/or severe hypothyroidism leading to myxedema coma.

4. D) Administer Lantus 30 units earlier in the evening

This is likely a Somogyi effect. The patient developed nocturnal hypoglycemia (40 mg/dL) at around 3 a.m., which then stimulated a surge of counterregulatory hormones that raise blood sugar, resulting in elevated early-morning (7 a.m.) glucose levels. The Lantus dosage is likely too high and will probably need to be decreased and/or adjusted to a shorter-acting basal regimen to avoid nocturnal hypoglycemic episodes. Appropriate steps would include decreasing the Lantus dosage and/or moving it to earlier evening or even switching to a shorter-acting agent such as Levemir. This is not dawn phenomenon. Dawn phenomenon occurs as a result of decreased sensitivity to insulin at night due to growth hormone, which spikes at night. There is usually progressive hyperglycemia, not a period of hypoglycemia nocturnally. Increasing the bedtime dose of Lantus could potentially worsen nocturnal hypoglycemia and may cause a worsening paradoxical rise in early-morning glucose. Unfortunately, this patient has DM1 and needs insulin (i.e., basal + rapid-acting) at all times, so this basal insulin should not be omitted; at most, its dosage can be decreased in half, even if the patient is nothing by mouth (NPO).

5. The adult gerontology acute care nurse practitioner (AGACNP) is called to evaluate a 38-year-old male patient with obesity and a previous medical history of hypertension who presents with fatigue, nausea, vomiting, polyuria, and unintentional 10-lb weight loss. Initial vital signs: blood pressure (BP) 80/50, heart rate (HR) 130 (sinus tachycardia), respiratory rate (RR) 24. Workup reveals glucose 628 mg/dL, pH 7.15, K^+ 5.4 mEq/L, HCO_3^- 12 mEq/L, elevated serum ketones. The AGACNP orders 2 L 0.9 NaCl bolus. Repeat vital signs: BP 120/70, HR 95, RR 22. The AGACNP should then order:

   A. Lantus 20 units subcutaneously (SQ) ×1 dose immediately (STAT)
   B. Novolog 10 units SQ ×1 dose STAT
   C. $NaHCO_3$ 50 mEq ampule ×1 dose STAT
   D. Novolin 10 units intravenous push (IVP) ×1 dose STAT

6. The AGACNP is called to evaluate a 60-year-old patient with previous medical history of type 2 diabetes mellitus (DM2) who presents to the ED after a 3-day history of polyuria, polydipsia, and progressive disorientation with increasing periods of lethargy. Workup: glucose 780 mg/dL, serum osmolarity 325 mOsm/kg, pH 7.32, HCO_3^- 17, $PaCO_2$ 28. Thyroid-stimulating hormone, free T_4, and morning cortisol levels are normal. There is no ketonuria. Which of the following is the *most* likely diagnosis?

   A. Diabetic ketoacidosis (DKA)
   B. Hyperosmolar hyperglycemic syndrome (HHS)
   C. Myxedema coma
   D. Adrenal crisis

7. A 45-year-old male patient with a previous medical history of type 1 diabetes mellitus (DM1) and nephrolithiasis presents with left-sided flank pain and hematuria. Workup reveals obstructing left ureteral stone. His sugars (ACHS) over the past 24 hours have been ranging from 80 to 200 mg/dL. His current insulin regimen includes Lantus 30 units daily, Novolog 4 units TID, Novolog sliding scale. He is NPO today for cystoscopy and ureteral stent placement. The nurse calls the AGACNP asking for orders regarding the patient's sugars and insulin regimen. The AGACNP should provide the nurse with which of the following orders?

   A. Hold Lantus and Novolog TID, continue Novolog sliding scale
   B. Hold Lantus, continue Novolog TID and sliding scale
   C. Continue Lantus, hold Novolog TID and sliding sale
   D. Administer half dose of Lantus, hold Novolog TID, continue Novolog sliding scale, start D5 0.9 NaCl at 50 mL/hr while NPO

8. A 55-year-old female patient with previous medical history of hypertension, hyperlipidemia, and type 2 diabetes mellitus (DM2) on metformin and Januvia presents with confusion and lethargy. Workup includes negative CT head, normal thyroid-stimulating hormone, vitamin B_{12}, folate, ammonia, and a noninfectious urinalysis. Chest x-ray (CXR) shows no acute pulmonary disease. The patient is found to have a blood sugar of 48 mg/dL. The AGACNP should then order which of the following?

   A. 1 ampule of D50 intravenous push (IVP)
   B. 8 ounces of orange juice (24 g of sugar)
   C. 2 graham crackers (10 g of sugar)
   D. D5W infusion at 100 mL/h

(See answers next page.)

5. D) Novolin 10 units intravenous fluid ×1 dose STAT

Given the metabolic acidosis (pH less than 7.30, HCO_3^- less than 15 mEq/L), hyperglycemia (600 mg/dL), and serum positive ketones with the clinical presentation, this patient is likely in diabetic ketoacidosis (DKA). DKA management initially involves attempting to replenish free water deficit and, in this case, restoring hemodynamics (which was accomplished). The next step would be to initiate glucose normalization. Glucose normalization typically involves parenteral insulin, typically with a bolus (0.15 unit/kg) followed by an infusion (0.1 unit/kg/hr), *not* subcutaneous insulin (e.g., Lantus, Novolog). The basal and rapid-acting insulin regimen (i.e., Lantus and Novolog) is typically initiated only after the anion gap has closed in patients with DKA after receiving parenteral insulin (i.e., Novolin or regular insulin). $NaHCO_3$ supplementation may be a consideration in patients with severe metabolic acidosis (pH less than 6.90), refractory hypotension, and/or hyperkalemia-induced arrhythmias. In this case, the patient had a pH greater than 6.90 with hyperkalemia that did not result in arrhythmias along with hypotension that resolved after fluid resuscitation. Therefore, the most appropriate next step is Novolin 10 units IVP ×1 dose STAT.

6. B) Hyperosmolar hyperglycemic syndrome (HHS)

Neurologic changes such as disorientation, lethargy, seizures, stupor, or even coma are usually the most obvious presenting signs often associated with HHS, more so than with DKA. Additionally, it is more likely to be HHS than DKA given the glucose greater than 600 mg/dL, pH greater than 7.30, HCO_3^- greater than 15 mEq/L, and lack of ketones in the urine. Myxedema coma and adrenal crisis are both unlikely given normal biochemical testing (thyroid function tests and cortisol, respectively).

7. D) Administer half dose of Lantus, hold Novolog TID, continue Novolog sliding scale, start D5 0.9 NaCl at 50 mL/hr while NPO

The patient has DM1 or insulin-dependent DM (IDDM). Those with DM1 or IDDM have absolute insulin deficiency and therefore require insulin at all times; otherwise, they are at high risk of going into diabetic ketoacidosis. Their basal or long-acting insulin (i.e., Lantus) should not be held, even if they are NPO and/or going for a procedure. The patient's rapid-acting insulin (i.e., Novolog) should be held as he is NPO. His Lantus dose should be halved. The rapid-acting sliding scale can be continued to prevent hyperglycemia. Fluids with dextrose can also be initiated to prevent hypoglycemia.

8. A) 1 ampule of D50 intravenous push

The patient has symptomatic hypoglycemia (glucose less than 50 mg/dL) with central nervous system symptoms. Treatment of hypoglycemia depends on level of consciousness. Enteral supplementation is appropriate if the patient is conscious and/or alert enough. However, given her lethargy and therefore high risk for aspiration, an enteral approach would not be appropriate. Administration of D5W infusion can be considered to prevent recurrence of hypoglycemia, but this needs to be treated more quickly because untreated hypoglycemia can progress to coma or even cardiac arrest. Administration of an ampule of D50 can normalize a patient's glucose levels and sensorium in minutes and mitigate any further deterioration.

9. A 70-year-old male patient with obesity and previous medical history of coronary artery disease (CAD) with stents, hypertension , and type 2 diabetes mellitus (DM2) is admitted for non-ST-segment elevation myocardial infarction (NSTEMI). A rapid response team is called around 4 p.m. for increasing confusion and difficulty speaking after a bout of diaphoresis and nausea. Per the patient's primary nurse's report, his last meal was likely before 12 midnight because he had to be NPO for his cardiac catheterization today. The AGACNP asks for a STAT glucose fingerstick and an ampule of D50 with the anticipation that the patient's glucose will be less than:

   A. 80 mg/dL
   B. 70 mg/dL
   C. 60 mg/dL
   D. 50 mg/dL

10. A 70-year-old female patient with unknown medical history was found unresponsive in her home. Her friend saw her the day before and states that she had exertional dyspnea. Upon arrival, she was obtunded, so she was intubated for airway protection. Pre-intubation vital signs: temperature 90°F, blood pressure (BP) 80/40 mm Hg, respiratory rate (RR) 10, SpO$_2$ 80% RA. Exam: sluggish but reactive pupils, absent deep tendon reflexes (DTR)s, and withdrawal to pain. Code sepsis was called so she was given intravenous (IV) fluids, cultured, and started on antibiotics. Workup: glucose 100 mg/dL, Na$^+$ 125, blood urea nitrogen 70, creatinine 2.6, HCO$_3$ 8, K$^+$ 5.4, lactate 5.0, white blood count (WBC) 20, thyroid-stimulating hormone (TSH) 146 (high), free T$_4$ (FT$_4$) less than 0.4 (low), plasma free metanephrines normal. Cortisol 10. CT head and urine drug screen are negative. The AGACNP's *most* appropriate next step would be to:

    A. Start 0.45 NaCl infusion at 150 mL/hr
    B. Place patient on warming blanket STAT to normalize temperature within 5 minutes
    C. Give levothyroxine (LT$_4$) 100 mcg IV STAT
    D. Give 10 units Novolin IV STAT

11. A 25-year-old female patient with a previous medical history of thyroiditis on levothyroxine is admitted to the hospital after a 2-month history of nausea, vomiting, decreased PO intake, and unintentional 20-lb weight loss. She is very thin with skin hyperpigmentation. Vital signs: blood pressure (BP) 80/50 mmHg, heart rate (HR) 120 bpm. Labs: glucose 100, blood urea nitrogen (BUN) 25, creatinine 1.4, Na$^+$ 129 mEq/L, K$^+$ 5.2 mEq/L. She is given 2 L of 0.9 NaCl. Repeat vital signs: BP 90/55 mmHg, HR 115 bpm. CT scan of abdomen is negative. Infectious workup is negative to date. Other pertinent labs include thyroid-stimulating hormone (TSH) 1.05 (normal), cortisol 2 (low), plasma metanephrines normal. The AGACNP's *most* appropriate next step would be to:

    A. Give hydrocortisone (HCT) 100 mg intravenous push (IVP) STAT
    B. Give levothyroxine (LT4) 100 mcg IVP STAT
    C. Give methimazole 60 mg PO STAT
    D. Initiate D5W infusion at 150 mL/hr

12. A 30-year-old male patient with previous medical history of depression and anxiety presents for further evaluation after a 4-month history of worsening fatigue, lack of concern, and social isolation. He was initially diagnosed by his primary care provider and psychiatrist with difficult-to-control depression as his symptoms worsened despite a trial of multiple antidepressants. He was then urged by his family to seek out another opinion. Exam relevant for thin-appearing male patient with areas of skin hyperpigmentation. Vital signs: blood pressure (BP) 90/50 mmHg, heart rate (HR) 110 bpm, afebrile. Workup: Na$^+$ 130 mEq/L, K$^+$ 4.9 mmol/L, thyroid-stimulating hormone (TSH) normal, plasma metanephrines normal, AM cortisol 2 mcg/dL, adrenocorticotropic hormone (ACTH) 200 pg/mL, aldosterone low, renin high. Based on these clinical findings, the AGACNP anticipates that this patient will require which of these medications in the long term?

    A. Spironolactone 25 mg PO twice per day (BID)
    B. Methimazole 10 mg PO twice per day (BID)
    C. Hydrocortisone 25 mg PO total daily dose, fludrocortisone 0.1 mg daily
    D. Hydrocortisone 15 mg PO total daily dose

(See answers next page.)

9. D) 50 mg/dL

Clinical manifestations of hypoglycemia are typically categorized into two subtypes: surge in autonomic activity and central nervous system (CNS) symptoms. Autonomic activity, such as adrenergic activation, increased cortisol, glucagon, and growth hormone secretion, as well as decreased insulin secretion, occurs once plasma glucose is less than 60 mg/dL. Clinical findings include nausea, diaphoresis, and tremulousness. On the other hand, CNS symptoms such as confusion and difficulty speaking occur due to insufficient glucose to the brain when plasma glucose is less than 50 mg/dL. This patient initially had a glucose of less than 60 mg/dL given findings of surge in autonomic activity resulting in nausea and diaphoresis. However, his glucose decreased to less than 50 mg/dL given his CNS symptoms of confusion and difficulty speaking.

10. C) Give levothyroxine (LT_4) 100 mcg IV STAT

Patient has profoundly elevated TSH and depressed FT4. In addition, she has objective data such as profound hypothermia, bradycardia, and encephalopathy (obtundation) that were likely precipitated by an infection. This patient has severe hypothyroidism—in this case, myxedema coma. Levothyroxine (LT_4) replacement is the most appropriate treatment. Clinical findings are not suggestive of hyperthyroidism. Her cortisol is also slightly lower than expected but is still within acceptable range. A cosyntropin or adrenocorticotropic hormone stimulation test can be completed for confirmation if there is concern for a concomitant adrenal crisis. Her presentation is less likely a pheochromocytoma given normal plasma free metanephrines. Those with myxedema crisis who are hypothermic should be warmed *slowly* because faster warming can precipitate cardiovascular collapse. Dextrose-filled solutions are appropriate in these patients because they tend to be hypoglycemic. This patient is euglycemic, so insulin would be inappropriate and would potentially make her hypoglycemic. These patients also tend to be hyponatremic; therefore, hypotonic solutions would *worsen* hyponatremia. The AGACNP would need to administer isotonic solution (0.9 NaCl) and in some cases hypertonic fluids (3% NaCl or D5W with $NaHCO_3$) to those who are severely hyponatremic.

11. A) Give hydrocortisone (HCT) 100 mg IVP STAT

The patient is in adrenal crisis. She has clinical manifestations consistent with adrenal insufficiency (AI) such as gastrointestinal (GI) symptoms, unintentional weight loss, skin hyperpigmentation, hyponatremia, and hyperkalemia. She also has hypotension that is partially responsive to isotonic fluid administration. Therefore, initiation of high-dose steroids such as HCT is the most appropriate next step. The patient is unlikely to have hypothyroidism given her physical exam findings and normal TSH, so LT_4 administration is not appropriate. Although clinical findings (i.e., weight loss, tachycardia) may be suggestive of hyperthyroidism, it is unlikely given the patient's normal TSH; therefore, methimazole administration is also inappropriate. The patient does have hyponatremia that is likely hypovolemic from her GI losses. Patients with AI, specifically adrenal crisis, are at risk for hypoglycemia, and therefore infusions with dextrose are appropriate. However, the patient is also hyponatremic, so a hypotonic infusion (i.e., 0.45% NaCl, D5W) would be inappropriate as it would worsen her clinical picture.

12. C) Hydrocortisone 25 mg PO total daily dose, fludrocortisone 0.1 mg daily

This patient likely has primary adrenal insufficiency (PAI). His clinical findings of worsening fatigue, difficult-to-control depression, thin frame, skin hyperpigmentation, and low-normal BP are suggestive of this. Biochemical confirmation of PAI was also confirmed with a low morning cortisol, high ACTH, low aldosterone, and high renin levels. It is less likely hyperthyroidism given the normal TSH, and therefore, methimazole would be inappropriate. Given the normal-high K^+, low aldosterone, and high renin with relative hypotension, primary aldosteronism (PA) is highly unlikely, and therefore, spironolactone would be inappropriate. First-line treatment for AI is hydrocortisone. Total daily dosing is typically higher in those with PAI than with SAI given absolute cortisol deficiency. Moreover, those with PAI may also have concurrent mineralocorticoid deficiency that contributes to hyperkalemia, hyponatremia, and hypovolemia, which is a possibility in this patient, warranting treatment with fludrocortisone. Therefore, hydrocortisone with fludrocortisone would be the most appropriate long-term treatment for this patient.

13. A 48-year-old female patient with obesity and previous medical history of coronary artery disease (CAD), essential hypertension (HTN), type 2 diabetes mellitus (DM2), and obstructive sleep apnea (OSA) on continuous positive airway pressure (CPAP) is admitted to the hospital for atypical chest pain and uncontrolled HTN (blood pressure [BP] greater than 220/110 mmHg) with associated headache and dizziness. She reports poorly controlled BP (systolic BP [SBP] greater than 160 mmHg) over the past month despite being controlled on four medications: HCTZ 50 mg daily, amlodipine 10 mg daily, lisinopril 20 mg daily, and labetalol 200 mg 2× daily. She reports medication, Na^+ restricted diet, and CPAP compliance. She denies any recent life stressors. She is started on a nicardipine drip that slowly controls her BP. Heart rate (HR) 45 to 55 bpm. Workup: creatinine 1.2, K^+ 3.0 mmol/L, HCO_3 30 mEq/L, plasma aldosterone concentration (PAC) 20 ng/dL (high), plasma renin activity 0.5 ng/mL/h (low), aldosterone–renin ratio (ARR) 40 ng/dL per ng/mL/hr (high), HbA1C 7.5, normal thyroid-stimulating hormone (TSH), cortisol, and plasma metanephrines. CT adrenal glands confirm bilateral adrenal hyperplasia. Given these findings, the AGACNP should order which of the following to improve her BP regimen?

A. Adding doxazosin 4 mg PO daily

B. Adding spironolactone 25 mg PO 2× daily

C. Surgical consultation for evaluation of adrenalectomy

D. Increasing labetalol to 400 mg 2× daily

14. A 60-year-old female patient with a previous medical history of hypertension presents with a 2-hour history of chest pain with palpitations, nausea, diaphoresis, and severe headache. Blood pressure (BP) is initially 160/90 mmHg. Initial workup shows elevated troponin, EKG with ST depression inferolateral leads. D-dimer, pro-B-type natriuretic peptide (BNP), renal and liver function tests, and electrolytes are all normal. The patient undergoes a cardiac catheterization without evidence of CAD. Post-procedure BP is 230/110 mmHg, HR 110 bpm. Nicardipine drip is started, resulting in improvement in BP to 180/90 mmHg. Computer tomograpgy angiography (CTA) of chest and abdomen is negative for dissection or pulmonary embolism but incidentally shows a right adrenal mass. Further biochemical workup: normal cortisol, thyroid-stimulating hormone, elevated plasma metanephrines. To safely wean the patient off the nicardipine drip, the AGACNP should order:

A. Propranolol 40 mg PO 2× daily

B. Labetalol 100 mg PO 3× daily

C. Doxazosin 4 mg PO daily

D. Metoprolol tartrate 50 mg PO 2× daily

15. A 75 year-old female with previous medical history of fibromyalgia on duloxetine, type 2 diabetes mellitus (DM2), and hypertension presents with abdominal pain and constipation. She has nausea but no emesis, and no dysuria, polyuria, polydipsia, or polyphagia. CT abdomen and pelvis are negative for any acute pathology. She appears euvolemic on exam. Lab workup: HbA1C 7.0, glucose 150, HCO_3 24, Na^+ 118 mEq/L, thyroid-stimulating hormone (TSH) 2.5 mIU/L, cortisol 20 mcg/dL, and serum osmolality 250 mOsm/kg. Arterial blood gas (ABG) pH 7.39, $PaCO_2$ 40. Urine studies: no ketones, trace glucose, Na^+ 75 mmol/L, and osmolality 400 mOsm/kg. Which of the following is the *most* likely diagnosis?

A. Diabetic ketoacidosis (DKA)

B. Diabetes insipidus (DI)

C. Syndrome of inappropriate antidiuretic hormone (SIADH)

D. Hyperosmolar hyperglycemic syndrome (HHS)

(See answers next page.)

13. B) Adding spironolactone 25 mg PO 2× daily

Given the patient's resistant hypertension requiring four medications for adequate control, hypokalemia, metabolic alkalosis (also known as the clinical triad for primary aldosteronism [PA]), elevated ARR and PAC with suppressed renin, the patient likely has PA. She also has confirmed bilateral adrenal disease based on CT findings. Bilateral adrenal disease is typically treated with mineralocorticoid receptor (MR) antagonists such as spironolactone or eplerenone, whereas unilateral disease involves a unilateral adrenalectomy. Adrenalectomy is not appropriate for this patient given the presence of bilateral disease; therefore, there is no need for a surgical consultation. Thus, adding spironolactone to her BP regimen would be the most appropriate step. Because this patient has normal plasma metanephrines, pheochromocytoma is unlikely, and therefore, a selective alpha-blocker is not appropriate. Increasing labetalol would be inappropriate because the patient has bradycardia, and it would further lower her HR.

14. C) Doxazosin 4 mg PO daily

Given the clinical triad of palpitations, diaphoresis, and severe headache along with severe (paroxysmal) hypertensive crisis requiring nicardipine infusion for BP control, the presence of an adrenal mass, and elevated plasma metanephrines, this patient likely has a pheochromocytoma. Her pheochromocytoma is likely contributing to her symptoms and will ultimately require a unilateral adrenalectomy for treatment. In the interim, BP optimization requires either alpha-blockers such as doxazosin or DH-CCBs such as amlodipine. Beta-blockers (e.g., labetalol, metoprolol) are helpful with arrhythmia control; however, their use is limited in those with pheochromocytoma given (a) increased risk for unopposed alpha-stimulation leading to worsening hypertension, (b) interference with biochemical testing, and (c) decreased tumor uptake of radioisotopes. Therefore, BP needs to be adequately controlled with alpha-blockers and/or DH-CCBs prior to initiating beta-blockers.

15. C) Syndrome of inappropriate antidiuretic hormone (SIADH)

Given the patient's history of chronic pain and being on a selective serotonin reuptake inhibitor (SSRI), she is more likely to develop SIADH. In addition to being clinically euvolemic, she has diagnostic findings consistent with SIADH: hyponatremia (Na^+ 118 mEq/L), hypo-osmolality (250 mOsm/kg), elevated urine Na^+ (75 mmol/L), and concentrated urine (urine osmolality 400 mOsm/kg) with urine osmolality greater than serum osmolality. Additionally, TSH and cortisol are normal, ruling out hypothyroidism and adrenal insufficiency as causes of her hyponatremia. She also has no polyuria or hypernatremia, making DI unlikely. Her glucose and acid-base are normal with lack of ketonuria and the 3P's of hyperglycemic emergencies (polyuria, polyphagia, and polydipsia), making DKA or HHS unlikely.

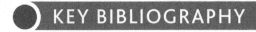

KEY BIBLIOGRAPHY

Only key resources appear in the print edition. Access the full bibliography for this chapter on ExamPrepConnect.com.

Else, T., & Hammer, G. D. (2019). Disorders of the adrenal cortex. In G. D. Hammer & S. J. McPhee (Eds.), *Pathophysiology of disease: An introduction to clinical medicine* (8th ed.). McGraw Hill.

Garg, R. K., Hennessey, J. V., Malabanan, A. O., & Garber, J. R. (2020). *Handbook of inpatient endocrinology.* Springer Publishing Company. https://doi.org/10.1007/978-3-030-38976-5

Llahana, S., Follin, C., Yedinak, C., & Grossman, A. (Eds.). (2019). *Advanced practice in endocrinology nursing.* Springer Publishing Company. https://doi.org/10.1007/978-3-319-99817-6

Papadakis, M. A., McPhee, S. J., & Rabow, M. W. (2021). *Current medical diagnosis & treatment.* McGraw-Hill Education.

Vanek, C., & Loriaux, L. (Eds.). (2021). *Endocrine emergencies: Recognition and treatment* (2nd ed.). Springer Publishing Company.

Musculoskeletal System Review

Karen Pawelek, Kelly Esborn, and Roxanne M. Buterakos

▶ INTRODUCTION

Orthopedic problems are a common reason patients seek care. Musculoskeletal problems are classified as traumatic or atraumatic and acute or chronic. A detailed history is essential to determining the etiology of the symptoms. Eliciting key symptom descriptions for musculoskeletal pain provides clues to the diagnosis. For example, a "locking" sensation of a joint suggests an internal joint problem, whereas a "give way" suggests a ligament injury.

A thorough musculoskeletal physical examination includes inspection, palpation, range of motion (active and passive), strength, and neurovascular exam. Document the presence or absence of swelling, erythema, atrophy, deformities, asymmetry, and/or surgical scars. This information assists in developing differential diagnoses.

The AGACNP should be familiar with specific tests that are key for evaluating the underlying cause of a patient's pain. For example, a positive ipsilateral straight leg raise test is consistent with sciatic pain. There are a variety of special tests for each musculoskeletal problem that can help to increase or decrease the likelihood ratio of a diagnosis if positive. These special tests are listed within each diagnosis in this chapter.

▶ UPPER EXTREMITY

DEQUERVAIN SYNDROME/TENOSYNOVITIS
DISEASE OVERVIEW
DeQuervain syndrome is a common tendonitis (also called tenosynovitis) of the two tendons of the first extensor compartment tendon sheath on the dorsal of the wrist. This sheath acts like a hollow straw that the tendons pass through. As these tendons slide back and forth within the sheath, they can rub against the distal edge of the extensor retinaculum, creating friction that leads to inflammation. Patients complain of pain on the thumb side of the wrist. This pain can radiate up the thumb side of the distal forearm. A sensitive and specific test, the Finklestein test, can be performed.

CLASSIC PRESENTATION
A 55-year-old woman presents to the urgent care center with a complaint of right-sided wrist and thumb pain at the base of the styloid of the radius. Pain is referred up her forearm. She states that she works in a shipping warehouse and has packaged boxes daily for the past 2 years. She described the pain as "achy" and "sharp" with certain movements. She denies any numbness or tingling but notes that her grip strength is weakened.

DIAGNOSTIC CRITERIA
Physical exam reveals a positive Finkelstein test on the right. This is performed by having the patient place their thumb in the palm of their hand and then wrap their fingers around their thumb to make a fist with their thumb tucked inside. Have the patient tilt their wrist toward their pinky finger. This will re-create the pain.

TREATMENT/MANAGEMENT

Standards of care are rest, nonsteroidal anti-inflammatory drugs (NSAIDs), and immobilization of the thumb and wrist (with a thumb spica splint). This conservative management often will cure the condition. In cases where symptoms persist, a cortisone shot into the first extensor tendon sheath is the next step and is almost always curative.

COMPLICATIONS

Ultimately, complications would be failure to improve with conservative management. At that time, surgical treatment is an option to release the sheath around the tendons. It is typically effective but not without the risks associated with surgery.

SCAPHOID FRACTURE
DISEASE OVERVIEW

Carpal bone fractures are often missed. The scaphoid carpal bone is the carpal bone most commonly fractured (Figure 16.1). The palmar branch of the radial artery supplies blood to the scaphoid's distal pole, so accurate assessment and management is imperative. The mechanism of injury is classically a fall on an outstretched hand.

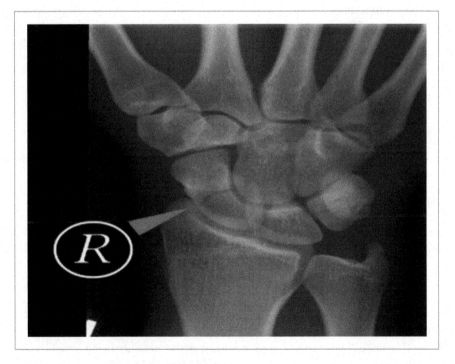

Figure 16.1 Scaphoid fracture

Source: Sjoehest, C. C. (2018). BY-SA 3.0 https://creativecommons.org/licenses/by-sa/3.0, via Wikimedia Commons. https://commons.wikimedia.org/wiki/File:Scaphoidfraktur_1_pfeil.jpg

CLASSIC PRESENTATION

A 23-year-old man presents approximately 24 hours after a mechanical fall on the outstretched right hand. Since the fall, the patient endorses that he has pain in the radial aspect of the right wrist proximal to the right thumb (snuff box). He also endorses decreased grip strength.

DIAGNOSTIC CRITERIA

Snuff box tenderness demonstrates sensitivity of 90% and specificity of 40% for a scaphoid fracture. Standard radiographs (posteroanterior [PA], lateral, oblique) plus scaphoid are typically performed. Standard x-rays may miss this fracture. Radiographs may be repeated in 7–10 days, or a CT scan or MRI can be performed. An MRI is considered the gold standard for definitive diagnosis.

TREATMENT/MANAGEMENT

Although this is the most common carpal fracture, up to 16% of initial radiographs fail to detect a fracture. Therefore, initial treatment is based on clinical suspicion. Suspected scaphoid fractures are immobilized in a thumb spica splint and referred to hand surgery. Rest, ice, and analgesia are staples following an acute injury as well.

COMPLICATIONS

A missed fracture can result in malunion, nonunion, and development of avascular necrosis, which can lead to debilitating arthritis.

CARPAL TUNNEL SYNDROME
DISEASE OVERVIEW

Carpal tunnel syndrome is increased pressure within the carpal tunnel due to swelling and inflammation compressing the median nerve. This creates the sensation of numbness and tingling classically on the palm side of the thumb, the index and middle fingers, and the lateral side of the ring finger. Increased carpal tunnel pressure can be the result of fluid retention as in pregnancy and thyroid dysfunction or of inflammation as seen in arthritis, overuse, and trauma.

CLASSIC PRESENTATION

The AGACNP cares for a 56-year-old patient who presents for evaluation of numbness and tingling on the palmar aspect of the thumb and index and middle fingers. The patient is an administrative assistant who spends most of the day typing. Symptoms started about 6 months ago but have gotten progressively worse.

DIAGNOSTIC CRITERIA

Patients will commonly complain of numbness/tingling in the median nerve distribution, but there are other expected physical exam findings. Tinel sign is performed by tapping over the palmar surface of the carpal tunnel. This test is considered positive if the tapping produces numbness and tingling in the median nerve distribution. Another physical exam test is Phalen test, which is performed by bending the wrist so that the carpal tunnel is "kinked."

TREATMENT/MANAGEMENT

Treatment is aimed at relieving the pressure in the carpal tunnel. Conservative management includes NSAIDs and a wrist brace that keeps the wrist straight. If symptoms are unrelieved with NSAIDs and bracing, the next step is a cortisone injection directly into the carpal tunnel. This typically provides temporary relief. If conservative measures do not provide adequate relief, the carpal tunnel release operation is a simple and safe surgical solution.

BOXER'S FRACTURE
DISEASE OVERVIEW

A *boxer's fracture* (Figure 16.2) is the most common fracture of the metacarpal. It is an injury to the neck of the fifth metacarpal and typically occurs from direct trauma from punching an object.

CLASSIC PRESENTATION

The AGACNP is assessing the right hand of 56-year-old male patient. The patient endorses that in anger he punched a wall earlier today. The hand is exquisitely tender to palpation over the fifth metacarpal. Ecchymosis and edema are noted as well.

DIAGNOSTIC CRITERIA

Patients typically present with swelling and tenderness over the dorsal aspect of the affected metacarpal. It is imperative to assess for any rotational injury by asking the patient to open and close the fist. Most metacarpal fractures are visible on lateral view of x-ray.

TREATMENT/MANAGEMENT

Boxer's fractures are immobilized in an ulnar gutter splint. The patient can be managed outpatient with sufficient analgesia and close orthopedic follow-up.

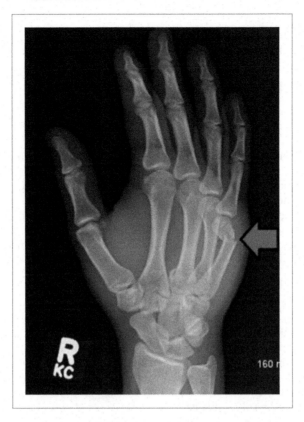

Figure 16.2 Boxer's fracture

Source: James Heilman, M. D. (2018). CC BY-SA 4.0 https://creativeco
mmons.org/licenses/by-sa/4.0, via Wikimedia Commons. https://
upload.wikimedia.org/wikipedia/commons/0/0d/Fractured5thMetaca
rpalHead2018.jpg

COMPLICATIONS
Patients typically have a great prognosis and good long-term function after this injury. Joint stiffness is the most common complication after a boxer's fracture.

CLAVICULAR FRACTURE
DISEASE OVERVIEW
Clavicular fractures are most commonly the result of a blow to the shoulder. Many times, the middle third of the clavicle is fractured. Typically, there is an obvious deformity of the affected clavicle, and patients endorse swelling and tenderness. Crepitus is noted.

CLASSIC PRESENTATION
An 18-year-old male patient presents after a football injury. He states that he was tackled and immediately felt pain in his left shoulder. The AGACNP notes a deformity of the left clavicle. The patient endorses tenderness with palpation to this area and difficulty with any range of motion of the left shoulder.

DIAGNOSTIC CRITERIA
Clavicular fractures are easily seen on x-rays.

TREATMENT/MANAGEMENT
A closed clavicular fracture typically heals uneventfully. Conservative management includes pain control and immobilization with a sling. An open clavicular fracture or those with skin tenting or neuromuscular compromise require consultation with orthopedics. Additionally, open fractures require immediate intravenous antibiotic treatment.

COMPLICATIONS

Most clavicular fractures are straightforward and heal well, but there is a risk of nonunion as well as infection with open clavicular fractures. Patients with open clavicular fractures require hospitalization.

▶ LOWER EXTREMITY

PELVIC FRACTURE

DISEASE OVERVIEW

Pelvic fracture is a broad term referring to fractures of the bones of the pelvis, including pelvic ring, iliac crest/wing, pubic bone, acetabulum, ischium, sacrum, and coccyx. Pelvic fractures most often occur in the setting of high-impact injuries and are commonly associated with additional abdominal and pelvic injuries. The most severe pelvic fractures most commonly result from motor vehicle collisions (MVCs), falling from a height, or being struck by a vehicle as a pedestrian or cyclist. Understanding the mechanism of injury can lead to the diagnosis of the fractures. Anterior compression, lateral compression, and vertical shear have distinct injury patterns. Damage to the pelvic ring is most concerning and leads to unstable fractures. The pelvic bones are highly vascular, and fractures can lead to significant bleeding and hemorrhagic shock.

CLASSIC PRESENTATION

The patient was the driver in an MVC where the car was "T-boned" on the driver's side. There was substantial intrusion into the vehicle, causing a prolonged extrication time. The patient presents with sluggish mentation but is oriented. They have pale skin and oral mucosa. Vital signs are temperature 36°C, heart rate (HR) 120, respiratory rate (RR) 26, blood pressure (BP) 70/50, O_2 Sat 90%. The patient complains of left hip pain with movement. Abdominal tenderness is noted. Pelvic x-ray reveals widened symphysis pubis. Focused abdominal ultrasound of the abdomen in trauma is positive for fluid in the pelvis. A mass transfusion protocol is initiated.

DIAGNOSTIC CRITERIA

Plain films are the first imaging to be done. Anteroposterior (AP) films should be performed immediately in the trauma bay for any unstable patient. Noncontrast CT scans may be needed by orthopedics to plan operative intervention. CT angiography (CTA) may be needed to assess for vascular involvement, denoted as a "blush" on the scan where contrast is extravasated into the tissues. CT urethrogram and/or CT with rectal contrast may be needed if urethral injury or rectal injuries are suspected.

TREATMENT/MANAGEMENT

Any patient who is in hemorrhagic shock with a pelvic fracture should immediately have a pelvic binder applied to control bleeding. Initial transfusion is according to the patient's vital signs, not hemoglobin. Massive transfusion protocol may be required for severe fractures with hemorrhagic shock. For severe bleeding, interventional radiology may need to embolize bleeding vessels to control hemorrhage. Once the patient is stabilized, standard transfusion guidelines should be followed.

Consultation with orthopedics is needed to determine treatment course and weight-bearing status. External fixation may be needed until surgical fixation can be accomplished. Skeletal traction may be needed for vertical shear injuries.

All patients should have mechanical deep vein thrombosis (DVT) prophylaxis. Chemical DVT prophylaxis should begin as soon as bleeding is controlled. For nonhemorrhagic fractures, chemical DVT prophylaxis should not be held prior to operative intervention. Prophylactic antibiotics are needed for open fractures, including fractures that invade the rectum or skin; otherwise, only perioperative antibiotics are needed for closed fractures. Patients will need physical therapy consultation to determine whether a rehabilitation is needed and what level of rehabilitation the patient can accommodate.

COMPLICATIONS

Complications of pelvic fractures depend on the area and extent of the fracture. Hematoma, hemorrhage, urethral or rectal injuries, and nerve root injury/damage are the most severe. Acute and chronic pain, and venous thromboembolism (VTE) are persistent concerns. Transfusion, including transfusion-related acute lung injury and transfusion-associated cardiac overload, can occur. Infection from pin sites or implanted hardware can occur.

HIP FRACTURE
DISEASE OVERVIEW
Hip fractures are common in the older adult population, but high-energy trauma may also cause an acute hip fracture in younger adults. Evaluating the underlying cause of a hip fracture is as important as managing the hip fracture. For example, a "fall" causing a hip fracture must be determined, whether it was a result of a syncopal or a mechanical fall. In the geriatric population, a pathological hip fracture from malignancy or osteoporosis is common.

CLASSIC PRESENTATION
- *Traumatic fracture:* A 70-year-old female patient presents with severe right hip pain after slipping on ice and landing on the right hip. She had immediate pain of the right hip and was not able to walk after falling. 911 was called, and the patient was transported to the emergency department (ED) for evaluation.
- *Pathological fracture:* An older adult with a history of breast cancer was turned while lying in bed, felt a "pop" in the hip turned onto, and noticed immediate 8/10 pain. X-ray reveals a fracture line extending through a lytic lesion in the bone.

DIAGNOSTIC CRITERIA
The classic physical exam of a patient with a hip fracture is a shortened and externally rotated limb of the affected lower extremity. Documentation of lower extremity sensation, circulation, and movement of distal digits is essential. A hip fracture is often seen on a plain anteroposterior view of the pelvis and lateral view of the affected hip. Occult fractures may not be visible on an x-ray; thus, a patient with persistent pain should have an MRI. For a patient who has a contraindication to MRI, a CT scan is a reasonable alternative.

TREATMENT/MANAGEMENT
The fracture pattern will determine surgical or conservative management. Pharmacological VTE prophylaxis is recommended during the postoperative period providing there are no contraindications. Postoperative blood transfusion is recommended only if the hemoglobin is below 8 g/dL or the patient is symptomatic with their anemia.

Postoperative rehabilitation is as important as the initial surgery. The aim of the surgery is to restore mobility; therefore, early mobilization should be commenced. Patients who have undergone arthroplasty or fixation of an extracapsular fracture can usually mobilize immediately after surgery without weight restrictions. Following fixation of an intracapsular fracture, protected weight-bearing is often recommended to reduce the risk of subsequent fracture displacement.

Regular intensive physiotherapy is required to encourage rapid progression of mobility to restore the patient's original mobility status. Medical management must also be optimized to reduce the risk of associated complications. Unfortunately, many patients do not regain their previous level of mobility or independence.

COMPLICATIONS
Complications from a hip fracture should be recognized early to decrease associated mortality. Patients with an extensive fracture are at risk for blood loss, neurovascular injuries, pain, acute kidney injury, infection, pneumonia, DVT or pulmonary embolism, delirium, or skin damage.

FEMUR FRACTURE
DISEASE OVERVIEW
One of the most common fractures treated by orthopedic surgeons, femur fractures are often a result of high-energy mechanisms of injury. The components of the femur include the femoral head, neck, intertrochanteric, subtrochanteric, shaft, supracondylar, and condylar regions. Younger patients generally experience high-energy mechanisms of injury such as MVCs, whereas older adult patients may sustain osteoporotic femur fractures from ground-level falls.

DIAGNOSTIC CRITERIA
Imaging includes plain radiographs and CT scans.

TREATMENT/MANAGEMENT

The gold standard for treatment of femoral shaft fractures is intermedullary nailing, whereas cephalomedullary nailing is done for subtrochanteric femur fractures. Nailing decreases blood loss, reduces operative time, has superior strength and fewer complications, and expedites time to weight-bearing. Operative fixation ideally should occur within the first 24 hours because this decreases pulmonary complications and mortality and reduces ICU stays.

COMPLICATIONS

Complications include neurovascular injury, fat emboli, pulmonary embolism, infection, compartment syndrome (less common than tibial/fibular fractures), and osteomyelitis.

TIBIAL AND FIBULAR FRACTURES, INCLUDING TIBIAL PLATEAU
DISEASE OVERVIEW

Tibial fractures occur in a bimodal pattern including low-energy and high-energy mechanism of injury. Low-energy injury is a result of a torsional force causing a spiral fracture with or without an associated fibular fracture occurring at a different level having minimal surrounding soft-tissue injury. Conversely, a high-energy mechanism injury typically results from direct trauma causing wedge or short oblique fractures. Fractures with significant comminution are associated with increased soft-tissue injury, which can lead to compartment syndrome (discussed later).

DIAGNOSTIC CRITERIA

Plain film x-rays of the tibia and fibula are the initial imaging. Additionally, the joint above and below should also be imaged; in this case, AP and lateral x-ray of the knee and ankle should be obtained as well.

TREATMENT/MANAGEMENT

Eternal fixation is used in damage control surgeries. Intramedullary nailing is the treatment of choice. Rarely, amputation may be a necessary intervention if the limb is not salvageable. A Mangled Extremity Severity Score greater than 7 has a higher likelihood of amputation (Table 16.1). Relative indications include significant soft-tissue destruction, warm ischemic time greater than 6 hours, and severe trauma to the ipsilateral foot. Consultation with vascular surgery may also be required to facilitate reperfusion. Prophylactic fasciotomies can prevent compartment syndrome or can be performed if symptoms develop.

Table 16.1 Mangled Extremity Severity Score

Criteria	Points
Skeletal/soft tissue	
Low energy (stab, simple fracture, civilian GSW)	1
Medium energy (open or multiple fracture, dislocation)	2
High energy (shotgun, rifle, or military GSW, crush injury)	3
Very high energy (high energy with soft-tissue avulsion, gross contamination)	4
Shock	
Stable (SBP consistently greater than 90 mmHg)	0
Transient hypotension	1
Persistent hypotension	2
Limb ischemia (double for ischemia greater than 6 hours)	
No ischemia (pulse present)	0
Mild ischemia (decreased or absent pulse but normal perfusion), paresthesia	1
Moderate ischemia (decreased capillary refill, cool)	2
Severe ischemia (no capillary refill, paralyzed, insensate)	3
Age	
Younger than 30 years	0
30–50 years	1
Older than 50 years	2
TOTAL	

GSW, gunshot wound; SBP, systolic blood pressure.
Source: Modified from Mommsen, P., Zeckey, C., Hildebrand, F., Frink, M., Khaladj, N., Lange, N., Krettek, C., & Probst, C. (2010). Traumatic extremity arterial injury in children: Epidemiology, diagnostics, treatment and prognostic value of Mangled Extremity Severity Score. *Journal of Orthopaedic Surgery and Research, 5*(1), 1–8. https://doi.org/10.1186/1749-799X-5-25

COMPLICATIONS

Complications include neurovascular injury, compartment syndrome, infection, and osteomyelitis.

▶ ACUTE LIMB COMPARTMENT SYNDROME

DISEASE OVERVIEW

Acute limb compartment syndrome is a surgical emergency. It occurs when pressures within a noncompliant compartment are greater than perfusion pressures, resulting in muscle ischemia and nerve injury and, if left untreated, contractures, loss of limb function, and loss of limb. It is commonly caused by crush injuries, fractures, static positioning, casting of an extremity, postoperative bleeding, peripheral arterial surgery, tourniquet use, and edema from injuries with or without fractures. Myofascial compartments mostly affected include calf, thigh, hand and forearms, and buttocks. Signs and symptoms include the 6P's (Table 16.2).

Table 16.2 Signs and Symptoms: The 6P's

Signs/Symptoms	Description
Pain	Pain is characteristically described as being out of proportion to the injury with passive stretching.
Pallor	Pale appearance
Paresthesias	Altered sensation distal to the affected compartment
Paralysis	Loss of function, ability to move
Poikilothermia	Change in temperature, presence of coolness
Pulselessness	A late finding and poor indicator

CLASSIC PRESENTATION

A 55-year-old patient is in hospital day 2 after being involved in an MVC with resultant right tibia and fibula fracture. The AGACNP examines the patient before rounds and notes the right lower extremity appears larger than the day before. On further examination, the patient has also lost the ability to move the right toes and is endorsing increased severe 10/10 pain with paresthesia.

DIAGNOSTIC CRITERIA

Clinical presentation is telling for acute compartment syndrome, including evaluation of the 6P's. Pain is progressive and severe, disproportionate to exam, and refractory to escalating treatments. The extremity is palpably tight and firm. Dorsiflexion of the fingers and great toe increase pain. Pressure measurements are an adjunct to aid diagnosis. Tissue pressures of greater than 30 mmHg suggest decreased capillary blood flow, which can result in muscle and nerve damage from anoxia. Loss of pulses is a very late sign.

TREATMENT/MANAGEMENT

Treatment includes removing all constrictive dressings, casts, and splints; elevating the affected extremity to reduce edema; and STAT consultation to surgery, which may be orthopedics, vascular, or trauma, depending on the institution. Fasciotomy is the standard of care to decrease compartment pressures and preserve limb function.

COMPLICATIONS

Complications include infection, muscle necrosis, rhabdomyolysis and acute kidney injury, ischemic contractures (Volkmann contracture), loss of limb function, and loss of limb. Sepsis secondary to wounds is usually the cause of mortality in these cases. Primary wound closure is preferred but may require skin grafting.

▶ OSTEOMYELITIS

DISEASE OVERVIEW

Osteomyelitis is an infection of the bone and is classified as either acute or chronic and bacterial, fungal, or mycobacterial. The infectious process involves the bone and its structures and is spread through blood, fracture site, or surgery. Malperfusion and diabetes place patients at higher risk for developing osteomyelitis. Patients can seed bones from the skin or gastrointestinal tract, although pressure-related skin breakdown is a common source. The sacrum, buttock, hips, and heels are at highest risk to contribute to pressure-related osteomyelitis.

DIAGNOSTIC CRITERIA

Laboratory data are usually nonspecific for osteomyelitis. Complete blood count (CBC) assesses for leukocytosis, elevation of erythrocyte sedimentation rate (ESR), and C-reactive protein; these may or may not be elevated. Index of clinical suspicion should guide additional studies. Plain x-rays are used to rule out other differential diagnoses such as fracture, metastasis, or osteoporotic lesions. MRI has the highest sensitivity and specificity to diagnose osteomyelitis. Obtain ankle-brachial index (ABI) to assess for adequate perfusion.

TREATMENT/MANAGEMENT

Treatment is specific to the organism and its sensitivities. Typically, a peripherally inserted central catheter (PICC) line is required for prolonged antibiotic use. A broad-spectrum empiric antibiotic regimen with activity against both gram-positive and gram-negative organisms, including methicillin-resistant *Staphylococcus aureus* (MRSA), is needed. Vancomycin (15 mg/kg intravenous [IV] every 12 hours) and ceftriaxone 2 g IV daily *or* piperacillin–tazobactam 3.375 IV every 8 hours is commonly used. When sensitivity data are available, then antibiotics are narrowed to target susceptible organisms. Consultation with the infectious disease team is recommended. This team will follow along on an outpatient basis. For patients with decreased ABIs, consult vascular surgery to ensure patients have adequate perfusion to enhance wound healing and resolution of infection.

COMPLICATIONS

Complications include surrounding soft-tissue infection, abscess, septic arthritis, sepsis, pathological fractures, squamous cell carcinoma, and bone deformities.

▶ SUMMARY

AGACNPs will diagnose or treat musculoskeletal injuries or infections. Interprofessional collaboration with orthopedic, vascular, and/or infectious disease specialists is common in the care of these patients. Early mobilization, physical therapy, and DVT prophylaxis are mainstays for preventing complications.

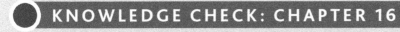

KNOWLEDGE CHECK: CHAPTER 16

1. An adult female patient presents with a history of numbness and tingling in her left hand. She states that it has gotten progressively worse over the past 6 months since she started her job as a unit clerk on a busy medical floor. She states the numbness and tingling are worse at night, and nothing seems to help with her symptoms. What is the most likely diagnosis?

   A. Carpal tunnel syndrome
   B. Ulnar neuropathy
   C. Diabetic neuropathy
   D. Osteoarthritis

2. Which of the following is associated with carpal tunnel syndrome?

   A. Rheumatoid arthritis
   B. Polycythemia vera
   C. Tendonitis
   D. Cervical radiculopathy

3. What is the most appropriate initial treatment for carpal tunnel syndrome?

   A. Steroid injection
   B. Short arm cast
   C. Thumb spica splint
   D. Nonsteroidal anti-inflammatory drugs (NSAIDs) and neutral position wrist splints

4. A 48-year-old female patient was involved in an MVC. She suffered multiple fractured ribs, right-sided pneumothorax, and an open compound fracture of the right radius and ulna. The patient was taken to the operating room for washout and reduction of the fracture and then casted. Postoperative day 2, the patient is complaining of severe pain in the right arm at the fracture site not relieved with pain medications, and her distal digits are swollen and numb with diminished capillary refill. Based on these subjective and objective findings, what should the AGACNP suspect, and what is the immediate treatment?

   A. The wound is infected; start antibiotics.
   B. This is postoperative swelling; elevate the extremity and encase it in ice packs.
   C. This is a compartment syndrome; remove the cast and perform compartment pressures.
   D. This is a postoperative complication; call the surgeon.

5. An 18-year-old male patient presents following a sports injury. He states that he was tackled and immediately felt pain in his left shoulder. The AGACNP notes a deformity of the left clavicle. The patient endorses tenderness with palpation to this area and difficulty with any range of motion of the left shoulder. The AGACNP should:

   A. Obtain CT scan
   B. Apply a sling
   C. Prepare for casting
   D. Consult orthopedics

(*See answers next page.*)

1. A) Carpal tunnel syndrome

Carpal tunnel syndrome is due to median nerve entrapment in the wrist. Symptoms include numbness, paresthesia, and pain on the palmar/radial aspect of the hand. Ulnar neuropathy classically affects the ulnar aspect of the hand, most notably in the fourth and fifth fingers. Diabetic neuropathy is classically seen in the feet. Osteoarthritis of the wrist does not typically cause nerve symptoms.

2. A) Rheumatoid arthritis

Rheumatoid arthritis is associated with erythema, pallor, or cyanosis. Conditions associated with carpal tunnel syndrome include pregnancy, menopause, obesity, end-stage renal disease, diabetes, hypothyroidism, rheumatoid and osteoarthritis, acromegaly, sarcoidosis, and amyloid infiltration of the carpal ligament. Polycythemia vera can cause erythromelalgia, which is a burning pain of the hands and feet. Tendonitis and cervical radiculopathy are also differential diagnoses.

3. D) Nonsteroidal anti-inflammatory drugs (NSAIDs) and neutral position wrist splints

Carpal tunnel syndrome is best initially treated with conservative therapy. Many patients respond well to NSAIDs and neutral position splints.

4. C) This is a compartment syndrome; remove the cast and perform compartment pressures.

Injuries with potential to swell that are constricted with items such as a cast put the patient at risk for compartment syndrome. The patient is experiencing pain (greater than expected), paresthesias, and decreased circulation to the limb, all of which are signs and symptoms of the 6P's related to compartment syndrome. The treatment is to remove the constrictive cast. Waiting for a surgeon risks damage to the patient with prolonged constriction and decreased perfusion to the limb.

5. B) Apply a sling

Treatment of a clavicle fracture is conservative in nature with a sling. An open clavicular fracture, fractures that tent the skin, or neuromuscular compromise require a consultation with orthopedics. A CT scan is not appropriate, and casting is not indicated.

6. A patient presents with a complaint of right-sided wrist and thumb pain at the base of the styloid of the radius. They report pain is referred up the forearm. They work for a large shipping company and have repetitively packaged boxes daily for the past 2 years. The pain is described as "achy" yet "sharp" with certain movements. They deny numbness or tingling but note that hand strength is weakened. The most likely cause of these symptoms is:

   A. Colles fracture
   B. Rheumatoid arthritis
   C. Carpal tunnel syndrome
   D. DeQuervain tenosynovitis

7. A young adult presents after falling while skiing. She reports having fallen on an outstretched arm and presents with a deformity of the wrist. The most likely cause of these symptoms is:

   A. Colles fracture
   B. Rheumatoid arthritis
   C. Carpal tunnel syndrome
   D. DeQuervain tenosynovitis

8. A patient with diabetes and peripheral arterial disease presents with a warm, erythematous, painful foot. White blood count (WBC) is 16.8. The patient reports having had cellulitis three times in the last 5 months. The great toe has an open wound that has not healed since the first infection. The ankle-brachial index (ABI) is 0.6 in the affected extremity. The AGACNP is *most* concerned that this is:

   A. Cellulitis
   B. Osteomyelitis
   C. Venous insufficiency
   D. Critical limb ischemia

9. A patient with diabetes and peripheral arterial disease presents with a warm, erythematous, painful foot. The white blood count (WBC) is 16.8. The patient reports having had cellulitis three times in the last 5 months. The great toe has an open wound that has not healed since the first infection. The ankle-brachial index (ABI) is 0.3 in the affected extremity. The AGACNP's *next* action should be to:

   A. Start cefazolin (Ancef)
   B. Consult vascular surgery
   C. Consult infectious disease team
   D. Start piperacillin/tazobactam (Zosyn)

10. An adult female patient presents after riding a horse who was spooked, reared up, and fell backward onto the patient. X-ray reveals open book pelvic fracture, and a binder has been applied. CTA shows extravasation into the pelvis. Vital signs are temperature 36.4°C, heart rate (HR) 120, respiratory rate (RR) 24, blood pressure (BP) 80/50, O_2 Sat 95%. The AGACNP should:

    A. Start 1 L intravenous (IV) fluid
    B. Page orthopedic surgery
    C. Transport to the operating room
    D. Consult interventional radiology

(See answers next page.)

6. D) DeQuervain tenosynovitis

The patient has right-sided wrist and thumb pain at the base of the styloid of the radius, indicative of DeQuervain tenosynovitis. Patients with carpal tunnel syndrome complain of numbness/tingling in the median nerve distribution. The Colles fracture is a distal radius fracture close to the wrist resulting in posterior displacement of the radius with obvious deformity. Rheumatoid arthritis presents as tender, warm, swollen joints and joint stiffness typically worse in the mornings and after inactivity.

7. A) Colles fracture

Colles fracture is a distal radius fracture close to the wrist resulting in posterior displacement of the radius with obvious deformity. Colles fractures most often occur with a fall onto an outstretched hand. Carpal tunnel syndrome occurs when the median nerve, which runs from the forearm into the palm of the hand, becomes pressed or squeezed at the wrist. Rheumatoid arthritis presents as tender, warm, swollen joints and joint stiffness typically worse in the mornings and after inactivity. Patients with carpal tunnel syndrome complain of numbness/tingling in the median nerve distribution. Tinel and Phalen signs will be positive.

8. B) Osteomyelitis

While this presents with signs similar to cellulitis, the AGACNP should be most concerned that the etiology is osteomyelitis due to the reinfections/recurrence. Osteomyelitis can be the nidus to reinfect the skin and soft tissues. Osteomyelitis requires adjustment to the treatment plan with a prolonged course of antibiotics. The ABI confirms arterial insufficiency, which is a likely contributor to osteomyelitis; however, it is not critical limb ischemia. An ABI less than 0.3 is considered severe peripheral arterial disease.

9. B) Consult vascular surgery

The ABI confirms critical limb ischemia. An ABI less than 0.3 is considered severe peripheral arterial disease and requires revascularization to enhance perfusion to heal the wound and adequately treat the infection. Infectious disease consult is likely required; however, it is not the highest priority. Cefazolin (Ancef) is not broad enough coverage as these wounds commonly are due to multiple organisms. Piperacillin–tazobactam (Zosyn) is not sufficient as vancomycin is also needed to cover for possible methicillin-resistant *Staphylococcus aureus* (MRSA).

10. D) Consult interventional radiology

The patient has uncontrolled hemorrhage. Cessation of bleeding is the highest priority, thus consulting interventional radiology for embolization is the priority action. The patient should be given blood products, not intravenous fluid (IVF), at this point. The patient may actually require a massive transfusion protocol. While orthopedic surgery needs to be consulted, stopping the bleeding is more urgently needed to stabilize the patient.

11. A young adult presents after a motor vehicle crash. His left leg was trapped under the car for several hours before he was freed. Upon examination of his left lower extremity, the AGACNP notes ecchymosis, edema, and tenderness. The patient reports severe pain and numbness to the calf. X-ray of the left leg is negative. The next step in the management of this patient is to:

    A. Consult surgery to evaluate the leg
    B. Apply a pressure dressing and ice to the leg
    C. Elevate the leg above the level of the heart
    D. Increase dosage of hydromorphone (Dilaudid)

12. A frail older patient with dementia presents following a fall and denies pain at rest but yells out during a turn. Upon assessment, the AGACNP notes a shortened externally rotated right leg. The AGACNP suspects the patient has:

    A. Hip fracture
    B. Pelvis fracture
    C. Patella dislocation
    D. Ankle sprain

13. A victim of a motor vehicle crash presents with bilateral femur fractures and a large left hemothorax. He declines a blood transfusion because of his religious beliefs (Jehovah's Witness). After the risks and benefits are explained, the patient continues to decline a transfusion. The most appropriate intervention is to:

    A. Contact the patient's family for consent
    B. Implement hemostasis measures
    C. Perform autotransfusion of blood from the chest tube
    D. Obtain an emergency court order to transfuse blood products

14. A football player presents after a playoff game with complaint of "ankle sprain." The right ankle is painful and edematous. The patient is unable to bear weight. X-rays are negative for fracture. The AGACNP suspects high ankle sprain. What test should be performed to confirm this diagnosis?

    A. Squeeze test
    B. Talar tilt test
    C. Anterior drawer test
    D. Hawkins test

15. A 70-year-old female patient with history of diabetes and hypertension complains of left shoulder pain persisting for 2 months. The pain is worse at night, and the patient has limited range of motion in the shoulder. The AGACNP diagnoses the patient with adhesive capsulitis. What is the best treatment for *immediate* pain relief?

    A. Oral nonsteroidal anti-inflammatory drugs (NSAIDs)
    B. Intravenous prednisone
    C. Oral opioids
    D. Intra-articular lidocaine and cortisone

(See answers next page.)

11. A) Consult surgery to evaluate the leg

This patient has likely developed compartment syndrome, which requires surgical consult. Elevating the leg will help with swelling but will not reduce the pressure from compartment syndrome. Applying a pressure dressing and ice would further compromise the extremity. Increasing hydromorphone will mask symptoms and delay diagnosis and definitive intervention.

12. A) Hip fracture

A shortened and externally rotated leg is highly suspicious for a hip fracture or femur fracture. The leg may be shortened with a pelvic fracture but not usually rotated. Patella dislocation or ankle sprain does not shorten the leg.

13. B) Implement hemostasis measures

The patient has the right to refuse a medical intervention, including a blood transfusion. The AGACNP must honor this wish. Thus, preventing additional blood loss is critical. There is no need to contact family if the patient is of legal age. Autotransfusion may be an option to consider; there are varying views within the religion, but autotransfusion is not accepted by all. A court order is not indicated.

14. A) Squeeze test

The squeeze test is a confirmatory provocative test for syndesmotic ankle sprain. The examiner supports the lateral fibula and tibia with one hand and gently forces external rotation with the other. Pain at the distal syndesmosis (at lateral malleolus) confirms distal syndesmotic ligamentous injury. The Talar tilt test is done to determine joint instability. Anterior drawer test of the ankle detects excessive anterior displacement of the talus on the tibia. Hawkins test is used to determine rotator cuff impingement.

15. D) Intra-articular lidocaine and cortisone

Adhesive capsulitis is very painful. Patients benefit most from lidocaine/cortisone injection in the shoulder. The patient will need to follow up with orthopedics for further evaluation. While oral NSAIDs, prednisone, and opioids would also provide pain relief, they would not take effect immediately.

KEY BIBLIOGRAPHY

Only key resources appear in the print edition. Access the full bibliography for this chapter on ExamPrepConnect.com.

Aziz, F., & Doty, C. I. (2017). Orthopedic emergencies. In C. Stone & R. I. Humphries (Eds.), *Current diagnosis & treatment: Emergency medicine* (8th ed.). McGraw Hill.

Collins, N., & Rose, J. (2017). Hand trauma. In C. Stone & R. L. Humphries (Eds.), *Current diagnosis & treatment: Emergency medicine* (8th ed.). McGraw Hill.

Gumbs, S. (2019). Acute compartment syndrome: A literature review and updates. *Clinical Journal of Surgery,* 2(2), 1–5. https://doi.org/10.33309/2639-9164.020201

Luke, A., & Ma, C. (2023). Musculoskeletal injuries of the hip. In M. A. Papadakis, S. J. McPhee, M. W. Rabow, & K. R. McQuaid (Eds.), *Current medical diagnosis & treatment 2023*. McGraw Hill. https://accessmedicine.mhmedical.com/content.aspx?bookid=3212&sectionid=269161280

McMillan, T. E., Gardner, W. T., Schmidt, A. H., & Johnstone, A. J. (2019). Diagnosing acute compartment syndrome—Where have we got to? *International Orthopaedics (SICOT), 43,* 2429–2435. https://doi.org/10.1007/s00264-019-04386-y

Parks, E. (Ed.). (2017). The hand, wrist, and elbow. In E. Parks (Ed.), *Practical office orthopedics.* McGraw Hill. https://accessmedicine-mhmedical-com.yale.idm.oclc.org/content.aspx?bookid=2230&sectionid=172778553

Integumentary System Review

Roxanne M. Buterakos*

▶ INTRODUCTION

The integumentary system includes the components of skin, hair, nails, and exocrine glands. Skin is a protective multilayer interface between internal body systems and the environment and is often said to be the body's largest organ. It protects the body from mechanical injuries, microorganisms, substances, and radiation in the environment. It also aids in regulation of temperature and water content. The integumentary system is involved in the functionality of the nervous system, as in detection of stimuli such as pressure, pain, heat, and cold. Any disruption of these functions can increase risk of disease and illness susceptibility and could result in life-threatening conditions. This chapter discusses skin issues seen in the care of acutely and critically ill patients.

▶ INFECTIOUS SKIN DISORDERS

SKIN AND SOFT TISSUE INFECTIONS
Acute care management of critically ill patients includes identification and management of multiple infectious skin disorders seen in the ICU. These include a variety of pathological conditions involving skin and tissues, including the subcutaneous and muscular layers. Skin and soft tissue infections (SSTIs) are divided between uncomplicated-superficial and complicated-deep tissue infections, as noted:

- *Uncomplicated-superficial infections:* cellulitis, simple abscesses, impetigo, carbuncles, furuncles, erysipelas, folliculitis
- *Complicated-deep soft tissue infections:* necrotizing infections, myonecrosis, infected ulcers, infected burns, major abscesses

CELLULITIS

Overview
Cellulitis is an infection characterized by warmth, erythema, edema, pain, lymphadenopathies, fever, and leukocytosis. It will often have a precursor lesion that presents a portal of entry for the invading microorganism.

Classic Presentation
A 39-year-old male patient with diabetes presents to the ED with complaints of worsening pain and tenderness over the anterior left thigh over the past 5 days. He states that he has had a persistent fever with chills that did not respond to Tylenol. Upon examination of the thigh, it is noted that the area is hyperthermic and edematous with an angry red, painful plaque that does not blanch upon touch.

Diagnostic Criteria
Diagnosis is made based on clinical signs and symptoms. Classic signs and symptoms of erysipelas include superficial soft tissue infection involving the upper dermis with distinct boundaries and a fiery-red, painful plaque. Erysipelas is commonly caused by streptococcal species. Cellulitis is a lower dermal infection that can involve the subcutaneous fat layer with ambiguous boundaries and is predominantly caused by beta-hemolytic streptococci. Signs and symptoms include local signs of

* The author gratefully acknowledges the support of Guillermo R. Ethier, BSN, RN, and Kathleen G. Mehall, BS, in the research for this chapter.

inflammation, induration, warmth, erythema, pain/tenderness, lymphangitis, and fever. The adult gerontology acute care nurse practitioner (AGACNP) can expect to see a mild leukocytosis with a left shift and a mildly elevated sedimentation rate. To differentiate cellulitis from abscess, an ultrasound can be obtained. Ultrasound can reduce unnecessary painful incision and drainage when no fluid is present.

Treatment/Management
The usual causative organisms for cellulitis are *Staphylococcus aureus* or beta-hemolytic streptococci. First-generation cephalosporins, nafcillin, ampicillin/sulbactam, or amoxicillin/clavulanate are used for treatment of cellulitis, and penicillin/amoxicillin treats erysipelas. If methicillin-resistant *S. aureus* (MRSA) is suspected, antibiotic coverage will need to be expanded to include anti-MRSA antibiotics like vancomycin. Empiric therapy for severe cellulitis in the immunocompromised patient includes combination therapy (vancomycin + piperacillin–tazobactam or vancomycin + imipenem or meropenem). Antibiotic duration of treatment of uncomplicated cellulitis can be 5 days but extended if needed. Treatment can also include warm compresses.

Complications
Complications range from lymphatic inflammation with potential permanent damage to lymphedema to sepsis or septic shock due to necrotizing fasciitis.

ABSCESSES

Overview
Abscess is pooling of purulent exudate within the dermis layer or lower, occurring from infectious infiltration of nearby skin or mucosal cells. It is a purulent SSTI predominantly caused by *S. aureus* but can be a polymicrobial infection depending on the site.

Classic Presentation
Classic presentation of abscess is influenced by its location (Table 17.1).

Diagnostic Criteria
Diagnosis is based on clinical presentation in combination with gram stain and bacterial cultures/sensitivities from samples of purulent exudates.

Treatment/Management
Treatment includes incision and drainage of the abscess. Use of antibiotics is recommended when multiple lesions or gangrene are present, in the immunocompromised patient, with extensive cellulitis near abscess, or with systematic symptoms (fever, hypotension, diaphoresis, and tachycardia). Empiric antibiotic therapy can include a first-generation cephalosporin, amoxicillin/clavulanate, or clindamycin. If there is previous MRSA colonization or infections or if the patient does not respond to primary treatment, then treat with anti-MRSA agents for the nonpregnant patient with normal hepatic and renal function (Table 17.2). Severe infections not responding to incision and drainage with oral antibiotic therapy warrant intravenous (IV) antibiotic therapy.

Complications
Complications include sepsis and septic shock, osteomyelitis, endocarditis, and development of multiple abscesses.

NECROTIZING FASCIITIS

Overview
Necrotizing fasciitis is a life-threatening infection of the subcutaneous tissues and a surgical emergency with a high mortality rate. Fournier gangrene is a subtype of necrotizing fasciitis of the perineal and perianal regions that often involves the genital regions. It progresses rapidly and may not be visible or easy to detect. It can progress to full toxic streptococcal syndrome or gas gangrene. Predisposing conditions include diabetes, arteriosclerotic vascular disease, venous insufficiency with edema, venous stasis or vascular insufficiency, ulcer, and injection drug use.

Table 17.1 Types and Presentation of Abscesses With Causative Organisms

Type of Abscess	Cutaneous	Hidradenitis Suppurativa	Breast	Bartholin Cyst	Pilonidal	Perianal	IVDU
Common site of infection	Head Neck Axillae Buttock Perineal	Axillae Pubic	Breast tissue	Vagina	Sacro-cocygeal pilonidal sinus	Anal crypt and anal sphincter	Thighs, buttocks, or forearms
Description	Arise from furuncles, red, fluctuant, tender tissues	Abscess with resultant scarring, recurrent formation risks tunneled fistula formation, often painful draining wounds	Associated with postpartem period, Mastitis is pre-abscess formation, abscesses occur in superficial or deep breast tissue. Pain, malaise, myalgia, fever/chills, warmth, firmness, swelling, erythema, enlarged axillary lymph nodes	Ductal occlusion of the Bartholin gland, red, swollen tender labia	Painful induration of the buttock crease	Can be associated with deeper abscesses for which patients complain of deep rectal, low back, perineal, buttock or pelvic pain, fistula in anus is common. May appear toxic with pain, fever, diaphoresis and tachycardia	Local complications: soft tissue necrosis Intra-arterial injection, septic arthritis, osteomyelitis High incidence of hepatitis, endocarditis, and HIV Persistent infections require evaluation for endocarditis or retained foreign bodies such as broken needle
Most common organism	MSSA, MRSA, *Proteus mirabilis*, and group A Strep	Coagulase-negative Staph and *S. aureus*	MRSA, MSSA, anaerobes, and mixed flora	*Neisseria, Chlamydia,* gram-positive and gram-negative, anaerobes	Gram-negative enteric organisms and anaerobes	*E. coli, Bacteroides* and Strep species	Strep, Staph, MSSA, MRSA, and anaerobes
Recommend consultant	No	Yes	Yes	No	No	Yes	Yes

E., *Escherichia*; IVDU, intravenous drug use; MRSA, methicillin-resistant; MSSA, methicillin-sensitive *Staphylococcus aureus*; S., *Staphylococcus*; *Staphylococcus aureus*; Strep, *Streptococcus*; Staph, *Staphylococcus*.

Source: Data from Trott, A. (2012). *Wounds and lacerations: Emergency care and closure* (4th ed.). Elsevier Saunders; Kwak, Y. G., Choi, S.-H., Kim, T., Park, S. Y., Seo, S.-H., Kim, M. B., & Choi, S.-H. (2017). Clinical guidelines for the antibiotic treatment for community-acquired skin and soft tissue infection. *Infection & Chemotherapy, 49*(4), 301. https://doi.org/10.3947/ic.2017.49.4.301; Burnham, J. P., Kirby, J. P., & Kollef, M. H. (2016). Diagnosis and management of skin and soft tissue infections in the intensive care unit: A review. *Intensive Care Medicine, 42*(12), 1899–1911. https://doi.org/10.1007/s00134-016-4576-0; Sartelli, M., Guirao, X., Hardcastle, T. C., Kluger, Y., Boermeester, Marja. A., Raşa, K., Ansaloni, L., Coccolini, F., Montravers, P., Abu-Zidan, F. M., Bartoletti, M., Bassetti, M., Ben-Ishay, O., Biffl, W. L., Chiara, O., Chiarugi, M., Coimbra, R., De Rosa, F. G., De Simone, B., & Di Saverio, S. (2018). 2018 WSES/SIS-E consensus conference: Recommendations for the management of skin and soft-tissue infections. *World Journal of Emergency Surgery, 13*(1), 58. https://doi.org/10.1186/s13017-018-0219-9; and Boakes, E., Woods, A., Johnson, N., & Kadoglou, N. (2018). Breast infection: A review of diagnosis and management practices. *European Journal of Breast Health, 14*(3), 136–143. https://doi.org/10.5152/ejbh.2018.3871.

Table 17.2 Antibiotic Regimens if Previous MRSA Colonization or Infection

Drug	Considerations
Clindamycin 300–350 mg PO TID	Associated with *Clostridioides difficile* infection
Trimethoprim-sulfamethoxazole (Bactrim) double strength PO BID	Use caution in older and renal-compromised populations Risk of hyperkalemia Contraindicated in pregnant and breastfeeding patients with megaloblastic anemia
Doxycycline 100 mg PO BID	Contraindicated in pregnant and breastfeeding patients
Minocycline 200 mg PO first dose, then 100 mg PO BID	Contraindicated in pregnant and breastfeeding patients
Linezolid 600 mg PO BID	Associated with thrombocytopenia and serotonin syndrome

Classic Presentation

A 65-year-old male patient with a past medical history of type 1 diabetes with severe neuropathies of the bilateral lower extremities presents to the ED with a history of embedded glass to the sole of his right foot. Blood glucose is 359, temperature is 30°C, blood pressure is 80/56, and heart rate is 110. Upon examination of the foot, erythema and swelling that extends to midtibia is noted. The extremity affected tissues are tense and extremely tender to palpation.

Diagnostic Criteria

A thorough history and physical examination is imperative to determine what exposures might have exacerbated this infection. It is important to consider a history of exposure to brackish seawater or raw oysters, traumatic lesions in freshwater, and gastrointestinal portal of entry. Abnormal physical and objective findings include disproportionate pain, tense edema, bullae, ecchymosis, crepitus, tenderness, cutaneous anesthesia, "wooden" induration of the subcutaneous tissue, and rapid progression of infection of the affected area. Signs of systemic toxicity are those of septic shock, including fever, tachycardia, leukocytosis, hypotension, and acute kidney injury. Diagnostic testing should include complete blood count with differential, coagulation studies, comprehensive metabolic panel, lactic acid, creatine phosphokinase, and blood cultures. Laboratory risk indicators for necrotizing fasciitis have been shown to help differentiate cellulitis/abscess from necrotizing fasciitis (Table 17.3).

Table 17.3 Laboratory Risk Indicators for Necrotizing Fasciitis

Lab Variable	Points			
	0	1	2	4
CRP	Less than 150 mg/L	n/a	n/a	≥150 mg/L
WBC	Less than 15/mm³	15–25/mm³	Greater than 25/mm³	n/a
Hgb	Greater than 13.5 g/dL	11–13.5 g/dL	Less than 11 g/dL	n/a
Sodium	≥135 mmol/L (135 mEq/L)	n/a	Less than 135 mmol/L (135 mEq/L)	n/a
Creatinine	≤1.6 mg/dL (141 mmol/L)	n/a	Greater than 1.6 mg/dL (141 mmol/L)	n/a
Glucose	≤180 mg/dL (10 mmol/L)	>180 mg/dL (10 mmol/L)	n/a	n/a
Maximum score is 13, a score of ≥6 correlates with increased risk of necrotizing fasciitis, a score of 8 or more is highly predictive.				

CRP, C-reactive protein; Hgb, hemoglobin; WBC, white blood count.
Source: Data from Wong, C., Khin, L., Heng, K., Tan, K., & Low, C. (2004). The LRINEC (Laboratory Risk Indicator for Necrotizing Fasciitis) score: A tool for distinguishing necrotizing fasciitis from other soft tissue infections. *Critical Care Medicine, 32*(7), 1536–1541. https://doi.org/10.1097/01.ccm.0000129486.35458.7d.

Time is of the essence, and point-of-care ultrasound can be crucial for early detection (100% sensitivity and 98% specificity) when performed by trained, credentialed, and experienced providers looking for thickened fascial planes with fluid accumulation in the fascial layers and distortion of fascial planes and presence of subcutaneous gas. MRI or CT scans commonly reveal gas within fluid collections tracking along fascial planes and fascial thickening.

Treatment/Management

Treatment involves early and aggressive surgical intervention. Repeated surgical debridement may be necessary to ensure all necrotic tissue has been removed. Empiric treatment is initiated with broad-spectrum antibiotics to cover various gram-positive organisms, gram-negative organisms, proteus species, and anaerobic organisms. In cases with suspected clostridial myonecrosis/gas gangrene, treatment with hyperbaric oxygen has been shown to be effective.

Complications

Complications include a mortality rate of about 12%. Risk of needing a limb amputation is 10%.

ECTHYMA GANGRENOSUM

Overview

Ecthyma gangrenosum (EG) is a cutaneous manifestation of *Pseudomonas aeruginosa*. Its lesions are bloodborne, are seeded metastatically to the skin, or exist as a primary lesion without bacteremia. EG occurs in patients with increased risk for infection, immunocompromised patients, burn patients, patients treated with penicillin, and patients with neutropenia or pancytopenia.

Classic Presentation

A 62-year-old patient with a recent kidney transplant presents with primary lesions that started as a small bunch of simple ingrown hairs and is now a large contiguous hemorrhagic bullae.

Diagnostic Criteria

It is important to identify the offending organism. This must include skin biopsy for histopathology and cultures, gram stain of lesions, and blood cultures.

Treatment/Management

Start broad-spectrum systemic antibiotics once cultures are obtained. Localized application options include silver nitrate 0.5%, 5% acetic acid wet compresses, and silver sulfadiazine cream.

Complications

Although rare, the death rate is high for bloodborne bacteremic patients and approximately 15% for nonbacteremic patients.

▶ EXFOLIATIVE SKIN DISORDERS

STEVENS–JOHNSON SYNDROME AND TOXIC EPIDERMAL NECROLYSIS
OVERVIEW

Stevens–Johnson syndrome (SJS) and *toxic epidermal necrolysis* (TEN) are severe mucocutaneous reactions of blistering and sloughing of the epithelium secondary to reactions to drugs or infections. SJS is less extensive than TEN; both are rare but devastating disease processes. The at-risk population includes those who are immunocompromised, have brain tumors and are undergoing radiation and receiving antiepileptics, or have slow acetylator genotypes. The Score of TEN scale evaluates severity and chance of survival.

CLASSIC PRESENTATION

A 37-year-old patient with epilepsy, currently controlled with Keppra and phenytoin, presents with fever, malaise, and mucositis of the mouth and nose.

DIAGNOSTIC CRITERIA

A delay of 4 to 28 days is common between initiation of drug use and onset of adverse reaction. Skin biopsy is needed if classic lesions are absent.

TREATMENT/MANAGEMENT

Stop the causative agent (Table 17.4). Patients should be admitted to a burn care unit for fluid resuscitation and electrolyte replacement. Treatment is largely supportive, including wound and pain management. There is potential for surgical debridement and skin grafting.

Table 17.4 Drugs Commonly Associated With SJS/TEN

Acetaminophen	Carbamazepine	Nevirapine	Phenytoin
Allopurinol	Ibuprofen	Penicillin	Sulfasalazine
Amoxicillin	Lamotrigine	Phenobarbital	Trimethoprim/sulfamethoxazole

SJS, Stevens–Johnson syndrome; TEN, toxic epidermal necrolysis.

COMPLICATIONS

Complications include secondary infections and systemic infections (septicemia and gram-negative pneumonia). Multisystem organ failure and death can result. Long-term sequelae debilitation includes ophthalmic, mucocutaneous, and psychological complications.

TOXIC SHOCK SYNDROME
OVERVIEW

Toxic shock syndrome is a rare, potentially life-threatening, multisystem illness associated with *Staphylococcus aureus* infection and production of superantigen toxins. Formerly associated with tampon use, most cases now are postoperative or associated with conditions such as HIV, allergic contact dermatitis, burns, cellulitis, sinusitis, influenza, and tracheitis, as well as IV drug use and the postpartum state.

CLASSIC PRESENTATION

A 32-year-old female patient is recently diagnosed with acute sinusitis. Despite starting antibiotic therapy, her symptoms have progressed with an elevated temperature of 38.7°C, blood pressure of 82/60, and complaints of persistent headache, nausea and vomiting, and rash with desquamation of bilateral palms and soles of the feet.

DIAGNOSTIC CRITERIA

The incubation period is typically 2 to 10 days. Risk factors include wound or vaginal colonization with toxin-producing bacteria, recent minor trauma with or without a break in the skin, previous surgery, and varicella infection or staphylococcal syndrome usually associated with menses. Patients can present with rash, fever, exanthem, mucositis, and strawberry tongue and progress to more severe symptoms, including skin desquamation, convalescent desquamation, and soft tissue infection. Hypotension and multiple organ dysfunction can be noted as the process progresses. Biopsy may be helpful in the early stages. Causative organisms include *S. aureus* and group A *Streptococcus pyogenes*.

TREATMENT/MANAGEMENT

Treatment is largely supportive with hydration, vasopressor support, removal of offending tampon, and incision and drainage of abscesses. Antibiotic therapy and surgery for necrotizing soft tissue infections and IV immunoglobulin may be indicated.

COMPLICATIONS

Complications may include severe local cellulitis, myonecrosis, or necrotizing fasciitis.

INTRAVENOUS INFILTRATION AND EXTRAVASATION
INFILTRATION

This occurs when a catheter either slips out of the vein or goes through the vein and/or the blood vessel wall, allowing fluid into the tissues.

EXTRAVASATION

Extravasation injury occurs when the infiltrate is a vesicant and is now a serious threat to the patient.

Overview

Vesicants are agents that can cause serious damage such as blistering, tissue sloughing, or necrosis.

Classification of vesicants includes hyperosmolar solutions (fluids and medications), nonphysiological pH (acidic and alkalotic), vasopressors, and cytotoxic drugs. Risk factors include sensory and/or cognitive deficits; obesity; lymphedema; patient movement; small and/or fragile veins; multiple venipunctures; inability to visualize insertion sites; prolonged IV therapy; and volume, pH, osmolarity, and chemical compositions of the infiltrate. Infiltrations are graded by severity (Table 17.5).

Table 17.5 Gradation and Treatment of Extravasation

Signs/Symptoms Peripheral IV	Grade			
	1	2	3	4
Pain at IV site	Painful	Painful	Painful	Painful
IV integrity	Difficulty flushing or running infusion, leakage of medication around needle	Difficulty flushing or running infusion, leakage of medication around needle	Difficulty/inability to flush cannula, leakage of medication around needle	Unable to flush cannula, leakage of medication around needle
Erythema/skin tone/blanches	None or pink	Erythema, skin is red, nonblanching	Blanched	Blackened
Skin temperature	Warm	Hot	Cool	Cool
Edema	Minimal	Mild	Marked	Very marked
Perfusion	Normal	Normal	Normal/decreased	Decreased or absent pulse/perfusion
Capillary refill	Brisk	Brisk	Sluggish	Capillary refill greater than 4 seconds
Mobility	Slight limitation	Very limited	Immobile	Immobile
Skin integrity	Blistered	Superficial skin loss	Tissue loss, exposed subcutaneous tissue	Tissue loss, exposed muscle/bone, deep crater or necrosis
If the drug is a vesicant	Grades 1 and 2		Grades 3 and 4	
	▪ Stop the infusion ▪ Remove the IV cannula ▪ Mark area with a pen ▪ Elevate limb for 48 hours ▪ Remove all constricting items ▪ Consider antidote ▪ Consult surgery for washout ▪ Warm/cold compresses ▪ Strict reevaluation of the site around the clock		▪ Stop the infusion ▪ Leave the IV cannula in situ until evaluated by surgery ▪ Aspirate fluid if possible ▪ Mark area with a pen ▪ Elevate limb ▪ Remove all constricting items ▪ Consider antidote ▪ Consult surgery for washout ▪ Warm/cold compresses ▪ Strict reevaluation of the site around the clock	
Signs/symptoms Central venous catheters	▪ Stinging pain ▪ Edema around the insertion site ▪ Medication leakage around the insertion site ▪ Chest wall, collarbone, or neck erythema ▪ No backflow of blood in the catheter			

IV, intravenous.

Treatment/Management

See Table 17.5.

WOUNDS
SURGICAL WOUNDS AND SURGICAL SITE INFECTIONS

Overview
Surgical site infections are the most prevalent soft tissue infection, accounting for 21.8% of the approximately 721,800 healthcare-associated infections reported annually. Surgical site infections usually result from contamination and colonization. Risk increases with impaired defense mechanisms secondary to aging, malnutrition, diabetes, prolonged hospitalization, shock states, and hypothermia.

Classic Presentation
A 55-year-old patient presents with a ruptured diverticula and undergoes emergent hemicolectomy. Postoperative day 3, the patient is febrile, and the abdominal incision is erythematous with peri-wound erythema. Upon further exam, there is induration of the peri-wound area and purulent exudates between the staples of the incision.

Diagnostic Criteria
Erythema, induration, and purulent drainage are commonly observed.

Treatment/Management
Opening the wound or incision and drainage are needed. Obtain wound cultures and sensitivities. Debride any necrotic tissue. Wound packing with wet-to-dry dressing is commonly needed. Use empiric antibiotic therapy initially when the pathogen is identified, then change to sensitivity-identified antibiotics.

Complications
Complications include delayed or no healing of the wound, osteomyelitis, cellulitis and/or abscess formation, and further wound breakdown.

ENTEROCUTANEOUS FISTULA

Overview
Enterocutaneous fistula is defined as any communication between the gastrointestinal tract and the abdominal wall.

Classic Presentation
A 20-year-old male patient suffered a gunshot wound to his abdomen. His injuries were severe, and he underwent a splenectomy and small bowel resection. His abdomen was unable to be closed initially as the surgeons needed to go back in 3 days for another evaluation of the injuries, and there was increased edema to the tissues. A closed wound vac system was in place for those 3 days. After the abdomen was closed, the patient developed multiple areas of draining purulence from the abdomen consistent with enteric content.

Diagnostic Criteria
Patients may present with an array of symptoms, from small, localized abscesses to florid septic shock. Patients present with suspected surgical site infection, frank bilious drainage, or initial purulent drainage followed by enteric contents during ensuing days. It should also be suspected if localized wound infection persists for several weeks postoperatively.

Fistulae are categorized as either low or high output. Low-output fistula is defined as effluent volume less than 200 mL/24 hr and has a higher likelihood of spontaneous closure with appropriate nutritional support and wound care. High-output fistula is characterized as greater than 500 mL/24 hr. Persistent fistulae have multiple contributors, including foreign body/material at the fistula site, prior radiation exposure to the involved bowel, active infection/unaddressed sepsis, inflammatory bowel disease, epithelization of the fistula tract, neoplasm, presence of a distal obstruction, and active steroid use. Surgical management is almost always required.

Treatment/Management
Identify and control underlying intra-abdominal septic source. Perform percutaneous or surgical drainage of abscess. Rapidly initiate broad-spectrum antibiotics covering enteric organisms. Resuscitate

in sepsis/septic shock. Consult the wound/ostomy continence nurse (WOCN) for proper skin and wound care as drainage may be caustic to the peri-wound area. Employ customized pouching systems and negative pressure wound therapy with fistula isolation. Ensure adequate nutritional intake; enteral nutrition is preferred but may lead to increased fistula output as it stimulates the production of intestinal secretions. Poor oral intake can result in issues with dehydration and electrolyte imbalances.

Complications
Complications include an impaired quality of life that requires several months or even years to resolve. Consider referral to specialty centers for complex wound closure.

SURGICAL WOUND DEHISCENCE

Overview
Surgical wound dehiscence (SWD) is often preceded by the presence of a surgical site infection and may affect only superficial tissues and/or may involve the muscle fascia. SWD can appear simultaneously with other complications such as surgical wound infection or peri-wound fluid collection, including seromas, and hematomas, which increase tension at the incision and are more prone to infection. Risk factors for SWD include surgical procedures and their characteristics, such as emergent procedures, prolonged surgical time, presence of edema, high-tension incision, contamination, aggressive undermining, and previous radiation treatments near the site. Patients at risk for SWD include patients with diabetes, advanced age, tobacco use, malnutrition, obesity, steroid use, alcohol, chronic kidney disease, and/or chronic obstructive pulmonary disease (COPD).

Classic Presentation
An 86-year-old patient admitted after a motor vehicle crash resulting in a high-grade splenic laceration who underwent exploratory laparotomy and splenectomy is now postoperative day 2. The AGACNP notes the patient's midline surgical incision has opened from the distal pole to the umbilicus.

Diagnostic Criteria
Classic signs include separated wound margins or sutures that are not holding the wound margins closed. Additionally, peri-wound erythema, tenderness, fluctuant induration, bleeding at the incision site, malodorous wound drainage, or hyperthermia of the peri-wound tissue may be noted.

Treatment/Management
Treatment depends on the complication, the type of surgery, and the underlying diagnosis for the operative intervention. SWDs that are deeper may heal by secondary intention or delayed skin closure. Consult the WOCN. Dressing options include negative pressure wound therapy, silver ion-impregnated dressings, or wet-to-dry dressings. If infection is present, treat with appropriate antibiotics and remove sutures, staples, drains, and any necrotic tissue via debridement.

Complications
SWDs require prolonged wound care, increase morbidity, increase length of stay, and delay hospital discharge, which imposes significant cost increases to both patients and healthcare providers.

▶ NONTRAUMATIC NONSURGICAL WOUND

CHRONIC SKIN ULCERS
Arterial ulcers, diabetic ulcers, and venous stasis ulcers are the most prevalent types of chronic skin ulcers.

ARTERIAL ULCERS
Arterial ulcers most commonly affect the lateral ankle, toes, base of fifth metatarsal head and heel, and the ball of the foot. Classic signs of arterial ulcers include resting pain. Signs of arterial insufficiency include pale atrophic skin, extremity hair loss, nail dystrophy, claudication, weak or absent peripheral pulses, or reduced ankle-brachial index.

DIABETIC ULCERS

Diabetic ulcers can be classed as ischemic or neurotrophic. Ischemic ulcers have diminished pulses and pale atrophic tissue, whereas arterial perfusion and pulses are present with neurotrophic ulcers. Sites affected include the forefoot and toes.

VENOUS STATIS ULCERS

Venous statis ulcers (VSUs) are most often located on the inner aspect of the distal leg and ankle along the saphenous venous system. Chronic venous insufficiency is caused by failure of the calf muscle to pump, venous valvular reflux, or venous flow obstruction. Risk factors include age, female sex, race, obesity, malnutrition, prolonged standing, impaired mobility, sedentary lifestyle, personal or family history of VSU, deep vein thrombosis (DVT), trauma to leg, pregnancy, and smoking.

Classic Presentation

An 83-year-old woman with a history of COPD who smokes tobacco (two packs per day for 70 years) presents with a large wound to her inner right ankle with dependent edema and decreased sensation. The wound is painful and has copious amounts of malodorous exudates clinging to the pant leg and stuck to the ankle.

Diagnostic Criteria

Assessment reveals ulcer formation, hyperpigmentation, edema, lipodermatosclerosis-inflamed subcutaneous fat beneath the skin (panniculitis), atrophic blanch scarring, abnormally dilated veins at the ankle/varicosities, and venous stasis dermatitis. The Venous Clinical Severity Scoring System is used to grade the VSU. Grading includes pain; varicosities; edema; skin pigmentation; inflammation; induration; number, duration, and size of active ulcers; and compliance with compression therapy. Scores range from absent (0) to severe (3). Diagnosis can include a dermatology consult with skin biopsy to rule out other differential diagnoses.

Treatment/Management

Treatment of VSU is complex and requires optimal nutrition, moderate exercise as tolerated, compression therapy, and local wound care with debridement, cleaning, irrigation, and use of wet-to-dry dressings to promote debridement of necrotic tissue. A variety of types of specialized wound dressings can be used to optimize moisture balance, for epimerization stimulation, for infection, and for inflammation control. Antibiotics are needed for infected wounds. Multiple pharmacologic agents such as pentoxifylline, aspirin, calcium channel blockers, and topical corticosteroids are used if needed. Surgical debridement or skin grafting may be needed. Adjunctive therapies can include laser and light treatments.

Complications

Complications include high recurrence rates, long-term (often lifelong) management, and reduced quality of life. VSU has a wound-related mortality rate of 2.5%.

PRESSURE INJURIES

Overview

In 2016, new terminology was developed to describe pressure ulcers. The term *pressure injury* was coined to replace *pressure ulcer* in the National Pressure Ulcer Advisory Panel Pressure (NPUAP) Injury Staging System. Pressure injuries are defined as any damage to the skin and/or underlying tissue that results from intense or prolonged pressure with or without shear. The most common sites for pressure injuries are the hip (60%) and the foot (17%). Other sites include the ischium, sacrum, and trochanter.

Classic Presentation

A 49-year-old man with a history of alcoholism fell from a horse while inebriated and suffered a fractured C5 vertebrae and spinal cord injury, rendering him quadriplegic. Prealbumin was 10, albumin was 1.9, and body mass index (BMI) was 17. Initially, it was noted in the ED that there was redness over the coccyx when the patient was removed from the backboard. Despite a specialized bed to alleviate pressure to that area, early nutritional intervention, scheduled repositioning, and consultation with the wound care team, the patient's coccyx developed an open wound with full-thickness skin loss with fat visible within the wound.

Diagnostic Criteria

There are now six recognized types of pressure injuries per the NPUAP (Table 17.6).

Table 17.6 Types of Pressure Injuries

Nomenclature	Description
Stage 1	Intact skin Nonblanchable erythema in lightly pigmented skin Darkly pigmented skin may appear differently
Stage 2	Partial-thickness skin loss with exposed dermis Pink or red, moist, viable tissue Fluid-filled blister (intact or ruptured)
Stage 3	Full-thickness skin loss with fat visible in the wound Granulation tissue may be present
Stage 4	Full-thickness skin and tissue loss Fascia, muscle, tendon, ligament, cartilage, or bone exposed or palpable
Unstageable	Slough or eschar in wound bed Obscured full-thickness skin and tissue loss
Deep tissue	Persistent nonblanchable deep red, maroon, or purple discoloration Blood-filled blister (intact or ruptured) Epidermal separation and dark wound bed

Treatment/Management

Prevention is the best treatment. It is imperative to take patients off backboard, remove cervical collars as soon as clinically able, turn patients frequently, optimize nutritional status, and use specialized dressings, surfaces, mattresses, and/or beds to minimize pressure to bony prominences. Early recognition of signs of breakdown permits earlier interventions. Implement measures to minimize shearing of skin and tissues when moving patients. Pad any splinting or bracing devices. Treatment should include consultation with wound care specialist and early debridement as needed.

Complications

Complications can include stretching, tearing/disruption, or occlusion of blood vessels leading to tissue ischemia and tissue death; disfigurement; and impaired body image.

▶ SUMMARY

Healthy skin is important to protect our body from radiation, infection, extreme heat or cold, injuries, and invasive microorganisms. It supports the life of all of the other organs encased within. When the skin is compromised, the patient is at risk for a host of infections and potentially life-threatening complications. For AGACNPs, prompt attention to any change in patients' skin integrity is warranted, and immediate action is required.

KNOWLEDGE CHECK: CHAPTER 17

1. Which of the following is an example of an exfoliative skin disorder?

    A. Gas gangrene
    B. Necrotizing fasciitis
    C. Ecthyma gangrenosum
    D. Toxic epidermal necrolysis

2. Which of the following best describes a stage 4 pressure injury?

    A. Full-thickness skin loss with fat visible in the wound
    B. Partial-thickness skin loss with exposed dermis
    C. Full-thickness skin loss with fascia, muscle, tendon, ligament, cartilage, or bone exposed or directly palpable
    D. Partial-thickness skin loss where granulation tissue may be present

3. A 36-year-old man is noted to have a red, fluctuant lesion on his leg that is very tense and painful to touch. He stops by urgent care to have it evaluated. He is diagnosed with a cutaneous fistula, and an incision and drainage are performed. The wound is packed, and the patient is asked to return in 3 days for reevaluation. The patient is empirically placed on Bactrim DS for 7 days. The wound appears to improve, and the patient does not follow up. On day 5 of the antibiotic, the wound continues to improve; however, the patient begins to feel feverish, and the next day awakens with diffuse rash that progresses to blisters in a few hours. The chest wall is involved as well as the oral mucous membranes. Which of the following is the most likely diagnosis?

    A. Acute allergic reaction
    B. Drug exanthem
    C. Toxic shock syndrome
    D. Stevens–Johnson syndrome

4. An 82-year-old man with a history of chronic diverticulitis has a severe episode of lower abdominal pain. Upon his arrival to the ED, an upright chest x-ray is done, and free air is noted below the diaphragm. The patient is taken urgently to the operating room and undergoes a partial colectomy. Postoperative day 3, the incision begins to appear reddened, indurated, warm to touch, and tender to palpation. The wound appears tense, and a small amount of purulent exudate is noted on the dressing when changed. Which of the following is the most likely diagnosis?

    A. Wound dehiscence
    B. Cellulitis
    C. Surgical site infection
    D. Enterocutaneous fistula

5. An 89-year-old patient presents to the unit for an acute exacerbation of chronic obstructive pulmonary disease. Upon admission history and physical, the AGACNP notices the patient has ulcers along the lateral ankle. The patient states that the ankle is more painful at rest. The nurse practitioner suspects arterial ulcerations. What other signs would the nurse practitioner expect to see to support this patient's condition?

    A. Complaints of hair loss and claudication
    B. Good arterial perfusion
    C. Hyperpigmentation
    D. Lipodermatosclerosis

(See answers next page.)

1. D) Toxic epidermal necrolysis

Toxic epidermal necrolysis is an example of a severe mucocutaneous reaction to drugs or infective processes that results in blistering and epithelial sloughing. Gas gangrene, necrotizing fasciitis, and ecthyma gangrenosum are all examples of infective skin disorders.

2. C) Full-thickness skin loss with fascia, muscle, tendon, ligament, cartilage, or bone exposed or directly palpable

Pressure injuries are the net result of external forces that lead to localized loss of integrity to the epidermis, dermis, and subcutaneous tissue secondary to decreased blood flow. If unchecked, this ulcerative process can involve deep fascia, muscle, and bone.

3. D) Stevens–Johnson syndrome

Trimethoprim/sulfamethoxazole is a causative agent for Stevens–Johnson syndrome. The rash can appear within 4 to 28 days from initiation of medication. A rash that rapidly progresses to blisters is one of the hallmarks of this syndrome. This case is not typical of the conditions associated with toxic shock syndrome. Drug exanthems do not usually involve mucous membranes.

4. C) Surgical site infection

With perforation of the diverticula, there is a high risk of contamination. This, coupled with the advanced age of the patient, can cause a surgical site infection. The symptoms of localized erythema, induration, warmth, pain at incision site, and purulent exudates are all consistent with surgical site infection.

5. A) Complaints of hair loss and claudication

The patient has signs of an arterial ulcer. The hallmark of arterial ulcers is resting pain most commonly found over the lateral ankle and toes in the base of the fifth metatarsal head and heel and the ball of the foot. Other signs consistent with arterial insufficiency include pale atrophic skin with hair loss and nail dystrophy. Claudication is common, and peripheral pulses can be either weak or absent. Diabetic ulcers have good arterial perfusion, and venous stasis ulcers have hyperpigmentation and lipodermatosclerosis.

6. A 61-year-old patient presents to the ED with altered mental status and fever. Vitals include heart rate of 112, blood pressure of 82/43, and respiratory rate of 21. The patient's caregiver reports the patient has had a perineal skin infection that has worsened over the past 24 hours. A CT is obtained and demonstrates air under the perineal skin infection. The *best* step to achieve source control is:

   A. Broad-spectrum antibiotics
   B. Surgical debridement
   C. Initiation of vasopressors
   D. 1 L normal saline bolus

7. Lesions associated with acne vulgaris are typically described as:

   A. Vesicular
   B. Bullous
   C. Papular
   D. Pustular

8. A 24-year-old patient with no past medical history and no known allergies presents with worsening redness, pain, and swelling to the left lower extremity. Initially, a small area of redness appeared just below the knee where the patient wears kneepads while wrestling. The area increased in size to what appeared to be a boil. The AGACNP notes an erythematous, warm, raised lesion with mild fluctuance to the skin distal to the left patella. Vital signs are unremarkable with the exception of a low-grade fever. Based on this assessment, the AGACNP performs an incision and drainage and orders:

   A. Cephalexin (Keflex) 1 g oral every 8 hours for 7 days
   B. Ciprofloxacin (Cipro) 500 mg oral every 12 hours for 7 days
   C. Amoxicillin/clavulanate (Augmentin) 875 mg oral every 8 hours for 7 days
   D. Sulfamethoxazole/trimethoprim (Bactrim DS) 1 tablet oral twice a day for 7 days

9. An 82-year-old patient is being cared for on the general wards for hospital-acquired pneumonia and is receiving broad-spectrum antibiotics. The nurse caring for the patient tells the AGACNP that upon removing the patient's brief, she noticed redness to the lower back. On assessment, the AGACNP notices diffuse erythematous patches to the lower back extending into the gluteal fold with small areas of pustules in a satellite pattern. The patient denies pain but states they can feel some irritation. Based on this assessment, the AGACNP orders:

   A. Acyclovir
   B. Nystatin powder
   C. Transparent film
   D. Hydrocortisone 1% cream

10. The AGACNP is completing an assessment of a 78-year-old woman who states that she has a painless area on her forehead. She is worried that she may have skin cancer. On exam, the AGACNP notes an isolated papule that is rough, poorly circumscribed, and erythematous with white scaling. The AGACNP suspects the lesion to be:

    A. Actinic keratosis
    B. Basal cell carcinoma
    C. Squamous cell carcinoma
    D. Melanoma

(See answers next page.)

6. B) Surgical debridement
Antibiotics, vasopressors, and a normal saline bolus are all indicated for this patient, but the best step to achieve source control is surgical debridement to remove the necrotic tissue.

7. D) Pustular
Acne vulgaris is associated with pustular lesions. These lesions are filled with yellow proteinaceous fluid. Herpes zoster lesions are vesicular (palpable elevations with fluid-filled cavities). Impetigo and pemphigoid are associated with bullous lesions; these lesions are 1.0 cm or larger and fluid filled. Papular lesions are slightly raised and nonfluid filled and are associated with basal cell carcinoma.

8. D) Sulfamethoxazole/trimethoprim (Bactrim DS) 1 tablet oral twice a day for 7 days
Community-acquired MRSA (CAMRSA) is the suspected organism causing the symptoms. The patient's risk factor is sports-related use of equipment with close skin contact. Sulfamethoxazole/trimethoprim, doxycycline, and clindamycin all have good sensitivity to CAMRSA bacteria and are first-line treatment for such a diagnosis. The patient would not meet admission criteria, and it is feasible to begin oral antimicrobials after the incision and drainage. Cephalexin, ciprofloxacin, and amoxicillin/clavulanate would provide adequate coverage for streptococcus- and methicillin-sensitive staphylococcal organisms.

9. B) Nystatin powder
The patient is at risk for fungal skin infection related to administration of broad-spectrum antibiotics and bedridden status while wearing a brief. Candidiasis is the most common fungal skin organism. Candida pustules can develop on the backs of bedridden patients and appear as red patches, sometimes with erosion, and peripheral satellite pustules. Nystatin powder is a topical polyene that is used to treat fungal skin infections. Acyclovir is prescribed for herpes zoster; these lesions are typically grouped vesicles on an erythematous base along a dermatome. Transparent film will protect the area from friction but will not decrease the fungal load. Topical steroids are used to decrease inflammation and itching but will not inhibit the synthesis of ergosterol (an essential component of the fungal cytoplasmic membrane).

10. A) Actinic keratosis
Actinic keratoses are benign precancerous lesions caused by chronic ultraviolet radiation and are characterized by tender, rough, poorly circumscribed, erythematous papules with white or yellow scaling. These lesions are typically found in older adults. They appear most often in areas with prolonged sun exposure. Basal cell carcinoma has three common appearances: (a) waxy translucent papule with overlying telangiectasias with central ulceration, (b) scar-like appearance, and (c) erythematous macule or papule with fine scale or superficial erosion, often surrounded by telangiectasia. Squamous cell carcinoma presents as an occasionally tender, erythematous papule, plaque, or nodule with keratotic scale. Melanoma is typically irregularly shaped with variations in tan, brown, and gray discoloration.

● KEY BIBLIOGRAPHY

Only key resources appear in the print edition. Access the full bibliography for this chapter on ExamPrepConnect.com.

Bhama, A. (2019). Evaluation and management of enterocutaneous fistula. *Diseases of the Colon & Rectum*, *62*(8), 906–910. https://doi:10.1097/DCR.0000000000001424

Blair, D., & Piccicacco, N. (2020). Management and treatment of necrotizing fasciitis. *AACN Advanced Critical Care*, *31*(2), 118–125. https://doi.org/10.4037/aacnacc2020467

Buterakos, R. (2023). Burns. In V. Fuller & P. McCauley (Eds.), *Textbook for the adult-gerontology acute care nurse practitioner: Evidence-based standards of practice*. Springer Publishing Company.

Clebak, K., & Malone, M. A. (2018). Skin infections. *Primary Care*, *45*(3), 433–454. https://doi.org/10.1016/j.pop.2018.05.004

Gabriel, A., Gupta, S., & Orgill, D. (2019). Challenges and management of surgical site occurrences. *Plastic and Reconstructive Surgery*, *143*(1S), 7S10S. https://doi.org/10.1097/PRS.0000000000005305

Psychosocial, Behavioral, and Cognitive Health Review

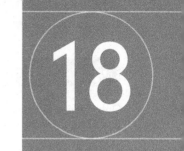

Kerri Ellis, Shari Harding, and Martha Ofeibea Agbeli

▶ INTRODUCTION

Annually in the United States, more than 130 million emergency department visits occur, with approximately 16.2 million patients admitted to the hospital and 2.3 million admitted to critical care. Critical illness is associated with a negative impact on patients' cognitive, physiological, and psychological well-being. Patients with prolonged hospital stays, specifically in the ICU, are at risk for an exacerbation of their psychological symptoms, development of post-ICU syndrome (PICS), and increase in morbidity and mortality. A call to action has been instituted to improve mental health care delivery during patients' ICU admission. An AGACNP's understanding of mental health in this patient population will likely lead to improved patient outcomes in acute care settings. This chapter discusses common mental health diagnoses affecting patients with critical illness.

▶ ANXIETY DISORDERS

DISEASE OVERVIEW
The term *anxiety disorder* encompasses many disorders, including generalized anxiety disorder, panic attacks, agoraphobia, panic disorder, social anxiety disorder, phobias, and anxiety disorders induced by substance exposure, substance withdrawal, or medical conditions. Anxiety disorders are some of the most common psychiatric disorders and are twice as common in female patients than in male patients but nonetheless are quite prevalent across all ages and sexes.

CLASSIC PRESENTATION: GENERALIZED ANXIETY DISORDER
A 24-year-old female patient presents with a history of "anxiety and worrying" with onset in the teen years. She describes an increase in anxiety over the past 2 months in the context of increased stressors, specifically starting graduate school and breaking up with her girlfriend of 2 years. She reports difficulty falling asleep, racing thoughts at night, decreased concentration, decreased appetite with weight loss of 5 lb in the past month, and fatigue.

DIAGNOSTIC CRITERIA
- Diagnosis is based on clinical interview and history.
- Screening tools include the general anxiety disorder-7 (GAD-7), Beck Anxiety Inventory, or Hamilton Anxiety rating scale (HAM-A).
- Elements include history of presenting illness (HPI), family history, presence of symptoms such as anxiety, fear, excessive worrying, racing thoughts, irritability, panic attacks, or disturbances in sleeping, appetite, concentration, or energy levels.
- Physical symptoms are common among people with anxiety disorders and can include muscle tension, headaches, nausea, dizziness, pounding heart, feeling of choking, numbness/tingling in extremities, sweating, shaking/chills, and gastrointestinal upset.
- Underlying medical causes for symptoms should be ruled out.
- Anxiety is a common emotion; to classify as a disorder, symptoms must cause clinically significant distress or impairment in functioning.

TREATMENT/MANAGEMENT

Psychotherapy is generally clinically indicated for anxiety disorders. Psychotherapy is provided by mental health clinicians such as psychologists, psychiatric mental health nurse practitioners, psychiatrists, and other licensed counselors. Multiple types of psychotherapy exist. Common modalities include cognitive behavioral therapy (CBT), supportive or "talk therapy," psychodynamic or psychoanalytic therapies, and exposure-based therapies. Common psychopharmacological treatments include one or more of the agents in Table 18.1.

Table 18.1 Anxiety Disorder Psychopharmacology

Drug Category	Examples
Selective serotonin reuptake inhibitors (SSRIs)	Prozac (fluoxetine) Paxil (paroxetine) Zoloft (sertraline) Celexa (citalopram) Lexapro (escitalopram) Luvox (fluvoxamine)
Serotonin-norepinephrine reuptake inhibitors (SNRIs)	Effexor (venlafaxine) Cymbalta (duloxetine)
Partial serotonin agonist	Buspar (buspirone)
Norepinephrine-dopamine reuptake inhibitor (NDRI)	Wellbutrin (bupropion)
Tricyclic antidepressants	Elavil (amitriptyline) Silenor (doxepin) Anafranil (clomipramine) Pamelor (nortriptyline) Tofranil (imipramine) Norpramin (desipramine)
Other antidepressants	Remeron (mirtazapine) Trintillex (vortioxetine) Serzone (nefazodone) Desyrel (trazodone) Viibryd (vilazodone)
Central alpha-agonists	Minipress (prazosin) Catapres (clonidine)
Benzodiazepines	Valium (diazepam) Klonopin (clonazepam) Ativan (lorazepam) Xanax (alprazolam)
Other anxiolytics	Vistaril (hydroxyzine pamoate) Neurontin (gabapentin)
Atypical antipsychotics (not first line, off-label use with a heavy side effect burden)	Seroquel (quetiapine) Zyprexa (olanzapine) Risperdal (risperidone) Abilify (aripiprazole)

COMPLICATIONS

Individuals with anxiety disorders often have other psychiatric disorders such as depression, substance abuse, or substance use disorders. Individuals with anxiety disorders may experience suicidal ideation or attempt suicide.

▶ MOOD DISORDERS

DISEASE OVERVIEW

The term *mood disorder* encompasses multiple disorders, including major depressive disorder, persistent depressive disorder, bipolar I disorder, bipolar II disorder, premenstrual dysphoric disorder, disruptive mood dysregulation disorder, and mood disorders induced by substance exposure, substance withdrawal, or medical conditions.

MAJOR DEPRESSIVE DISORDER

- Major depressive disorder has a lifetime prevalence of nearly 17% and a past-year prevalence of 7.1%.
- Onset is typically at least after puberty, peaking during the 20s, but it can occur at any age, with first episodes occurring even among older adults.
- It is about twice as common among female patients.

BIPOLAR DISORDER

- Bipolar disorder is less prevalent than depression: bipolar I lifetime prevalence of up to 2.4% and bipolar II up to 4.8%, annual incidence less than 1%.
- Mean age of onset is approximately 18 years; literature is mixed on possible "second wave" with menopause.
- It has roughly equal prevalence among male and female patients.

CLASSIC PRESENTATION: MAJOR DEPRESSIVE DISORDER

A 48-year-old male patient presents with a chief complaint of feeling "empty and tired" over the past month. He endorses difficulty with sleep onset and early morning awakening, increased appetite, low energy, and decreased ability to make decisions. He has low self-esteem and has missed work twice in the past 2 weeks because he could not get out of bed. He reports sometimes thinking he would "be better off dead."

DIAGNOSTIC CRITERIA

- Bipolar disorder is diagnosed on clinical interview.
- Screening tools for depression include Patient Health Questionnaire-9, Beck Depression Inventory, or Hamilton Depression rating scale (HAM-D).
- Screening tools for bipolar disorder include Mood Disorder Questionnaire and Composite International Diagnostic Interview.
- Major depressive symptoms include depressed mood or feeling empty/hopeless, anhedonia, low energy, decreased concentration, increased or decreased sleep or appetite, low self-esteem, guilt, and/or suicidal thoughts.
- Bipolar I disorder is diagnosed when a person has had at least one depressive episode and one manic episode.
- Manic symptoms include distractibility, increased energy and activities, decreased need for sleep, grandiosity, pressured speech, flight of ideas, hallucinations or delusions, and disinhibition/ engaging in excessive pleasurable activities with high potential for painful consequences, such as overspending, risky sex practices, risk-taking behaviors, and overuse of ethyl alcohol (ETOH) or illicit drugs.
- Bipolar II disorder is diagnosed when a person has had at least one depressive episode and one hypomanic episode.
- Hypomanic episodes are less severe than manic episodes and may even present as periods of high productivity with fewer or no negative consequences.

TREATMENT/MANAGEMENT

- Psychotherapy is generally clinically indicated for mood disorders.
- Common psychopharmacological treatments for depression include one or more of the following: selective serotonin reuptake inhibitors (SSRIs), selective serotonin-norepinephrine reuptake

inhibitors (SNRIs), other antidepressants (e.g., mirtazapine, tricyclic antidepressants [TCAs], trazodone, bupropion, monoamine oxidase inhibitors [MAOIs]), atypical antipsychotics, and anticonvulsant mood stabilizers (e.g., lamotrigine).

- Common psychopharmacological treatments for bipolar disorder include one or more of the following: lithium carbonate, atypical antipsychotics, or anticonvulsant mood stabilizers (e.g., valproic acid, lamotrigine, carbamazepine).

COMPLICATIONS
Individuals with mood disorders often have other psychiatric disorders such as anxiety, substance abuse, or substance use disorders. Individuals with mood disorders may experience suicidal ideation or attempt suicide.

▶ POSTTRAUMATIC STRESS DISORDER

DISEASE OVERVIEW
Posttraumatic stress disorder (PTSD) has a lifetime prevalence of 8.7%; past-year prevalence is 3.5%. PTSD is common among veterans and ICU patients during hospitalization and after discharge.

CLASSIC PRESENTATION
A 35-year-old female patient has a history of childhood physical abuse and a history of intimate partner violence in her 20s. She presents with a chief complaint of mood swings and trouble sleeping. She endorses intrusive thoughts about past trauma and nightmares every night. She often has trouble falling and staying asleep. She feels irritable "all the time" and has gotten into trouble at work for "having a bad attitude." She avoids romantic relationships, crowds, and enclosed spaces.

DIAGNOSTIC CRITERIA
- PTSD is diagnosed on clinical interview.
- Screening tools for PTSD include Primary Care PTSD and Trauma Screening Questionnaire.
- Elements include HPI, family history, trauma history, and the presence of symptoms such as reexperiencing past trauma (e.g., intrusive thoughts, nightmares, flashbacks), hyperarousal symptoms (sleep disturbance, irritability/anger, hypervigilance), negative or numb mood, and avoidance behaviors (e.g., avoiding triggers, isolating self).

TREATMENT/MANAGEMENT
- Psychotherapy is generally clinically indicated for PTSD.
- Common psychopharmacological treatments include one or more of the following:
  - Central alpha-agonists
  - SSRIs
  - SNRIs
  - Other antidepressants (e.g., mirtazapine, TCAs, trazodone, bupropion, MAOIs)
    - ❑ MAOIs are not first-line options due to many significant drug–drug interactions as well as food–drug interactions.
    - ❑ MAOIs inhibit the enzyme that breaks down monoamines including serotonin, dopamine, and norepinephrine; interactions with other medications can lead to toxicity.
    - ❑ Consumption of tyramine-rich foods can precipitate hypertensive crisis.
  - Atypical antipsychotics such as quetiapine (off-label use and heavy side effect burden)
  - Anticonvulsant mood stabilizers (e.g., lamotrigine)

COMPLICATIONS
Individuals with PTSD may experience suicidal ideation or attempt suicide.

▶ OBSESSIVE-COMPULSIVE DISORDER

DISEASE OVERVIEW

Obsessive-compulsive disorder (OCD) is characterized by severe anxiety, worry, or distress as well as obsessions and/or compulsions that lead to distress or impairment, including odd behaviors or significant portions of the day occupied with compulsive behaviors. Obsessions are unwanted/intrusive and recurrent thoughts, images, or urges. Common themes for obsessions include contamination fears; taboo thoughts involving sex, aggression, or religion; and symmetry/order. Compulsions are the behaviors or mental acts that are repetitive that the person feels driven to perform either in response to the obsession or according to a set of mental rules. Common compulsions include excessive washing/cleaning, arranging, checking, counting, or praying. OCD has a 2.5% lifetime prevalence and a 1.2% past-year prevalence. Mean age of onset is 19.5 years; age 6 to 15 years for male and 20 to 29 years for female patients. Female patients are affected at a slightly higher rate than in adulthood, and male patients are more commonly affected in childhood.

CLASSIC PRESENTATION

A 25-year-old male patient presents with his spouse, who has observed "odd" behaviors, including the patient tapping his foot a certain number of times before crossing the threshold of any door. The spouse has also witnessed excessive concerns about germs and refusal to eat raw fruits or vegetables. The patient endorses both obsessions and compulsions related to germs/contamination fear, as well as a belief that if he does not tap his foot "until it feels just right" before crossing a threshold, then something bad will happen to his spouse. He has had difficulty with arriving at work on time due to this behavior and has experienced constipation related to limiting of certain foods.

DIAGNOSTIC CRITERIA

- OCD is diagnosed on clinical interview.
- Screening tools include Yale–Brown OCD Scale (Y-BOCS; adult and child versions are available).
- Elements include HPI, family history, presence of symptoms such as anxiety, excessive worrying, obsessions, and/or compulsions.
- Physical signs of compulsions may be present (e.g., irritated skin from excessive washing).
- The content of obsessions is often embarrassing to those with OCD because it is incongruent with their actual preferences, beliefs, and values; normalizing and direct inquiry with examples of common obsessions can be helpful.

TREATMENT/MANAGEMENT

Psychotherapy is generally clinically indicated for OCD, especially exposure and response prevention and CBT. Common psychopharmacological treatments include one or more of the following: SSRIs and clomipramine (a TCA).

COMPLICATIONS

Individuals with OCD often have other psychiatric disorders such as substance abuse or substance use disorders. Individuals with OCD may experience suicidal ideation or attempt suicide. Individuals with OCD may experience complications related to compulsive behaviors (e.g., skin irritations, repetitive movement–induced injuries, nutritional excesses/deficiencies).

▶ SEROTONIN DISCONTINUATION SYNDROME

DISEASE OVERVIEW

Serotonin discontinuation syndrome occurs when serotonergic agents are tapered or stopped too quickly. Symptoms include flu-like symptoms (fatigue, lethargy, myalgias, chills, headache), insomnia (sleep disturbances, vivid dreams), nausea (gastrointestinal symptoms, vomiting, diarrhea), imbalance (dizziness, vertigo, ataxia), sensory disturbances (sensation of electric shocks in the arms, legs, or head), and hyperarousal (anxiety, agitation).

TREATMENT/MANAGEMENT

Reintroduce a serotonergic agent; consider a longer-acting agent such as fluoxetine.

▶ SEROTONIN SYNDROME

DISEASE OVERVIEW

Serotonin syndrome is serotonin toxicity; it occurs when there is too much serotonergic action and can occur from the use or misuse of one or more serotonergic medications or substances. Symptoms include altered mental status, delirium, agitation, confusion, autonomic hyperactivity, shivering, hyperreflexia, increased body temperature, vital sign abnormalities, restlessness, and sweating.

TREATMENT/MANAGEMENT

Serotonin syndrome can be a medical emergency. Immediately discontinue all serotonergic agents. Consider use of benzodiazepines or an antiserotonergic agent (e.g., cyproheptadine). Manage hyperthermia with acetaminophen, cooling blankets, and so on.

▶ NEUROLEPTIC MALIGNANT SYNDROME

DISEASE OVERVIEW

Neuroleptic malignant syndrome (NMS) occurs as an adverse event among people taking antipsychotic medication. Symptoms can include elevated core body temperature, moderate to severe muscle rigidity, diaphoresis, tachycardia, elevated or labile blood pressure, dysphagia, incontinence, tremor, changes in level of consciousness, mutism, leukocytosis, elevated serum creatine kinase (CK), and electrolyte abnormalities.

TREATMENT/MANAGEMENT

- NMS is a medical emergency.
- Treatment includes intravenous (IV) fluids, dopamine agonists, and muscle relaxants.

▶ BENZODIAZEPINE WITHDRAWAL

- Benzodiazepine withdrawal occurs if benzodiazepines are tapered or stopped too quickly
- Symptoms include seizures, tremors, anxiety, altered mental status, psychosis or other perceptual disturbances, and autonomic instability.

TREATMENT/MANAGEMENT

Treatment includes long-acting benzodiazepines (e.g., diazepam), often given IV, and titrated to effect.

▶ DELIRIUM

DISEASE OVERVIEW

Delirium is characterized by acute/rapid disturbance of consciousness and change in cognition. Patients have reduced ability to focus, sustain, or shift attention. Delirium occurs in 25% to 65% of hospitalized older patients and often goes unrecognized. It can develop over a short period of time (hours to a few days) and tends to fluctuate over the course of the day (waxes and wanes). Classic features include altered level of consciousness from baseline; memory impairment; perceptual disturbance (e.g., hallucinations); altered sleep–wake cycles; change in psychomotor activity; disorientation to time, place, and/or person; and alteration in mood. Three types of delirium exist (Table 18.2). Risk factors for delirium are presented in Table 18.3.

Table 18.2 Subtypes of Delirium

Hypoactive	"Quiet type": decreased psychomotor activity, drowsiness, lethargy, and stupor
Hyperactive	"ICU psychosis": psychomotor agitation, mood lability, and uncooperativeness
Mixed	Fluctuation of psychomotor activity and mental status changes

Table 18.3 Risk Factors for Delirium

■ Advanced age ■ Severe illness ■ Cognitive impairment ■ Dehydration (high urea–creatinine ratio suggestive of dehydration) ■ Use of medications such as sedatives, narcotics, anticholinergics, psychotropic drugs ■ Acute illness such as infection or organ impairment	■ Biochemical disturbances (abnormal electrolytes or glucose) ■ Presence of comorbid diseases ■ Functional impairment ■ Alcohol or drug intoxication/withdrawal ■ Use of physical restraints ■ Malnutrition ■ Polypharmacy ■ Consequence of a general medical condition

COMPLICATIONS

Increased mortality, poor prognosis: 40% mortality rate in 1 year, longer length of hospital stays, increased hospital-acquired infections and complications, and persistent cognitive deficits increased when discharged to long-term care.

CLASSIC PRESENTATION

An 81-year-old male patient recently underwent an elective knee replacement. Two days postoperative, he is confused, restless, urinating on the floor, and unable to follow directions and has poor safety awareness (attempting to climb out of bed). The registered nurse (RN) reports that despite administering Haldol 2 mg and Ativan 1 mg as needed (PRN) for agitation, the patient's behaviors seem to have worsened over time.

ETIOLOGY OF DELIRIUM

The etiology of delirium can be summarized by the mnemonic D-E-L-I-R-I-U-M-S:

■ *D*rugs (e.g., anticholinergics, neuroleptics, opioids, benzodiazepines, alcohol)
■ *E*lectrolyte imbalance (e.g., hyponatremia)
■ *L*ow oxygen; *L*ack of drugs (i.e., withdrawal from substances such as alcohol)
■ *I*nfection (e.g., urinary tract infection, pneumonia)
■ *R*etention of urine or feces; reduced sensory input
■ *I*ctal or postictal state
■ *U*ndernutrition: vitamin deficiencies
■ *M*etabolic: uncontrolled diabetes, hypo- versus hyperthyroidism; *M*yocardial problems
■ *S*ubdural hematoma

DIAGNOSTIC CRITERIA

Screening/diagnosis includes comprehensive health and physical examination to identify and treat etiology. Diagnosis is based on clinical symptoms; however, the confusion assessment method can be used to assess for the presence, severity, and fluctuation of nine delirium features and can be completed at the bedside within a few minutes.

Diagnostic testing can include complete blood count (CBC) with differential, chemistries, hepatic enzymes, vitamin B_{12}/folate levels, thyroid stimulating hormone (TSH) with reflex T_4 and T_3, urinalysis (UA) and urine culture and sensitivity, EKG and others as directed by patient presentation such as computerized tomography (CT) scan and PET scan, toxic screen, chest x-ray, erythrocyte sedimentation rate (ESR), and HIV panel.

TREATMENT/MANAGEMENT
- Addressing of underlying cause(s)
- Symptom management
- Prevention of complications
- Education of patient, family, and caregivers
- Family presence
- Avoidance of restraints
- Optimal mobility and self-care
- Nutritional supplements when indicated
- Supportive care to prevent physical and cognitive decline

Clinical Pearls

Behavioral symptoms associated with delirium (e.g., agitation, aggression, calling out, wandering) are often challenging to manage.

- Nonpharmacologic approach includes calmly approaching the patient, offering reassurance, addressing any unmet needs (toileting, hunger/thirst, pain), optimizing vision and hearing, reorienting patient, optimizing sleep, and using one-to-one sitter if needed.
- Pharmacologic interventions can include the D2 antagonist haloperidol, which can be administered PO, intramuscular (IM), or IV; however, it can exacerbate extrapyramidal symptoms. Atypical antipsychotics include Risperdal 0.5 to 4 mg daily, olanzapine 2.5 to 10 mg daily, and quetiapine 50 to 200 mg. The advantage of using atypical agents is a lower incidence of adverse reactions and side effects (e.g., extrapyramidal effects).

Clinical Pearls

- There is a U.S. Food and Drug Administration boxed warning for antipsychotic medication use in the geriatric population due to increased risk of cardiovascular and cerebrovascular events and sudden death.
- Extensive treatments of non-alcohol-related delirium may worsen delirium given the anticholinergic side effects.
- Restraints can worsen agitation and cause injury but may be used in the short term.

CLASSIC PRESENTATION
An 80-year-old female patient was recently started on Ativan 0.5 mg at bedtime secondary to insomnia. Today, the nursing home staff report incoherence, lethargy, unsteady gait, and urinary incontinence. This morning, the patient refused her medications due to paranoia that the nurse was attempting to poison her.

▶ NEUROCOGNITIVE DISORDERS

DEMENTIA
DISEASE OVERVIEW
Neurocognitive disorders are a broad categorization of chronic loss of intellectual or cognitive function. Cognitive decline is a gradual deterioration over 5 to 10 years leading to death and interfering with social and occupational function. Neurocognitive disorders present with an insidious onset (over months or years with a gradually worsening course). Cognitive changes do not fluctuate. The etiology of neurocognitive disorders includes Alzheimer type, vascular dementia, Lewy body dementia, frontotemporal degeneration, Parkinson disease, HIV infection, Huntington disease, and prion disease (Table 18.4).

Table 18.4 Comparison of Types of Dementia

Type of Dementia	Alzheimer Disease	Vascular Disease	Lewy Body Disease	Frontotemporal Degeneration (Pick Disease)
Background information	▪ Most common (60%–90%) ▪ Diagnosis is often made after age 65 years	▪ Second most common cause of neurocognitive disorder		▪ Typically presents between ages 35 and 65 years ▪ More common in men
Clinical manifestation	▪ Insidious onset ▪ Gradual progressive decline in cognitive function ▪ Aphasia (language disturbance ▪ Apraxia (impairments of motor activity despite intact motor function) ▪ Agnosia (failure to recognize objects despite intact sensory function) *Note:* Personality changes, mood swings, and paranoia are very common. Death often occurs within 10 years of diagnosis.	▪ Sudden onset ▪ Stepwise deterioration corresponding with occurrence of micro-infarcts ▪ May be an acute onset with partial improvement ▪ May have an insidious onset with gradual decline *Note:* Clinical manifestations depend on the area of infarction.	▪ Waxing and waning cognition ▪ Well-formed and detailed visual hallucinations and delusions ▪ Excessive sleepiness ▪ Postural instability and recurrent falls ▪ Development of extrapyramidal signs (parkinsonism) at least 1 year after cognitive decline becomes evident	Personality and behavioral changes and early-stage behavioral symptoms ▪ Disinhibited behaviors ▪ Oral exploration ▪ Lack of sympathy, empathy ▪ Apathy ▪ Limited insight ▪ Social misconduct ▪ Repetitive speech, behaviors, and rituals ▪ Difficulties with speech and comprehension (decrease in speech production and word finding) *Note:* Cognitive changes later in the disease. ▪ Klüver–Bucy syndrome: hypersexuality, hyperorality, and placidity

(*continued*)

Table 18.4 Comparison of Types of Dementia (*continued*)

Type of Dementia	Alzheimer Disease	Vascular Disease	Lewy Body Disease	Frontotemporal Degeneration (Pick Disease)
Etiology	▪ Hypoactive acetylcholine and norepinephrine ▪ Accumulation of extraneuronal beta-amyloid plaques and intraneuronal tau protein tangles ▪ 1% from an autosomal dominant single gene mutation ▪ Definitive diagnosis made postmortem *Note:* Age of onset is earlier in patients with family history.	▪ Cardiovascular and cerebrovascular disease (hypertension, diabetes, smoking, obesity, hyperlipidemia, atrial fibrillation, coronary artery disease, advanced age) ▪ Associated with multiple infarctions	Lewy bodies and Lewy neurites in the brain	▪ Atrophy and hyperactivity of the frontal and temporal lobes ▪ Accumulations of Pick bodies
Treatment	No cure ▪ Cholinesterase inhibitors ▪ NMDA receptor antagonists *Note:* Serotonergic agents, mood stabilizers, and antipsychotics are used for behavioral disturbances.	No cure ▪ Treat underlying cause such as such as management of vascular disease	Antipsychotic sensitivity ▪ Cholinesterase inhibitors ▪ Quetiapine or clozapine for psychotic symptoms ▪ Melatonin and/or clonazepam for REM sleep behavior disorder	Symptom focused ▪ Consider serotonergic agents to help reduce disinhibition, anxiety, repetitive behaviors and eating disorders

NMDA, *N*-methyl-D-aspartate; REM, rapid eye movement

TREATMENT/MANAGEMENT

▪ Pharmacologic interventions:
  ● Cholinesterase inhibitors: donepezil (Aricept), rivastigmine (Exelon), and galantamine (Razadyne):
    ❑ Slows clinical deterioration: Mild to moderate
    ❑ Reduces agitated behaviors
    ❑ Rivastigmine available as transdermal patch
    ❑ Common side effects: nausea, diarrhea, vomiting, weight loss, insomnia
    ❑ *Does not alter the course of the disease process*
    ❑ *N*-methyl-D-aspartate (NMDA) receptor antagonist: memantine (Namenda)
    ❑ Moderate to severe disease
    ❑ Common side effects: nausea, vomiting
    ❑ Promotes neuroplasticity
    ❑ Often prescribed in combination with cholinesterase inhibitors
    ❑ Antipsychotic medication
      ○ Used to treat agitation and aggression
      ○ High risk of extrapyramidal symptoms
      ○ Lowest effective dose used
      ○ Should be used after weighing the benefits versus risk
▪ Supportive care with psychosocial interventions
▪ Neurological consult
▪ Referral to psychotherapy if appropriate

SCREENING TOOLS
- Mini-Mental State Examination
- Montreal Cognitive Assessment
- Mini-Cog
- Saint Louis University Mental Status (SLUMS) exam

LAB TESTING
Testing includes CBC with differential, chemistries, TSH, and vitamin B_{12} and folate levels.

DISEASE PROGRESSION
Progression is increased agitation, emotional outbursts, poor sleep, then wandering.

▶ SUICIDE

SUICIDE OVERVIEW
Suicide is a leading cause of death in the United States. The rate of suicide deaths has continued to increase in incidences across all ages, with the highest increase in ages 18 to 25 years. Suicide is highest among non-White males, with highest incidence in ages 75 years and older. The most common method of suicide is by firearm, followed by suffocation in male patients and poisoning in female patients. For every suicide death, there are 25 suicide attempts with in-hospital suicide of less than 65 incidents per year. In 2020, more than 405,000 patients were hospitalized after a suicide attempt. Care of a patient after a suicide attempt varies and is based on the individual's planning of the self-injurious behavior.

CLASSIC PRESENTATION
A 48-year-old male patient presented to the emergency department after a self-inflicted gunshot wound to the right temporal area of the head. Emergency medical services reported multiple alcohol bottles at the scene; no bottles of medications or other paraphernalia were noted. Vital signs stable; Glasgow Coma Scale score: 3. Patient was intubated for airway protection.

INDIVIDUALS AT RISK
Individuals at risk include those with mental health diagnoses, previous suicide attempt, unexpected loss of a loved one, loss of employment, loss of housing, incarceration, recent discharge from a psychiatric faculty, and access to firearms. Also at risk are those who have recently learned of a new, potentially fatal diagnosis.

DIAGNOSTIC CRITERIA
- If suicide attempt is suspected, the initial evaluation is to stabilize life-threatening medical conditions. Once the individual is identified to be medically stable, the focus will be on the patient's mental health stabilization and recovery.
- Diagnostic abnormalities will be dependent on suicide attempt method. If suspected overdose or toxic ingestion, order CBC, comprehensive metabolic panel (CMP), liver function tests (LFTs), prothrombin time (PT)/international normalized ratio (INR), EKG, and drug screen and levels.

TREATMENT/MANAGEMENT
Medical clearance to ensure clinical stability. Prevention of additional self-harm while hospitalized by initiating 1:1 observation by a trained sitter. Removal of any means of self-harm, keeping personal items outside the room, and limiting visitors to family.

SCALE
The SAD PERSON Scale (Table 18.5) was developed to assist providers in identifying patients at risk of suicide.

Table 18.5 The SAD PERSONS Scale

S = Sex (male) A = Age (younger than 19 years or older than 45 years) D = Depression P = Previous attempt E = Ethanol abuse R = Rational thinking loss S = Social supports lacking O = Organized plan N = No spouse S = Sickness (new diagnosis or chronic illness)	Each item, if present, receives 1 point. 0–2: Provider able to send home with follow-up 3–4: Consider hospitalization versus close follow-up 5–6: Hospitalization advised if follow-up not certain 7–10: Commit or hospitalize

COMPLICATIONS

Complications include ongoing suicide ideation or suicide attempt.

▶ POST-ICU SYNDROME

DISEASE OVERVIEW

Patients who survive a critical illness may experience cognitive, emotional, and physical symptoms after hospital discharge. Up to 50% of patients will not be able to return to their previous employment due to symptoms of PICS. These symptoms may last for months to years. Symptoms of PICS vary and are quite individualized based on the individual's experiences. See Table 18.6 for possible symptoms of PICS.

Table 18.6 Symptoms of PICS

Cognitive	Emotional	Physical
◼ Difficulty with focus, concentration, and attention ◼ Loss of memory ◼ Speech may be affected	◼ Anxiety ◼ Depression ◼ Posttraumatic stress disorder ◼ Decreased energy and motivation	◼ Fatigue ◼ Muscle weakness ◼ Decreased breathing ◼ Decreased mobility

PICS, post-ICU syndrome.

CLASSIC PRESENTATION

A 54-year-old female patient was admitted to the medical ICU for management of hypoxic respiratory failure secondary to viral pneumonia. She was intubated for 10 days. During this time, she received IV sedation with fentanyl and versed, as well as a paralytic to improve oxygenation and ventilation. She was transferred to a rehab facility and required 2 weeks to regain her strength. She had been discharged home, but her family is concerned about her progress. She is having difficulty remembering recent events and managing her activities of daily living. She is also struggling with going up and down stairs and is complaining of ongoing fatigue. She has not been able to sleep through the night due to nightmares and feeling anxious. She is scheduled to go back to work in 2 weeks.

RISK FACTORS

They include age older than 65 years, critical illness requiring ICU admission, and decreased functional status prior to critical illness.

TREATMENT/MANAGEMENT

There is no specific treatment for PICS at this time. Preventive measures to reduce time in ICU are the key to avoiding PICS. Implement the ABCDEF bundle for all critically ill patients (Table 18.7).

Table 18.7 The ABCDEF Bundle

Acronym	Meaning
A = Analgesia	A: Assess and Manage Pain
B = Breathing	B: Spontaneous: Awaking Trials (SAT) and Breathing Trials (SBT)
C = Choice	C: Choice of Analgesia and Sedation
D = Delirium	D: Assess, Prevent, and Treat Delirium
E = Early	E: Early Mobility and Exercise
F = Family	F: Family Engagement and Foley removal

Note: Family meetings held within 72 hours of admission can improve patient outcomes.

COMPLICATIONS

Cognitive, emotional, and physical symptoms post hospital discharge can persist and impact activity of daily life and reduce quality of life.

▶ SUMMARY

Patients who are admitted to the hospital for management of acute illness or exacerbation of chronic illness symptoms may have a preexisting psychiatric condition. It is important for the AGACNP to be knowledgeable on mental health conditions to improve patient experience and outcomes. Restarting or continuing home psychiatric medications in the acute care setting should be a priority when it is medically safe to do so.

KNOWLEDGE CHECK: CHAPTER 18

1. An individual has a history of two major depressive episodes and now presents meeting criteria for hypomania in the absence of any medications or other substances. The individual can be diagnosed with:

   A. Bipolar I disorder
   B. Bipolar II disorder
   C. Major depressive disorder
   D. Major depressive disorder with anxious distress

2. Serotonin syndrome symptoms include:

   A. Shivering, hyperreflexia, sweating, tachycardia, increased temperature
   B. Shivering, hyperreflexia, inability to sweat, increased temperature
   C. Flu-like symptoms, insomnia, nausea, hyperarousal
   D. Flu-like symptoms, hypersomnia, nausea, sensory disturbance

3. Benzodiazepines cannot be suddenly stopped because of the risk of:

   A. Seizures
   B. Alcohol use disorder relapse
   C. Serotonin syndrome
   D. "Brain zaps"

4. A 24-year-old female patient presents with flu-like symptoms, insomnia, nausea, sensory disturbance including "brain zaps," and anger. The nurse practitioner suspects:

   A. Benzodiazepine withdrawal
   B. Neuroleptic malignant syndrome
   C. Selective serotonin reuptake inhibitors discontinuation syndrome
   D. Serotonin syndrome

5. It is a priority to assess for which of the following symptoms in an individual with major depressive disorder (MDD)?

   A. Feelings of emptiness
   B. Increased appetite
   C. Difficulty with sleep
   D. Suicidal ideation

6. Which of the following medications carries the highest risk for serotonin syndrome?

   A. Clonazepam
   B. Bupropion
   C. Fluoxetine
   D. Quetiapine

7. Which of the following patients is at the *greatest* risk for a suicide attempt?

   A. 76-year-old man newly diagnosed with metastatic lung cancer
   B. 45-year-old man who just started a new job
   C. 56-year-old woman who participates in Alcoholics Anonymous
   D. 35-year-old woman who was fired from her job as a server

(See answers next page.)

1. B) Bipolar II disorder

The *DSM-V* diagnostic criteria for bipolar II disorder require a history of one or more depressive episodes plus one hypomanic episode. The patient has not met the criteria for a manic episode. Major depressive disorder and major depressive disorder with anxious distress are not appropriate diagnoses for this patient because the individual meets the criteria for a hypomanic episode.

2. A) Shivering, hyperreflexia, sweating, tachycardia, increased temperature

Shivering, hyperreflexia, sweating, tachycardia, and increased temperature are signs and symptoms of serotonin syndrome. An inability to sweat is not a symptom of serotonin syndrome. Flu-like symptoms, insomnia, nausea, and hyperarousal are symptoms of serotonin discontinuation syndrome. Flu-like symptoms, hypersomnia, nausea, and sensory disturbance are not symptoms of serotonin syndrome.

3. A) Seizures

Sudden or abrupt cessation of benzodiazepines can cause seizures. Alcohol use disorder relapse is not a direct risk of stopping benzodiazepines. Benzodiazepines are not serotonergic agents. "Brain zaps" are a symptom of serotonin discontinuation syndrome.

4. C) Selective serotonin reuptake inhibitors discontinuation syndrome

The patient's symptoms occur with the abrupt cessation of serotonergic antidepressants. Symptoms of neuroleptic malignant syndrome include elevated core body temperature, moderate to severe muscle rigidity, diaphoresis, tachycardia, elevated or labile blood pressure, dysphagia, incontinence, tremor, changes in level of consciousness, mutism, leukocytosis, elevated serum CK, and electrolyte abnormalities. Benzodiazepine withdrawal symptoms include seizures, tremors, anxiety, altered mental status, psychosis or other perceptual disturbances, and autonomic instability. Serotonin syndrome symptoms include altered mental status, delirium, agitation, confusion, autonomic hyperactivity, shivering, hyperreflexia, increased body temperature, vital sign abnormalities, restlessness, and sweating.

5. D) Suicidal ideation

Individuals with MDD are at increased risk of suicide, and suicidal ideation is a symptom of MDD. Feelings of emptiness, increased appetite, and difficulty with sleep can all be symptoms of major depressive disorder but do not carry the same risk or priority level as assessing suicidal ideation.

6. C) Fluoxetine

Fluoxetine is a selective serotonin reuptake inhibitor and increases serotonin; clonazepam, bupropion, and quetiapine do not directly increase serotonin.

7. A) 76-year-old man newly diagnosed with metastatic lung cancer.

Recent diagnosis with a serious illness is a risk factor for suicide attempt. In addition, men older than 75 years have the highest risk of suicide attempts. While loss of a job can be a risk factor for suicide attempt, being a 35-year-old woman is not a risk factor.

8. A 27-year-old man was found on the ground with empty containers of acetaminophen and lorazepam. Emergency medical services bring him to the emergency department with C-spine precautions in place. He is intubated for airway protection. The Glasgow Coma Scale score is 3. What will the AGACNP order for diagnostic workup?

   A. Complete blood count (CBC), comprehensive metabolic panel (CMP), liver function tests (LFTs), prothrombin time (PT)/international normalized ratio (INR), acetaminophen level
   B. thyroid stimulating hormone (TSH), folic acid, CMP, CBC, urine drug screen
   C. C-reactive protein, D-dimer, LFTs, PT/INR
   D. TSH, folic acid, lorazepam level, LFTs

9. A 64-year-old female patient is admitted for management of hypoxic respiratory failure secondary to pneumonia. She required intubation and sedation to improve oxygenation and ventilation. It is now hospital day 5. Which of the following interventions will decrease the likelihood of her developing post-ICU syndrome (PICS)?

   A. Daily awakening trials
   B. De-escalating antibiotics after 3 days
   C. Increasing sedation daily
   D. Holding tube feeds after midnight and resuming at 6 a.m. daily

10. Which of the following is a key diagnostic feature that aids in differentiating delirium and dementia?

   A. Acute and rapid onset
   B. Laboratory tests that are pathognomonic for delirium
   C. No alterations in attention
   D. None; there is no need to differentiate the two conditions

11. Which medication or drug class poses the greatest risk for causing or precipitating delirium in older adults?

   A. Antihypertensives
   B. Antibiotics
   C. St. John's wort
   D. Anticholinergics

12. According to the Beers criteria, which of the following drugs or drug classes should be avoided in the treatment of delirium?

   A. Rivastigmine
   B. Olanzapine
   C. Sedative-hypnotics
   D. Haloperidol

(See answers next page.)

8. **A) Complete blood count (CBC), comprehensive metabolic panel (CMP), liver function tests (LFTs), prothrombin time (PT)/international normalized ratio (INR), acetaminophen level**

The patient's situation suggests possible polypharmacy drug overdose. Assessing electrolytes and ruling out infection, acute anemia, toxic level of acetaminophen, and end organ damage will assist the provider in next steps of the patient's care. There is no benefit to testing for benzodiazepine level. TSH, C-reactive protein, and D-dimer are not the highest priority.

9. **A) Daily awakening trials**

If safe to do so, all sedation should be stopped daily and, if needed, restarted at half the dose with ongoing assessment to meet the patient's needs. Daily interruption of sedation has been shown to decrease the number of days of required mechanical ventilation and duration of ICU admission. Changing antibiotics should be guided by clinical presentation and microbiology results. Increasing amounts of sedation and undernutrition are linked to the development of PICS.

10. **A) Acute and rapid onset**

When differentiating dementia from delirium, delirium is characterized by an acute/rapid disturbance of consciousness and change in cognition, whereas dementia is a chronic loss of intellectual or cognitive function.

11. **D) Anticholinergics**

According to the acronym D-E-L-I-R-I-U-M, drugs with anticholinergic properties pose the greatest risk for causing or precipitating delirium in older adults. Because of pharmacokinetic and pharmacodynamic changes, this population is sensitive to medications.

12. **C) Sedative-hypnotics**

The Beers criteria were developed by the American Geriatric Society with the goal to decrease inappropriate medication prescribing and adverse drug events in patients 65 years and older. According to the Beers criteria, benzodiazepines and nonbenzodiazepine receptor agonist hypnotics (i.e., the "Z drugs:" zolpidem, eszopiclone, and zaleplon) should be avoided in older adults with delirium.

13. An older female patient is admitted for sepsis due to a urinary tract infection. She is pulling her IV out and climbing out of bed despite redirection. The best approach to this patient is:

    A. Physical restraints
    B. Normalization of sleep–wake cycle
    C. Nonpharmacological approaches
    D. Pharmacological management

14. A 68-year-old man presents with early dementia, fluctuating level of consciousness, parkinsonism, and visual hallucinations. Which of the following is the most likely diagnosis?

    A. Dementia with Lewy bodies (DLB)
    B. Dementia due to Alzheimer disease
    C. Dementia due to a medical condition
    D. Frontotemporal dementia

15. If an AGACNP needed to administer an antidote for a suspected benzodiazepine overdose, what would they order?

    A. Flumazenil (Romazicon)
    B. Naloxone (Narcan)
    C. Fentanyl (Sublimaze)
    D. Phenytoin (Dilantin)

(See answers next page.)

13. C) Nonpharmacological approaches

In patients with delirium, nonpharmacological interventions such as approaching the patient calmly, reorientation, optimizing sleep, and addressing unmet needs are considered first-line. Pharmacologic interventions such as antipsychotics can be considered to address safety concerns such as agitation and aggression. Physical restraints are not recommended and should be used only as a last resort and for a short time if warranted.

14. A) Dementia with Lewy bodies (DLB)

This patient has DLB. With DLB, cognitive symptoms tend to wax and wane. Patients experience well-formed, detailed visual hallucinations, excessive sleepiness, and postural instability. Extrapyramidal signs tend to develop at least 1 year after cognitive decline. These patients are sensitive to antipsychotic medications. Cholinesterase inhibitors, clozapine, and quetiapine are generally well tolerated.

15. A) Flumazenil (Romazicon)

Patients with suspected overdose usually will recover with supportive management; however, if the provider decides to reverse the benzodiazepine overdose, the medication of choice is flumazenil (Romazicon). The provider needs to be aware that when flumazenil (Romazicon) is administered to a patient with routine use of a benzodiazepine, the patient will develop acute benzodiazepine withdrawal that can be fatal. Naloxone is for opioid overdose. Fentanyl is an opioid receptor agonist. Dilantin is for the management of seizures.

KEY BIBLIOGRAPHY

Only key resources appear in the print edition. Access the full bibliography for this chapter on ExamPrepConnect.com.

American Psychiatric Association. (2013). *Diagnostic and statistical manual of mental disorders* (5th ed.). https://doi.org/10.1176/appi.books.9780890425596

Boland, R., Verduin, M., & Ruiz, P. J. (2021). *Kaplan & Sadock's synopsis of psychiatry* (12th, North American ed.). LWW.

Holroyd-Leduc, J., & Reddy, M. (2012). *Evidence-based geriatric medicine: A practical clinical guide*. BMJ Books.

Marra, A., Ely, E. W., Pandharipande, P. P., & Patel, M. B. (2017, April). The ABCDEF bundle in critical care. *Critical Care Clinics*, 33(2), 225–243. https://doi.org/10.1016/j.ccc.2016.12.005

Sadock, B. J., Sadock, V.A., & Ruiz, P. (2021). *Kaplan and Saddock's synopsis of psychiatry: Behavioral sciences/clinical psychiatry* (12th ed.). Wolters Kluwer.

Multisystem Review

Dawn Carpenter, Alexander Menard, Johnny Isenberger,
Roxanne M. Buterakos, and Gail Lis

▶ INTRODUCTION

This chapter covers problems that span multiple systems. These are some of the most complex problems AGACNPs will manage. Many of the problems reviewed in this chapter can and do lead to death. Prompt recognition and early interventions by the AGACNP will save patients' lives.

▶ ACID-BASE IMBALANCES

DISEASE OVERVIEW
Acid-base disturbances are common in acutely ill patients. AGACNPs must be able to interpret arterial blood gases (ABGs) and chemistries, identify underlying etiologies, and implement appropriate actions.

INTERPRETATION
- Step 1. Evaluate the pH: Is the patient acidemic (pH less than 7.38) or alkalotic (pH greater than 7.42)?
- Step 2. Evaluate the PCO_2 and HCO_3:
  - If the pH is acidemic and the PCO_2 is greater than 45, then it is a respiratory acidosis.
  - If the pH is acidemic and the HCO_3 is less than 22, then it is a metabolic acidosis.
  - If the pH is alkalotic and the PCO_2 is less than 35, then it is a respiratory alkalosis.
  - If the pH is alkalotic and the HCO_3 is greater than 26, then it is a metabolic alkalosis.
- Step 3. Evaluate the level of compensation (Table 19.1).
- Step 4. Evaluate the anion gap (AG): AG = (Sodium [Na] + Potassium [K]) − (HCO_3 + chloride [Cl]).
  - Anion gap metabolic acidosis (AGMA) exists when AG is greater than 12 (with albumin correction).
- Step 5. If there is a metabolic acidosis, evaluate for another metabolic disturbance:
  - For AGMA, calculate a delta gap, which is (AG-12) − (24-HCO_3).
    - ❏ If greater than 6, then there is an additional metabolic alkalosis.
    - ❏ If less than 6, then there is an additional normal gap metabolic acidosis.

Table 19.1 Acid-Base Disorder and Additional Evaluation

Primary Disorder	Evaluation
Respiratory acidosis	If there is a change in HCO_3 of: ■ 1 mmol/L increase per 10 mmHg $PaCO_2$ above 40 mmHg, then it is an "acute" respiratory acidosis ■ Less than 1 mmol/L increase per 10 mmHg $PaCO_2$ above 40 mmHg, then there is an additional metabolic acidosis ■ 4–5 mmol/L increase per 10 mmHg $PaCO_2$ above 40 mmHg, then it is a "chronic" respiratory acidosis ■ Greater than 5 mmol/L increase per 10 mmHg $PaCO_2$ above 40 mmHg, then there is an additional metabolic alkalosis

(continued)

Table 19.1 Acid-Base Disorder and Additional Evaluation (*continued*)

Primary Disorder	Evaluation
Respiratory alkalosis	If there is a change of HCO_3 of: ■ 2 mmol/L decrease per 10 mmHg decrease in $PaCO_2$ below 40 mmHg, then there is an "acute" respiratory alkalosis ■ Less than 2 mmol/L decrease per 10 mmHg decrease in $PaCO_2$ below 40 mmHg, then there is an additional metabolic alkalosis ■ 4–5 mmol/L decrease per 10 mmHg decrease in $PaCO_2$ below 40 mmHg, then there is a "chronic" respiratory alkalosis ■ Greater than 5 mmol/L decrease per 10 mmHg decrease in $PaCO_2$ below 40 mmHg, then there is an additional metabolic acidosis
Metabolic acidosis	Expected $PaCO_2 = 1.5 \times [HCO_3] + 8 (\pm2)$ ■ If $PaCO_2$ is lower than expected, then there is an additional respiratory alkalosis. ■ If $PaCO_2$ is higher than expected, then there is an additional respiratory acidosis.
Metabolic alkalosis	Expected $PaCO_2 = 0.7([HCO_3]-24) + 40 (\pm2)$ ■ If $PaCO_2$ is lower than expected, then there is an additional respiratory alkalosis. ■ If $PaCO_2$ is higher than expected, then there is an additional respiratory acidosis.

For classic presentations of each disorder, see Table 19.2. Evaluation and management of each acid-base disorder is noted in Table 19.3.

Table 19.2 Classic Presentations of Acid-Base Disorders

Disorder	Classic Presentations
Respiratory acidosis	A 64-year-old female patient is post-ORIF of her hip fracture and is in acute pain. She received 10 mg morphine and now she is sleepy but arouses to voice. Her ABG reveals pH 7.18, $PaCO_2$ 70 mmHg, PaO_2 60 mmHg, HCO_3 of 27.
Respiratory alkalosis	A 23-year-old male patient is admitted after a motor vehicle crash resulting in a femur fracture. He says his pain is 10/10, and he is hyperventilating. His ABG reveals pH 7.53, $PaCO_2$ 22 mmHg, PaO_2 100 mmHg, HCO_3 22. He is started on a PCA regimen and is much more comfortable.
Metabolic acidosis	A 64-year-old female patient is admitted with CAP. She is hypotensive and requires IV fluid resuscitation and vasopressors. Her ABG reveals pH 7.2, $PaCO_2$ 22 mmHg, PaO_2 52 mmHg, HCO_3 16. Lactic acid is 10.4.
Metabolic alkalosis	A 72-year-old female patient with a history of HFrEF is admitted to the hospital with a heart failure exacerbation. She is aggressively diuresed. Her ABG reveals pH 7.54, $PaCO_2$ 55 mmHg, PaO_2 72, HCO_3 38.

ABG, arterial blood gas; CAP, community-acquired pneumonia; HFrEF, heart failure with reduced ejection fraction; IV, intravenous; ORIF, open reduction internal fixation; PCA, patient-controlled analgesia.

Table 19.3 Evaluation and Management of Acid-Base Disorders

Disorder	Evaluation and Management
Respiratory acidosis	■ Determine if acidosis is acute or chronic. ■ Calculate A-a gradient which is $150-PaO_2-(1.25 \times PaCO_2)$: ● If greater than 10, then cause is hypoventilation with intrinsic lung disease, V/Q mismatch, or both. ● If less than 10, then cause is hypoventilation without intrinsic lung disease. ■ Causes of hypoventilation include CNS depression (medications, neurologic injury), airway occlusion, thoracic disease (post-thoracic procedures, rib fractures, hemothorax, pneumothorax), abdominal disease (postsurgical procedures, abdominal compartment syndrome), and myopathies. ■ Treatment involves reversing cause of hypoventilation. For those with intrinsic lung disease, noninvasive ventilation may be helpful but should not delay intubation.

(*continued*)

Table 19.3 Evaluation and Management of Acid-Base Disorders (*continued*)

Disorder	Evaluation and Management

Respiratory alkalosis	▪ Determine if alkalosis is acute or chronic.
	▪ Calculate A-a gradient which is $150 - PaO_2 - (1.25 \times PaCO_2)$:
	  ● If greater than 10, then cause is hyperventilation with intrinsic lung disease, V/Q mismatch, or both.
	  ● If less than 10, then cause is hyperventilation without intrinsic lung disease.
	▪ Causes of hyperventilation include fever, pregnancy, pulmonary embolism, pneumonia, pain, anxiety, CNS disease, hypoxia, and inappropriate ventilator settings.
	▪ Treatment involves reversing the cause of hyperventilation.

Metabolic acidosis	▪ Determine if it is AGMA or NGMA. **AGMA** Think MUDPILERS: Methanol Uremia DKA/Alcoholic KA Paraldehyde Isoniazid Lactic acid Ethanol/ethylene glycol Rhabdomyolysis or renal failure Salicylate **NGMA** Think HARDUPS: Hyperalimentation Acetazolamide Renal tubular acidosis Diarrhea Uretero-pelvic shunt Post-hypocapnia Spironolactone and saline ▪ Management involves reversing the cause of the metabolic acidosis and providing specific therapy. For instance, dialysis is indicated for ethylene glycol poisoning, and aggressive IV fluid resuscitation is needed for rhabdomyolysis. ▪ Bicarbonate infusion is helpful to keep the pH greater than 7.2 in the setting of renal failure.
Metabolic alkalosis	▪ Think CLEVER PD: Contraction Licorice Endocrine Vomiting Excess alkali Refeeding alkalosis Post-hypercapnia Diuresis ▪ Management involves removing the cause of the metabolic alkalosis. ▪ Acetazolamide may be used.

AGMA, anion gap metabolic acidosis; CNS, central nervous system; IV, intravenous; NGMA, non-anion gap metabolic acidosis; V/Q, ventilation/perfusion.

▶ SHOCK

DISEASE OVERVIEW

Shock is an imbalance of oxygen delivery and consumption, not just hypotension. The AGACNP must be able to diagnose and manage all types of shock states. Older adult, medically frail, and immunocompromised patients do not always have classic signs and symptoms, making diagnosis of shock challenging. Measurement of lactic acid and mixed venous oxygen saturation (SvO_2) can help with the diagnosis. Additionally, patients can experience two or more types of shock simultaneously, such as neurogenic and hemorrhagic, as in a trauma patient or a patient in cardiogenic shock who develops septic shock. Table 19.4 reviews the hemodynamics associated with each shock state. Table 19.5 reviews classifications of hemorrhagic shock.

Table 19.4 Hemodynamics by Type of Shock

Type of Shock	CVP/PCWP Preload	CO	SVR Afterload	SvO$_2$
Hypovolemic	↓	↓	↑	↓
Cardiogenic	↑	↓	↑	↓
Distributive: Septic	↓	↑	↓	↑
Distributive: Neurogenic	↓	↓	↓	↓
Distributive: Anaphylactic	↓	↓	↓	↔
Obstructive	↑	↓	↔	↔
Adrenal insufficiency	↔	↓	↔	↓

CVP, central venous pressure; PCWP, pulmonary capillary wedge pressure; SVR, systemic vascular resistance; CO, carbon monoxide; SvO$_2$, venous oxygen saturation.

Table 19.5 Classification of Hemorrhagic Shock

	Class I	Class II	Class III	Class IV
Blood loss	750	750–1,500	1,500–2,000	Greater than 2,000
Percentage (%) blood volume	15%	15%–30%	30%–40%	Greater than 40%
HR	Less than 100	Greater than 100	Greater than 120	Greater than 140
BP	Normal	Normal	Decreased	Decreased
Capillary refill	Normal	Decreased	Decreased	Decreased
RR	14–20	20–30	30–40	Greater than 35
U/O	Greater than 30 mL/hr	20–30 mL/hr	5–15 mL/hr	Negligible
Mental status	Slightly anxious	Anxious	Anxious/confused	Confused/lethargic

BP, blood pressure; HR, heart rate; RR, respiratory rate; U/O, urine output.

TREATMENT

Treatment of shock depends on the type of shock and its etiology (Table 19.6). Treat the underlying etiology. Vital signs and hemodynamic monitoring should be dynamic in nature and may include measurements from arterial lines, pulmonary artery catheters (PACs), FloTrac/Vigileomonitors, esophageal Doppler monitors, and/or bioimpedance monitors. Fluid resuscitation is commonly used in all types of shock except for left-sided heart failure. In septic shock, guidelines recommend fluid bolus of 30 mL/kg, with ongoing dynamic evaluation of clinical response. Multiple volume assessment modalities exist, including passive leg raises, pulse pressure variation, ultrasound of inferior vena cava (IVC) variability, and PACs. Vasopressors and inotropes may be needed to support hemodynamics (Table 19.7). End points of resuscitation should be continually evaluated, including urine output, capillary refill, lactate clearance, and tissue perfusion.

TABLE 19.6 Treatments by Type of Shock

Type of Shock	Treatments
Hypovolemic: Nonhemorrhagic	■ IVF boluses and maintenance fluids
Hypovolemic: Hemorrhagic	■ PRBCs, plasma, platelets, cryoprecipitate ■ Serial CBC, INR, fibrinogen, TEG/ROTEM

(*continued*)

Table 19.6 Treatments by Type of Shock (*continued*)

Type of Shock	Treatments
Cardiogenic	▪ Rhythm control ▪ Reperfusion strategies: PCI, CABG ▪ Vasopressor support (norepinephrine) ▪ Inotropic support (milrinone, dobutamine) ▪ Mechanical support: IABP, Impella, VAD
Distributive: Septic	▪ Culture and obtain lactate ▪ Source control (e.g., debridement, surgery, line removal) ▪ Broad-spectrum antibiotics ▪ Fluid bolus 30 mL/kg ▪ Vasopressor support (norepinephrine, vasopressin, epinephrine) ▪ Consider steroids (hydrocortisone)
Distributive: Neurogenic	▪ Spine immobilization ▪ Fluids, ensure not hemorrhaging simultaneously ▪ Vasopressors (norepinephrine, phenylephrine, dopamine) ▪ + Chronotrope for severe bradycardia (dopamine, Isuprel)
Distributive: Anaphylactic	▪ Secure airway ▪ Epinephrine IM ▪ IV steroids
Obstructive: PE	▪ Systemic TPA ▪ Thrombectomy ▪ Open heart surgery for open embolectomy
Obstructive: Tamponade	▪ Pericardiocentesis ▪ Pericardial window ▪ Emergent thoracotomy
Obstructive: Tension ptx	▪ Needle decompression: second ICS MCL; followed by: ▪ Chest tube insertion: fourth or fifth ICS MAL
Obstructive: Tumor	▪ Cardiothoracic surgery consult
Adrenal insufficiency	▪ IV steroids (hydrocortisone)

CABG, coronary artery bypass grafting; CBC, complete blood count; IABP, intra-aortic balloon pump; ICS, intercostal space; IM, intramuscular; INR, international normalized ratio; IV, intravenous; IVF, Intravenous fluid; MAL, midaxillary line; MCL, midclavicular line; PCI, percutaneous coronary intervention; PE, pulmonary embolus; PRBC, packed red blood cells; ptx, pneumothorax; tPa, tissue plasminogen activator; TEG/ROTEM, thromboelastography; VAD, ventricular assist device.

Table 19.7 Vasoactive Infusions, Dosing, Receptor Activity, and Cardiovascular Effects

Drug and Doses	Mechanism of Action	Main Effects
Inopressors		
Dopamine (Inotropin) ▪ 0.5–5 mcg/kg/min ▪ 5–10 mcg/kg/min ▪ 10–20 mcg/kg/min	b-1+, DA++++ a+, b-1++, DA+++ a+++, b-1++, DA+	VD +, I ++, CH + VD +, I ++++, CH ++ VC +++, I +++, CH +++, HR ++, MAP +, CO +
Epinephrine 0.01–0.05 mcg/kg/min Greater than 0.05 mcg/kg/min	a+, b-1+++, b-2++ a+++, b-1++, b-2++	VD +, VC +, I++++, CH++, HR+, MAP+, CO++ VC +++, I+++, CH+++, HR++, MAP++, CO++
Norepinephrine (Levophed) 0.5–30 mcg/min or 0.01–0.04 mcg/kg/min	a++++, b-1++	VC++++, I+, CH++, HR +-, MAP+++
Pure Vasopressors		
Angiotensin II (Giapreza) 0.125–40 ng/kg/min	Angiotensin II	VC+++,

(*continued*)

Table 19.7 Vasoactive Infusions, Dosing, Receptor Activity, and Cardiovascular Effects (*continued*)

Drug and Doses	Mechanism of Action	Main Effects
Inopressors		
Phenylephrine (Neosynephrine) 2–300 mcg/min or 0.1–1 mcg/kg/min	a++++	VC++++, HR Ø/-
Vasopressin (Pitressin) 0.01–0.06 units/min	Vasopressin +++	VC++++, MAP+++
Inodilators		
Dobutamine (Dobutrex) ■ 2–10 mcg/kg/min ■ 10–20 mcg/kg/min	a+, b-1++++	VD+, VC+, I+++, CH+, HR+, MAP+, CO+ VD++, VC+, I++++, CH++, HR++, MAP v, CO+
Milrinone (Primacor) 0.375–0.75 mcg/kg/min	cAMP	VD++, I+++, CH+++, HR++, CO+
Isoproterenol (Isoprel) 2–10 mcg/min	b-1++++	VD+, I++++, CH++++, HR ++++, MAP v, CO +++
Vasodilators		
Nitroglycerine ■ 1–50 mcg/min ■ Greater than 50 mcg/min	Increases cGMP production	Venous vasodilation Arterial vasodilation
Nitroprusside (Nipride) 10–200 mcg/min or 0.2–4 mcg/kg/min	Increases cGMP production	Systemic vasodilation

CH, chronotropy; CO, cardiac output; HR, heart rate; I, inotropy; MAP, mean arterial blood pressure; v, variable effects dependent on clinical status; VC, vasoconstriction; VD, vasodilation; Ø, no change; +, slight; ++, mild; +++, moderate; ++++, maximum; -, slight decrease.

MEDICAL SEQUELAE OF SHOCK AND RESUSCITATION

Patients in shock are at risk for complications, including organ ischemia, that can lead to organ failure. Ischemic complications include myocardial infarction (MI), ischemic cerebrovascular accident (CVA), and gastrointestinal ischemia. Organ failure can include acute kidney injury (AKI), acute respiratory distress syndrome (ARDS), and acute liver failure. Sequalae of shock also includes abdominal compartment syndrome, disseminated intravascular coagulation (DIC), venous thromboembolism (VTE), ventilator-associated pneumonia, other hospital-acquired infections with or without multidrug-resistant organisms, multisystem organ failure, pressure ulcers, ICU-acquired weakness, myopathy or neuropathy, and post-ICU syndrome. The AGACNP must be able to identify these sequelae, institute preventive measures, and treat these sequelae.

▶ POLYTRAUMA

DISEASE OVERVIEW

Trauma care starts at the site where the injury occurs. Hospitals and emergency medical personnel must have a good working relationship to ensure optimal care for the injured individual. *Polytrauma* is when a patient has multiple traumatic injuries at one time. Polytrauma increases the complexity of patient care for the AGACNP. Initial management of the trauma patient is complex given the multiple and competing priories to be considered. Initial management must include assessment of airway, breathing, and circulation.

Trauma activations are called into the ED before hospital arrival. Trauma facilities have a standard nomenclature to describe the acuity of the trauma patient (Table 19.8). This nomenclature is crucial to ensure appropriate resources are available in the trauma bay, give the trauma team a sense of acuity of the patient, and allow for adequate institutional preparation.

Table 19.8 Example of Trauma Levels

Trauma Level	Description—Meet Any of These Criteria
Level 1 Trauma	Serious or immediate threat of death or amputation ■ Intubated or unstable airway ■ RR less than 10 or greater than 40, HR less than 60 or greater than 120 ■ Penetrating trauma ■ Total or near amputation ■ Focal paralysis
Level 2 Trauma	Less serious ■ Loss of consciousness (witnessed) ■ HR greater than 100 ■ Burns greater than 20% ■ Pregnancy greater than 20 weeks with traumatic injury
Level 3 Trauma	Multisystem injuries ■ Burns less than 20% ■ No symptoms from level 1 or 2

COMPLICATIONS OF TRAUMA
CARDIAC TAMPONADE

The AGACNP must know *Beck triad* for cardiac tamponade (hypotension, jugular venous distension [JVD], and muffled heart sounds). This triad can represent a medical emergency: cardiac tamponade. It can be a result of blunt-force trauma to the chest. To make a definitive diagnosis of cardiac tamponade, an echocardiogram is required. The key to treatment is relief of pressure on the heart by means of a pericardiocentesis.

TENSION PNEUMOTHORAX

Tension pneumothorax is a condition that typically occurs in the setting of mechanical ventilation of resuscitative efforts. A tension pneumothorax generates positive pleural pressure that is transmitted to the mediastinum, which decreases venous return to the heart, resulting in reduced cardiac output. Typical findings in a patient with a tension pneumothorax include cardiovascular collapse, cyanosis, respiratory distress, and a sudden increase in peak pressures in the mechanically ventilated patient. The diagnosis can be made with a combination of chest radiograph or ultrasound with the clinical features outlined earlier. The treatment is relief of the pressure by means of needle decompression or tube thoracoscopy.

HEMORRHAGE

Hemorrhage must always be suspected in the polytrauma patient. With the presentation of hemodynamic instability, the patient can be brought directly to the operating room for intervention. For the hemorrhaging patient, direct pressure can be applied to the bleeding area, tourniquets can be applied, and pelvic binders can be used. Interventional radiologists can also explore methods like embolization to stop bleeding. The highest priority in treating the bleeding patient is to stop the bleed and replace blood as clinically warranted. It is important to note that replacing blood is not always a decision made based on a patient's hemoglobin and hematocrit but rather based on a constellation of clinical indicators.

If a cause for hemodynamic instability can be immediately identified, it can then be fixed. It is not always possible to completely fix the cause of the hemodynamic instability. In those cases, damage control surgery is done. Damage control surgery is a technique to avoid time-consuming definitive repair and instead focus on avoiding physiobiological derangements and reassessing the optimal time for definitive repair.

TRAUMA-INDUCED COAGULOPATHY AND MASSIVE TRANSFUSION PROTOCOLS

Coagulation abnormalities are common after major/polytraumas. Systemic tissue hypoperfusion seems to be a key factor in the development of trauma-induced coagulopathy (TIC). The physical damage to body tissues causes a biochemical reaction that sets off a cascade of events that cause TIC. The mainstay of treatment is supportive care. A randomized controlled study (the CRASH II study) showed a significant reduction in death from hemorrhage when tranexamic acid therapy was initiated within the first 3 hours following the trauma.

Much of the literature for hemostatic resuscitation and TIC comes from the military and the experience of treating combat-wounded soldiers. Massive transfusion protocols (MTPs) have developed from the literature for treating the trauma patient with TIC and hemorrhage. Administering blood products (packed red blood cells, platelets, plasma, cryoprecipitate) in equal ratios is a widely accepted approach for preventing or correcting TIC. The AGACNP must know institution-based protocols for TIC and MTPs, because these will vary. Depending on the institution, thromboelastography testing can assist in optimal resuscitation, aiding in the identification of specific deficiencies and allowing the AGACNP to tailor product replacement.

MTPs have been shown to reduce mortality in the trauma patient. Current MTPs use a ratio of 1:1:1 or 1:1:2 (plasma:platelets:red blood cells), although institutional protocol will determine exact ratios.

INTERDISCIPLINARY APPROACH

The trauma patient requires an interdisciplinary approach to care. With the polytrauma patient, it is infrequent that only one body system will be impacted. This requires consultation with specialists within each body system. An example is a patient involved in a motor vehicle crash (MVC) who suffers bilateral rib fractures and a femur fracture and sustains a moderate-to-severe traumatic brain injury. This patient will be a trauma activation, and the trauma service will be the primary team coordinating care but will also have consultation with the orthopedic service as well as neurosurgical service at a minimum. To obtain optimal outcomes for patients, an interdisciplinary approach is required.

▶ BURNS

DISEASE OVERVIEW

The AGACNP must know how to evaluate and treat a patient with a burn injury. The first 48 hours of burn care are critical and offer the greatest influence on morbidity and mortality. Most burn injuries are a result of thermal injury, while less than 10% of burns are a result of electrical or chemical burns. Flame and scald burns, considered thermal burns, are the leading cause of burns in adults. The extent of the burn injury is usually expressed as a percentage of total body surface area (TBSA) involved (Table 19.9). Burn injuries are classified into several categories (Table 19.10).

Table 19.9 Estimating TBSA

Method	Description	
Rule of Nines	Head = 9% Each arm = 9% Anterior chest and abdomen = 18%	Posterior chest and back = 18% Each leg = 18% Perineum = 1%
Lund and Browder chart	Each arm = 10% Anterior trunk = 13% Posterior trunk = 13% Head and legs percentage varies based on patient's age	
Palmar surface	For small burns, the patient's palm surface (excluding the fingers) represents approximately 0.5% of their body surface area, and the hand surface (including the palm and fingers) represents about 1% of their body surface area.	

TBSA, total body surface area.

Table 19.10 Classification of Burns

Classification of Burn	Description of Burn Injury	Signs and Symptoms
Superficial burns	Epidermis only	▪ Red ▪ Blanch with light pressure ▪ Painful and tender ▪ No vesicles or bullae

(continued)

Table 19.10 Classification of Burns (*continued*)

Classification of Burn	Description of Burn Injury	Signs and Symptoms
Superficial partial-thickness burns	Papillary dermis	■ Blanch with pressure ■ Painful and tender ■ Vesicles and bullae develop within 24 hours. ■ Bases of the vesicles and bullae are pink and develop fibrinous exudate.
Deep partial-thickness burns	Reticular dermis Involves hair follicles and sweat glands	■ May be white, red, or mottled white and red ■ No blanching with pressure and are less painful and tender than the more superficial burns ■ Will have difficulty discerning pinprick as will be described as pressure instead of sharp ■ Vesicles or bullae may develop ■ Burns are usually dry.
Full-thickness burns	Below the dermal layers of the skin into adipose	■ May be white or pliable, black or charred, brown or leathery, or bright red secondary to fixed hemoglobin in the subdermal region ■ Pale full-thickness burns may appear to be normal skin except that the skin does not blanch to pressure. ■ Can be anesthetic or hypo-esthetic ■ Hairs can be pulled easily from follicles. ■ Vesicles and bullae do not usually develop.
Subdermal burns	Extends through the skin and subcutaneous tissue into the fascia, muscle, or bone	■ Goes through both layers of skin. Underlying adipose, muscle, and/or bone are involved. ■ Hypoesthesia exists in the area since the nerve endings are destroyed.

INHALATION INJURY

The AGACNP must know that *inhalation injuries* can be a result of smoke inhalation or chemical inhalation as well as thermal injury. Confirmation of an inhalation injury requires direct visualization. The AGACNP must have high suspicion of an inhalation injury with any burn patient. Soot around the mouth and/or nose, facial burns, and singed nasal passages or hairs are highly suggestive of a thermal inhalation injury.

Aside from the airway and lung parenchymal injury that can occur, the AGACNP can evaluate for systemic toxicity like carbon monoxide (CO) poisoning and cyanide poisoning. CO poisoning can be excluded by a normal blood carboxyhemoglobin level. Signs and symptoms of CO and cyanide poisoning include headache, dizziness, weakness, upset stomach, vomiting, chest pain, and confusion and can progress to depressed mental status, cardiac arrest, or not otherwise explained cardiac decompensation. Cyanide poisoning is more difficult to detect as it cannot be measured in the blood quickly enough. Treatment options for those at risk of cyanide poisoning include oxygen, sodium thiosulfate, amyl nitrite, sodium nitrite, hydroxocobalamin, and dicobalt edetate (Kelocyanor).

TREATMENT

The American Burn Association recommends patients be referred to a burn center if they meet any of the criteria in Table 19.11. Minor burns can be treated with cooling, cleaning, covering, and comfort (Table 19.12).

Table 19.11 Criteria for Referral to Burn Center

■ Partial-thickness burns greater than 10% TBSA ■ Full-thickness burns ■ Burns to face, hands, feet, genitalia, major joints ■ Circumferential burns of an extremity ■ Chemical burns	■ Electrical or lightning strike injuries ■ Significant inhalation injuries ■ Burns in patients with multiple medical disorders ■ Burns in patient with associated traumatic injuries

TBSA, total body surface area.

Table 19.12 Minor Burn Treatment

Treatment	Use/Description
Cooling	Small areas of burn can be cooled with tap water or saline solution.
Cleaning	Mild soap and water or antibacterial wash can be used to clean a burn.
Covering	Topical antibiotic ointments or cream with absorbent dressing or specialized burn dressing materials can be used to cover a burn.
Comfort	Over-the-counter pain medications or prescription pain medications can be used when needed. Splints can also provide support and comfort for certain burned areas.

Severe burns, classified as greater than 20% TBSA, require more intensive treatment and management. Fluid resuscitation is a major component of burn care, particularly within the first 24 to 48 hours. Fluid resuscitation is focused on maintaining an adequate urine output of greater than 0.5 mL/kg/hr. The Parkland formula is commonly used to achieve this:

Total fluid to be given in the first 24 hours = 4 mL of LR x Paient weight (kg) x % TBSA.

Half of the total fluid to be given in the first 24 hours needs to be given over 8 hours from when the burn occurred, with the remaining fluid being given evenly over the remaining 16 hours. *Note:* The Parkland formula is a guide to resuscitation, and individual patient needs for resuscitation may vary. Additional treatments can include escharotomies, debridement, skin grafting, dressing changes, pain control, bronchoscopy, inhaled heparin, and Mucomyst (Table 19.13).

Table 19.13 Additional Burn Treatments

Treatment	Use/Description
Dressing changes	Most common with second- and third-degree burns
Topical ointments	Antimicrobial agents Chemical debridement
Pain control	Can range from over-the-counter medications to continuous IV infusions and should address background, breakthrough, procedural, perioperative, and chronic pain
Debridement	Sloughed or necrotic skin, including ruptured blisters, should be debrided before applying a dressing.
Bronchoscopy, inhaled heparin, and Mucomyst	Used for inhalation injuries
Skin grafting	*Split-thickness autografting:* includes epidermis and varying amounts of dermis *Full-thickness autografting:* includes entire thickness of skin (epidermis and dermis) *Skin substitutes:* primarily used to treat full-thickness burns

IV, intravenous.

COMPLICATIONS

Burn patients frequently develop complications, including infection, AKI, acute respiratory failure, cardiovascular failure, compartment syndrome, and multisystem organ failure. Survivors commonly experience ICU weakness, neuropathies, tolerance to opioids, and possibly contractures. Contractures can be minimized with early initiation of physical and occupational therapies.

NUTRITION

Nutritional support is critical to burn recovery and wound healing. Burn patients have exceptionally high caloric needs, specifically for extra protein. Nutritionist consultation should be obtained upon admission. Nutrition support should be started enterally (if able) as early as possible. Protein supplements should be provided if the patient can take an oral diet; the patient may still need nocturnal enteral support to meet caloric needs. Postpyloric feedings should be used to minimize holding tube feedings during repeated operations. Severely burned patients are challenged by hypermetabolism, which increases oxygen consumption and is associated with substantial increases in resting energy expenditure.

▶ MORBID OBESITY

Patients with obesity may have increased comorbidities and may require additional healthcare resources. Patients in the obese and extremely obese (formerly morbidly obese) categories have increased risks of hypertension, hyperlipidemia, coronary artery disease, vascular diseases, diabetes, infections, and obstructive sleep apnea. Patients with central obesity (men with waist circumference greater than 40 inches and women with waist circumference greater than 35 inches) have increased disease risk beyond what is listed in Table 19.14.

Table 19.14 BMI Classifications

	Classification	BMI	Disease Risk
Underweight		Less than 18.5	
Normal		18.5–24.9	
Overweight		25–29.9	Increased
Obesity	Class I Class II	30–34.9 35–39.9	High Very high
Extreme obesity	Class III	Greater than 40	Extremely high

BMI, body mass index.

For patients with BMI ≥30, document obesity classification and BMI in the assessment and plan section of notes. Documenting obesity increases the patient and hospital case mix index (CMI). CMI is a measure of the severity of illness and complexity of the inpatient population. The higher the CMI, the more complex is the hospital population, with higher acuity levels, greater use of resources, and higher risk of death. Documenting all comorbidities, including obesity classification, directly impacts the expected-to-observed mortality ratio for the hospital.

▶ INTRA-ABDOMINAL HYPERTENSION AND ABDOMINAL COMPARTMENT SYNDROME

DISEASE OVERVIEW
Intra-abdominal hypertension (IAH) can progress into abdominal compartment syndrome, a vicious cycle of inflammation with third spacing of fluids that results in organ ischemia, leading to superior vena cava (SVC) compression that impedes venous return to the heart, worsening preload and progressive shock state, and eventually leading to death if not intervened upon in a timely manner. It can occur in any patient who requires large volume resuscitation, including those with multisystem trauma, bowel injury, burns, pancreatitis, or septic shock.

SYMPTOMS
Symptoms of abdominal compartment syndrome include oliguria, hypotension, and tachycardia, with subsequent high-volume fluid resuscitation, followed by distended firm abdomen, increased peak and plateau ventilator pressures, decreased JVD, persistent hypotension, worsening hypotension despite escalating doses of vasopressors, progressive hypoxia, and metabolic acidosis.

DIAGNOSTIC CRITERIA
Abdominal compartment syndrome is a clinical diagnosis. Monitoring of abdominal compartment pressures can aid in the diagnosis. IAH can be diagnosed with intra-abdominal pressures of greater than 12 mmHg, whereas abdominal compartment syndrome is diagnosed with intra-abdominal pressures of greater than 20 mmHg with progressive organ dysfunction. Accurate measurement requires the patient to be supine. Acute bladder trauma is a contraindication to performing bladder pressures.

TREATMENT

Treatment of IAH and abdominal compartment syndrome includes interventions to decompress the abdominal cavity. Remove any excess volume that consumes space, including gastric decompression with a nasogastric tube, decompression of colon with a rectal tube or enema, and paracentesis, as applicable. Paralytics can decrease abdominal muscular resistance. Definitive treatment includes surgical decompression with laparotomy and opening of the fascia. Tertiary abdominal compartment syndrome can occur if the abdomen is not fully decompressed. Application of negative pressure wound therapy or VAC dressing temporizes the abdomen until diuresis or renal replacement therapy can remove excess volume. Primary closure can typically be accomplished in one to three operations, or secondary closure may be required if the fascia cannot be approximated.

CLASSIC PRESENTATION

A young adult man is 48 hours post-MVC with multiple injuries, including pelvic fracture, bowel injury, and splenic injury. He is status post-splenectomy and small bowel resection. He has a pancreatic injury as well. He received 10 L of IVF for ongoing oliguria. Vital signs currently are temperature 98.6°F, heart rate (HR) 120, respiratory rate (RR) 24, blood pressure (BP) 84/48, O_2 sat 90% on 60% 12PEEP. Plateau pressures have trended up to 30 cm.

▶ PAIN MANAGEMENT

OVERVIEW

Identify the type of pain (Table 19.15) to ensure appropriate and effective treatment. Determine whether the pain is acute or chronic. Chronic pain is defined as pain that persists longer than 3 to 6 months. Many hospitalized patients have acute and chronic pain simultaneously, which must be managed concurrently. Use caution to avoid oversedating, especially in older adults and medically frail persons.

Table 19.15 Types of Pain

	Description	Localization	Example
Neuropathic: ■ Central or peripheral nerves	■ Burning ■ Pins/needles ■ Tingling ■ Stabbing ■ Shooting ■ Severe	■ Stocking/glove pattern ■ Radiates down nerve	■ Peripheral neuropathy (diabetes, HIV, chemotherapy) ■ Neuralgia ■ Spinal cord or nerve root compression
Somatic: ■ Skin ■ Subcutaneous tissue ■ Joints ■ Connective tissue ■ Muscle ■ Fascia	■ Aching ■ Deep ■ Cramping ■ Throbbing ■ Constant ■ Dull ■ Gnawing ■ Sore	■ Localized ■ Sometimes radiates to surrounding areas	■ Joints ■ Tendonitis ■ Bursitis ■ Gout ■ Incisional pain ■ Wounds ■ Bone ■ Bone metastasis
Visceral ■ Organs ■ Organ capsule ■ Connecting structures	■ Cramping ■ Squeezing ■ Heaviness ■ Stabbing ■ Deep ■ Squeezing	■ Diffuse ■ Radiates to adjacent or supporting structures	■ Angina ■ Bowel obstruction ■ Pancreatitis ■ Cholecystitis

Pain management strategies should always include nonpharmacologic and pharmacologic interventions:

■ Nonpharmacologic strategies include rest, ice, heat, elevation, compression, and stretching.
■ Multimodal pain management strategies should be used to target multiple receptors, potentiate other agents, and minimize the use of narcotics.

■ Nonopioid medications include (as appropriate) nonsteroidal anti-inflammatory drugs (NSAIDs), acetaminophen, Lidoderm patch, muscle relaxants such as methocarbamol (Robaxin) or cyclobenzaprine (Flexeril), gabapentin (Neurontin) or pregabalin (Lyrica), peripheral nerve block, or epidural catheter.

■ Opioids are commonly required to manage acute pain in surgical and trauma patients, along with other acute pain syndromes such as sickle cell crisis, nephrolithiasis, and pancreatitis. Opioids are highly addictive; thus, develop a plan to taper off opioids at the initiation of the agent. Start with oral narcotics (as able); use IV medications for breakthrough pain. Avoid morphine in patients with AKI as metabolites can accumulate, causing oversedation.

■ Older adult patients have physiologic changes that make them less sensitive to pain. The aging process and chronic conditions can change pharmacodynamics and pharmacokinetics. Extreme caution must be used when prescribing pain medications in older adult patients. Older adults, especially frail older adults, can tolerate only very small doses of narcotics. Start low, go slow; it is easier to give more than to have to rescue a patient.

MANAGEMENT OF PAIN IN THE ICU

Management of pain in the ICU also requires the AGACNP to focus on sedation, delirium prevention, and mobility. Use of the ABCDE bundle is critical to improving ICU outcomes:

■ A = assessing, preventing, managing pain
■ B = both spontaneous awakening and breathing trial
■ C = choosing proper sedation and analgesia: intermittent dosing decreases drug accumulation, avoid benzodiazepines, use propofol
■ D = delirium monitoring and prevention
■ E = early mobility and exercise = physical therapy (PT)/occupational therapy (OT) within 72 hours of ICU admission

▶ TOXIC INGESTION/INHALATIONS

DISEASE OVERVIEW

AGACNPs will care for patients with overdose and toxic ingestions/inhalations. Initial steps are to quickly identify the agent to initiate treatments/antidotes. Second, inquire if the ingestion was accidental versus intentional. If intentional, a 1:1 sitter and psychiatric evaluation are needed to keep the patient safe during hospitalization and may impact discharge destination. A comprehensive physical exam is needed. Specifically, review vital signs, skin and temperature, mental status, pupils, bowel and bladder function, reflexes, muscular tone, and odors, which can be clues to a specific toxidrome or chemical agent.

TOXIDROMES

A *toxidrome* is a pattern of clinical signs and symptoms associated with toxicity from a specific classification of chemical agents. Prescription medications, illicit drugs, household chemicals, poisons, and chemical warfare agents can be encountered in clinical settings. Physical examination can provide clues to the substance ingested. Table 19.16 outlines toxidromes.

Table 19.16 Common Toxidromes

Toxidrome	Examples	Vital Signs	Mental Status	Pupils	Other
Anticholinergic	Atropine, antihistamines, TCAs, scopolamine, antispasmodics, Jimson weed, psychedelic mushrooms	Hyperthermia, tachycardia, hypertensive, tachypnea	Hypervigilant, agitated, hallucinating	Mydriasis	Dry flushed skin, urinary retention

(*continued*)

Table 19.16 Common Toxidromes (*continued*)

Toxidrome	Examples	Vital Signs	Mental Status	Pupils	Other
Cholinergic	Organophosphates, carbamate pesticides, cholinesterase inhibitors, nerve agents, physostigmine	Bradycardia, tachycardia, hypertension	Confused, coma	Miosis	SLUDGE (salivation, lacrimation, urination, diarrhea, GI upset, emesis)
Opioid	Opioids (morphine, oxycodone, hydrocodone, hydromorphone, fentanyl, codeine, methadone, heroin)	Hypothermia, bradycardia, hypotension, bradypnea	CNS depression, coma	Miosis	Hyporeflexia, pulmonary edema
Sedative/hypnotic	Benzodiazepines, nonbenzodiazepine GABA agonists, barbiturates, chloral hydrate, alcohols	Hypothermia, bradycardia, hypotension, bradypnea	CNS depression, confusion, coma	Miosis	Hyporeflexia
Sympathomimetic	Cocaine, amphetamines, pseudoephedrine, phenylephrine, ephedrine	Hyperthermia, tachycardia, tachypnea	Agitated, hyperalert, paranoia	Mydriasis	Diaphoresis, tremors, hyperreflexia, seizures
Serotonergic	MAOIs, SSRIs, buspirone, tramadol, dextromethorphan	Hyperthermia, tachycardia, hypertension, tachypnea	Confused, agitated, coma	Mydriasis	Tremor, myoclonus, diaphoresis, hyperreflexia, trismus, rigidity, muscular hypertonicity
Neuroleptic	Haloperidol, olanzapine, quetiapine, chlorpromazine, promethazine, prochlorperazine, fluphenazine, perphenazine	Hypotension, arrhythmias			Trismus, dystonia, ataxia, parkinsonism, neuroleptic malignant syndrome

CNS, central nervous system; GABA, gamma-aminobutyric acid; GI, gastrointestinal; MAOI, monoamine oxidase inhibitor; SSRIs, selective serotonin reuptake inhibitor; TCA, tricyclic antidepressant.

TREATMENT

Treatment of overdose is specific to the agent ingested (Table 19.17). Consultation with a toxicologist or poison control center can be helpful in diagnosing and treating overdoses and ingestions.

Table 19.17 Specific Toxin and Adult Dosing of Antidotes

Drug/Agent	Antidote	Dose
Acetaminophen	N-Acetylcysteine	140 mg/kg PO or IV over 1 hour, then 70 mg/kg over 1 hour q4h × five doses, then reassess toxin clearance, PT/INR and transaminases
Anticholinergics	Physostigmine	2 mg over 4 minutes, may repeat every 1–2 hours prn
Benzodiazepine	Flumazenil	0.5 mg over 30 seconds; may repeat every 30–60 minutes
Beta-blockers	Glucagon	5 mcg/kg IV over 1–2 minutes up to 10 mg max; follow with infusion of half to full initial dose
Calcium-channel blockers	10% calcium chloride Dextrose and insulin	1–2 g over 5 minutes (CVC preferred); may repeat 25 g IV as D50% (50 mL) and 0.5–1 unit/kg bolus followed by 0.5–1 unit/kg per hour infusion
Cholinergic	Atropine Pralidoxime	0.02 mg/kg IV or IM 1–2 g IV infusion (10–20 mg/mL) over 15–30 minutes, repeat in 1 hour if necessary and q12h PRN
Coumadin	Phytonadione Fresh frozen plasma PCC	10 mg IV daily × 3 days 15 mL/kg (roughly 3 units FFP for therapeutic INR) INR 2 to less than 4 = 25 units/kg, maximum 2,500 units; INR 4–6 = 35 units/kg, maximum 3,500 units; INR greater than 6 = 50 units/kg maximum 5,000 units
Cyanide	Hydroxocobalamin*	70 mg/kg over 15 minutes
Digoxin	Digibind	10–20 vials over 30 minutes for acute empiric dosing or base on serum digoxin levels
Ethylene glycol, methanol	Fomepizole (preferred) Ethanol	15 mg/kg/dose IV load over 30 minutes, then 10 mg/kg q12h × four doses, then 15 mg/kg q12h prn till nontoxic 10 mL/kg of 10% vol/vol solution, then continuous infusion of 1.5 mL/kg until nontoxic; double rate during dialysis
Heparin	Protamine sulfate	1–1.5 mg per 100 USP units of heparin; not to exceed 50 mg; monitor APTT 5–10 minutes after dose then in 2–8 hours
Insulin	Glucose	D50% 50 mL bolus IV; consider D10% infusion and titrate to glucose levels
Iron	Deferoxamine	5 mg/kg/hr continuous infusion and titrate to 15 mg/kg/hr as tolerates total daily dose 6–8 g
Isoniazid, hydrazine	Pyridoxine	5 g IV
Lead	Dimercapol $CaNa_2$ EDTA Succimer (DMSA)	75 mg/m² q4h, first dose to precede edetate calcium disodium ($CaNa^2$ EDTA) 1,500 mg/m² by continuous infusion 10 mg/kg PO q8h for 5 days, then 12 hours for 14 days
Methemoglobinemia	Methylene blue 1%	1–2 mg/kg IV over 5 minutes with 30 mL flush; may repeat 1 mg/kg ×1
Methotrexate	Folinic acid (leucovorin)	100 mg/m² over 15–30 min q3–6h with resolution of bone marrow toxicity
Neuroleptics	Bromocriptine Dantrolene	5 mg q12h per gastric tube, increase as high as 10 mg q6h 3–10 mg/kg over 15 minutes with oral doses of 25–600 mg/day to maintain response
Opioids	Naloxone	0.5 mg IV with repeat dosing every 15 minutes to reversal of respiratory depression (can be given IM or ETT)

(continued)

Table 19.17 Specific Toxin and Adult Dosing of Antidotes (*continued*)

Drug/Agent	Antidote	Dose
Organophosphates	Atropine Pralidoxine (2-PAM)	1–2 mg IV, double every 3–5 minutes until bronchorrhea resolves 1–2 g over 30 minutes, then up to 500 mg/hr; alternatively, 30 mg/kg IV (IM, SC if no IV access) over 20 minutes; follow by 4–8 mg/kg/hr maintenance IV infusion IM: 600 mg IM × three doses; administer each dose 15 minutes apart for mild symptoms, or in rapid succession for severe symptoms
Sulfonylureas	Octreotide	50 mcg SC q6–12h
TCAs	Sodium bicarbonate	50 mEq per dose to address acidemia and/or signs of sodium channel blockade (150 mEq and KCl 40 mEq in 1 L D5W; serum pH 7.5–7.55
Valproic acid	L-Carnitine	Clinically ill: 100 mg/kg IV over 30 min (max 6 g), then 15 mg/kg q4h Clinically well: 100 mg/kg PO per day (max 3 g) divided q6h

APTT, activated partial thromboplastin time; CVC, central venous catheter; ECG, electrocardiogram; ETT, endotracheal tube; IM, intramuscular; INR, international normalized ratio; IV, intravenous; PCC, prothrombin complex concentrate; PT, prothrombin time; SC, subcutaneous; TCA, tricyclic antidepressant.
*Antidote of choice for cyanide poisoning.

AGACNPs must know the reversal agents for narcotics (Naloxone/Narcan) and benzodiazepines (Flumazenil/Romazicon), which are commonly used for conscious sedation.

▶ SOLID ORGAN TRANSPLANT

DISEASE OVERVIEW

Solid organ transplant (SOT) can be a lifesaving and life-changing procedure for a patient. It is a therapy for end-stage organ failure. In the United States, the most common organ transplant is the kidney followed by the liver, heart, and lung. The AGACNP must have general knowledge about SOT as well as the common post-transplant medication regimens and complications this patient population is at risk for. The most challenging part of SOT is that demand greatly surpasses supply. Therefore, the U.S. Congress passed the National Organ Transplant Act in 1984, which established the Organ Procurement and Transplantation Network under the United Network for Organ Sharing to maintain a national registry for organ matching.

HEART TRANSPLANT

Despite advances in medical treatment for heart failure, transplantation remains the most effective and long-lasting treatment for advanced heart failure in terms of mortality and quality of life. Heart transplants are done for patients with refractory acute and chronic heart failure. These patients have disabling symptoms despite optimal medical management.

LUNG TRANSPLANT

Lung transplantation is the optimal treatment for patients with end-stage lung disease and is the best treatment to improve quality of life. Some of the more common reasons for lung transplantation include idiopathic pulmonary fibrosis, chronic obstructive pulmonary disease, cystic fibrosis, and alpha-1 antitrypsin deficiency emphysema.

KIDNEY TRANSPLANT

Kidney transplantation is done to prolong and improve the lives of the patients with end-stage renal disease. One-year survival rates for deceased-donor recipients are greater than 92% and for living-donor recipients are greater than 97%.

PANCREAS TRANSPLANT

Pancreas transplantation is most often performed together with or after kidney transplantation but can be performed alone. Pancreas transplantation performed with or after kidney transplantation can prolong the life of the kidney transplant, offering protection against recurrent diabetic neuropathy.

LIVER TRANSPLANT

Liver transplantation is indicated for end-stage liver cirrhosis. The most common reasons for transplant are hepatitis C infection and alcoholic liver disease. One-year survival rates have increased since the 1980s (about 70%) to now (85%–90%), and 5-year survival rates exceed 60%.

IMMUNOSUPPRESSIVES

All SOT recipients will be on some form of immunosuppression (Table 19.18). The goal of immunosuppression is to prevent graft rejection. Immunosuppressive therapy is largely attributable to increased survival rates due to immunosuppressive drugs preventing allograft rejection.

Table 19.18 Common Immunosuppressive Drugs and Side Effects

Drug	Side Effects	Notes
Antithymocyte globulins ▪ Thymoglobulin	Cytokine release syndrome (fever, chills, rigors, dyspnea, nausea, vomiting, diarrhea, hypo- or hypertension, malaise, rash, and headache)	Patients can be premedicated with steroids, acetaminophen, and diphenhydramine 30 minutes prior to the infusion to treat symptoms associated with cytokine release syndrome
Glucocorticoids ▪ Prednisone ▪ Methylprednisolone	Neurotoxicity (headache, insomnia, psychosis) Glucose intolerance Leukocytosis	Mainstay of immunosuppression since SOT began
Calcineurin inhibitors ▪ Tacrolimus ▪ Cyclosporine	Nephrotoxicity Electrolyte disturbances Hypertension Neurotoxicity	Can increase drug levels of: ▪ Amiodarone ▪ Nicardipine ▪ Diltiazem ▪ Verapamil Can decrease drug levels of: ▪ Rifampin ▪ Phenytoin ▪ Carbamazepine
Antiproliferatives ▪ Mycophenolate mofetil ▪ Azathioprine (not commonly used)	Diarrhea Pancytopenia	Mycophenolic acid derivatives are associated with first trimester loss of pregnancy and congenital malformations.
mTOR Inhibitors ▪ Sirolimus	Hypercholesterolemia Hypertriglyceridemia Leukopenia Anemia Thrombocytopenia Mouth ulcers Impaired wound healing	Sirolimus has been associated with hepatic artery thrombosis, increased mortality, and graft failure in liver transplant and bronchial anastomotic dehiscence in lung transplant.

INFECTION

Patients who receive a transplant are at higher risk for infection given their immunocompromised state (see Table 19.19 for infections associated with respective transplanted organs). SOT patients are on longer periods of immunosuppression (possibly lifelong), so the infection risk remains. During the early period (less than 1 month), post-transplant infections are most often caused by extracellular bacteria.

Table 19.19 Organ Transplanted and Common Infections

Organ	Infection	
Heart	Mediastinitis *Toxoplasma gondii* Endocarditis	CMV infection EBV infection
Lung	Pneumonia Mediastinitis CMV infection	Pneumonitis EBV infection
Kidney	Cystitis Pyelonephritis BK virus	JC virus CMV infection EBV infection
Pancreas	Urinary tract infections Intra-abdominal infections	CMV infection EBV infection
Liver	Cholangitis CMV infection	EBV infection

CMV, cytomegalovirus; EBV, Ebstein–Barr virus.

PROPHYLACTIC REGIMENS TO DECREASE RISK INFECTION

Patients who are post transplant will be on prophylactic regimens due to their immunocompromised state. See Table 19.20 for examples of potential regimens and possible side effects.

Table 19.20 Commonly Used Prophylactic Regimens

Prophylactic Regimens				
Risk Factors	Organism Addressed	Prophylactic Drug	Workup	Medication Side Effects
Travel to or known endemic area for fungal infections	*Histoplasma Blastomyces Coccidioides*	Triazoles Ex. Fluconazole	CXR Antigen testing serology	■ Nausea ■ Vomiting ■ Diarrhea ■ Loss of appetite
Latent herpes virus	HSV, VZV, CMV, EBV	Ganciclovir Acyclovir	Serologic tests for HSV, VZV, CMV, EBV,	■ Nausea ■ Vomiting ■ Diarrhea
Latent fungi or parasites	*Pneumocystis jirovecii, Toxoplasma gondii*	Trimethoprim–sulfamethoxazole	Serologic tests for *Toxoplasma*	■ Nausea ■ Vomiting ■ Diarrhea ■ Thrombocytopenia
Hx of exposure to active or latent TB	*Mycobacterium tuberculosis*	Isoniazid	Chest imaging TST QuantiFERON gold	■ Nausea ■ Vomiting ■ Diarrhea ■ Paresthesias in extremities

CMV, cytomegalovirus; CXR, chest x-ray; EBV, Epstein–Barr virus; HSV, herpes simplex virus; Hx, history; TB, tuberculosis; TST, tuberculin skin test; VZV, varicella-zoster virus.

REJECTION

Organ rejection can occur days to months after a transplant and occurs because the recipient's body identifies the organ as foreign and attacks the organ. The diagnosis of acute rejection is made based on patient symptoms, laboratory blood data, and a tissue biopsy. Early detection can lead to intervention and salvaging of the organ, but repeated rejection can lead to chronic rejection.

▶ OBSTETRIC CONDITIONS

DISEASE OVERVIEW

Pregnant patients may be admitted to the hospital for pregnancy-related conditions, medical or surgical reasons not related to pregnancy, and underlying diseases that worsen. Manage acute and critical care needs including neurologic concerns, respiratory or cardiac failure, or exacerbations. AGACNPs possess knowledge and expertise to swiftly respond to patient deterioration. AGACNPs must know the physiologic changes related to pregnancy to best respond to these conditions (Table 19.21).

Table 19.21 Physiologic Changes in Pregnancy

System	Changes	Impact
Cardiovascular	■ Peripheral vascular resistance ■ Heart rate ■ Arterial pressure Increased cardiac output	Masks initial signs of sepsis ■ Hypoperfusion Uteroplacental circulation cannot autoregulate, thus dependent on maternal circulation
Blood	■ Plasma volume and ■ Red cell volume Anemia	Greater reduction of oxygen supply to tissues
Respiratory	■ Tidal volume and ■ Respiratory rate ■ Minute-ventilation by 30%–40% ■ Residual volume	Decreased ability to respond to metabolic acidosis Impaired oxygenation
Renal	■ Renal blood flow, GFR ■ Creatinine levels ■ Ureteral dilation and ureteral pressure d/t smooth muscle relaxation ■ Intravesical pressure d/t pregnant uterus weight ■ Vesicoureteral reflux ■ Glomerular filtration rate ■ Urea and creatinine ■ Asymptomatic bacteriuria	Even normal levels can signify renal compromise Delays identification of renal injury secondary to sepsis Favorable to pyelonephritis
Gastrointestinal	■ Tone of lower esophageal sphincter ■ Muscle tone across the GI tract ■ Perfusion of gastric mucosa ■ Delayed gastric emptying ■ Diaphragm elevation by the uterus ■ Changes in bile composition ■ Production of pro-inflammatory cytokines by Kupffer cells	■ Risk of aspiration ■ Risk of bacterial translocation ■ Risk of aspiration pneumonia ■ Risk of cholestasis, hyperbilirubinemia, and jaundice
Hematologic	■ Leukocyte count ■ Platelet count ■ Factors VII, VIII, IX, X, XII, von Willebrand, and fibrinogen ■ Protein S ■ Fibrinolytic activity	■ Leukocytosis is unreliable indicator of sepsis ■ Risk of thrombotic events Increased risk of DIC
Genital	■ Uteroplacental circulation cannot autoregulate ■ Vaginal pH ■ Glycogen in vaginal epithelium	■ Maternal infection can easily affect the fetus. ■ Risk of chorioamnionitis

DIC, disseminated intravascular coagulation; GFR, glomerular filtration rate; GI, gastrointestinal.

GENERAL PRINCIPLES

A multidisciplinary approach to acutely and critically ill pregnant patients is essential to ensure the best outcome for the patient and the fetus. Treatment focuses on stabilization and management of both the patient and the fetus. When the fetus is over 24 weeks' gestation, prepare for emergent delivery. The AGACNP will manage the pregnant patient, while the obstetrical team manages the delivery.

MEDICATIONS

Carefully weigh risks and benefits of all drugs used in pregnant patients. The U.S. Food and Drug Administration (FDA) narrative classification summarizes evidence to guide prescribing practices. The FDA classifies medications into three categories (pregnancy, lactation and, female and male patients of reproductive potential) and provides a description of the risks and clinical considerations. Collaborate with obstetricians and pharmacy for safe prescribing.

SPECIFIC RISKS
VENOUS THROMBOPROPHYLAXIS

Obstetrical patients are at a higher risk for venous thromboembolism (VTE). Recommendations include use of mechanical thromboprophylaxis for all patients needing Cesarean delivery and pharmacologic prophylaxis with low-molecular-weight heparin or unfractionated heparin (UFH) for high-risk thrombophilia, any prior VTE event, or family history of VTE thrombophilia. Warfarin causes teratogenic effects and should be avoided. Patients with a high risk of VTE may be converted to UFH infusions to manage the risks of bleeding and thrombosis during delivery.

SEPSIS/SEPTIC SHOCK IN OBSTETRICAL PATIENTS

Sepsis in the pregnant patient can be challenging to recognize due to physiologic changes associated with pregnancy. Septic shock most commonly occurs due to pyelonephritis, chorioamnionitis, and endometritis. Management of sepsis and septic shock follows the sepsis clinical practice guidelines. Therapy should continue for 7–10 days. De-escalation can be challenging due to the polymicrobial nature of these infections. Outcome of sepsis in pregnant patients is typically better because this is generally a healthy and younger population without significant comorbid conditions.

CRITICAL CARE OBSTETRICAL EMERGENCIES

Obstetrical emergencies routinely require admission to critical care units for ongoing management. Conditions the AGACNP may co-manage are highlighted in Table 19.22. For severe preeclampsia, eclampsia, HELLP (hemolysis, elevated liver enzymes and low platelets) syndrome, and any fetal distress, urgent delivery is indicated.

Table 19.22 Obstetrical Emergencies, Diagnostic Criteria, and Treatments

Obstetric Emergency	Diagnostic Criteria	Treatment

Severe preeclampsia	Eclampsia:
	■ BP greater than 140/90 on two readings over 4 hours apart or greater than 160/110 on two readings minutes apart, proteinuria greater than 300 mg/24 hr
	Severe preeclampsia is preeclampsia with any of the following:
	■ Platelet count less than 100,000 mcL
	■ Creatinine greater than 1.1 mg/dL or twice the patient's baseline
	■ AST or ALT greater than twice upper limit of normal or RUQ pain
	■ Pulmonary edema
	■ CNS symptoms: headache, changes in vision
		■ BP control with IV pushes of labetalol or hydralazine or infusion of labetalol or nicardipine
		■ IV magnesium
		  ● Load of 4–6 g IV over 15–30 minutes followed by 2 g/hr
		  ● Recurrent seizures 2 g over 10–15 minutes
		■ Watch for signs of magnesium toxicity: patellar reflexes, somnolence, respiratory difficulty, cardiac dysrhythmias
		■ To reverse magnesium: calcium gluconate 1 gram over 10 minutes

(continued)

Table 19.22 Obstetrical Emergencies, Diagnostic Criteria, and Treatments (*continued*)

Obstetric Emergency	Diagnostic Criteria	Treatment
Eclampsia	Severe preeclampsia (as earlier) plus seizures or coma.	■ BP control as above ■ IV magnesium ■ Monitor for signs of magnesium toxicity and treat as earlier ■ Deliver the fetus
Hemorrhagic shock (can be due to uterine atony, placenta previa, accreta, increta, or percreta, uterine rupture, surgical and urogenital tract trauma)	*Note:* Overt signs of bleeding may be absent or misinterpreted as normal physiologic changes with pregnancy. Shock signs: ■ Sinus tachycardia ■ Tachypnea ■ Anxiousness, restlessness ■ Pallor, cool skin, diaphoresis ■ Oliguria or anuria ■ Hypotension	■ Volume resuscitate with blood, plasma, platelets and cryoprecipitate ■ Warm the patient ■ ABG to assess acid-base status ■ Place a urinary catheter ■ Bimanual massage ■ Uterotonics: oxytocin infusion ■ Manual exploration to remove retained products of conception ■ Weight risk/benefit of tranexamic acid or recombinant factor VIIa ■ Interventions: balloon tamponade, uterine artery embolization, operative interventions

HELLP syndrome (hemolysis, elevated liver enzymes and low platelets)	Subjective but not specific: nausea, vomiting, headache, general malaise; requires laboratory evaluation:
	■ Hemolysis:
	  ● Schistocytes on blood smear
	  ● Elevated indirect bilirubin
	  ● LDH greater than 600 IU or bilirubin greater than 1.2 mg/dL
	  ● Low serum haptoglobin (≤25 mg/dL)
	■ AST greater than 70 U/L
	■ Platelets less than 100,000/mm³
		■ Deliver the fetus

Amniotic fluid embolism	Abrupt onset with rapid deterioration ■ Dyspnea ■ Profound hypoxemia ■ Profound hypotension ■ Cardiac dysrhythmias ■ Cyanosis ■ Pulmonary edema or ARDS ■ Altered mental status and/or seizures ■ DIC and hemorrhage	■ Immediate delivery of the fetus ■ Treatment depends on the severity of illness and capabilities of the institution ■ Intubate and mechanically ventilate ■ Vasopressor and inotropic support ■ Consider inhaled nitric oxide or prostacyclins ■ Intra-aortic balloon pump, ventricular assist devices; ECMO or cardiopulmonary bypass
Peripartum cardiomyopathy	■ Idiopathic cardiomyopathy ■ Develops near the end of pregnancy/within months of delivery ■ Absence of an identifiable cause ■ LV systolic dysfunction (dilated or nondilated) ■ EF less than 45%	■ Urgent cardiology consultation for workup, co-management, device therapy, transplantation evaluation ■ IV furosemide for preload reduction ■ Vasodilators for afterload reduction ■ With shock: inotropic support with dobutamine or milrinone ■ For compensated state beta blockade ■ For low EF or evidence of VTE: anticoagulate ■ ACEI are contraindicated during pregnancy; recommended in postpartum period

ABG, arterial blood gas; ACEI, angiotensin-coverting enzyme inhibitor; ARDS, acute respiratory distress syndrome; AST, aspartate aminotransferase; BP, blood pressure; CNS, central nervous system; DIC, disseminated intravascular coagulation; ECMO, extracorporeal membrane oxygenation; EF, ejection fraction; IV, intravenous; LDH, lactate hydrogenase; LV, left ventricular; RUQ, right upper quadrant; VTE, venous thromboembolism.

POSTPARTUM COMPLICATIONS

Postpartum complications can be challenging to identify due to the physiologic changes of pregnancy, causing delays in diagnosis and treatment. These delays are associated with increased maternal morbidity and mortality, thus increasing the need for training related to post-birth events.

Postpartum patients are at high risk for VTE up to a month after delivery. Maintain a high index of suspicion for any patient who presents with shortness of breath, leg swelling, and/or tachycardia. Patients can also develop sepsis and/or septic shock due to endometritis from retained placenta during birth. Mastitis can also complicate recovery of patients admitted during the postpartum period.

▶ MULTISYSTEM ORGAN DYSFUNCTION SYNDROME

DISEASE OVERVIEW

Multisystem organ dysfunction syndrome (MODS) refers to critical illness with two or more systems failing simultaneously. It is commonly caused by severe trauma or septic shock with medical sequelae of severe and prolonged inflammatory process and/or shock resulting in progressive and multiple organ systems failing simultaneously. Commonly, the patient experiences multiple physiologic insults or episodes of malperfusion. Patients with MODS have increased mortality. MODS is not recognized as an ICD-10 Code and thus is not a billable diagnosis; rather, the AGACNP should document the individual systems that are failing, including the clinical indicators and lab values supporting the diagnosis of the organs failing along with the management of each.

▶ PALLIATIVE CARE, HOSPICE, END OF LIFE, AND TRANSITION TO COMFORT

OVERVIEW

Palliative care is specialized care for patients with serious illness and life-limiting illness and can be incorporated during any stage of an illness and also provide curative treatment. The focus of palliative care is to provide patients with symptom management and to support caregiver/family needs. Palliative care consultations are appropriate for many hospitalized patients; thus, AGACNPs should discuss palliative care with patients and families when death within a year would not be surprising.

Hospice care is a specialized form of palliative care for patients with a limited life expectancy and does not support curative treatment. Hospice care incorporates medical, psychosocial, and spiritual support in caring for patients and family members as death nears. The aim of hospice care is not to shorten or prolong life, but rather to adequately treat symptoms. Consider hospice when patients decline such that death is likely within 6 months.

Patients admitted to the hospital should have a goals-of-care discussion at the time of admission and any time there is a change in their condition. Explore the patient's health status over the last year or two. Were there multiple admissions? Has the patient returned to their previous level of health each time, or has there been stepwise regression in overall health? Start discussions broadly to elicit the patient's perspective and then narrow the discussion to specifics relevant to the patient's case. Asking permission and offering the healthcare team's recommendations as the best course of treatment is part of a shared decision-making process. Interventions should be decided based on a risk–benefit analysis.

COMMUNICATION SKILLS

Patients and families are commonly stressed during hospitalizations, especially if the course is tenuous and the patient is unstable or decompensating. Tips for communicating with families include:

- *Regularly communicate:* daily communication from the same person if possible. Communicate changes in condition and reassure the family you will call if things change.
- *Listen:* Assess the patient's and family's understanding of the situation. Listening helps to establish trust and allows families to vent frustrations and fears. Ask about the patient's life and their values.
- *Provide psychological support:* Acknowledge emotions. Validate emotions with supportive statements: "You seem distressed/angry/sad," or "This must be very difficult for you."
- *Inform:* Inform the patient/family about the diagnoses, treatments, and response to treatments.
- *Convey uncertainty:* It is appropriate to say, "I don't know," and then find the answer.

- *Always continue care:* Caring for the patient never stops, even if the focus changes from curative to comfort measures. Withdraw interventions, not care!
- *Do not ask the family to decide:* Families are surrogate decision-makers, giving voice to the patient when the patient cannot speak. Ask, "If (the patient) could know everything we just talked about, what would they choose for themselves?" This relieves the family from making decisions.

BREAKING BAD NEWS

AGACNPs commonly communicate bad news, including explaining new diagnoses, describing treatments and interventions, notifying families of changes in conditions, explaining poor prognosis, and/or discussing code status. It is helpful to use a protocol to ensure a consist pattern to conversations. The SPIKES mnemonic (Table 19.23) is a way to break news to patients or families.

Table 19.23 SPIKES Protocol

S = Set up	■ Prepare for the discussion ■ Arrange for private area ■ Involve family/significant others with patient permission ■ Sit down during meeting, maintain eye contact ■ Manage interruptions (e.g., hand off pager or phone to colleague)
P = Perception	■ Ask about family or patient's perception or understanding of medical condition
I = Invitation	■ Ask how much the patient wants to know ■ Ask who else would the patient like to be engaged in the conversation
K = Knowledge	■ Share your knowledge with the patient/family ■ Prepare them to hear bad news: "I'm sorry, I need to share some bad news." ■ Avoid medical jargon ■ Give information in small amounts, and check understanding before proceeding
E = Emotions	■ Address patient's/family's emotions with empathetic responses
S = Summarize/strategize	■ Assess understanding ■ Ask if patient is ready to discuss any decisions and treatment plan ■ Create a treatment plan based on goals

Consistent messages about the patient's status among healthcare team members is crucial to developing trust with the patient and family. Ensure messages from all team members are aligned. When patients and families receive mixed messages, they can become frustrated and distrustful.

▶ PRONOUNCEMENT OF DEATH, BRAIN DEATH, AND DONATION

PRONOUNCEMENT OF DEATH

Pronouncing a patient deceased, identifying the cause of death, and attesting the death are within the scope of the AGACNP role. States and institutions may regulate this activity. The process of pronouncing a patient dead involves assessment for absence of respirations, pulse, pupil reactivity, and spontaneous movement. A pronouncement note should be written documenting the exam findings, time and date of death, manner of death (natural), and cause of death. Review the state requirements for referral to the medical examiner or coroner. If the case is accepted by the medical examiner, they will determine the manner (e.g., homicide, suicide) and cause of death.

The cause of death should never be listed as cardiac or pulmonary arrest. Seek the immediate cause of the cessation and link to what triggered this cause and the previous cause of it (e.g., cause of death: acute hypoxic respiratory failure due to adult respiratory distress syndrome due to pneumonia). Also, document any associated or contributing factors such as chronic obstructive pulmonary disease, tobacco use, and heart failure.

BRAIN DEATH

Pronouncement of brain death, in most states, signifies that a patient has legally died despite continuing to have a pulse. Notify the organ procurement center early when a patient has a significant brain injury, or when goals-of-care discussions are being planned with the family. Hospitals determine their respective requirements for brain death testing and can designate specific people who are authorized to perform brain death testing. Commonly, neurocritical care intensivists, neurologists, neurosurgeons, or other intensivists can declare a patient brain dead. Brain death requires cessation of all brain functions, including the brainstem, and documentation includes:

■ an irreversible and proximate brain injury, excluding other confounding medical conditions
■ absence of current drug intoxication or poisoning
■ absence of sedatives/CNS depressants, neuromuscular blocking agents, alcohol level less than 80
■ normotensive (not hypotensive based on patient's normal blood pressure)
■ normothermic (not hypothermic)
■ not hypoxic
■ absence of severe metabolic abnormalities
■ a period of observation (commonly 24 hours) without clinical improvement
■ both clinical and ancillary testing (Table 19.24)

Table 19.24 Clinical Testing for Brain Death

Brainstem Reflexes	Apnea Testing
Absence of: ■ Cerebral motor response ■ Pupillary response to light ■ Corneal, cough, and gag reflexes ■ Oculocephalic reflex (doll's eyes) ■ Oculovestibular reflex (ice water calorics) ■ Respiratory drive ● $PaCO_2$ greater than 60 mmHg or 20 mmHg above patient's baseline	■ Adjust ventilator to normalize $PaCO_2$ (~40 mmHg) ■ Preoxygenate with 100% FIO_2 for 10 minutes ■ Obtain baseline ABG to establish $PaCO_2$ ■ Change ventilator to CPAP at 100% FIO_2 ■ Observe patient's chest and abdomen for respiration for 10 minutes Draw ABG: to evaluate $PaCO_2$: ■ If $PaCO_2$ is greater than 60 mmHg (or greater than 20 mmHg above baseline) and no respiratory effort, patient has confirmed apnea ■ If $PaCO_2$ is less than 60 mmHg or less than 20 mmHg above baseline, continue test, repeat ABG in 2 minutes
Ancillary Testing Options (not always required):	
EEG, nuclear scan, transcranial doppler, CT angiogram and/or MRI/MRA. Four-vessel cerebral angiography is commonly a definitive test.	

ABG, arterial blood gas; CPAP, continuous positive air pressure; MRA, magnetic resonance angiography.

DONATION AFTER CARDIAC DEATH

The decision to withdraw life-sustaining treatments should be made before and separately from discussion of any consideration of donation after cardiac death (DCD). This sequencing avoids the perception that patients are being removed from life support to become an organ donor. DCD can be considered if patients are expected to die within close proximity (30–60 minutes) of withdrawal of life support. Key tenets to caring for a patient who is a candidate for DCD include the following:

■ Separate care teams are required to care for the donor and any potential recipients to avoid a conflict of interest.
■ The provider who is caring for the dying patient should pronounce the patient, not the transplant team.
■ Discuss specific medications needed to preserve organ function that can be given before death and that these medications cannot hasten death.
■ Discuss the process for consent for procedures needed for organ procurement (e.g., lines, bronchoscopy).
■ A time interval between pronouncement and organ recovery should be predetermined by policy (typically 2–5 minutes) to ensure the patient has not had spontaneous recovery.
■ If family desires, ensure family can be present at the time of death.
■ Clearly define a timeframe between withdrawal of life-sustaining treatments and duration of patient survival that precludes organ procurement.

ORGAN AND TISSUE DONATION

AGACNPs commonly interact with organ procurement organizations (OPOs) and manage patients who will become organ and tissue donors. Management of these donors is guided by OPO guidelines. Additional testing may include transthoracic or transesophageal echocardiogram, bronchoscopy, and additional laboratory testing. Typically, hemodynamic targets maintain mean arterial blood pressure (MAP) greater than 65, systolic blood pressure (SBP) greater than 100, urine output (UOP) greater than 0.5 mL/kg/hr, and PaO_2 greater than 100 to ensure organ perfusion.

▶ SUMMARY

Many of the patients the AGACNP will care for will present with multisystem disease and involvement. Understanding the interconnectedness of the human body and its respective systems is integral to being a competent AGACNP.

KNOWLEDGE CHECK: CHAPTER 19

1. A 65-year-old male patient with chronic obstructive pulmonary disease arrives to the ED with shortness of breath and somnolence. An arterial blood gas is obtained and reveals pH 7.15, $PaCO_2$ 70, PaO_2 50, HCO_3 38. What should be instituted immediately?

   A. Noninvasive ventilation
   B. Intravenous (IV) fluid resuscitation
   C. Acetazolamide
   D. Oxygen via nasal cannula

2. A 70-year-old female patient arrives to the unit following a motor vehicle crash resulting in left-sided rib fractures. She is somnolent. Which of the following acid-base abnormalities would the AGACNP expect on an ABG?

   A. Metabolic alkalosis
   B. Metabolic acidosis
   C. Respiratory acidosis
   D. Respiratory alkalosis

3. A 54-year-old male patient is admitted to the ICU for respiratory distress. He is tachypneic, and oxygen is applied via a high-flow device. Arterial blood gas (ABG) reveals a pH 7.20, $PaCO_2$ 22, PaO_2 78, HCO_3 14. Other labs are notable for sodium 145, potassium 3.3, chloride 110, CO_2 14, blood urea nitrogen (BUN) 25, creatinine 1.5, white blood count (WBC) 18, hemoglobin (Hgb) 12, hematocrit (Hct) 33, platelet 79. Which of the following labs should the AGACNP obtain?

   A. International normalized ratio (INR)
   B. Urine sodium
   C. Lactate
   D. D-dimer

4. A 65-year-old male patient is admitted to the hospital with an acute kidney injury. His labs are notable for blood urea nitrogen (BUN) 100, creatinine 4.3, CO_2 12, potassium 5.2, pH 7.14, PCO_2 30, PaO_2 65. Which of the following should the AGACNP administer?

   A. Acetazolamide
   B. Sodium bicarbonate
   C. Lactated Ringer solution
   D. Lasix

5. A 65-year-old female patient is admitted to the hospital with an acute exacerbation of heart failure. She is started on Lasix 80 mg IV twice a day, and the AGACNP notes that the CO_2 has been increasing daily and is now at 44. An ABG reveals pH 7.6, PCO_2 56, PaO_2 80, HCO_3 44. Which one of the following should the AGACNP order?

   A. Hydrochloric acid
   B. Sodium bicarbonate
   C. Hydrochlorothiazide
   D. Acetazolamide

(See answers next page.)

1. A) Noninvasive ventilation

The patient has acute on chronic respiratory acidosis, and the treatment to prevent intubation is noninvasive ventilation. IV fluid resuscitation would not reverse the hypercarbia, and acetazolamide may make the pH more acidotic. Oxygen via nasal cannula would not provide ventilatory support.

2. C) Respiratory acidosis

The patient has a thoracic injury that would impede breathing and cause hypoventilation, leading to respiratory acidosis.

3. C) Lactate

The patient has an anion gap metabolic acidosis (AGMA), and a common cause of AGMA is elevated lactate. INR, urine sodium, and D-dimer would not determine the cause of the metabolic acidosis.

4. B) Sodium bicarbonate

Sodium bicarbonate is beneficial in treating metabolic acidosis in the setting of renal failure. It would also help in stabilizing potassium levels. Acetazolamide would make the metabolic acidosis worse. Lactated Ringer solution may help; however, the patient is already hypoxic, and additional fluids may be detrimental. Lasix can be tried, but it would not help with the metabolic acidosis acutely.

5. D) Acetazolamide

The patient has contraction metabolic alkalosis and should be treated with acetazolamide. Hydrochloric acid should not be given. Sodium bicarbonate and hydrochlorothiazide may worsen the alkalosis.

6. A 65-year-old male patient is in the ICU for a small bowel obstruction and has significant nasogastric tube output. Which one of the following IV fluids should the AGACNP use for this patient?

   A. 0.9% sodium chloride
   B. Lactated Ringer solution
   C. 1.26% sodium acetate
   D. Albumin

7. A 23-year-old female patient is found unresponsive with empty acetaminophen bottles nearby. She is in a coma and is intubated but remains tachypneic. Arterial blood gas (ABG) reveals pH 7.6, $PaCO_2$ 15, PaO_2 240, HCO_3 20. International normalized ratio (INR) is 2.3. The AGACNP should be concerned for which of the following?

   A. Salicylate overdose
   B. Cerebral edema
   C. Sepsis
   D. Pulmonary embolism

8. A 54-year-old male patient is on mechanical ventilation for community-acquired pneumonia. His vital signs are temperature 39°C, heart rate (HR) 120, blood pressure (BP) 130/76, SpO_2 90% on 50% FIO_2. Arterial blood gas (ABG) reveals pH 7.55, PCO_2 20, PaO_2 60, HCO_3 20. Which of the following should the AGACNP do to improve the patient's ABG?

   A. Administer an antipyretic
   B. Increase the FIO_2
   C. Increase positive end-expiratory pressure (PEEP)
   D. Give acetazolamide

9. The AGACNP is caring for a 42-year-old patient who presents after falling into a campfire. The patient has burns to both arms, the anterior chest, and the abdomen. The burns extend through the epidermis to the dermis. The AGACNP knows this patient will require:

   A. Fluid resuscitation targeting a urine output greater than 0.5 mg/kg/hr
   B. Fluid resuscitation targeting 30 mL/kg
   C. STAT echocardiogram
   D. Intubation

10. The AGACNP is caring for a 68-year-old patient who presents after an explosion at their workplace. The patient has burns to the face, bilateral hands, and anterior chest. The burns extend through the epidermis to the dermis. The AGACNP knows this patient has which degree of burns?

    A. Superficial (first degree)
    B. Partial-thickness (second degree)
    C. Full-thickness (third degree)
    D. Complete-thickness (fourth degree)

11. A female older adult patient from an assisted-living facility presents to the ED following a fall. The patient complains of fever, malaise, cough, nausea, and vomiting for 2 days. She is found to be febrile to 101.5°F with blood pressure to 85/40 and heart rate to 120. A fluid bolus is given. Which of the following should the AGACNP do *first*?

    A. Place the patient in airborne precautions with respiratory viral panel (RVP) testing.
    B. Order metronidazole (Flagyl) 500 mg IV TID due to concern for bowel perforation.
    C. Place a central line and order norepinephrine (Levophed) due to concern for septic shock.
    D. Order loperamide (Imodium) 2 mg by mouth to treat acute viral gastroenteritis.

(*See answers next page.*)

6. A) 0.9% sodium chloride

The patient has significant gastric fluid losses, which include chloride and acid. The patient will develop metabolic alkalosis and should be treated with normal saline. Lactated Ringer solution and sodium acetate would not replace the gastric loss. Albumin should not be given.

7. B) Cerebral edema

The patient has evidence of acute liver failure, likely from acetaminophen overdose. She is in a coma and is at risk for cerebral edema. The respiratory alkalosis is in response to the cerebral edema. Salicylate overdose would also include metabolic acidosis. Sepsis is a concern, but not the primary one. Pulmonary embolism is not on the differential.

8. A) Administer an antipyretic

The respiratory alkalosis is driven by the patient's fever and would improve with an antipyretic.

9. A) Fluid resuscitation targeting a urine output greater than 0.5mg/kg/hr

Severe burn resuscitation guidelines state that targeting a urine output greater than 0.5 mg/kg/hr is recommended. Fluid resuscitation targeting 30 mL/kg is the recommendation for patients with sepsis. A STAT echocardiogram is not indicated at this point, and there is no evidence this patient requires intubation.

10. B) Partial-thickness (second degree)

Partial-thickness burns involve the epidermis to the dermis. First-degree burns involve only the epidermis, while third-degree burns surpass the dermis and reach into subcutaneous fat or deeper.

11. A) Place the patient in airborne precautions with respiratory viral panel (RVP) testing.

Knowing older adult populations in long-term facilities are at increased risk for exposure to communicable disease, the AGACNP chooses to place the patient in airborne precautions to limit the risk of transmission of viruses and sends for a screening test. Bowel perforation is on the differential, but there is no history to support this. While a central line and norepinephrine are appropriate for use in the setting of septic shock, it is not known if the patient received sufficient fluids of if she responded to the fluids; thus, this may be premature. Imodium is the correct treatment for suspected gastroenteritis from an unknown etiology; however, acute gastroenteritis does not normally present with respiratory components.

12. Using the rule of nines, calculate the percentage of total body surface area (TBSA) burned in a 60-kg male patient with burns covering the entire right leg, anterior thorax including the abdomen, and entire surface of both arms.

    A. 18%
    B. 35%
    C. 54%
    D. 44%

13. Which of the following is part of the secondary survey in a trauma patient?

    A. Head-to-toe exam
    B. Airway assessment
    C. Pulse exam
    D. Urine drug screen

14. Which of the following types of thoracic trauma can be managed with a pigtail catheter pleural chest tube?

    A. Flail chest
    B. Cardiac tamponade
    C. Hemothorax
    D. Pneumothorax

15. During a focused assessment with sonography for trauma examination in an acute trauma patient, fluid is noted in the left upper quadrant. The patient's vital signs continue to downtrend despite administration of warmed 2 L of lactated Ringer solution, and vital signs are now blood pressure (BP) 70/50, heart rate (HR) 120 sinus tachycardia, and Glasgow Coma Scale (GCS) 12. Laboratory analysis reveals complete blood count (CBC): hemoglobin (Hgb) 10, hematocrit (HCT) 30, platelets (PLT) 100k, international normalized ratio (INR) 3.0. Chemistries reveal: K^+ 3.4, Cr 2.0, lactate 3.0, Ca 8.5. A type and crossmatch are obtained for this patient. What is the *best* intervention for the AGACNP to perform?

    A. Initiate massive transfusion protocol and transport the patient to the operating room.
    B. Order 2 units of packed red blood cells (PRBCs) and 1 unit fresh frozen plasma (FFP).
    C. Replace potassium and obtain an arterial blood gas to assess for metabolic acidosis.
    D. Attempt to contact the patient's family members to ascertain code status.

16. Which of the following parameter(s) is an end point in the resuscitation of a patient in septic shock?

    A. Central venous pressure 4–8 mmHg
    B. Lactate less than 2
    C. Urine output less than 0.25 mL/kg/hr
    D. Oxygen saturation greater than or equal to 95%

17. In caring for an older adult male patient who has had a motor vehicle crash, sustaining a suspected traumatic subarachnoid hemorrhage, which supportive measure is the AGACNP likely to order?

    A. Targeted temperature management to 34°C
    B. Levetiracetam (Keppra)
    C. Nimodipine (Nimotop)
    D. Norepinephrine (Levophed) for cerebral perfusion pressure (CPP) less than 50 mmHg

(See answers next page.)

12. C) 54%

In the rule of nines calculation, a leg is 18%, anterior thorax is 18%, and each arm is 9% for a total of 54% TBSA burn.

13. A) Head-to-toe exam

A head-to-toe exam is part of the secondary survey. The primary survey focuses on airway, breathing, circulation, disability (neurologic exam), exposure, and environmental control. Urine drug screen is part of trauma care to seek an etiology/contributor to the trauma.

14. D) Pneumothorax

Pneumothorax can be managed with a small-bore chest tube or pigtail catheter. A hemothorax requires a larger chest tube to prevent the smaller tube from being clotted off. A flail chest may require internal stabilization with intubation and positive pressure ventilation. Cardiac tamponade requires pericardiocentesis or pericardial window.

15. A) Initiate massive transfusion protocol and transport the patient to the operating room.

The patient is in hemorrhagic shock, likely due to a splenic laceration. Initiate a massive transfusion protocol and transport to the operating room immediately. Recognize that a lag time exists between time of hemorrhage and hemoglobin changes. Although it is important to recognize that the patient likely has metabolic acidosis (likely secondary to lactic acidosis resulting from hypoperfusion) and the patient has mild hypokalemia, this is not the highest priority. Ordering 2 units of packed red blood cells (PRBC) and 1 fresh frozen plasma (FFP) may help initially to control bleeding, but the exact degree of resuscitation cannot be predicted, and it is imperative to order more products. It is extremely important to attain the code status of the patient; however, the initial action of the AGACNP is to ensure an appropriate resuscitation.

16. B) Lactate less than 2

The end points of resuscitation include lactate clearance, central venous pressure (CVP) 8 to 12, urine output (UOP) greater than 0.25 mL/kg/hr, and mixed venous oxygenation of 70% to 85%.

17. B) Levetiracetam (Keppra)

Anticonvulsive medications are indicated to prevent and treat seizures, which helps prevent secondary brain injuries that can exacerbate primary injuries and increase mortality. The goal is to keep cerebral perfusion pressure at 50 to 70 mmHg. Targeted temperature management is indicated to keep patients with traumatic brain injury from being hyperthermic, not to induce hypothermia, which can worsen cerebral bleeding.

18. An adult male patient presents as an unrestrained driver status post motor vehicle crash. He reports hitting his chest on the steering wheel. The patient is noted to have an anterior chest wall hematoma. His blood pressure (BP) changes include BP at the end of expiration 135/90 mmHg and at the end of inspiration 110/92 mmHg. Which of the following conditions is *most* likely?

    A. Aortic insufficiency
    B. Cardiogenic shock
    C. Left ventricular failure
    D. Cardiac tamponade

19. In caring for patients with chronic illnesses, it is important for the AGACNP to integrate palliative care into the overall management of patients to:

    A. Assist patients toward understanding their illness trajectory
    B. Provide seamless care coordination into hospice
    C. Prepare the family for the dying process and death
    D. Aid patients and families to comprehend the illness trajectory and dying process

20. Which of the following burn patients can be safely managed outside a level I trauma center?

    A. 44-year-old patient with diabetes with second-degree burn to leg
    B. 35-year-old patient with inhalation injury
    C. 29-year-old patient with 15% third-degree burns
    D. 25-year-old patient with 30% first-degree burns

(See answers next page.)

18. D) Cardiac tamponade

This patient has sustained a steering wheel injury and blunt cardiac trauma, most likely causing a tamponade as evidenced by variations in BP during inspiration and expiration. There is no evidence of any new-onset murmurs; thus, aortic insufficiency is not likely, nor is there evidence of any symptoms of left ventricular failure. The patient has a paradoxical BP, which is typical of cardiac tamponade. A BP of 135/90 is atypical of cardiogenic shock.

19. D) Aid patients and families to comprehend the illness trajectory and dying process

Palliative care provides a structured foundation for delivery of healthcare to meet several outcomes. These outcomes include assisting *both* patients and families to obtain information related to their current health condition that includes the illness trajectory. The information should be provided in such a manner that the patient is able to comprehend the treatment plan and possible outcome. Palliative care is delivered by an interdisciplinary team that assists with seamless care coordination, not just transition into hospice. Ultimately, palliative care provides the opportunity for *both* patient and family to prepare for death in a manner that allows for personal reflection and growth, hospice, and bereavement.

20. D) 25-year-old patient with 30% first-degree burns

The patient with first-degree burns can be managed and discharged from a non-burn center. The American Burn Association criteria for transfer to a burn center includes 10% partial-thickness burns; any full-thickness burn; electrical, chemical or inhalation injuries; and burns of the hands, feet, perineum, face, or major joints; as well as increased risk for mortality, including preexisting medical conditions. Patients with diabetes, inhalation injury, and third-degree burns would require transport to a burn center.

KEY BIBLIOGRAPHY

Only key resources appear in the print edition. Access the full bibliography for this chapter on ExamPrepConnect.com.

Allison, T. L. (2016). Immunosuppressive therapy in transplantation. *Nursing Clinics of North America, 51*(1), 107–120. https://doi.org/10.1016/j.cnur.2015.10.008

Kaur, M., Singh, P. M., & Trikha, A. (2017). Management of critically ill obstetric patients: A review. *Journal of Obstetric Anaesthesia and Critical Care, 7*(1), 3. https://doi.org/10.4103/joacc.JOACC_21_17

Kraut, J. A., & Madias, N. E. (2014). Lactic acidosis. *New England Journal of Medicine, 371*(24), 2309–2319. https://doi.org/10.1056/nejmra1309483

Kummerfeldt, C. E., Pastis, N. J., & Huggins, J. T. (2017). Pleural diseases. In S. C. McKean, J. J. Ross, D. D. Dressler, & D. B. Scheurer (Eds.), *Principles and practice of hospital medicine* (2nd ed.). McGraw-Hill Education.

Seifter, J. L. (2014). Integration of acid-base and electrolyte disorders. *New England Journal of Medicine, 371*(19), 1821–1831. https://doi.org/10.1056/nejmra1215672

Part IV: Professional Role

Scope and Standards of Professional Practice

20

Jennifer Lakeberg, Christina Vest, and Jody Beckington

▶ INTRODUCTION

This chapter describes the origins of the nurse practitioner (NP) role, the Consensus Model for Licensure, Accreditation, Credentialing, and Educational requirements to become an NP. The Consensus Model provides a framework for the regulation of all four advanced practice registered nurse (APRN) groups and indicates that the education and practice of an NP must be aligned with a specific population rather than a specialty. AGACNPs must also be familiar with and adhere to the AGACNP scope and standards of practice to protect patient safety, promote effective high-quality care, and limit risks to the NP's license. This chapter also reviews the ethical standards that are foundational to all nurses as well as advanced practice nurses.

▶ HISTORY OF THE NURSE PRACTITIONER ROLE

The role of the NP was created in the 1960s. Dr. Loretta Ford and Dr. Henry Silver developed the first NP program in pediatric primary care. These two clinicians saw a need to improve care for rural and underserved populations and to supplement the services of primary care physicians. The original focus of the first NP role was to provide health promotion, disease prevention, and primary care services. As healthcare evolved and the quality of care provided by NPs was recognized, employers began to hire NPs to provide care to acutely and critically ill and hospitalized adults. This led to the development of the acute care nurse practitioner (ACNP) role. Factors contributing to the development of the ACNP role were changing healthcare delivery models; increased patient and care complexity; demand for high-quality, cost-effective acute care services; increased demand for access to care; and reduction in medical trainee services due to work-hour limitations.

▶ CONSENSUS MODEL FOR ADVANCED PRACTICE REGISTERED NURSE REGULATION: LICENSURE, ACCREDITATION, CERTIFICATION, AND EDUCATION

The *Consensus Model for APRN Regulation: Licensure, Accreditation, Certification, and Education* (the Consensus Model) was published in 2008 after lengthy collaboration with more than 70 national nursing organizations. The model serves as a guide for standardization of APRN recognition and regulation across the United States. Baccalaureate-prepared registered nurses can obtain graduate preparation in a several kinds of advanced nursing practice. Only those who have completed a formal graduate-level academic program (masters or higher) with advanced preparation required to diagnose and prescribe are referred to as APRNs. Nurse managers and executives, advanced public health nurses, nurse informaticians, nurse educators, and others may complete an advanced graduate-level program, but they are not APRNs. The Consensus Model clarified this differentiation in advanced nursing practice.

Leading up to development of the Consensus Model, colleges were developing new and uniquely focused, highly specialized educational programs leading to NP practice (e.g., school health, oncology, holistic care). However, there were sometimes no certification examinations for graduates of these programs to complete. Boards of nursing (BONs) were left with many questions regarding which kinds of NPs to recognize. One of the goals of the Consensus Model was to clarify to BONs which NPs should be licensed. The Consensus Model addressed this issue by differentiating broad NP preparation for practice (based on a patient population) from specialty practice. It clarified that state recognition (licensure) should occur after broad preparation at the population foci level and that specialty practice should be recognized after licensure and managed by professional organizations rather than the state.

In addition, clarifying criteria that differentiate APRNs from other nurses with advanced nursing skills, the Consensus Model supported the four previously identified APRN roles—certified registered nurse anesthetist, certified nurse midwives, clinical nurse specialist, and certified nurse practitioner (CNP)—and adopted eight of the existing nine NP population foci (Pediatric Nurse Practitioner [PNP], Adult Nurse Practitioner [ANP], Family Nurse Practitioner [FNP], Women's Health Nurse Practitioner [WHNP], Neonatal Nurse Practitioner [NNP], Psychiatric-Mental Health Nurse Practitioner [PMHNP], Acute Care Nurse Practitioner [ACNP], Pediatric Nurse Practitioner-Acute Care [PNP-AC]). Those population foci were governed by nationally vetted NP population competencies, as well as formal educational programs, existing certification examinations, and state recognition (licensure) in all 50 states. Recognizing the shortage of APRNs with expertise to address the complex needs of a growing number of older adults, the limited pipeline preparing APRNs for geriatric care, and the small number of APRNs seeking certification in geriatrics, the Consensus Model proposed that all APRNs whose population included older adults (family, adult, acute care, women's health) should be better educated for that practice. It proposed that gerontologic NP (GNP) preparation be fully integrated with the existing education and certification for adult NPs and ACNPs, and that family and women's health NP education related to care of older adults be enhanced. The resulting new populations for NPs would be adult-gerontology primary care and adult-gerontology acute care. This meant that preparation and certification as a GNP would be phased out, six of the original nine NP population foci (PNP, FNP, WHNP, NNP, PMHNP, PNP-AC) would be retained, and AG-PCNP and AG-ACNP would be added to replace the previous ANP and ACNP populations. Today, the eight NP population foci are family primary care, adult-gerontology primary care, adult-gerontology acute care, neonatal, pediatric primary care, pediatric acute care, women's health, and psychiatric mental health. APRNs may develop a depth of expertise in a "specialty," but that specialization does not extend the APRN's role or population foci. Examples of NP specialties for which certification exists include oncology, cardiology, and palliative care.

The CNP is educated and certified at an advanced level to provide care in a variety of settings within their patient population. The population focus defines NP scope of practice for a specific patient population that is congruent with the NP's formal graduate educational program and certification.

The Consensus Model prompted the development of new adult-gerontology acute care NP competencies and scope and standards of practice documents (American Association of Critical-Care Nurses [AACN] critical care, National Organization of Nurse Practitioner Faculties [NONPF] primary and acute care statement) and the revision of ACNP program curricula to create adult-gerontology acute care programs; it also led to the retirement of the original ACNP-BC and ACNPC acute care certifications and the creation of the AGACNP-BC and the ACNPC-AC certification examinations in 2014. NPs educated and certified as ACNP-BC and ACNPC continue to practice along with their acute care colleagues who completed the associated adult-gerontology processes.

▶ ACCREDITATION

The AGACNP must obtain their graduate advanced education from an accredited educational program. Nursing accreditors (e.g., Commission on Collegiate Nursing Education [CCNE], Accreditation Commission for Education in Nursing [ACEN], National League for Nursing [NLN], and Commission for Nursing Education Accreditation [CNEA]) are recognized by the U.S. Department of Education (USDE). Accreditation ensures the quality of the academic programs in nursing at institutions of higher education, ensures a culture of quality improvement, and raises academic standards at these institutions. Accreditation requires that educational institutions meet quality standards related to their mission and governance, institutional resources, curriculum and teaching-learning practices, and program effectiveness. CCNE and ACEN accreditation also requires NP programs use the National Task Force on Quality Nurse Practitioner Education: Criteria for Evaluation of Nurse Practitioner Programs (2016) to ensure that the programs they deliver provide students with appropriate preparation for practice. To obtain accreditation, NP program faculty complete a comprehensive self-study and undergo an accreditation visit in which compliance with accreditation standards is independently verified. Graduation from an accredited program is required for NP certification examination eligibility.

▶ EDUCATION

AGACNP educational preparation is at the graduate level and results in either a master's degree in nursing, a postgraduate certificate, or a Doctor of Nursing Practice degree. Through their *Essentials* documents, the American Association of Colleges of Nursing establishes general requirements for educational programs in nursing: until 2021, *The Essentials of Master's Education in Nursing* (2011) and *The Essentials of Doctoral Education for Advanced Nursing Practice* (2006). Patient needs and healthcare systems continue to evolve, and to ensure AGACNP program graduates are prepared to meet those needs, the most recent *Essentials* documents were replaced by *The Essentials: Core Competencies for Professional Nursing Education* (2021). AACN also supports use in NP programs of the Consensus Model and its guidance regarding the APRN role and population foci. AGACNP educational programs should also base their curriculum on the AACN Scope and Standards (2017; 2021) and the NONPF AGACNP Competencies (2016). In 2004, AACN recommended that all APRNs be prepared at the doctoral level; however, in 2022, AACN published a statement indicating continued support of master's degree programs. In 2015, the NONPF recommended all NPs receive their preparation at the doctoral level, and in 2018 it set 2025 as the target for transitioning NP education for nurses entering advanced practice from a master's degree to the Doctor of Nursing Practice. Postgraduate preparation continues to be available to master's and doctorally prepared NPs and other APRNs, especially those whose practice has evolved, and those who wish to expand either their APRN role or their population foci. Many adult and family primary care NPs have expanded their credentials to match the patients they are serving by completing a postgraduate AGACNP program and earning the associated certification.

NP curriculum includes but is not limited to content to "ensure attainment of the APRN core, role core and population core competencies." APRN core curriculum includes separate graduate courses in advanced physiology/pathophysiology, advanced health assessment, and advanced pharmacology. Verification of completion of these courses is required to be eligible to take a NP population-focused certification exam.

The educational preparation of an AGACNP is also guided by the AACN through its scope and standards documents. Since 2017, AGACNP curricula, certification, and practice have been based on the AACN Scope and Standards for Acute Care Nurse Practitioner Practice. In 2021, a new document, the AACN Scope and Standards for Adult-Gerontology and Pediatric Acute Care Nurse Practitioners, which encompasses information important to both adult-gerontology and pediatric acute care NPs, was published. Nursing education must remain elastic, as this document reflects explicit expectations that span all levels of nursing and all NP education programs. The latest edition to be implemented includes new or enhanced competencies in social determinants of health; diversity, equity, and inclusion; person-centered care; care coordination and interprofessional practice; palliative and end-of-life care; accountability for care outcomes; professional identity; disaster preparedness; and nurse health, self-care, and healthy work environments.

The educational preparation of an AGACNP encompasses all the knowledge, skills, and attitudes required to diagnose and safely manage acute, complex, chronic, and critical illnesses. The AGACNP is prepared to provide comprehensive care, from health promotion and disease prevention to palliative and end-of-life care, to individuals who are "physiologically unstable, technologically dependent, require frequent monitoring and intervention and who are highly vulnerable to complications." This includes an understanding of the scientific basis of health and disease, advanced health assessment, and clinical decision-making, evaluation, and application of evidence-based practice (EBP) to deliver and improve care processes and ensure optimal patient and system outcomes, prescription of pharmacologic and nonpharmacologic interventions, care coordination, and patient and family education for self-care management and advanced care decision-making. Educational programs for the AGACNP provide both clinical and didactic coursework.

▶ CERTIFICATION

Before licensure, the AGACNP graduate must pursue certification from either the American Nurses Credentialing Center (ANCC) or the AACN. Both examinations are accepted for licensure by BONs in all 50 states. Before the certification examination, the AGACNP graduate should again review documents foundational to their practice (AACN Scope and Standards, NONPF AGACNP Competencies) and review the most recent examination role delineation study (also called a study of practice) and the associated certification examination test blueprint for the exam they will complete (see Chapter 1 for more information).

▶ SPECIALTY PRACTICE

Specialty practice is placed at the top of the Consensus Model triangle. Specialty certification does not expand an NP's scope of practice beyond their role and population boundaries. Specialty certification is a voluntary process managed by professional organizations to recognize individuals who demonstrate a depth of expertise in a functional or clinical area of nursing. Certification in a specialty validates an individual's knowledge base for practice in a narrowly defined area of nursing. NP certifications are available for oncology, orthopedics, dermatology, hospice and palliative care, nephrology, and cardiology.

▶ LICENSURE

Upon graduation from an accredited program and population-based NP certification, an AGACNP graduate must apply for licensure in the state in which they intend to practice. BON requirements for NP recognition and licensure vary by state. AGACNPs who plan to include invasive procedures, such as endotracheal intubation, insertion of arterial or central venous catheters, thoracentesis or tube thoracostomy, lumbar puncture, or wound care and suturing, need to meet BON requirements to authorize these procedures. In addition, after obtaining licensure, the AGACNP must also be credentialed by the hospital or other practice site before practice and will need to be credentialed by insurance payers before billing for services.

▶ STATE REGULATIONS

BONs oversee the NP scope of practice based on broadly written state statues. They define more specifically within regulations what the NP is authorized to do, under what conditions, and the limits or boundaries for practice. Scope of practice, practice authority and autonomy, and practice requirements vary dramatically across the 50 states. NPs in 26 states have what is referred to as full practice authority, and in the remaining 24 states, NPs lack autonomous authority over their practice and are required to work under the oversight or supervision of physicians.

NPs may manage only patients who match the population focus of the NP's formal graduate education and certification. Patient setting and nursing experience do not determine the NP's scope of practice. When evaluating the match between a patient's needs and the NP's capacity to provide the patient care, NPs should consider the focus of their APRN education and certification in terms of role, population as well as state-authorized scope of practice, age and level of care required by a patient, types of therapies that may be indicated, and risks for complications from needed care.

▶ NURSE PRACTICE ACTS

All U.S. states and territories have a *Nurse Practice Act* (NPA) that is broadly written to authorize and guide nursing practice. NPAs were first developed in the early 1900s to protect the public; before that, states did not define or recognize nursing practice, and anyone could engage in the delivery of nursing care without formal education or training. Over the years, NPAs evolved to define nursing practice, authorize practice through licensure, set educational standards for licensure, and establish standards for practice through regulations. Elements of NPAs include definitions, composition and authority of the BON, educational program requirements, scope and standards of practice, titling and licensure definitions and protection, licensure requirements, and grounds for disciplinary action. NPAs vary by state, and thus NP scope of practice will vary based on state laws.

▶ INSTITUTIONAL POLICIES AND PROCEDURES

Individual practice environments have their own policies and procedures that dictate clinical practice. As scope of practice can vary for the NP from state to state, it can also vary from organization to organization within a state. Individual organizations may not expand NP scope of practice beyond that defined by statutes and BON regulations, but they may restrict practice of NPs. It is the responsibility of the NP to understand and practice within their institution's policies, procedures, and by-laws related to NP practice. Institutions are also responsible for credentialing and privileging providers who practice in their facilities.

Credentialing is the process by which a healthcare delivery organization determines an NP's eligibility for appointment to the medical or nursing staff and privileges to provide healthcare services. Their credentials–verification personnel collect and independently verify information regarding the NP's identity, education, certification, licensure, and professional practice, including information regarding practice before APRN licensure. Credentialing ensures that the individual provider meets all federal and state requirements to safely practice. During the credentialing process, the National Practitioner Data Bank is queried regarding the provider's practice history. The National Practitioner Data Bank, a national repository of data related to malpractice claims, licensure actions, and other adverse actions reported about an individual provider, was created by Congress in 1986 to prevent practitioners from moving from state to state without disclosing previous damaging performance.

After the initial credentialing process, provider credentials are periodically reevaluated before reappointment to the institutional medical or nursing staff. This periodic review and reappointment allow the organization to stay informed of any major changes (disciplinary action with the BON, failure to maintain certification, legal action) that may impact the provider's ability to safely deliver care to patients and the potential risks to the institution. It is the responsibility of the NP to provide all information required to complete the credentialing process and make a determination regarding clinical privileges.

Privileging refers to the clinical activities within a healthcare facility that the provider has the right to perform. Privileges should match the APRN's education and certification. An APRN should not apply for privileges to manage the care of patients beyond their education and certification-based population foci or to perform procedures outside their scope of practice. For example, an APRN should not apply for privileges to read and interpret an electroencephalogram unless they have documentation of completion of didactic education and supervised practice and perhaps other credentials to do so. Some institutions have a "core" set of privileges for all NPs, but an AGACNP should be sure that any request for privileges that they submit is based on their formal education and certification.

To obtain independent privileges to perform invasive procedures, institutions may require a provider to submit evidence of successful performance under the supervision of a credentialed individual of a specific number procedures and perhaps documentation of the individual's successful management of any common complications of that procedure. An example is central line placement. During AGACNP education, an NP completes didactic and task trainer instruction and performs this procedure under supervision, placing several central lines during student clinical rotations. After graduation and passing boards, the NP accepts a position in a medical ICU. The NP is not immediately granted privileges to place central lines until they have successfully placed 10 central lines under direct supervision by a provider with privileges for this procedure. The NP keeps track of the medical-record numbers for these patients and submits to the credentialing committee a request for independent privileges for central line insertion. The NP also needs to determine if they need authorization from the BON in their state to perform this procedure and ensure their medical malpractice policy includes coverage for the procedure.

▶ ADULT-GERONTOLOGY ACUTE CARE NURSE PRACTITIONER

This section reviews specific details pertinent to the AGACNP role, scope of practice, population, and practice environment and outcomes, including AGACNP standards for clinical practice and standards for professional practice. AGACNPs must have intimate knowledge of these elements and be able to articulate these details to people and organizations that may not have a full understanding. Adhering to the scope and standards of practice and population are key to minimizing exposure to medicolegal issues.

AGACNPs are registered nurses who have completed a graduate degree from an accredited school and program specifically focused on the AGACNP role. The educational program for AGACNPs prepares them to care for late adolescent through geriatric patients with acute, complex, chronic, and critical illness and injury. NP scope of practice generally includes obtaining and documenting comprehensive health assessments, ordering and interpreting diagnostic tests, performing procedures, formulating differential diagnoses, developing and implementing a plan of care for the patient's identified diagnoses and problems, prescribing medications and biological agents, ordering or prescribing therapies, providing symptom management, evaluating outcomes and interventions, providing health promotion and disease prevention services, providing patient and family education, collaborating as part of an interprofessional team, and billing for health services delivered. The goal of the AGACNP is to provide care to stabilize life-threatening conditions, restore health, minimize complications, and provide palliative and end-of-life care.

PRACTICE POPULATION

The practice population for AGACNPs is clearly outlined by the AACN in the AACN Scope and Standards for Acute Care Nurse Practitioner Practice and the AGACNP Competencies. The AGACNP population focus includes diagnosis and management of patients "with acute, critical, and complex chronic, physical, and mental illnesses across the entire adult age spectrum from young adults through older adults (including frail adults)." AACN similarly defines the AGACNP population to include "late adolescents, young adults, adults, and older adults and focuses on the care of patients who are: physiologically unstable, technologically dependent, and highly vulnerable to complications."

Patients may present with or develop episodic acute or critical illnesses, stable chronic illnesses, acute exacerbation of chronic illness, acute injury, and palliative and end-of-life problems that require high-intensity nursing intervention or continuous nursing vigilance.

PRACTICE ENVIRONMENT

The practice setting or environment is not specified by education, certification, or state BONs. Rather, the needs of the patient and the match with the NP's competencies, education, and certification determine whether care of a patient is within the NP's scope of practice. In simpler terms, the practice environment of the AGACNP is not setting-specific but rather determined by the needs of the patients in that practice environment.

The AGACNP may care for patients in any practice environment in which patients with acute, chronic, and/or complex chronic illnesses are found, which incorporates a variety of different practice settings/environments. AGACNPs can provide comprehensive care to patients across the continuum of acute care. These settings may include but are not limited to the ED, ICU, and inpatient hospital services. The AGACNP is not limited to working in a hospital setting; they can provide care in a patient's home, ambulatory care, urgent care, long-term care, rehabilitative care, and palliative and/or hospice care. Further extensions of the practice environment for the AGACNP include mobile health environments such as advanced air and ground ambulance services and virtual locations using telehealth, including tele-ICUs and other areas using telehealth services. The AGACNP fills a critical role as communicator, facilitator, and collaborator during the intersections of care processes where care transitions occur, ensuring appropriate and safe care across providers and patient care environments.

OUTCOMES

Many studies show the value-added and significant impact of ACNPs and AGACNPs on patient care processes and patient as well as systems outcomes. These data show that ACNPs/AGACNPs contribute to decreases in length of stay, nosocomial infection, duration of mechanical ventilation, and adverse events; improve care consistency; and reduce hospital and ICU readmissions.

AGACNP STANDARDS OF PRACTICE

The *Standards of Practice* (Table 20.1) address entry-level skills for AGACNP practice, including advanced assessment, differential diagnoses, patient outcomes, patient management, and evaluation.

Table 20.1 Standards of Clinical Practice for the AGACNP

Standard	Description
Standard 1: Advanced Assessment	The AGACNP can obtain a thorough history and review all pertinent data for patients with acute, critical, or complex illnesses. The AGACNP will also be able to perform a complex physical examination and know the significance of the findings.
Standard 2: Differential Diagnosis	The AGACNP can analyze and synthesize the history, physical exam findings, and diagnostic information to formulate differential diagnoses and a working diagnosis list.
Standard 3: Outcomes Identification	The AGACNP can develop appropriate goals and outcomes for acutely ill patients. They engage in shared decision-making with patients and families for optimum outcomes. They can modify goals as a patient's illness progresses, and they can also facilitate care coordination.
Standard 4: Care Planning and Management	The AGACNP can develop an outcomes-focused plan of care that can be implemented across the continuum of care. This includes interpreting diagnostic imaging, collaborating with other members of the care team, and clearly communicating with patients and families regarding treatment and potential adverse effects of treatment.
Standard 5: Implementation	The AGACNP has the ability to implement evidence-based treatments and therapies to patients with acute or complex illness; perform diagnostic and therapeutic interventions consistent with the AGACNP's education, training, and state laws; perform consultations; utilize technology, including telehealth technology; and clearly communicate with all members of the care team.
Standard 6: Evaluation	The AGACNP can evaluate the patient's progress toward previously identified goals and outcomes and adjusts the plan according to patient's needs.

STANDARDS OF PROFESSIONAL PERFORMANCE

The *Standards of Professional Performance* (Table 20.2) address entry-level skills related to professional practice, including collaboration, advocacy, education, leadership, EBP, and clinical inquiry.

Table 20.2 Standards of Professional Performance

Standard	Description
Standard 1: Professional Practice	Professional practice involves maintaining professional certification and state licensures. It also refers to the ability to monitor patient care and to hold oneself accountable for the care that one provides. It also includes evaluating patient outcomes and participating in peer review to promote a culture of transparency and excellence.
Standard 2: Education	This standard involves a commitment to being a lifelong learner and staying up to date on the latest evidence-based practice through formal and informal means. It also includes keeping documentation of educational activities and meeting the requirements for national certification renewal and state licensure. Healthcare is an ever-evolving landscape, and new medications, treatments, and diagnostic tests are constantly improving. It is imperative to continue to build on foundational knowledge and keep practice current.
Standard 3: Collaboration	The AGACNP collaborates with all members of the healthcare team and engages in shared decision-making with patients. The AGACNP also acts as mentor and teacher to other members of the healthcare team. They also work with other disciplines to advance professional activities like research and technology use.
Standard 4: Ethics	Ethical care is based on the American Nurses Association Code of Ethics. Ethical care includes reporting unethical or illegal practices, ensuring protected health information is kept confidential, and respecting the autonomy of patients. It also means maintaining a high level of accountability for practice and delivering care in an equitable and inclusive manner. When an ethical dilemma arises, the AGACNP will serve as a leader in ethical principles and will engage an ethics consultation when appropriate.

(continued)

Table 20.2 Standards of Professional Performance (*continued*)

Standard	Description
Standard 5: Advocacy	Advocacy relates to the AGACNP serving as a spokesperson for the profession, patients, and patient families. It involves valuing the full spectrum of human perspectives and identities and working at local, state, and federal levels to ensure all people have access to high-quality, equitable care. Advocacy can be thought of as "speaking up for people who cannot speak up for themselves." This advocacy can be achieved on the immediate level by participating at the organizational level to identify and overcome barriers to patient care. Membership and participation in professional organizations allow the AGACNP to be educated on legislative issues related to professional practice and regulation. The AGACNP can also serve as an expert and spokesperson for the profession when legislation related to access to care and models of care is in congressional committees or up for congressional votes.
Standard 6: Systems/ Organizational Thinking	Systems and organizational thinking relate to the overall healthcare delivery system and ways to improve it. The AGACNP should play an integral role in the development and design of quality improvement initiatives to promote excellence in patient care. The AGACNP should also be able to evaluate system projects through quality improvement models to ensure they are meeting the identified outcomes they were designed to address. It is also important to bear in mind the financial implications to patients and to systems and to promote stewardship of resources.
Standard 7: Resource Utilization	Resource utilization involves efficiently using resources without compromising quality and evidence-based care. This includes the appropriate and judicious use of testing and guiding the healthcare team in selecting therapies that consider risk, benefit, quality, safety, and fiscal responsibility. One way to think of resource utilization is to ask, "How will this test change patient management?"
Standard 8: Leadership	Leadership is a vital part of the AGACNP's role. It involves educating the public and the interdisciplinary team on the AGACNP role. It also means that the AGACNP leads teams and committees at the organizational level and with professional organizations. The AGACNP promotes the profession of nurses and the advancement of the profession. In addition, the AGACNP serves as a leader in the implementation of the APRN Consensus Model at the local, state, and national levels.
Standard 9: Collegiality	Collegiality refers to the professional interaction of the AGACNP with their colleagues. The AGACNP leads by example by fostering an atmosphere of open communication between all members of the interdisciplinary team. In addition, the AGACNP is respectful and professional in their communication with patients, families, and colleagues. The AGACNP also serves as a teacher and mentor and shares their skills and knowledge with others.
Standard 10: Quality and Evidence-Based Practice	Quality improvement and evidence-based practice are the hallmarks of excellence in patient care. The AGACNP works with patients, families, and colleagues to ensure quality patient outcomes. The AGACNP will remain a lifelong learner to stay up to date on current evidence related to patient care. As part of the quality process, the AGACNP will also engage in frequent self-reflection, performance appraisal, and peer review to improve the quality of care they provide.
Standard 11: Clinical/ Practice Inquiry	Clinical/practice inquiry relates to participation in research, translating research into clinical practice, and promotion of evidence-based practice. In addition to implementing evidence-based care, practice inquiry also involves dissemination of best practices at local, state, and national levels with scholarly work such as publications, journal clubs, formal presentations, and community presentations.

▶ ETHICS

Ethics relate to the moral tradition that forms the basis of the nursing profession and the care provided to patients. All nurses and advanced practice nurses are held to the same ethical standards. AGACNPs commonly encounter a variety of ethical situations centering on patients' autonomy for self-determination. Dilemmas frequently emerge related to patients who have impaired decisional capacity (temporary or permanent) and situations in which family members or loved ones struggle to honor the individual patient's pre-stated wishes. AGACNPs must be familiar with key ethical terminology (Table 20.3) and readily identify ethical dilemmas, guide family and staff to ethically accepted standards of care, and identify resources when ethical dilemmas arise.

Table 20.3 Ethical Terms and Their Definitions

Term	Definition
Autonomy	Right to self-govern and to make decisions about one's own healthcare
Beneficence	Moral obligation to promote goodness or benefit to the patient and provide care that maintains or improves health, decreases disability, and eases pain and suffering. It refers not just to removing harm but to providing benefit as well.
Nonmaleficence	Obligation of the provider to not do harm to the patient. It also includes weighing the risks and benefits of all testing and treatments.
Justice	Striving for fair distribution of resources
Veracity	Being honest and telling the truth
Fidelity	Keeping one's promises. Nurse practitioners must be faithful and true to professional codes of conduct and standards of care and responsibilities.
Accountability	Obligation to accept responsibility or to account for one's actions

INFORMED CONSENT

Informed consent is a process of communication between a provider and a patient that leads to consent for diagnostic testing or services. Patients have the right to obtain information and ask questions before procedures and treatments. There are five requirements of informed consent for a procedure or for research:

1. The patient must be competent and able to make decisions.
2. The patient must receive a full disclosure of risks and benefits.
3. The patient must understand the disclosure of the risks and benefits.
4. The patient must be deciding voluntarily (not under coercion).
5. The patient must consent to the treatment or research.

DECISIONAL CAPACITY

Capacity is the ability to understand information relevant to a decision. It also means understanding the foreseeable consequences of a decision. Capacity can change throughout the course of a day. For example, a patient with fever and sepsis may initially lack capacity to make their own medical decisions because of the way their illness affects their thinking. However, after several days of antibiotics and antipyretics, they are once again able to make treatment decisions that are in line with their own values and preferences.

In the acute care setting, it is often necessary for the APRN to determine if a patient has capacity to make their medical decisions at any given time. They can use the Aid to Capacity Evaluation (ACE) as a guide for determining capacity.

COMPETENCY

Competency is a legal term that is the key to rational decision-making. Laws assume every adult is mentally competent until a court decides otherwise. Thus, only a judge can deem a person incompetent to make their own decisions. This typically requires a series of neurologic and psychologic tests to be performed by a neuropsychologist prior to a person being deemed legally incompetent. APRNs do not determine a patient's competency.

ETHICS COMMITTEES AND CONSULTANTS

Ethics committees in a hospital or facility exist to assist in the decision-making processes for helping institutions create policies and procedures that align with ethical standards. They can also assist providers and other members of the healthcare team in navigating ethical dilemmas that arise in clinical practice.

▶ SUMMARY

AGACNPs must have a complete understanding of the history behind the development of the NP role's and specifically the AGACNP role's scope of practice. In transitioning from the RN role to the APRN role, additional responsibilities and regulations come into play. Keeping these in mind will better inform AGACNP practice and prevent violations of federal, state, or institutional rules and regulations.

KNOWLEDGE CHECK: CHAPTER 20

1. An AGACNP recently moved to New Mexico and will be working in a small community-based ED. What will determine the AGACNP's scope of practice in this new state?

   A. New Mexico State Practice Act
   B. AGACNP's informal education
   C. Needs of the emergency department
   D. 10 years of nursing practice in an ED

2. An AGACNP is practicing in North Carolina. What document by this state governs the nurse practitioner's legal right to practice?

   A. Nurse Practice Act
   B. Nurse practitioner's certification
   C. State licensure
   D. Consensus models

3. An AGACNP has recently graduated from an accredited nurse practitioner program. They are discussing the concept of prescribing narcotics with a group of colleagues. Which agency is responsible for overseeing this?

   A. State Boards of Nursing
   B. American Nurses Credentialing Center (ANCC)
   C. U.S. Drug Enforcement Agency
   D. American Association of Critical-Care Nurses (AACN)

4. The ethical principle that concerns the right of a person to make decisions about their own healthcare and the right to self-govern their body is:

   A. Beneficence
   B. Nonmaleficence
   C. Autonomy
   D. Veracity

5. The AGACNP is caring for a patient with limited English proficiency and notices that the patient's family member is acting as a translator for the care team. The AGACNP knows that access to a qualified medical interpreter is a patient right because there may be medical issues that they would like to keep private from their family. The AGACNP encourages the team to use the organization's medical interpreter services in further communications with the patient to respect the patient's privacy and maintain patient autonomy. Promoting use of interpreter services to maintain patient privacy and patient autonomy relates to what standard of professional practice?

   A. Differential diagnosis
   B. Advocacy
   C. Resource utilization
   D. Clinical/practice inquiry

6. Which of the following terms best identifies the organizational activities that are implemented to monitor, evaluate, and improve healthcare at a facility?

   A. Quality improvement program
   B. Credentialing committee
   C. Hospital by-laws and policies
   D. Licensing and certification

(See answers next page.)

1. A) New Mexico State Practice Act

Previous years of nursing experience do not apply when determining a nurse practitioner's scope of practice. The State Practice Act, formal education, certification, and the institution all help to determine a nurse practitioner's allowed scope of practice.

2. A) Nurse Practice Act

The Nurse Practice Act is the legal document that determines a nurse practitioner's legal right to practice in each state.

3. C) U.S. Drug Enforcement Agency

The U.S. Drug Enforcement Agency is responsible for regulating the manufacture and distribution of controlled pharmaceuticals. Individual state boards of nursing are responsible for creating, regulating, and enforcing their state's Nurse Practice Act. AACN and ANCC offer national certification exams to ensure graduates have safe entry into practice.

4. C) Autonomy

Autonomy is the ethical principle that relates to a patient's right to self-govern their own health and body. Beneficence is the moral obligation to do good. Nonmaleficence means to "do no harm." Veracity is the ethical principle related to truth telling.

5. B) Advocacy

Ensuring that patients are receiving the highest quality of care and that they receive the services they are entitled to receive is advocacy. In this case, the patient is unable to advocate for themselves due to a language barrier. The AGACNP acts as an advocate for the patient by encouraging the team to use appropriate interpreter services. Differential diagnosis refers to analyzing and synthesizing patient history, physical examination, and laboratory tests to determine a diagnosis of illness. Although it may seem as if use of interpretive services is resource utilization, this principle relates more to the judicious use of testing and therapies. Clinical/practice inquiry relates to translating research into clinical practice and promotion of evidence-based care.

6. A) Quality improvement program

Quality improvement is a structured organizational program that relates to the systematic review and implementation of quality improvement initiatives within a healthcare system. Credentialing refers to the process of verifying education, licensure, and experience before a provider can gain privileges to practice at an organization. Hospital by-laws are the formal self-governance structure of healthcare providers within an organization. Licensing is the process by which the board of nursing grants permission for an individual to engage in nursing practice.

7. The entity responsible for licensing an advanced practice registered nurse (APRN) for practice is:

   A. American Nurses Credentialing Center
   B. American Association of Critical-Care Nurses
   C. Individual hospital systems
   D. State Board of Nursing

8. The AGACNP is being recruited for a new position. During the interview, the AGACNP is informed that claims-made malpractice insurance coverage will be part of their compensation package. This means that the AGACNP:

   A. Will be protected from any claim made related to any incident during employment
   B. Will be covered for any claim made from their date of hire
   C. Should request a copy of the policy listing the AGACNP as an insured provider
   D. Will need to consider obtaining tail coverage insurance

9. What agency or organization enforces the protections safeguarded by the Health Insurance Portability and Accountability Act (HIPAA)?

   A. Office for Civil Rights (OCR)
   B. U.S. Department of Health and Human Services (HHS)
   C. American Medical Association (AMA)
   D. Agency for Healthcare Research and Quality (AHRQ)

10. The AGACNP is rounding in the ICU on a patient with a traumatic brain injury who has a Glasgow Coma Scale score of 12. The nurse asks the AGACNP to write an order for restraints to keep the patient from trying to get out of bed. Which of the following must occur to prevent the AGACNP from being held liable?

    A. AGACNP is not allowed to order restraints on patients and will not do so.
    B. AGACNP must document safety checks and exact reason and rationale for use of restraints.
    C. AGACNP must notify the medical director of the unit and obtain permission for the order.
    D. AGACNP must notify the family members and obtain their permission for use of restraints.

11. The AGACNP is working in an ICU when a critically ill patient is admitted in septic shock, requiring a central venous catheter (CVC) to be placed urgently. The AGACNP has completed the required training and has submitted credentialing paperwork to add this procedure to their institutional credential procedure list but has not yet received notification of approval. The AGACNP's best action is to:

    A. Proceed with the CVC placement
    B. Request supervision for the CVC placement
    C. Manage the patient with peripheral vasopressors until day shift arrives
    D. Obtain approval from the ICU attending to proceed with CVC placement

12. The AGACNP has been hired to work with a group of pulmonologists. This role will incorporate unique differences in both inpatient and outpatient clinic activities and responsibilities. This position:

    A. Will require the AGACNP to obtain credentialing privileges for hospital practice
    B. Will encompass substitutive care traditionally provided by physicians
    C. Is a fee-for-service–based practice model
    D. Must be supervised by a physician in the inpatient setting

(See answers next page.)

7. D) State Board of Nursing

State Boards of Nursing are the licensing bodies for nurses and APRNs. Both the American Nurses Credentialing Center and the American Association of Critical-Care Nurses offer board certification for AGACNPs. Individual hospital systems provide practice privileges and credential providers for practice at their institutions.

8. D) Will need to consider obtaining tail coverage insurance

Claim-made insurance will protect the AGACNP who has the policy only when the claim is made, which could happen after the AGACNP leaves their current employment. Tail coverage insurance would ensure protection if a claim was brought when the AGACNP was not employed.

9. A) Office for Civil Rights (OCR)

The OCR enforces the protections safeguarded by HIPAA. The HHS is the administrative agency that developed the regulations for HIPAA. The AMA is not involved in enforcement. AHRQ is an independent organization concerned with reporting research of quality measures.

10. B) AGACNP must document safety checks and exact reason and rationale for use of restraints.

The AGACNP, to avoid being held liable in a state of law, must document rea son for restraints, rationale, appropriate safety checks, and neuro checks, and must notify the attending physician. It is part of the scope of practice for AGACNP to order restraints, but restraints should be used only as a last resort. The medical director or patient's primary care provider should be notified of the need for patient restraints. The family should also be notified of restraint use, particularly if it involves a change in condition, but they do not need to give permission.

11. B) Request supervision for the CVC placement

The AGACNP requires supervision with procedures until the proper credentialing process is completed and the AGACNP has documentation that the additional procedure has been approved and added to their institutional credentials. The attending physician does not have the authority to override the credentialing process. This patient may have untoward outcomes by managing the patient with peripheral vasopressors.

12. A) Will require the AGACNP to obtain credentialing privileges for hospital practice

Credentialing privileges are required to practice in the acute care setting. Credentialing demonstrates that the AGACNP has the required education, licensure, and certification to practice. Care provided by an AGACNP may or may not always substitute for care provided by a physician, involve a fee for service, or require physician supervision.

13. Informed consent includes the patient's ability to:

    A. Comprehend information, contemplate options, and evaluate risks and consequences
    B. Make decisions based on written information that is provided about acceptable care
    C. Answer questions about information that is provided to the patient
    D. Successfully complete a full competency evaluation of the patient

14. The AGACNP contacts the healthcare proxy of an incapacitated patient. The healthcare proxy is expected to be able to make a decision in concordance with the patient's wishes. The ethical principle describing the concept of a person's right to self-determination is:

    A. Justice
    B. Autonomy
    C. Beneficence
    D. Veracity

15. The AGACNP is providing care in a busy ICU and is preparing to intubate a patient using rapid sequence intubation. The AGACNP tells the nurse to pull and administer 2 mg/kg succinylcholine. After the nurse gives the medication, the AGACNP remembers that the patient has a family history of malignant hyperthermia, and succinylcholine is contraindicated with this disease process. The AGACNP immediately calls the critical care team to tell them of the mistake. The action of calling the team demonstrates which ethical principle?

    A. Beneficence
    B. Nonmaleficence
    C. Veracity
    D. Autonomy

(See answers next page.)

13. **A) Comprehend information, contemplate options, and evaluate risks and consequences**

The patient needs a chance to ask questions, not rely solely on written materials. The patient does not need to be able to answer questions but does need to be able to ask questions about a potential procedure. A full competency evaluation is not required.

14. **B) Autonomy**

Autonomy or self-determination means that patients have the moral and legal right to determine what will be done with their own person. Justice is striving for fair distribution of resources. Beneficence is the moral obligation to promote goodness or benefit to the patient, and veracity is being honest and telling the truth.

15. **C) Veracity**

Veracity refers to telling the truth. The AGACNP exemplifies the ethical principle of veracity when they call the neurology team to tell them of the administration of succinylcholine during intubation, which may exacerbate the patient's myasthenia gravis. Beneficence is the moral obligation to do good. Nonmaleficence means to "do no harm." Autonomy is the ethical principle concerning the patient's right to make their own healthcare decisions.

KEY BIBLIOGRAPHY

Only key resources appear in the print edition. Access the full bibliography for this chapter on ExamPrepConnect.com.

Adult-Gerontology NP Competencies Work Group. (2016). *Adult-gerontology acute care and primary care NP competencies.* https://www.aacn.org/~/media/aacn-website/certification/advanced-practice/adultgero acnpcompetencies.pdf

American Association of Colleges of Nursing. (2006). *The essentials of doctoral education for advanced nursing practice.* https://www.aacnnursing.org/Portals/42/Publications/DNPEssentials.pdf

American Association of Colleges of Nursing. (2011). *The essentials of master's education in nursing.* https://www.aacnnursing.org/portals/42/publications/mastersessentials11.pdf

American Association of Colleges of Nursing. (2021b). *The essentials: Core competencies for professional nursing education.* https://www.aacnnursing.org/Portals/42/AcademicNursing/pdf/Essentials-2021.pdf

American Association of Critical-Care Nurses. (2021a). *AACN scope and standards for adult-gerontology and pediatric acute care nurse practitioners 2021.* https://www.aacn.org/~/media/aacn-website/nursing excell ence/standards/acnpscopeandstandards.pdf

American Association of Nurse Practitioners. (2019). *Scope of practice for nurse practitioners.* https://www.aan p.org/advocacy/advocacy-resource/position-statements/scope-of-practice-for-nurse-practitioners

APRN Consensus Work Group & National Council of State Boards of Nurses APRN Advisory Committee. (2008). *Consensus model for APRN regulation: Licensure, accreditation, certification and regulation.* https://www.ncsbn.org/public-files/Consensus_Model_for_APRN_Regulation_July_2008.pdf

Healthcare Policy and Systems Review

Keri Draganic and Moneé Carter-Griffin

▶ INTRODUCTION

AGACNPs have the responsibility and capacity to influence current and future healthcare practices within their community, at the state level, nationally, and globally. The 2010 Institute of Medicine (IOM) report, *The Future of Nursing: Leading Change, Advancing Health*, highlights the value and importance of including the nursing perspective and presence in advanced decision-making roles, including policy development. AGACNPs have the education, experiences, and unique health perspectives that equip them to actively participate in health policy. Despite these skills, AGACNPs are underrepresented in public health and policy discussions, which can lead to critical oversights impacting healthcare delivery. For example, nurses were excluded from the Trump administration's Coronavirus Task Force as well as Biden's Transition COVID-19 Advisory Board. This omission of nurses creates a lack of interdisciplinary perspectives on a national and global health problem that can affect patient outcomes, as well as community and national health.

The Future of Nursing 2020–2030 calls on nurses to participate, inform, and implement policies that will affect the greatest number of people in the most profound ways. Although there are four times as many nurses as physicians in the United States, currently only three members of Congress are nurses, compared with 17 physicians. The International Council of Nurses continues to support nurses around the world to contribute their expertise by advocating health-related public policy agendas through a nurse's perspective. AGACNPs must speak with a united voice on health issues that affect nursing practices and the health outcomes of patients. AGACNPs need to increase their visibility and influence regarding their perspectives to shape public health policy at the academic, health system, and research levels. AGACNPs can influence health policy by engaging in the policy process on various levels, which includes interpreting, evaluating, and leading policy change.

▶ THE POLICY PROCESS

According to the Centers for Disease Control and Prevention, health policy is the laws, rules, and/or regulations of institutions or governments used to achieve specific healthcare goals and/or determine access to and delivery of care. Policy is one of the most effective tools for directly and indirectly improving health and access. While an effective strategy with nurses as advocates and influencers, the policy process at all levels remains limited. AGACNPs have the capacity to affect policy development, whether creating an institutional policy to improve patient care or championing a policy at the state or national level. It is imperative that AGACNPs have foundational knowledge of the policy process and how policy development is used to promote individual, community, and national health.

POLICY DEVELOPMENT

Policy development is a multifaceted process involving many variables such as feasibility, sustainability, cost, and stakeholder interests. Often, policy originates from the need to address a broader issue. Once a problem is identified, the developmental process can vary depending on the policy level; however, there are key principles that should be considered for policy development at all levels (e.g., institutional, state, national). These principles include using evidence to plan and develop policies, designing clear policies with detailed regulations or procedures that promote successful implementation, and considering health equity.

POLICY FRAMEWORKS

The policy process can seem chaotic and confusing. However, several conceptual models have been developed to provide structure and predictability to the policy-making process. These models include the Kingdon's Policy Streams Model, Longest's Policy Cycle Model, Stages Model of Policymaking, and the Linear Model of Policymaking. Each model attempts to generalize and highlight the steps of the policy process from policy identification to implementation.

POLICY PROCESS

Policy development follows this process: (a) problem and/or challenge is identified; (b) solutions are introduced by interested parties, including AGACNPs; (c) agenda, which is usually based on stakeholder and/or policy maker interest or presumed policy need, is set; (d) policy is formulated, which poses an opportunity for AGACNPs to advocate for a solution influencing their practice and/or patient care; and (e) policy is implemented, which represents another hugely influential part of the policy process for AGACNPs. It is during the policy formulation and implementation phase that nurses can use their numbers and grassroots efforts to influence regulations, or rules, impacting practice, health, and access to care.

Regardless of the policy level, current and high-yield evidence should inform the identified solutions for policy development. It is imperative that the AGACNP influence and educate stakeholders during all phases of the policy process. Ideally, the policy appeals to policy makers and other stakeholders. The greater the appeal of the policy, the more likely it is that policy formulation, adoption, and implementation will occur.

BILLS, LAWS, AND REGULATIONS

AGACNPs must understand the terminology used during the policy-making process. Prior to any policy becoming a law, it starts as a bill and/or resolution. A bill is a proposed law based on a problem and an identified solution. Bills are mainly introduced through the legislative branch of government. Bills that pass in the legislative branch can become laws. Laws are the adopted and enforced rules intended to affect outcomes at the individual and/or population level. Regulations are rules adopted by those affected by a law, and they outline how the law will be enforced.

FROM A BILL TO A LAW

The process for a bill to become a law can vary from state to state and at the federal level. However, there are commonalities at both the state and the federal levels. Once a bill is drafted, it will be introduced in the legislative branch. Within the legislative branch, the bill will be referred to a committee for review. Some bills may be referred to more than one committee or referred to a subcommittee pending the provisions within the bill and/or the bill's focus. Committee review provides an opportunity for AGACNPs to give testimony as to why the bill should or should not progress. Throughout the committee process, further deliberation may occur until a final draft is presented to committee members for a vote. During this process, AGACNPs have yet another opportunity to continue their efforts through lobbying, meeting with legislators or legislative staff, phone calls, and/or emails.

Once a committee votes, if the bill is approved to progress, the bill will be placed on calendars for floor consideration. If the bill makes it to the legislative floor, legislative members will debate and vote to approve or deny the bill. For any bill that completes this process, it will be delivered to the governing official (e.g., president, governor) to sign or veto.

FACTORS INFLUENCING POLICY

The policy process is influenced by many factors, including individual, political, and societal. For example, more policy makers are using evidence-based practice and research as a strategy to highlight the significance of a problem and also as a strategy to identify a proposed solution. Additionally, policy makers are using evidence to inform their debates and guide their policy choices. Other influential factors include personal, population, and societal values; the current political climate; interest groups, professional organizations, and lobbyists; and the media. The degree to which these influence policies often depends on the significance of the identified problem and proposed solution.

AGACNPs engaging in the policy process must understand the importance of factors determining their current and/or future practice. For those pursuing or hoping to improve legislation governing their current practice, individual, and/or population outcomes, it is vital to gain a sense of the political feasibility of the proposed solution, the stakeholders affected by the policy, the economic implications, and potential resource allocation.

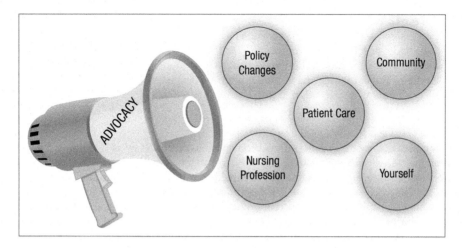

Figure 21.1 AGACNP advocacy topics that impact healthcare.

▶ ADVOCACY

For AGACNPs and master's- or doctorate-prepared nurses, it is imperative to engage in advocacy. Per the American Nurses Association's (ANA) Code of Ethics, the nurse will promote, advocate for, and protect the rights, health, and safety of the patient. Providing quality, affordable, and ethical care to patients is the epicenter of nursing and advocating. The World Health Organization has emphasized that a key role of nurses within health policy development is to ensure high-quality care for patients. Figure 21.1 elicits the various topics that AGACNPs can advocate for and become involved in when changing health policies.

Per the American Association of Colleges of Nursing (AACN) *The Essentials: Core Competencies for Professional Nursing Education*, advanced practice nurses are able to advocate for professional nursing to ensure optimal outcomes, advocate for policy at all levels, analyze the effect and efforts of policy, and participate in the policy implementation process. Nurses are committed to ensuring high-quality, humane, and respectful patient care that values all people holistically. Because of this commitment, as well as the experience and knowledge that AGACNPs possess regarding patient care, they must advocate for continual improvement. Lawmakers across the country need to be apprised of the issues that affect patients and the AGACNP role. This requires grassroots efforts by AGACNPs and various nursing organizations to come together with one voice to provide meaning and understanding to issues that affect healthcare. Nurses together can influence policy and healthcare delivery at a societal level. AGACNPs offer their knowledge and experience with nursing skills such as communication, clinical experience, empathy, and ability to manage conflict, which are transferrable skills to policy development and public advocacy. This skillset allows AGACNPs to participate as policy experts and analysts and to work with elected officials and partners within the political arena.

PATIENT ADVOCACY

Figure 21.2 highlights the topics that AGACNPs should advocate for within the acute care setting. Patient care issues include protecting patients from harm, encouraging patient autonomy, fostering collaboration, and providing patients and family with information for informed decision-making. Within the acute care setting, AGACNPs need to evaluate and advocate for their patients' informed decision-making capacity. Informed decision-making capacity includes the patient's ability to understand risks and benefits of treatment and alternatives to a proposed treatment or intervention, including no treatment. The AGACNP can assess and advocate for their patient's capacity for informed decision-making or consent when the patient understands their situation and consequences, elicit the reasoning within their thought process, and communicate their wishes. Some common risk factors of impaired medical decision-making capacity include older age, chronic psychiatric or neurologic condition, lower education level, or cultural or language barriers, as well as reversible causes of incapacity including infection, medications, illicit drugs, hypoxia, metabolic derangements, delirium, and critical illness. AGACNPs will need to be attuned to these patient conditions and advocate for patients who lack capacity. If there is uncertainty as

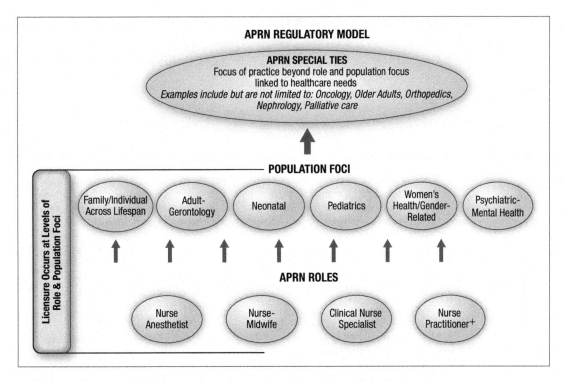

Figure 21.2 Advanced Practice Registered Nurse (APRN) regulatory model.

+The certified nurse practitioner (CNP) is prepared with the acute care CNP competencies and/or the primary care CNP competencies. At this point in time the acute care and primary care CNP delineation applies only to the pediatric and adult-gerontology CNP population foci. Scope of practice of the primary care or acute care CNP is **not setting specific** but is based on patient care needs. Programs may prepare individuals across both the primary care and acute care CNP competencies. If programs prepare graduates across both sets of roles, the graduate must be prepared with the consensus-based competencies for both roles and must successfully obtain certification in both the acute and the primary care CNP roles. CNP certification in the acute care or primary care roles must match the educational preparation for CNPs in these roles.

to a patient's capacity, the final judgment should err on the side of protecting the patient. The AGACNP should be mindful of their state's definition of capacity, as this can vary across the United States.

PROFESSIONAL ADVOCACY: COMMUNITY, STATE, AND FEDERAL

AGACNPs can participate in policy changes by learning about the legislative process, contacting or meeting elected officials, and providing expert testimony to assist with and inform policy decisions. The ANA has an advocacy toolkit that is composed of the various strategies that nurses can use to become more politically involved. The ANA recommends knowing who represents you within Congress and emailing, calling, or scheduling a meeting with the representative to investigate where they stand on specific healthcare issues. Attending town halls gives constituents an opportunity to offer insight on ideas and interact with elected officials within their community, state, or nation.

Common federal healthcare policies or acts that the AGACNP should be mindful of include the Emergency Medical Treatment and Labor Act, the Health Insurance Portability and Accountability Act (HIPAA), and the Patient Safety and Quality Improvement Act. Table 21.1 lists these acute care acts with definitions and implications for the AGACNP. Again, AGACNPs need to be aware of these laws and how they affect the patients they care for and treat.

Advocating for and within the community can involve economic matters, educational issues, and healthcare system issues, but it can also represent the creation of organizations in which the constituents share a common goal. AGACNPs can assess and advocate for issues when a need is apparent. This can include sharing healthcare costs within a community, providing information on available community resources, improving access to care, and providing expertise within public forums. Examples of possible community-specific acute care political issues include infectious

Table 21.1 Acute Care Health Acts: Definitions and Implications for AGACNPs

Healthcare Acts	Definition	Implications
EMTALA	A federal law that requires any patient who seeks treatment in an emergency room must be stabilized, and treated regardless of their insurance status or ability to pay	Ensures access to healthcare and reduces financial barriers. EMTALA requires providers to screen and treat emergency medical conditions of patients in a nondiscriminatory manner, regardless of the person's ability to pay, insurance status, national origin, race, creed, or color.
HIPAA	A federal law that requires the creation of national standards to protect sensitive patient health information from being disclosed without the patient's consent or knowledge	Individually identifiable health information including names, geographic identifiers including street address, city, zip code; dates related to an individual like birth date, admission date; telephone numbers; FAX numbers; email addresses; social security numbers; medical record numbers; health plan beneficiary numbers; and account numbers; must not be disclosed without the patients' authorization or legal authority.
PSQIA	Federal act that establishes a voluntary reporting system designed to enhance the data available to assess and resolve patient safety and healthcare quality issues, and to encourage the reporting and analysis of medical errors	Federal legal privilege and confidentiality protections to information that is reported by providers and limits the use of this information in criminal, civil, and administrative proceedings. There are provisions for monetary penalties for violations of confidentiality or privilege protections.

EMTALA, Emergency Medical Treatment and Labor Act; HIPAA, Health Insurance Portability and Accountability Act; PSQIA, Patient Safety and Quality Improvement Act.

diseases like COVID-19 or HIV, human trafficking, violence, substance use including use of medical cannabis, and contaminated water, all of which can affect the health of patients. The AGACNP can impact policy and procedures at the institutional level as well. There is a constant need for policies to be evaluated, refined, and developed as hospital-based care and the role of the AGACNP evolve. An example of policy work with which the AGACNP can be involved in a hospital setting is triaging policies and practices.

AGACNPs can also be active members of various nursing and healthcare organizations within their community, at the state level, nationally, or globally. Nursing organizations include the American Association of Nurse Practitioners, the Gerontological Advanced Practice Nurses Association, and state nurse practitioner organizations. Becoming a member of these organizations allows for educational opportunities, mentorship, connection, legislative support, up-to-date information, marketability, and role advancement. The National Occupational Research Agenda (NORA) Healthcare and Social Assistance Sector Council is another organization that brings together a community of individuals and organizations to share information, form partnerships, and promote adoption and dissemination of solutions that work. Many of these organizations support the active participation of AGACNPs within health policy to improve healthcare access, cost of care, health equality, health legislation, and nursing's scope of practice.

AGACNPs also have a duty to advocate for the nursing role and practice at the full scope of their practice, certification, and licensure in order to influence regulation and legislation. Advanced practice nurses should know their state's laws regarding AGACNP scope of practice. At the national level, some of the federal agencies that impact AGACNP practice include the Centers for Medicare and Medicaid Services (CMS), the Centers for Disease Control and Prevention, the Federal Employees Health Benefits program, the Federal Trade Commission, the U.S. Food and Drug Administration, the National Institutes of Health, and Veterans Affairs (see Chapter 20 for additional details on local, state, and national topics related to role development, delineation, and regulation).

PERSONAL ADVOCACY

Finally, it is imperative that AGACNPs advocate for themselves. This can include safety concerns within the workplace, professional wellness and well-being, and the highly skilled role AGACNPs fill within the healthcare system. AGACNPs can advocate through participating in activities that influence decision-making, joining practice committees, and collaborating with nurse leaders. Skills required to advocate for self include communicating effectively, knowing the scope of practice, knowing who to go to, and getting involved. An example of advocating for self, which can happen in the acute care setting, is when a provider needs to terminate their professional relationship with a patient for numerous reasons, including aggressive behavior, tampering with prescriptions, lying, and drug-seeking behavior. The AGACNP should be aware of the potential liability, including patient abandonment. To avoid the liability for abandonment, the provider must terminate the patient relationship by giving the patient notice, reasonable opportunity to find substitute care, and information on how to obtain their medical records.

With the rapidly changing and developing healthcare environment, AGACNPs need to engage and take on an active role to influence this change. AGACNPs are key stakeholders and therefore should influence policy and not simply implement the change. This requires AGACNPs to maintain an active practice to influence healthcare within their institutions, locally, regionally, nationally, and globally. It is ethically imperative to advocate for patients, profession, communities, policies, and self to continue to improve healthcare practices and legislature.

▶ QUALITY AND SAFE PATIENT CARE

The IOM provides a framework to assess and guide quality initiatives within the private and public sectors throughout healthcare, which includes providing safe, effective, person-centered, timely, efficient, and equitable care. Table 21.2 lists the aims provided within the framework, as well as the definitions and implications for acute care.

SAFE

According to the Agency for Healthcare Research and Quality (AHRQ), providing safe care includes avoiding harm to patients from care that is intended to help them. For example, the Joint Commission created a universal protocol that was designed to improve safety and reduce the occurrence of procedural

Table 21.2 IOM Health System Aims and Acute Care Implications

Aims for Health Systems	Definition	Examples in Acute Care
Safe	Avoiding harm to patients from the care that is intended to help them	Medication errors; time-out procedures
Effective	Providing services based on scientific knowledge to all who could benefit (avoiding underuse or misuse)	Overuse of antibiotics or CT scans (radiation exposure)
Patient centered	Providing care that is respectful of and responsive to individual patient preferences, needs, and values; ensuring the patient's values guide all clinical decisions	Patient–family advisory councils
Timely	Reducing waits and harmful delays for both those who receive and those who give care	Discharge planning begins at admission.
Efficient	Avoiding waste, including waste of equipment, supplies, ideas, and energy	Inflation Reduction Act to reduce excess and inflated costs; reduce unnecessary services, inefficient care, prevention failures, fraud
Equitable	Providing care that does not vary in quality because of personal characteristics such as gender, ethnicity, geographic location, and socioeconomic status	Obtaining and reporting patient demographic variables

IOM, Institute of Medicine.

errors. This protocol requires organizations to perform a time-out for all procedures, which requires the team to confirm the patient's identity, the procedure for which the patient was consented, and the site where the procedure will be performed before the procedure can begin. This time-out also allows any team members to voice concerns about the patient's safety before beginning the procedure.

EFFECTIVE

Providing services based on scientific knowledge to all who could benefit and refraining from providing services to those not likely to benefit is considered effective care. It includes avoiding underuse and misuse of care. The IOM defines overuse as the use of healthcare resources and procedures in the absence of evidence that the service could help the patient, and misuse is defined as failure to execute clinical care plans and procedures properly.

PERSON CENTERED

According to ECRI (founded as the Emergency Care Research Institute), an essential element of person-centered care is the shared decision-making between the provider and the patient concerning the patient's preferences and goals for their own healthcare and well-being. This is becoming ingrained within federal and state reimbursement policies, so the patient can choose what is right for them as well as achieve cost savings. The U.S. CMS require shared decision-making as a condition of reimbursement for certain cardiovascular and stroke prophylaxis procedures and lung cancer screenings.

Person-centered care means that physicians work collaboratively with patients and other healthcare providers to do what is best for patients' health and well-being. By collaboratively working together with the patient and various healthcare providers, they are better equipped to develop care plans that include empathy, dignity, and respect for patients and their families. One way hospitals do this is by forming patient–family advisory councils that consist of patients and families who have received care at an organization, along with administrators, providers, and staff. The goal of this council is to learn from the patient and family perspective; promote a culture of patient-centered care; collaborate to improve programs, services, and policies; and enhance the delivery of high-quality and safe patient care.

TIMELY

According to the AHRQ, timeliness includes reducing waits and harmful delays for both those who receive and those who give care. Within acute care, there can be three types of delays: input delays, which are delays in access to services such as a hospital bed once a decision is made to admit; throughput delays, which are delays affecting the length of time between a patient's admission and the time they are ready to be discharged from the hospital; and output delays, which are delays in the amount of time it takes to get a patient discharged from the hospital, such as a delay caused by a lack of availability of beds at a transitional care facility.

EFFICIENT

Care provided also needs to be efficient, meaning that it avoids waste, including waste of equipment, supplies, ideas, and energy. According to the IOM report, six areas of major healthcare waste are unnecessary services, inefficient delivery of care, excess administrative costs, inflated prices, prevention failures, and fraud. Attention must be observed to these six forms of waste to conserve scarce health resources and funds. In 2022, the U.S. House of Representatives passed the Inflation Reduction Act. This act provides subsidies for more consumers to purchase health coverage under the Affordable Care Act, and it also reduces the cost of healthcare by authorizing Medicare to negotiate with drug companies to lower the costs of prescription drugs. This act will provide more efficient and cost-saving care for millions of Americans.

EQUITABLE

Care that does not vary in quality because of personal characteristics such as gender, ethnicity, geographic location, and socioeconomic status is equitable. Equity is about fairness and justice in that everyone should have an equal opportunity to use and obtain healthcare. Many social factors contribute to one's ability to achieve healthy outcomes, including ethnicity, language, religion, socioeconomic status, gender, and sexuality. Providers need to recognize when and how a person's social determinants can impact their health outcomes for specific populations. If a health outcome varies between populations, there is

Table 21.3 Healthy People 2030: Social Determinants, Goals, and Acute Care Implications

Social Determinant	Goal	Implication in Acute Care
Economic stability	Help people earn steady incomes that allow them to meet their healthy needs	Cost of medications; chronic conditions that limit their ability to work or follow up; healthy food options
Education access and quality	Increase educational opportunities for all	Adults living with disabilities are less likely to get preventive care, as well as have challenges in finding a job, getting to school, and getting around their homes
Health access and quality	Increase access to comprehensive, high-quality healthcare services	Lack of health insurance and no preventive care for cancer screenings/blood pressure monitoring/diabetes; lack of drug and substance abuse treatment
Neighborhood/environment	Create neighborhoods and environment that promote health and safety	Violence; unsafe air or water; secondhand smoke; environmental or work exposures to harmful substances; lack of transportation options
Social and community context	Increase social and community support	Unsafe neighborhoods or home life; discrimination; lack of community resources with rural health

disparity, or lack of equity. An example of a health disparity is the COVID-19 pandemic. In the United States, Black, Hispanic, and Native American individuals were three times more likely to be hospitalized and twice as likely to die from COVID-19 as White individuals.

To reduce health disparities, the CMS created the Accountable Health Communities Model. This model addresses gaps in care by identifying and addressing social needs through screening, referral, and community navigation services to reduce healthcare use and costs. Identification and solving of a person's unstable housing situation or food insecurity, for example, may reduce the risk of the person developing a chronic condition that can lead to increased healthcare costs and avoidable healthcare use. Under the Affordable Care Act section 4302, it is a requirement to collect and report race, ethnicity, primary language, and disability status variables to understand the causes of health disparities and create effective solutions to ensure health equity.

▶ SOCIAL DETERMINANTS OF HEALTH

The Healthy People 2030 initiative released their Social Determinants of Health, which are the conditions within the environment where people live, learn, work, and age that can affect a range of health, functioning, and quality life outcomes and risks. Table 21.3 shows the five social determinants, goals, and their implications within the acute care environment.

▶ SUMMARY

AGACNPs are leading the changes that focus on professional ethics, healthcare delivery and financing, social determinants of health, and advancement of the AGACNP role to practice at their full scope of practice. AGACNPs can advocate for change that will influence future practice and legislation. The AACN Competencies and Curricular Expectations for Clinical Nurse Leader Education and Practice identify the AGACNP skillset and training, which include effective communication, interprofessional collaboration, conflict resolution, active listening, emotional intelligence, strategic thinking, compassion, accountability, stewardship, lifelong and reflective learning, nursing knowledge and expertise, and implementation of evidence-based practices.

Nursing organizations support active participation of AGACNPs in healthcare policy to improve healthcare access, cost of care, health equality, and health legislation. The AGACNP's training emphasizes nursing and healthcare policy involvement, advocacy, and improvement of healthcare practices for all. AGACNPs need to develop and acquire the skills needed to lead the change and become influential regarding the process for policy innovation and transformation. To do this, AGACNPs must know and understand the fundamentals of policy development, the stakeholders, resources, policy agendas, and their scope of practice. AGACNPs have an invaluable duty to advise educators, policy makers, and lobbyists to create legislation that improves patient safety, nursing practice, and access to care.

KNOWLEDGE CHECK: CHAPTER 21

1. How does applying for membership to a professional organization promote change within the role as an AGACNP?

   A. Professional organizations create a collective voice to lobby on behalf of nurses and AGACNPs, which can be heard at local, state, or national levels.

   B. Professional organizations promote safety, health, and wellness, as well as advocate for important health issues that affect AGACNPs.

   C. Professional organizations provide networking opportunities as well as access to experts or mentors, which can advance the nursing profession.

   D. All of the above

2. The AGACNP is admitting a patient to the ICU for acute-on-chronic hypoxemic respiratory failure from an interstitial lung disease exacerbation. The patient's spouse states that they recently filled out paperwork stating that the patient did not want to be intubated. What is this written statement of the patient's intent regarding medical care and treatment called?

   A. Living will

   B. Advance directive

   C. Do not resuscitate (DNR)

   D. Healthcare directive

3. A patient who is homeless comes to the ED for the fourth time this week complaining of chronic right ankle pain. The AGACNP indicates that the patient needs to go to another hospital to seek treatment because they have not paid for their previous visits. This action is likely a violation of which law?

   A. Patient Safety and Quality Improvement Act

   B. Health Insurance Portability and Accountability Act

   C. Emergency Medical Treatment and Labor Act (EMTALA)

   D. Patient Self-Determination Act

4. The AGACNP is preparing a presentation for fellow AGACNPs and plans to use case studies of patients cared for in the past. The AGACNP knows that including which of the following information will be in compliance with the Health Insurance Portability and Accountability Act (HIPAA)?

   A. Medical record number

   B. Birth date

   C. Admission date

   D. De-identified patient history

5. Which of the following diseases is reportable to the Centers for Disease Control and Prevention (CDC)?

   A. Methicillin-resistant *Staphylococcus aureus* (MRSA) infection

   B. *Clostridioides difficile* infection

   C. Vancomycin-resistant enterococcus (VRE) infection

   D. Tuberculosis

(See answers next page.)

1. D) All of the above

Becoming a member of a professional nursing or nurse practitioner organization provides a multitude of benefits.

2. B) Advance directive

An advance directive is a written statement of the patient's intent regarding medical care and treatment. A living will is a written compilation of statements in a document format that specifies which life-prolonging measures one does and does not want to be taken if they become incapacitated. A DNR is a code status. A healthcare directive is a type of advance directive that may or may not include a living will and/or specifications regarding durable power of attorney in one or two separate documents.

3. C) Emergency Medical Treatment and Labor Act (EMTALA)

According to the Centers for Medicare and Medicaid Services, EMTALA is a federal law that requires that any patient who seeks treatment in an ED be stabilized and treated regardless of their insurance status or ability to pay. The AGACNP should not tell the patient to go to another hospital when the patient chose to seek care at this facility.

4. D) De-identified patient history

The HIPAA identifiers that make health information protected include names, dates, telephone numbers, geographic data, fax numbers, Social Security numbers, email addresses, medical record numbers, account numbers, health plan beneficiary numbers, certificate or license numbers, vehicle identifiers and serial numbers including license plates, web URLs, device identifiers and serial numbers, internet protocol addresses, full-face photos and comparable images, biometric identifiers like retinal scans or fingerprints, and any unique identifying number or code. Protected health information does not include patient history or their current medical situation when there are not any HIPAA identifiers.

5. D) Tuberculosis

Clostridioides difficile infection, VRE, and MRSA are healthcare-associated infections that are not mandatory for reporting to the CDC. Each state lists various reportable infectious diseases, so AGACNPs should be knowledgeable of their state's practices regarding reportable medical conditions.

6. The AGACNP is obtaining a patient's consent for surgery tomorrow. What component is needed for the patient's informed consent?

   A. The consent must be involuntary.
   B. The patient must not have mental capacity to consent.
   C. The patient is informed of the benefits of surgery.
   D. The consent is translated by an interpreter of the patient's native language.

7. The U.S. Department of Health and Human Services has released their goals entitled *Healthy People 2030*. These goals include which of the following?

   A. Prevent healthy, thriving lives and well-being, free of preventable disease, disability, injury, and premature death
   B. Identify system facilitators and barriers to achieving a workforce that is diverse, including gender, race, and ethnicity, across all levels of nursing education
   C. Continue health disparities, achieve health equity, and attain health literacy to improve the health and well-being of all
   D. Engage leadership, key constituents, and the public across multiple sectors to act and design policies that improve the health and well-being of all

8. The AGACNP is aware that which of the following is an example of a social determinant that may lead to health disparities?

   A. Higher socioeconomic status
   B. Identifying as gay
   C. White Anglo-Saxon heritage
   D. Living in the suburbs of a major city

9. Providing care that does not vary in quality because of personal characteristics such as gender, ethnicity, geographic location, and socioeconomic status is:

   A. Efficient
   B. Equitable
   C. Patient centered
   D. Effective

10. The AGACNP is caring for a patient with a right lower extremity wound that was debrided in the operating room. Cultures from the operating room are growing pseudomonas. The AGACNP wants to discharge the patient today and prescribes ciprofloxacin for 7 days. The patient informs the AGACNP that they live on a fixed income and have no health insurance. What is the AGACNPs best intervention?

    A. Write the prescription and discharge the patient.
    B. Consult social services for assistance.
    C. Keep the patient admitted to complete the course of antibiotics.
    D. Transfer the patient to a skilled nursing facility.

(See answers next page.)

6. D) The consent is translated by an interpreter of the patient's native language.

Valid informed consent must include three major elements: disclosure of information including risks and benefits, competency or capacity of the patient or surrogate to decide, and voluntary nature of the decision. The information given to the patient, which could include information provided orally during the consent interview or as written information in the consent form, must be in language understandable to the potential patient or legally authorized representative.

7. D) Engage leadership, key constituents, and the public across multiple sectors to act and design policies that improve the health and well-being of all

We should aim to attain (not prevent) healthy, thriving lives and well-being, free of preventable disease, disability, injury, and premature death, as well as prevent (not continue) health disparities, achieve health equity, and attain health literacy to improve the health and well-being of all. Identifying system facilitators and barriers to achieving a workforce that is diverse, including gender, race, and ethnicity, across all levels of nursing education is not a goal for *Healthy People 2030* but is a goal of *The Future of Nursing 2020–2030: Charting a Path to Achieve Health Equity*. Other goals of *Healthy People 2030* include creating social, physical, and economic environments that promote attainment of the full potential for health and well-being for all and promote healthy development, healthy behaviors, and well-being across all life stages.

8. B) Identifying as gay

If a health outcome is seen to be a greater or lesser extent between populations, there is disparity. Race or ethnicity, gender, sexual identity, age, disability, socioeconomic status, and geographic location all contribute to an individual's ability to achieve good health. It is important to recognize the impact that social determinants have on health outcomes of specific populations. The Healthy People 2030 initiative strives to improve the health of all groups.

9. B) Equitable

The Institute of Medicine's aims for the health system include providing care that is safe, effective, patient centered, timely, efficient, and equitable. Providing care that does not vary in quality because of personal characteristics such as gender, ethnicity, geographic location, and socioeconomic status is equitable. Efficient care avoids waste, including waste of equipment, supplies, ideas, and energy. Patient-centered care is care that is respectful of and responsive to individual patient preferences, needs, and values and ensures that the patient's values guide all clinical decisions. Effective care includes providing services based on scientific knowledge to all who could benefit and avoiding underuse or misuse of treatments.

10. B) Consult social services for assistance.

This patient's socioeconomic health disparity should not preclude them from receiving appropriate care and treatment. The AGACNP should consult with social services, who can find resources available for the patient to receive the standard of care.

11. The AGACNP is working with a legislator on developing a policy to increase access to care for rural communities within the state. What is a key consideration that should be accounted for during policy development?

    A. Structure and predictability of the policy-making process
    B. Advocacy strategies to use during committee review
    C. Using evidence to describe the problem and the proposed solution
    D. Professional organization support before, during, and after development

12. A recently proposed bill to increase access to care in low-income communities has gained a lot of media attention and professional organization support for its innovative approach to care despite the economic cost of the program. Which of the following variables would be a barrier for bill support?

    A. Stakeholders
    B. Economic implications
    C. Media attention
    D. Problem significance

13. With the help of the advanced practice registered nurse (APRN) community, H.B. 41 Opioid Prescribing by the APRN was drafted and introduced during a recent legislative session. The policy was referred to committee; however, it did not receive enough votes to pass out of committee. What is the appropriate terminology when referring to this policy?

    A. Regulation
    B. Law
    C. Statute
    D. Bill

14. A recent bill, S.B. 80 Removal of Delegation for Advanced Practice Registered Nurses (APRNs), has unanimously passed committee. What is the next step for S.B. 80 according to the policy process?

    A. The bill will be signed into law.
    B. The bill will be placed on calendars.
    C. The bill will go to the subcommittee.
    D. The bill will go to the Senate floor.

15. A new AGACNP wants to actively engage in health policy but is unfamiliar with the policy process. What grassroots effort could the new AGACNP use to influence and/or educate their legislator?

    A. Volunteering to help a legislator at the state level
    B. Co-drafting a bill with a legislator
    C. Calling and/or emailing the legislator on a stance toward a specific bill
    D. Joining a professional organization that supports legislative initiatives

(See answers next page.)

11. C) Using evidence to describe the problem and the proposed solution

Current literature highlights the importance of evidence-based literature to describe the problem and the proposed solution to fully illustrate why a particular policy may be needed. Other variables are important; however, they are not necessarily needed as part of policy development.

12. B) Economic implications

The policy process can be positively or negatively influenced by many variables. Here, the significant economic implications (e.g., cost) may prove to hinder legislative support. The policy seems to have stakeholder support and positive media attention, and the significance of the problem should positively influence the fate of the proposed bill.

13. D) Bill

Bills are proposed policies with the goal of becoming a law. Bills are drafted based on an identified problem and proposed solution. If the bill passes, it becomes a law. Statutes and regulations are also formally passed laws or acts with legislative authority.

14. B) The bill will be placed on calendars.

Before a bill can be signed into law or go to the Senate floor, it must receive enough votes to progress out of committee, including the subcommittee. If the bill receives enough votes to pass out of the committee, it will be placed on calendars for a possible hearing on the Senate floor.

15. C) Calling and/or emailing the legislator on a stance toward a specific bill

Grassroots efforts are focused on action at the local level with the aim to impact change at the local, state, and/or national level. They are associated with bottom-up rather than top-down decision-making. Common efforts include calling and/or emailing legislators, gathering signatures, and attending meetings. Volunteering to help a legislator at the state level and co-drafting a bill with a legislator are active involvement, but they do not traditionally qualify as grassroots efforts. Joining a professional organization that supports legislative initiatives is not an active strategy for engaging in policy.

KEY BIBLIOGRAPHY

Only key resources appear in the print edition. Access the full bibliography for this chapter on ExamPrepConnect.com.

Agency for Healthcare Research and Quality. (2018). *Six domains of healthcare quality*. https://www.ahrq.gov/talkingquality/measures/six-domains.html

American Association of Colleges of Nursing. (2021). *The essentials: Core competencies for professional nursing education*. https://www.aacnnursing.org/Portals/42/AcademicNursing/pdf/Essentials-2021.pdf

American College of Emergency Physicians. (2022). *EMTALA fact sheet*. https://www.acep.org/life-as-a-physician/ethics--legal/emtala/emtala-fact-sheet/#:~:text=The%20Emergency%20Medical%20Treatment%20and,has%20remained%20an%20unfunded%20mandate

American Nurses Association. (2021). *ANA advocacy toolkit*. https://ana.aristotle.com/SitePages/toolkit.aspx

American Nurses Association. (2022). *Nurses serving in Congress*. https://www.nursingworld.org/practice-policy/advocacy/federal/nurses-serving-in-congress/

APRN Consensus Work Group and the National Council of State Boards of Nursing APRN Advisory Committee. (2008). *Consensus model for APRN regulation: Licensure, accreditation, certification & education. APRN Joint Dialogue Group Report*. https://www.nursingworld.org/~4aa7d9/globalassets/certification/aprn_consensus_model_report_7-7-08.pdf

Centers for Disease Control and Prevention. (2021). *Health insurance portability and accountability act of 1996 (HIPAA)*. https://www.cdc.gov/phlp/publications/topic/hipaa.html#:~:text=The%20Health%20Insurance%20Portability%20and,the%20patient's%20consent%20or%20knowledge

Quality Improvement

Alexander Menard and Margaret Emmons

▶ OVERVIEW

Two major papers published by the Institute of Medicine, *To Err Is Human* and *Crossing the Quality Chasm: A New Health System for the 21st Century*, are often cited when discussing quality improvement (QI). *To Err Is Human* is regarded as a turning point in quality and safety in healthcare. This report brought to light the shocking numbers of Americans who die because of medical error. *Crossing the Quality Chasm* was viewed as the initial response to *To Err Is Human*, recommending changes to redesign the healthcare system. Quality and safety continue to evolve since these publications.

The U.S. Agency for Healthcare Research and Quality (AHRQ) defines *quality healthcare* as "doing the right thing, at the right time, in the right way, for the right person—and having the best possible results." QI can also be described as a systematic continuous approach that aims to solve problems in healthcare, improve service provision, and ultimately provide better outcomes for patients. High-quality healthcare should be safe, effective, efficient, timely, patient centered, and equitable. QI is an integral aspect of the AGACNP's professional role.

QI represents a valuable opportunity for AGACNPs to be involved in leading and delivering change, spanning from improving individual patient care to transforming services across complex health and care systems. Improvement often requires deliberate redesign of processes based on knowledge of human factors (how people interact with products and processes) and tools known to assist improvement. This process is taught throughout AGACNP programs and is linked to the American Association of Colleges of Nursing (AACN) essentials and National Organization of Nurse Practitioner Faculties competencies. The QI process is outlined in this chapter.

▶ COLLABORATION

Collaboration is a key component of QI because a team approach is optimal. *Collaborate* is derived from the Latin *collabore*, which means "to labor together." Kraus, as cited in the work of Hennemann, Lee, and Cohen in a concept analysis of collaboration, has described collaboration as "a cooperative venture based on shared power and authority. It assumes power based on a knowledge or expertise as opposed to power based on role or function."

Collaboration is characterized by mutual goals and requires competence, confidence, and commitment on the part of all concerned participants. Respect and trust of all parties involved in the process are necessary. When determining what the QI team will look like, one must look at defining attributes, antecedents, and consequences.

INTERPROFESSIONAL AND INTRAPROFESSIONAL COLLABORATION

QI work requires interprofessional and intraprofessional collaboration. The AGACNP must be prepared to work within the nursing profession as well as with other healthcare providers to achieve QI. Compiling the team, or collaborating, requires the right people to be involved, and this is best achieved during the planning and implementation phases of QI. It is not uncommon to see a patient or a patient's family member as part of the QI team. After all, the end users (patients and families) ultimately benefit from QI.

AGACNPs with a Doctorate in Nursing Practice (DNP) are well situated to lead collaborative teams. Scientific knowledge and skills, as well as knowledge of organizational and systems improvement, outcome evaluation processes, and healthcare policy, provide a foundation for taking on QI leadership roles. This skill set of the DNP-prepared AGACNP is essential in the complex healthcare environment.

AACN's *Essentials of Doctoral Education for Advanced Nursing Practice* states that collaborative teams must be fluid to meet the needs of the population, and the DNP-prepared advanced practice nurse must be prepared to play a central role on the interprofessional team.

▶ QUALITY IMPROVEMENT APPROACH

OVERVIEW
The QI approach is a systematic data-guided activity to evaluate and improve outcomes of an intervention. Successful QI projects require forward planning. Careful consideration of the goal of the project and obtaining management and stakeholder support are crucial. Without leadership and stakeholder support, the project may not get past the planning stage. This section of the chapter briefly reviews the QI process.

QUALITY IMPROVEMENT PROJECT PROCESS
QI is a process, and following a standard format will help ensure success (Figure 22.1).

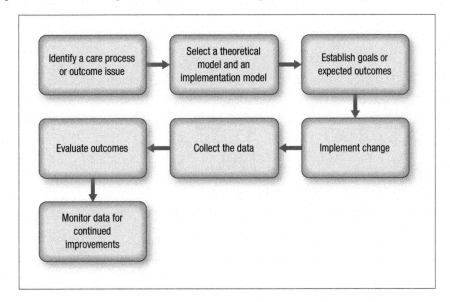

Figure 22.1 The quality improvement project process.

IDENTIFY A CARE PROCESS OR OUTCOME ISSUE
The practitioner's clinical experience may provide ideas for a QI project. Consider whether there is a problem in clinical practice or the patient care setting that has been observed. For example, why are daily weights not done or recorded in inpatient heart failure patients? Or, do critically ill mechanically ventilated patients receive the prescribed enteral feeding? Keeping one's eyes and ears open in the clinical setting can identify a phenomenon of interest. Consider problems, patient complaints, near misses, delays in care, and so on, that have been noted in the clinical environment, and determine what could be improved. Seek input from peers and management for project ideas. Explore the literature to assess best practice and compare to current practice. Then define the problem using the PICOT format:

- *P* = Population
- *I* = Intervention
- *C* = Comparison
- *O* = Outcome
- *T* = Timeframe

The Institute for Healthcare Improvement has a model, The Model for Improvement, to guide this process. The Model for Improvement is a core strategy for QI efforts and can accelerate the process.

First, the AGACNP must ask three questions:

1. What are we trying to accomplish?
2. How will we know that a change is an improvement?
3. What changes can we make that will result in improvement?

Question 1 represents the project aim. Aim statements are best written in SMART format (Table 22.1). A fishbone diagram (Figure 22.2) is a useful method for better understanding the problem. It identifies possible causes and effects for problems.

Table 22.1 SMART Format

Element	Description
S = Specific	One goal
M = Measurable	Improvement can be measured over time
A = Actionable	Barriers can be overcome
R = Realistic	With available resources
T = Timely	Date to achieve goal

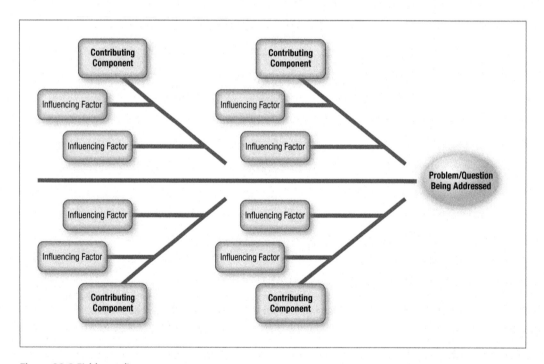

Figure 22.2 Fishbone diagram.

SELECT A THEORETICAL/CONCEPTUAL MODEL AND AN IMPLEMENTATION MODEL

Many factors influence the selection of an implementation model and a theoretical model to guide the QI project. They are outlined next.

Theoretical/Conceptual Framework

A theoretical or conceptual framework with its interrelated statements can help to predict, explain, and describe a phenomenon. The purpose of a framework is to help select variables and guide interventions. Use a theoretical framework to guide the project, which will help strengthen the results.

Examples of theoretical/conceptual frameworks are as follows:

- The *Health Belief Model* specifies a discrete set of commonsense beliefs that appear to explain, or mediate, the effects of demographic variables on health behavior patterns and are amenable to change through educational intervention. The model can be applied to a range of health behaviors and so provides a framework for shaping behavior patterns. The four essential ingredients of the model are (a) perception of susceptibility to disease, (b) belief that the impact of this disease will affect one biologically and/or psychosocially, (c) belief that the potential benefits of the regimen outweigh the risks of the disease and its treatment, and (d) ability to surmount barriers to treatment.
- The *American Association of Critical-Care Nurses Synergy Model's* main concept is that the needs or characteristics of patients and families influence and drive the characteristics or competencies of nurses. Synergy results when the needs and characteristics of a patient, clinical unit, or system are matched with a nurse's competencies.
- *Watson's Theory of Human Caring* focuses on how nursing practice, knowledge, and values interact with the patient's own healing processes and experiences. The theory includes 10 curative factors. The major concepts include the 10 curative factors, transpersonal caring relationship, caring moment, and caring-healing modalities.
- *Donabedian's Quality Framework* is a conceptual model that provides a framework for examining health services and evaluating quality of healthcare. According to the model, information about quality of care can be drawn from three categories: structure, process, and outcomes.
- Team reflexivity is the extent to which teams collectively reflect on and adapt their operating methods and ways of working. This research explores the fundamental belief that highly reflexive teams will be more innovative than teams low in reflexivity, especially when faced with demanding work environments. It is an important predictor of team outcomes and innovation. The researchers explore why teamwork is better and more effective than individual acts and innovation.

Implementation Models

Implementation models are meant to guide the implementation of the project by breaking it down into steps. An implementation model allows for evaluating the outcome, improving on it, and testing again. Examples of implementation models are as follows:

- The *Plan-Do-Study-Act* method is a way to test a change that is implemented. The prescribed four steps guide the thinking process and break down the task into steps. Having the steps written down often helps with focus and increases learning.
- *Lewin's Theory of Change* has three major concepts: driving forces, restraining forces, and equilibrium. Driving forces are those that push in a direction that causes change to occur. They facilitate change because they push the patient in a desired direction. They cause a shift in the equilibrium toward change. Restraining forces are those forces that counter the driving forces. They hinder change because they push the patient in the opposite direction. They cause a shift in the equilibrium that opposes change. Equilibrium is a state of being where driving forces equal restraining forces, and no change occurs. It can be raised or lowered by changes that occur between the driving and restraining forces.
- *Iowa Model of Evidence-Based Practice* (EBP) guides clinical decision-making and the evidence-based process from both clinician and systems perspectives. There are seven steps to follow in this model: (a) selecting a topic, (b) forming a team, (c) retrieving evidence, (d) grading the evidence, (e) developing an EBP standard, (f) implementing the EBP, and (g) evaluating.
- The *Gibbs Reflective Model* was developed by Graham Gibbs in 1988 to give structure to learning from experiences. It offers a framework for examining experiences and, given its cyclic nature, lends itself particularly well to repeated experiences, allowing one to learn and plan from things that either went well or did not go well. This model has six principal elements: (a) description, (b) feeling, (c) evaluation, (d) analysis, (e) conclusion, and (f) action plan.

ESTABLISH GOALS OR EXPECTED OUTCOMES

Once a care process or outcome issue has been identified and a theoretical model and an implementation model have been selected, the next step is to establish goals and expected outcomes. Refer to the care process or outcome issue, and the PICOT question will define the goals and expected outcomes. It is common for a QI project to shift direction(s) during the development phases. Evolution and revision are expected to occur.

IMPLEMENT CHANGE USING THE SELECTED IMPLEMENTATION MODEL

Before implementing a change process, gather baseline data to define the problem and then spend time planning the intervention. Many factors need to be considered when planning to implement a change. For example, consider any competing changes scheduled to occur concurrently. Consider whether the leadership team and essential support staff are available (i.e., avoid peak vacation or holiday times). Ensure any necessary equipment is available. Consider how the change will be communicated and reinforced. An email is not usually sufficient; rather, it may require discussion at a staff meeting or even the team leader's presence to answer questions and troubleshoot challenges during implementation. Project success can be augmented by identifying early adopters in the group and inviting them to participate in the project in some way. Engagement of front-line staff is crucial to success. Work toward getting a few people to "try it" to win a few more over. The selected implementation model will be instrumental in framing and guiding the actual rollout of the QI project. Then, implement the project at the preselected date and time.

IDENTIFY AND COLLECT DATA

After the change has been determined and the goals and specific aims of the project are decided upon, the collection method can be chosen. Collect both baseline data (preintervention) and postintervention data, so that improvement can be measured. This is a crucial point in any QI project. There are many data points and collection methods (Table 22.2).

Table 22.2 Examples of Types of Data and Collection Methods

Data Points	Collection Methods
■ Demographic data ■ Pre- and posttests ■ Physiologic measures ■ Established surveys that have documented reliability, validity, and sensitivity ■ Efficiencies in workflow (e.g., time savings) ■ Financial/cost savings ■ Reduction in waste or redundant work ■ Knowledge ■ Skills ■ Attitudes	■ Observation ■ Surveys (self-report) ■ Interviews (structured, individual, and focus groups) ■ Chart reviews ■ State or national registries ■ Reports

These methods result in both qualitative and quantitative data. Qualitative data describes qualities or characteristics; is often collected by means of survey, observation, and interviews; and is often presented in narrative form. Quantitative data are measures of certain quantities or ranges and are data about numeric variables.

Data collection methods must be congruent with the purpose of the project and the project design. Data collected should encompass measurement of the outcome (dependent variable) as well as the independent and confounding factors related to the outcome variables. Process flow diagrams and cause-and-effect diagrams are often used to guide QI project data collection. The data collection method should be feasible, practical, and able to be completed in the clinical setting and with the population impacted.

EVALUATE OUTCOME(S)

Evaluation of outcomes should be related back to the intended goal of the QI project. Was the intended goal achieved, or not? Further evaluation will be done to understand successes or barriers to then include in future iterations of the QI project or a complete redesign. Statistical analyses can organize and transform data that represent project outcomes into a meaningful form that can be interpreted and shared.

Structure measures capture components to include manpower and use of a specific specialty unit for patient management.

Process measures allow for individuals to quantify the methods used to provide care and to determine fidelity in the use of standards of care. Examples of process measures include time to treatment of antibiotics in sepsis care, delivery of reperfusion treatment in patients with stroke and myocardial infarction, and measurement of ejection fraction in patients with heart failure.

Outcome measures capture results and are meant to aid understanding of how healthcare processes affect patient results. Examples of outcome measures include disease severity, functional status, quality of life, mortality, and readmissions.

The data analysis plan will depend on the QI project and can include a variety of outcome measures:

- distribution of dependent and independent variables using histograms and frequency distributions
- descriptive analysis (mean, median, mode) and variation (range and standard deviation)
- relationships (Chi-square tests)

MONITOR DATA FOR SUSTAINED/CONTINUED IMPROVEMENT

Projects should have methods preplanned for how to ensure sustainability of the change. Project monitoring is essential for long-lasting change and improvement. The monitoring process includes problem-solving, decision-making, and managing issues that arise with the continued project. It is also a time to be continuously ensuring that project goals are being addressed and met.

DISSEMINATION

The final part of QI is dissemination or sharing of what has been learned with a broader audience. Dissemination can occur in many forms, such as peer-reviewed publications and poster or podium presentations. At a minimum, this information must be shared with the community that was impacted by the project and the leadership team that supported and/or funded the project. For example, if a QI project focused on addressing nursing perceptions of communication with mechanically ventilated patients, dissemination must include the specific ICU nurses and respiratory therapists as well as the leadership team. Consideration must be made for sharing this QI project with the broader ICU communities outside that specific ICU. Examples include presenting the QI project at a regional conference or publishing the results in a journal. Sharing successes and failures surrounding QI work will ultimately lead to better outcomes.

▶ SUMMARY

The AGACNP must be prepared to participate in and lead QI efforts. The Institute for Healthcare Improvement (IHI) has extensive resources to aid in development, implementation, and follow-through for QI projects and initiatives. The AGACNP brings a unique perspective to QI and incorporating QI into practice.

⬤ KNOWLEDGE CHECK: CHAPTER 22

1. Which clinical scenario would the AGACNP evaluate as a potential area for a quality improvement (QI) process?

    A. Expected decrease in mortality due to a new liver transplant technique

    B. New onset of central line–associated bloodstream infections

    C. Projected decrease in COVID-19 emergency department visits

    D. Expected increase in admission for seasonal influenza

2. The U.S. Agency for Healthcare Research and Quality (AHRQ) defines quality healthcare as:

    A. Providing good care at the right time

    B. Offering good care at the lowest possible cost

    C. Doing the right thing, at the right time, in the right way, for the right person, and having the best possible results

    D. Providing optimal care at the right time and for the right person while increasing healthcare costs

3. Which clinical scenario would the AGACNP evaluate for a quality improvement policy?

    A. Projected increases in admissions for the upcoming influenza season

    B. Case of *Clostridioides difficile* in an immunocompromised patient with recent antibiotic use

    C. Recent increase in the frequency of catheter-associated urinary tract infections

    D. Projected decrease in norovirus presentation to the emergency department

4. The AGACNP has started to embark on a quality improvement project. While developing the aims for the project, the AGACNP ensures that the project aims are in the SMART format and are:

    A. Specific, measurable, actionable, realistic, timely

    B. Special, measurable, attainable, rational, tough

    C. Specific, meaningful, attainable, relative, timely

    D. Specific, measurable, attainable, reactionary, timely

5. The AGACNP is starting to develop a quality improvement project and is seeking to predict, explain, and describe a phenomenon. What framework does the AGACNP need to shape this process?

    A. Implementation model

    B. Theoretical/conceptual framework

    C. Implementation framework

    D. SMART aims framework

6. The AGACNP is collecting data for a quality improvement project by means of interviews and is compiling the data for evaluation in a narrative form. What type of data is the AGACNP collecting?

    A. Quantitative

    B. Qualitative

    C. Expressional

    D. Informal

(See answers next page.)

1. B) New onset of central line–associated bloodstream infections

A new onset of central line–associated bloodstream infections indicates that something has changed, and this is an opportunity to improve quality of care with a QI project. Expected and projected changes have explanations and would not fit the build of a QI project.

2. C) Doing the right thing, at the right time, in the right way, for the right person, and having the best possible results

Doing the right thing, at the right time, for the right person, for the best possible result is how the AHRQ defines quality. Offering good or optimal care, lowering or increasing care costs, and providing care to the right person do not fully address AHRQ's definition.

3. C) Recent increase in the frequency of catheter-associated urinary tract infections

Catheter-associated urinary tract infection rates are used for quality markers. The recent increase indicates that something has changed and can therefore be evaluated for a quality improvement project. A recent case of *C. difficile* in an immunocompromised patient is an isolated case and in a patient at high risk for developing the infection. Increase in flu admissions and decrease in norovirus presentations are projected.

4. A) Specific, measurable, actionable, realistic, timely

SMART stands for specific, measurable, actionable, realistic, and timely.

5. B) Theoretical/conceptual framework

A theoretical or conceptual framework with its interrelated statements can help to predict, explain, and describe a phenomenon. An implementation model is about the process. SMART aims are not a framework.

6. B) Qualitative

Qualitative data describe qualities or characteristics and are often collected by means of survey, observation, and interviews and presented in narrative form. Quantitative data are measures of certain quantities or ranges and are data about numeric variables.

7. Descriptive data analysis includes all of the following *except:*

    A. Mean
    B. Median
    C. Range
    D. Total

8. The AGACNP is collecting data for a quality improvement project that includes the number of cases of ventilator-associated pneumonia compared with total ventilator days. What type of data is the AGACNP collecting?

    A. Quantitative
    B. Qualitative
    C. Expressional
    D. Informal

9. Which statement is *true* regarding implementation models for a Doctorate in Nursing Practice (DNP) project?

    A. Implementation models are meant to guide the thinking process and break it down into steps, evaluate the outcome, improve on it, and retest it.
    B. Implementation models are only a suggestion when conducting a DNP project and are generally not helpful.
    C. Implementation models are requirements that must be followed.
    D. Implementation modules increase the complexity of quality improvement projects.

10. Which statement is *true* regarding theoretical models in the Doctorate in Nursing Practice (DNP) project?

    A. A theoretical or conceptual framework with its interrelated statements can help to predict, explain, and describe a phenomenon.
    B. The purpose of a framework is to aid in selecting variables and guiding interventions.
    C. Using a theoretical framework to guide a project helps to strengthen the findings.
    D. All of the above are true.

11. The AGACNP recognizes which of the following as an example of evidence-based practice (EBP)?

    A. Obtaining daily chest x-rays on all intubated patients
    B. Prescribing broad-spectrum antibiotics within 1 hour to patients who present in septic shock
    C. Ordering stress ulcer prophylaxis for all older patients who are admitted to the hospital
    D. Ordering blood, urine, and sputum cultures for all hospitalized patients who spike a fever

12. When evaluating the effectiveness of a new protocol related to reducing rates of newly documented pressure ulcers, the AGACNP expects which of the following outcomes to indicate that the new protocol is successful?

    A. Increase in patient satisfaction scores
    B. Reduction in staff injuries when repositioning patients
    C. Reduction in rate of newly documented pressure ulcers
    D. Increase in job satisfaction among new staff members

(See answers next page.)

7. **D) Total**
Descriptive analysis includes mean, median, mode, and variation (range and standard deviation).

8. **A) Quantitative**
Quantitative data are measures of certain quantities or ranges and are data about numeric variables. Qualitative data describes qualities or characteristics and are often collected by means of survey, observation, and interviews and are often presented in narrative form.

9. **A) Implementation models are meant to guide the thinking process and break it down into steps, evaluate the outcome, improve on it, and retest it.**
Implementation models are designed to aid and guide in the quality improvement process.

10. **D) All of the above are true.**
A theoretical framework guides the DNP project. The purpose of a theoretical framework is to provide a context for selecting variables to include how they relate to one another and to guide in the development of an intervention.

11. **B) Prescribing broad-spectrum antibiotics within 1 hour to patients who present in septic shock**
Ordering and administering broad-spectrum antibiotics to a patient presenting in septic shock within 1 hour of presentation to the ED is EBP. Daily chest x-rays are not indicated on all intubated patients. Stress ulcer prophylaxis is not indicated for all admitted older patients. Hospitalized patients have reasons to become febrile other than infection, and thus not all require an infectious workup.

12. **C) Reduction in rate of newly documented pressure ulcers**
Data on reduction in the rate of newly documented pressure ulcers directly assess the intervention's effectiveness. Increased patient satisfaction scores, reduction in staff injuries when repositioning patients, and increased job satisfaction among new staff members may be results of the new protocol but do not directly assess the effectiveness of the protocol and its ability to reduce newly documented pressure ulcers.

13. The Centers for Medicare and Medicaid Services (CMS) uses quality measures in its quality improvement, public reporting, and pay-for-reporting programs for specific healthcare providers. What set of goals does CMS intend these quality measures to address?

    A. Effective, safe, efficient, patient-centered, equitable, and timely care
    B. None because the CMS is not concerned with quality
    C. Safe, equitable, and efficient care
    D. Effective, evidence-based, and timely care

14. After the initiation of a quality improvement process to decrease the number of central line–associated bloodstream infections (CLABSIs) through educating staff members about proper application of sterile drapes, the AGACNP will evaluate its effectiveness by:

    A. Polling nurses to see if drapes are being applied properly
    B. Comparing preintervention CLABSI rates to postintervention CLABSI rates
    C. Counting the number of sterile drapes used compared with the number of central lines placed
    D. Polling providers who insert central lines regarding proper sterile techniques

15. There have been an increased number of complaints from patients regarding a medical-surgical floor's noise level at night. The AGACNP has been asked to be a member of a new interprofessional team to address this quality improvement project. At the first meeting, the AGACNP identifies the team's *first* task as:

    A. Identifying the night staff members causing the excess noise
    B. Installing noise meters to collect data
    C. Identifying the interprofessional team's project goals
    D. Terminating the nurse manager for not intervening on the noise complaints

(See answers next page.)

13. A) Effective, safe, efficient, patient-centered, equitable, and timely care

The CMS does have a large focus on quality care. Safe, equitable, and efficient care, or effective, evidence-based, timely care address only some of the goals CMS intends to address with quality measures.

14. B) Comparing preintervention CLABSI rates to postintervention CLABSI rates

Polling nurses and providers on proper draping as well as counting drapes and comparing to the number of lines placed can provide data to assess the effectiveness of the training but will not directly measure the desired outcome, which is to decrease the number of CLABSIs.

15. C) Identifying the interprofessional team's project goals

The priority task is to identify the interprofessional team project goals. Any time a team is developed, it is crucial to identify and outline the project goals before starting to work on the problem/project. Identifying the night staff members causing the excess noise or installing noise meters may be effective interventions, but goals must first be defined to have a successful intervention. Terminating the nurse manager is not a rational intervention at this time; no data have been collected, and no interventions have been attempted.

KEY BIBLIOGRAPHY

Only key resources appear in the print edition. Access the full bibliography for this chapter on ExamPrepConnect.com.

Melnyk, B., & Fineout-Overholt, E. (2019). *Evidence-based practice in nursing and healthcare*. Wolters Kluwer.

Moran, K., Burson, R., & Conrad, D. (2020). *The doctor of nursing practice project*. Jones and Bartlett Learning.

Zaccagnini, M., & Pechack, M. (2021). *The doctor of nursing practice essentials*. Jones and Bartlett Learning.

Evidence-Based Practice and Research Review

Helen Miley and Al-Zada Aguilar

▶ INTRODUCTION

At times, there is confusion about evidence-based practice (EBP), research, and quality improvement (QI). EBP and research lie on the same continuum of scholarship. *Research* is the systematic investigation of a problem that generates new knowledge; it is a process of inquiry. First coined by a group in Ontario, Canada, led by Dr. David Sackett in 1990, the term *evidence-based practice* was then modified to apply to the nursing profession by Melnyk and Fineout-Overholt in 2010. EBP integrates best evidence from well-designed studies and healthcare data with professional expertise and patient preferences and values into clinical practice to optimize healthcare delivery. As an umbrella term, it transcends across all disciplines, emphasizing interdisciplinary professional collaboration. EBP clinical guidelines are founded based on research, specifically, meta-analyses and systematic reviews of available data related to that specific topic used to improve patient outcomes and enhance patient care. QI is the process that uses the *Plan, Do, Study, Act* model. QI evaluates the status quo, ensuring that quality is being maintained and, if not, identifying and implementing the necessary steps to ensure that barriers to procedure or protocol are identified and addressed.

▶ EVIDENCE-BASED PRACTICE BARRIERS AND FACILITATORS

Globally, nurses across the professional spectrum are responsible for the implementation of EBP into practice. EBP implementation involves the integration of quality evidence and clinical expertise, while considering patient and family preferences as well as available resources, to develop evidence-based organizational policies used to inform clinical practice. AGACNPs value EBP and its translation into clinical practice. After all, not only is EBP implementation associated with achieving high-reliability organizational status, it also empowers staff through enhanced autonomy in clinical practice, fosters teamwork, and leads to higher levels of job satisfaction and employee retention rates.

Unfortunately, barriers to EBP implementation exist. In fact, such barriers may lead to the antiquated implementation of treatments that are not only unnecessary but potentially harmful (Table 23.1). Fortunately, facilitators also exist for EBP implementation (Table 23.2).

Table 23.1 Barriers to EBP Implementation

Barriers	Description
Lack of organizational support	Lack of support from colleagues, upper management
Collaborative practice issues	Communication failures, lack of respect
EBP competence and knowledge deficits	Inadequate knowledge and skills Lack of EBP mentorship
Resource limitations	Finance (e.g., limited financial patient resources, prohibitive costs of tests and medications, insurance-related costs) Information technology (e.g., clinical decision support software programs) Time constraints Staffing-ratio issues

EBP, evidence-based practice.

Table 23.2 Facilitators to EBP Implementation

Facilitators	Description
Supportive organizational culture	Support from colleagues and leadership in the value of EBP and its integration into the organization Ongoing EBP knowledge and skills-building workshops
Spirit of inquiry	Ongoing curiosity about evidence and literature to guide clinical decision-making
Financial incentivization	Insurance pay-for-performance programs offering incentives to clinicians who follow evidence-based guidelines
EBP mentorship	Integration of clinicians into the organization with expertise in EBP and its implementation and can work directly with bedside clinicians for its implementation (i.e., EBP champions)
Feasibility	Easy, user-friendly, and free practical guidelines Dedicated resources for implementation (e.g., in-person education, models such as Iowa Model Revised 2015)
Technological support	Clinical decision support software programs Accessible, up-to-date resources and clinical tools

EBP, evidence-based practice.

Another facilitator is a stepwise approach that allows for the evaluation and integration of evidence-based research into healthcare delivery. One example is the Iowa Model of Research-Based Practice to Promote Quality Care. The Iowa Model is an algorithmic model developed to integrate evidence and implement practice changes (Figure 23.1).

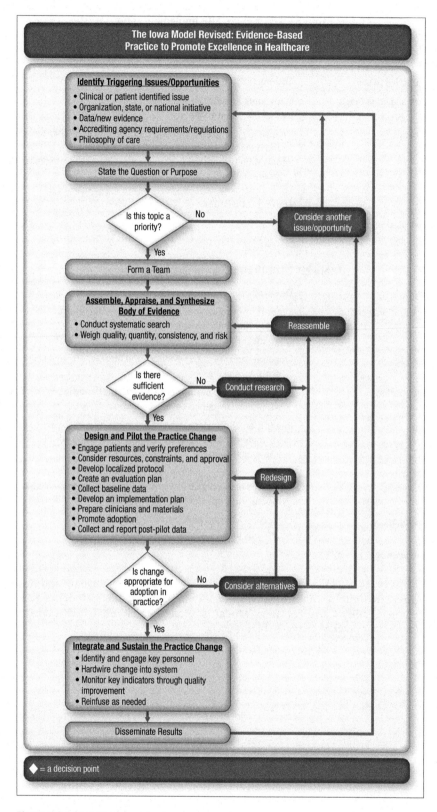

Figure 23.1 Iowa Model, revised.

Source: Used/reprinted with permission from the University of Iowa Hospitals and Clinics, copyright 2015. For permission to use or reproduce, please contact the University of Iowa Hospitals and Clinics at 319-384-9098.

▶ EVIDENCE-BASED PRACTICE IMPLEMENTATION

Implementation of EBP requires a stepwise approach (Table 23.3).

Table 23.3 Steps of EBP Implementation

Steps		Description
Step 1	Identify (potential) problems or issues	▪ Personal and/or professional experiences ▪ Existing literature ▪ *Socioeconomic and/or healthcare issues:* chronic illness (e.g., metabolic syndrome), epidemic (e.g., opioid, COVID-19), increased needs of the gerontologic population ▪ *Professional research priorities:* National Institutes of Health, National Institute of Nursing Research
Step 2	Determine significance of the problem	▪ *Stakeholder priorities:* patients, community, research ▪ *Applicability:* practice, education, administration ▪ Theory support or development ▪ Practice and/or policy support or change ▪ Build on prior findings
Step 3	Determine feasibility of addressing the problem	▪ *Cost:* need support from stakeholders (benefit of improved outcomes and/or value of evidence *must* outweigh costs) ▪ *Time:* complete within time constraints ▪ Collaboration with other disciplines ▪ Team interest and expertise
Step 4	Ask the clinical (or research) question in PICOT format	▪ *Clinical question:* describe and/or examine relationships among variables (see Table 23.14) ▪ *Population, Intervention, Comparison* (or control group), *Outcome* (effectiveness or results of intervention), *Time* ▪ *Subtypes 1:* (a) foreground (specific, relevant to clinical issue; determine which intervention is most effective in improving outcomes); (b) background (broader; provide general knowledge) ▪ *Subtypes 2:* (a) causation (or etiology), (b) diagnosis, (c), prevention, (d) prognosis, (e) treatment

Step 5	Search for the best evidence using (electronic) databases	▪ Identify type of PICOT question (see subtypes 1 and 2 in step 4) and use key words from the PICOT question to search databases
		▪ Select relevant databases to search (see Table 23.6) and streamline search with the following:
		  ● Database-controlled vocabulary ("MeSH terms")
		  ● Combined searches with Boolean connector "AND"
		  ● Search limited by defining parameters (e.g., language, data published, characteristics of subjects)

Step 6	Critical appraisal of the evidence	▪ Appraise evidence for (a) validity, (b) reliability, (c) relevance, and (d) applicability ▪ Determine level of evidence (design) that answers clinical question (see Table 23.7) ▪ Strength of evidence = level of evidence (design) + quality of evidence (validity of methods) ▪ Strength of evidence will determine clinical application of the evidence (i.e., EBP implementation)
Step 7	Integrate evidence with clinical expertise and patient preferences and values	▪ Integrate evidence with (a) clinical expertise, (b) patient preferences and values, and (c) objective data (e.g., diagnostics, clinical and institutional variables) prior to EBP implementation

(continued)

Table 23.3 Steps of EBP Implementation (*continued*)

Steps		Description
Step 8	Implementation	■ Use resource guide (e.g., ARCC model) ■ Assess for organizational culture and readiness for EBP implementation ■ Identify key stakeholders (active and passive) and facilitate ongoing stakeholder engagement and buy-in ■ *Develop team:* maintain consistent communication with frequent assessment ■ Include educational and outcomes measurement plan, implementation timeline (with use of dashboard) ■ *IRB submission:* ensure safety and confidentiality of subjects ■ Successful data collection = measurability + user-friendliness + accessibility ■ *Data analysis:* decide on support and program to use
Step 9	Monitoring and evaluation	■ Monitor and evaluate implementation process as well as healthcare quality outcomes or changes based on evidence ■ *Purpose:* (a) support positive effects; (b) remedy negative effects; (c) remedy process issues related to implementation; (d) identify patients who can most benefit from implementation ■ Address barriers (e.g., resistance to change) and incorporate facilitators (e.g., EBP champions) of implementation process, if present
Step 10	Dissemination of EBP findings	■ *Purpose:* others can learn about the EBP project's implementation, evaluation, and outcomes or endpoints ■ *Examples:* presentations at conferences, publications in professional journals or newsletters, hospital-based policy development or modification

ARCC, Advancing Research and Clinical Practice Through Close Collaboration; EBP, evidence-based practice; IRB, Institutional Review Board.

Step 1: Identify existing issues. The first step involves the identification of existing issues. Issues can be identified by drawing from personal and/or professional experiences, existing literature, or priorities of the community, institution, or the profession.

Step 2: Determine significance of the problem. The second step asks if the problem is worth addressing. It is important to take note of its (a) applicability to administration, education, or practice; (b) ability to support or develop theory; (c) ability to support or change current practice and/or policy; (d) ability to build upon prior findings while considering the most important facilitator or barrier to addressing this problem; and (e) stakeholder priorities.

Step 3: Determine feasibility of addressing the problem. The third step involves how feasible it would be (or not) in addressing the problem. Variables that need to be considered to evaluate for feasibility include cost, time, resources, collaboration and support, and interest and expertise of the team. Cost can serve as a barrier if not supported by stakeholders and/or funding bodies. Stakeholders are persons or groups that can influence or may be affected by the EBP implementation process.

Step 4. Ask the clinical (or research) question in PICOT format. Once the problem has been identified and is deemed significant and feasible, the next step is to form the clinical question. The clinical (or research) question can describe variables and/or examine relationships among the variables being studied through testing. There are two types of clinical questions: foreground and background. Foreground questions are specific and relevant to the clinical issues to inform clinical decisions or actions. Often, foreground questions compare two interventions to determine which is more effective in improving outcomes. Background questions, on the other hand, are broader and provide basic information or general knowledge.

A helpful strategy used by clinicians to extract critical parts from the clinical issue is to develop the PICOT mnemonic. PICOT provides a consistent and systematic way to identify and clarify components of the clinical issue and operationalize the clinical question, while guiding the search for evidence. The PICOT mnemonic is as follows:

- [P] *Population of interest:* accurately describe group or patient(s) of interest
- [I] *Intervention (or area of interest):* treatment or therapy provided or being considered
- [C] *Comparison (or reference or control group):* alternative to compare with intervention
- [O] *Outcome:* what is being measured to examine effectiveness or result of intervention
- [T] *Time:* duration of data collection

Clinical questions can be formulated based on subtypes in a PICOT format (Tables 23.4 and 23.5).

Table 23.4 Subtypes of PICOT-Formatted Clinical Questions

Type	Population (*P*)	Intervention (*I*)	Comparison (*C*)	Outcome (*O*)	Time (*T*)
Causation	Risk factors, disease or condition	Severity of risk factor, duration of exposure	Not applicable	Rates of disease progression, morbidity, mortality, and/or survival rates	
Diagnosis	Disease or condition	Diagnostic tests and/or procedures	Current standard (i.e., reference or "gold" standard)	Measures of test utility (e.g., positive or negative predictive value, sensitivity, specificity)	
Prevention	Risk factors (e.g., weight, hypertension)	Preventive measure (e.g., lifestyle change, medication)	Placebo, another intervention	Quality of life, complications, mortality or morbidity rates	*Optional:* Months, years
Prognosis	Main (prognostic) factor affecting severity and/or duration of disease or condition	Time (e.g., "watchful waiting")	Not applicable	Rates of disease progression; morbidity, mortality, and/or survival rates	
Treatment	Disease or condition	Treatment (e.g., medication, procedure or surgery, lifestyle change)	Placebo, another intervention, standard of care	Quality of life, complications, mortality or morbidity rates	

Table 23.5 Examples of PICOT-Formatted Clinical Questions Based on Subtypes

Subtype	PICOT Questions
Causation or etiology	- Are young men without known chronic lung diseases (*P*) who vape (*I*) compared with those who do not vape (*C*) at increased risk for respiratory tract infections (*O*)? - Are male patients (*P*) with parents who have substance use disorders (*I*) at increased risk for depression (*O*) compared with male patients with parents who do not have substance use disorders (*C*) in their lifetime (*T*)?

(continued)

Table 23.5 Examples of PICOT-Formatted Clinical Questions Based on Subtypes (*continued*)

Subtype	PICOT Questions
Diagnosis	▪ In patients with confirmed ischemic stroke (*P*), is an MRI (*I*) more accurate in determining the severity of injury (*O*) when compared to a dedicated cerebral perfusion scan (*C*)? ▪ Is the procalcitonin (*I*) more accurate in diagnosing bacterial infection (*O*) than the C-reactive protein (*C*) in patients with neutropenic sepsis (*P*)?
Prevention	▪ For patients with a family history of colon cancer (*P*), does early screening at 40 years old with colonoscopy (*I*) reduce the future risk of colon cancer (*O*) compared with screening at 50 years old (*C*)? ▪ Will a plant-based diet (*I*) decrease the risk for cardiovascular disease (*O*) when compared to the Mediterranean diet (*C*) in patients with a BMI greater than 30 (*P*) over 1 year (*T*)?
Prognosis	▪ Does prescribing a prophylactic dosage of oral vancomycin (*I*) in patients being treated for an acute bacterial infection with prior history of *Clostridioides difficile* infection (*P*) decrease the risk for severe *C. difficile* colitis (*O*)? ▪ For patients 65 years of age and older and/or immunocompromised (*P*), how does the use of the COVID-19 vaccine (*I*) compared to not receiving the vaccine (*C*) influence the risk of developing a COVID-19 infection requiring hospitalization (*O*) annually (*T*)?
Treatment	▪ In patients with diabetes mellitus (*P*), what is the effect of metformin (*I*) on HgbA$_{1c}$ (*O*) when compared with sitagliptin (*C*) over 3 months (*T*)? ▪ What is the effect of angiotensin II (*I*) on mean arterial pressure (*O*) when compared with norepinephrine (*C*) over 24 hours (*T*) in patients with septic shock (*P*)?

BMI, body mass index.

Step 5. Search for the best evidence (i.e., articles) using (electronic) databases. The next step would be to input the variables used in the PICOT format into electronic databases to search for the best evidence (i.e., articles). If written well, the PICOT mnemonic can identify key phrases or words in databases that can retrieve the best evidence to answer the clinical question and inform practice (Table 23.6). The search process can be streamlined to narrow results by (a using database-controlled vocabulary ("MeSH terms"); (b) combining searches with the Boolean connector "AND"; and (c) setting limits or defining parameters such as language, date published, and characteristics of subjects (e.g., age, sex).

Table 23.6 Databases

Databases	Website	Description
Primary		
PubMed (e.g., MEDLINE)	https://www.ncbi.nlm.nih.gov/pubmed	Medical and life sciences literature
Cumulative Index to Nursing and Allied Health Literature (CINAHL)	https://connect.ebsco.com/s/article/CINAHL-Databases-Basic-Searching-Tutorial?language=en_US	Nursing and allied health literature
PsycINFO	https://www.apa.org/pubs/databases/psycinfo	Comprehensive library of the psychological sciences
ERIC	https://eric.ed.gov	Sponsored by the Institute of Education Sciences
EMBASE	https://embase.com	8,000 journals referenced for biomedical literature
OVID	https://ovidsp.ovid.com	Medical research database for all healthcare professionals
Web of Science	https://www.webofscience.com	Estimated 1.6 billion sources

(*continued*)

Table 23.6 Databases (*continued*)

Databases	Website	Description
Secondary: References From Primary Sources or Filter		
Cochrane Library ▪ Cochrane Database of Systematic Reviews (CDSR)	https://www.cochrane.org	Systematic reviews and meta-analyses ***strongest level of evidence for intervention questions (most rigorous, best study designs)
Database of Abstracts of Reviews of Effects (DARE)	https://www.crd.york.ac.uk/CRDWeb/HomePage.asp	*DARE (Database of Abstracts of Reviews of Effects),* located on the University of York Centre for Reviews and Dissemination platform, is an index of over 35,000 systematic reviews of health and social care interventions.
Johanna Briggs Institute	https://jbi.global/	Over 5,000 EBP resources and best practice information
UpToDate	https://www.uptodate.com	Many institutions have this database; costly for an individual
DynaMed	https://www.dynamed.com	Point-of-care clinical reference tool
Hybrid		
TRIP	https://www.tripdatabase.com	Similar to the primary databases, but it organizes them according to evidence type; may charge a fee
Google Scholar	https://scholar.google.com	Effortless way to get started for a broad search of literature

Step 6. Critical appraisal of the evidence. Once the best evidence has been selected from the database search, the chosen articles should then be appraised for (a) validity; (b) reliability; and, most importantly, (c) relevance and (d) applicability to the clinical question. After all, the level of evidence (i.e., design) and the quality of evidence (i.e., validity of methods) will help determine the strength of the evidence, which will determine its clinical application. This can be done by looking for evidence with the highest level of evidence through a hierarchal classification (Table 23.7). To minimize bias or eliminate confounding variables, control or intervention groups should share key characteristics. After all, any difference in these groups could affect the outcome, potentially skewing results and increasing the risk that the outcome may be related to these differences rather than to the intervention itself. Moreover, tools being used to measure outcomes should have established acceptable validity and reliability. Once this has been confirmed, the next step would be to evaluate the relevance of the articles and their results.

Table 23.7 AACN Levels of Evidence and Study Descriptions

Level of Evidence	Study Type	Description
A	Meta-analysis	Process of using quantitative methods to summarize results from multiple similar studies addressing the same topic or research question
	Systematic review (quantitative studies)	Rigorous synthesis of research findings on a particular research question obtained by experts in the field or topic using systematic sampling and data collection with a formal protocol

(*continued*)

Table 23.7 AACN Levels of Evidence and Study Descriptions (*continued*)

Level of Evidence	Study Type	Description
B	RCT	An experimental test of a specific action, intervention, or treatment that involves random assignment (i.e., researchers blinded to which participants are receiving an intervention) to treatment groups *Strongest design: examines cause and effect of an intervention and greatly reduces bias*
C	Systematic review (qualitative studies)	Rigorous synthesis of research findings on a particular research question obtained by experts in the field or topic using systematic sampling and data collection with a formal protocol
	Cohort study	Nonexperimental design in which cohort (i.e., group) is followed over time to study outcomes Example: prospective longitudinal study
	Case-controlled study	Nonexperimental design involving comparison of a case and matched control Retrospective longitudinal study in which characteristics of a participant with certain type of condition (not very common) and often used to identify variables that may predict etiology and/or disease course
	Integrative review	Reviews of qualitative studies, taking the form of meta-synthesis (or compilation of studies reviewed and summarized), which are sources for EBP May integrate research and nonresearch articles
	Meta-synthesis	Interpretive translations produced from compilation of qualitative studies on a specific topic looking for common themes
	Qualitative research	Investigation of topic through the collection of narratives using a flexible research design such as interview or observation
	Others: descriptive studies, correlational studies, RCTs with inconsistent results	
D	Peer-reviewed professional and organizational standards with the support of clinical study recommendations	
E	Multiple case reports, theory-based evidence from expert opinions, or peer-reviewed professional organizational standards without clinical studies to support recommendations	
M	Manufacturer's recommendations only	

AACN, American Association of Colleges of Nursing; EBP, evidence-based practice; RCT, randomized controlled trial.

Step 7. Integrate evidence with clinical expertise and patient preferences and values. Once the evidence has been appraised thoroughly for reliability, validity, relevance, and applicability, one must then integrate it with clinical expertise along with objective data (e.g., diagnostics, clinical and institutional variables) and patient preferences prior to EBP implementation.

Step 8. Implementation. Implementation is a complex, multistep process warranting interdisciplinary collaboration for its success.

1. First and foremost, it would be prudent to use a resource guide for the implementation process. One such guide is the Advancing Research and Clinical Practice Through Close Collaboration (ARCC) model. It provides healthcare systems with an organized framework for system-wide EBP implementation and sustainability.
2. Second, organizational culture and readiness for EBP implementation should be assessed. Barriers need to be identified and mitigated, whereas facilitators need to be implemented.
3. Third, the team needs to be developed. Team composition can be determined after thinking about the project in an organizational context and after key stakeholders have been identified. An example of a team is the EBP implementers along with the EBP mentor(s). Throughout this process, the team members must maintain consistent communication with each other while progress is assessed at consistent, frequent intervals. More importantly, stakeholders should be kept engaged throughout the process.

4. Subsequently, the purpose of the project should be clearly defined with an educational and outcomes measurement plan as well as an implementation timeline to set the process in motion. This can be conceptualized with use of a dashboard, a tool that can be used to display quality initiatives with their progress and goals.
5. Next, the implementation plan should be submitted to the internal review board (IRB), also known as the ethics review board, human subjects or ethics committee, for approval, especially if it is a research study. The IRB will emphasize the safety and confidentiality of the subjects while ensuring that the study is conducted in a way that the findings are generalizable.
6. Once a team has been developed and the project has been approved by the IRB, baseline data collection should start prior to implementation because existing problems would then be recognized and addressed sooner. Moreover, deciding on who will help, which data analysis programs will be used, and how it will be managed earlier on will help facilitate the process of data collection and analysis.
7. Data can be internal evidence or data generated within the hospital from quality or risk management, the finance department, clinical or operational systems, and electronic medical records. Successful data collection involves measurability, user-friendliness, and accessibility.
    i.   *Measurability:* Data must be measurable or able to be counted. Specific tools or mechanisms, with established validity and reliability, should be used to help operationalize (i.e., define and measure) specific outcomes being looked at. For instance, use of the critical care pain observation tool may be useful in determining whether a ketamine infusion is superior or noninferior to fentanyl infusion in alleviating pain in critically ill intubated patients.
    ii. *User-friendliness:* Data should be user-friendly or understandable with ease of use. For instance, data are more user-friendly when uploaded in one place with regularly available updates and documented in a systematic yet comprehensive fashion (e.g., chart format) so that others (e.g., higher management) can readily interpret the data from the beginning and after the implementation process.
    iii. *Accessibility:* Data should be accessible to the EBP team. To ensure confidentiality of potentially private and/or restricted healthcare information, ability to access stored data should require specific clearances or restrictions, such as passwords.

Step 9. Monitor and evaluate the implementation process and healthcare quality and outcomes or changes based on evidence. During and after implementation, monitoring and evaluation of the process itself (e.g., fidelity of the intervention) and the process and healthcare quality outcomes (e.g., how well the project was implemented) are important. Such processes will then be able to (a) continue supporting positive effects, (b) remedy negative effects or process issues related to implementation, and (c) identify which patients are most likely to benefit from implementation.

In addition, barriers and facilitators to the implementation process should be identified and, if possible, addressed. For example, a common barrier to the implementation process is resistance to changing a routine. Addressing this would be effective in mitigating this barrier and keeping the process going. A facilitator to this would be the use of EBP champions, especially during initial implementation. After all, EBP champions have the ability to provide expertise, education, feedback, and support while mitigating barriers (e.g., speak with resisters and work with leadership to address resistance) as well as identifying and addressing other process issues.

Step 10. Dissemination of EBP findings. The last step of the EBP implementation process is to disseminate the findings. It is important to disseminate findings so that others can learn about the process (e.g., implementation, evaluation) and whether or not similar outcomes identified in the literature were obtained. Examples include presentations at conferences, publications in professional journals or newsletters, and hospital-based policy development or modification. Examples of specific formats of EBP implementation worthy of review include Johns Hopkins Evidence-Based Practice Model (https://www.hopkinsmedicine.org/evidence-based-practice/ijhn_2017_ebp.html) and Melnyk and Fineout-Overholt's collaborative efforts including EBP in Nursing and Healthcare and "Evidence-Based Practice: Step by Step" publications in the *American Journal of Nursing*.

▶ RESEARCH PROCESS

If there are no studies that can provide an answer to a specific question in mind, then research may be indicated. In this case, it is important to take note of the research process. Factors affecting the research process include the type of research design, the resources available, and the context in which it is conducted (Table 23.8).

Table 23.8 Stages in the Research Process

Steps		Description
Stage 1	Developing the research question	▪ Based on issues and/or questions worth addressing ● Based on experiences, existing literature, socioeconomic and/or healthcare issues, or professional research priorities/funding ▪ Develop research question with a hypothesis (statement predicting a specific outcome) either negative (i.e., null) or positive terms in a PICOT format ▪ Typically, more common in quantitative than qualitative research

Stage 2	Searching and appraising the evidence	▪ Search for the evidence via (electronic) database search
		   ● See Table 23.6
		   ● Use database-controlled vocabulary ("MeSH terms")
		   ● Combine searches with Boolean connector "AND"
		   ● Limit search with defining parameters
		▪ Appraise the evidence
		   ● Use academic and/or professional journals
		   ● Appraise for validity, reliability, relevance, and applicability along with level of evidence (see Table 23.7)

Stage 3	Determining methodology or research design	▪ Research design = most important stage in the research process ▪ Need to establish conceptual framework ▪ Subtypes: (a) qualitative and (b) quantitative (see Table 23.12)
Stage 4	Preparing and submitting a research proposal	▪ *What:* detailed written statement highlighting the who, what, why, when, and how ▪ *Purpose:* gain approval ± funding, guide implementation ▪ *Minimum requirements in format:* (a) maintain ethical standards; (b) develop Gantt chart; (c) list and explain resources needed ▪ *IRB submission:* maintain ethical standards and patient safety
Stage 5	Accessing data	▪ Obtain permission and clearance from data "gatekeepers" (e.g., audit department, research committee)
Stage 6	Sampling	▪ Data collection from sample rather than entire population ▪ Type and size of sampling as well as number of resources required depend on research design (see Table 23.12)
Stage 7	Pilot study	▪ *Purpose:* better understand research processes (e.g., subject recruitment) ▪ Psychometric testing of specific tool(s)
Stage 8	Data collection	▪ Successful data collection = measurability + user-friendliness + accessibility ▪ *Examples:* self-reports, questionnaires, interviews, clinical measurement, observation ▪ Ensure confidentiality of participant information and meticulous record keeping
Stage 9	Data analysis	▪ *Data analysis:* decide on support and program to use ▪ *Quantitative research:* statistical analysis (e.g., SPSS) ▪ *Qualitative research:* detailed description (e.g., NVivo)
Stage 10	Dissemination of the results	▪ *Purpose:* disseminate information, promote discussion, evaluate clinical and future implications ▪ *Methods:* presentations at conferences, publications in professional journals or newsletters, internet
Stage 11	Implementation of research findings	▪ *Purpose:* improve clinical practice, enhance knowledge, evaluate effects of innovation, and/or implement findings from a trial

IRB, internal review board; SPSS, Statistical Package for the Social Sciences.

Stage 1: Developing the research question. Similar to steps 1 and 2 of EBP implementation, developing a research question can be accomplished by identifying issues that may need to be addressed or questions that may need to be answered while taking into consideration if such issues or questions are worth addressing. Issues can be identified from personal and/or professional experiences (e.g., professional discussions, issues in the media), existing literature, or priorities of the community, institution, or profession. Additionally, a specific issue may be worth addressing if it can support or develop theory, support or change current practice and/or policy, and/or build upon prior findings. For instance, the research question may arise from a funding body calling for proposals and asking healthcare researchers to develop a proposal on a specific matter.

Once a specific issue or question has been identified, a research question can then be developed. An example of a research question would be a hypothesis. A hypothesis is a statement, often used in quantitative (i.e., experimental) research, that predicts whether a relationship exists in negative (i.e., null hypothesis) or positive terms. Parts of the hypothesis parallel those of the PICO(T) format, which includes the population of interest, independent and dependent variables, and comparisons leading to the study outcome (Table 23.9).

Table 23.9 Types of Hypotheses

Types	Description
1. Research (or testable)	Predict relationship between two or more variables in population of interest
a. Directional	Predict direction or path of relationship (e.g., decrease or increase)
b. Nondirectional	Predict relationship without direction or path
c. Null	Also known as statistical Predict no relationship among or between variables
2. Simple or complex	
a. Simple	Relationship between two variables
b. Complex (or multivariate)	Relationship between two or more variables
3. Associative or causal	Describe relationship among variables in hypothesis
a. Associative	Hypothesis state variables exist side by side with change in one variable accompanied by a change in another Variables change in association with each other
b. Causal (or directional)	One variable causes or brings about change in one or more other variables

Stage 2. Searching and appraising the evidence. Similar to steps 5 and 6 of EBP implementation, the next stage involves searching for and appraising the existing evidence. The evidence can be searched for using key phrases or words that can retrieve literature, typically academic or professional journals, relevant to the research question using multiple electronic databases (see Table 23.6). The search process can be streamlined to narrow results by (a) using database-controlled vocabulary ("MeSH terms"), (b) combining searches with the Boolean connector "AND," and (c) limiting final search by setting limits or defining parameters. Once the best evidence has been selected from the database search, the chosen articles should then be appraised for (a) validity, (b) reliability, and, most importantly, (c) relevance and (d) applicability to the research question. Not all content published is of good quality, nor can it be generalized or extrapolated into clinical practice. The appraisal process of these publications includes determining their validity and reliability based on the highest level of evidence (see Table 23.7). After all, the level of evidence (i.e., design) and the quality of evidence (i.e., validity of methods) will help determine the rigor or strength of evidence, which will determine its clinical application.

Stage 3. Determining methodology or research design. Next, the research design or methodology—the most important stage of the research process—should be determined. Research designs can be categorized as quantitative or qualitative. Qualitative studies are descriptive, often providing a detailed description or narrative of the phenomena of interest perceived by the study subjects. They are not concerned with relationships among variables. The purpose of qualitative studies is to explore new concepts and ideas about which little is known and to use the narrative for data analysis to identify concepts, relationships, and themes related to the human experience and even to develop theory. Because little is known about these concepts, a hypothesis cannot be developed. Examples of qualitative research include phenomenology, grounded theory, ethnography, and narrative inquiry (Table 23.10). On the other hand, quantitative studies investigate and attempt to answer research questions from an existing problem of interest or evaluate relationships among variables. Quantitative studies are explanatory in nature, which differs from their qualitative counterparts, which are exploratory. Examples include experimental, observational (e.g., questionnaire- or survey-based), and epidemiological (Table 23.11). Comparisons between qualitative and quantitative research are noted in Table 23.12.

Table 23.10 Qualitative Research

Study Type	Description
Phenomenology	Research method looking at the lived experience of the subjects
Grounded theory	Rich data by immersion in the topic of interest or group to develop a theory inductively
Ethnography	Descriptive study of culture looking at the aspects that impact their experiences
Narrative inquiry	Develop in-depth information, such as a case study

Table 23.11 Quantitative Research

Study Type	Description
Experimental	Involve hypotheses requiring statistical testing
Questionnaire based (i.e., surveys)	Include format with answers structured in box format to be checked, enabling data coding and translation into numerical format (e.g., survey involving number of hospitalized patients on a ventilator)
Epidemiologic	Determine incidence and distribution of diseases (e.g., number of hospitalized patients in the ICU and in non-ICU settings with COVID-19)

Table 23.12 Comparing Quantitative and Qualitative Research Methods

Element	Quantitative Research	Qualitative Research
Purpose/approach	Explanatory Investigate and attempt to answer questions from existing problem of interest → test hypotheses and theories	Exploratory Descriptive narrative and exploration of new ideas and concepts → identify concepts, relationship, and themes to develop theory
Viewpoint	Researcher's own to form prediction about study outcome	Participant viewpoint
Sample size	Large	Few
Variables	Evaluate relationships among variables	Does not evaluate relationships among variables
Hypothesis	Used; can be developed and tested	Not used; cannot be developed or tested
Format	Numbers, graphs, charts, and/or tables	Words
Data analysis	Statistical analysis	Interpretation and categorization to identify concepts, relationships, and themes
Description of quality of research	Validity, reliability	Credibility, trustworthiness, transparency
Examples	Experimental, observational, epidemiologic (see Table 23.11)	Phenomenology, grounded theory, ethnography, narrative inquiry (see Table 23.10)

Stage 4. Preparing and submitting a research proposal. The next step is preparing and submitting a research proposal. A research proposal is a written statement describing what the research intends to do with details clearly highlighting the who, how, when, and why. It is written to gain approval, to guide the research process during its implementation, and, if required, to secure funding. Although a specific format varies according to the purpose and nature of the research, there are some components

mandatory for successful submission and approval. They are (a) maintenance of ethical standards (e.g., confidentiality, informed consent) and (b) Gantt chart; and (c) list and explanation of resources needed. The Gantt chart shows a projected timeline used to identify tasks or milestones with associated dates and/or stages. Similar to step 8 of EBP implementation, this research proposal warrants submission to an advisory board such as the IRB to ensure that (ethical) standards and safety of the subjects are maintained.

Stage 5. Gaining access to the data. Gaining access to data (e.g., health-protected patient records) is the next step, involving formal permission and clearance from the "gatekeepers," such as the institution's audit department and the institution's ethical and research governance committees.

Stage 6. Sampling. Once the research proposal and data access have been approved, the next step involves selecting the sample. Research requires data collection from a sample, or selected group, rather than an entire population. The type and size of sampling depend on research design. Quantitative studies involving a comparison between two groups tend to require a power calculation, a statistical technique to estimate minimal sample size that is typically larger, whereas qualitative studies tend to have smaller sample size. Surveys, a form of quantitative research, warrant random sampling, whereas theoretical sampling is more appropriate for grounded theory, a form of qualitative research.

Stage 7. Pilot study. Sometimes referred to as a "dummy run," pilot studies are often conducted initially to have a better understanding of processes (e.g., subject recruitment processes), reduce waste of resources, or perform psychometric tests on a specific tool. For instance, questionnaires may be piloted to a small sample of subjects with traits paralleling those in a full study to identify questionnaire items that may need to be modified in order to limit waste of resources from premature distribution.

Stage 8. Data collection. The next step is data collection. Examples include self-reports, questionnaires, interviews, clinical measurement, observation, and use of documents. As a part of this stage, data collection tools will be used and, if necessary, refined. Similar to step 8 of EBP implementation, deciding on who will help, which data analysis programs will be used, and how it will be managed earlier on will help facilitate the process of data collection and analysis. Similar to EBP implementation, characteristics of successful data collection include measurability, user-friendliness, and accessibility. Ensuring confidentiality of potentially private and/or restricted healthcare information is mandatory; therefore, ability to access stored data should require specific clearances or restrictions (e.g., passwords).

Stage 9. Data analysis. The next most crucial and resource-intensive phase of the research process is data analysis. Once data are collected, they need to be organized and analyzed in such a way that conclusions and clinical implications can be drawn from them. Data are analyzed differently, depending on the type of research method. For instance, quantitative data are analyzed statistically, usually by a statistician, whereas qualitative data are analyzed through a detailed description of how the results were obtained. Data can be analyzed using software programs such as Statistical Package for the Social Sciences (SPSS) for quantitative analysis and NVivo for qualitative analysis. Sometimes, some research may use mixed methods involving both quantitative and qualitative approaches.

Stage 10. Dissemination of the results. The next step is the dissemination of the results. It is important to disseminate findings so that others can learn about the process (e.g., implementation, evaluation) and whether or not similar outcomes identified in the literature were obtained. Examples of disseminations include presentations at conferences and even dissemination over the internet. Although the internet allows for mass and feasible dissemination, there is no guarantee of quality. Therefore, publications in professional journals or newsletters remain the most widely accepted form of dissemination.

Stage 11. Implementation of the results. The final stage in the research process is the implementation of the results. Again, the purpose of research is to improve clinical practice in some way by enhancing knowledge, evaluating the effects of an innovation, and implementing findings from a trial.

▶ STATISTICS

Statistics are fundamental to presenting data in a scientific manner. Two basic types of statistics are descriptive and inferential. Descriptive statistics will "describe" the subjects or sample under investigation. Inferential statistics focus on making generalizations about a population or large group of subjects based on a sample. Table 23.13 lists some common statistical terms to become familiar with.

Table 23.13 Important Statistical Terms

Terms	Description
Significance level	*Definition:* probability of incorrectly rejecting a true null hypothesis Also known as alpha (α; 0.01, 0.05, 0.10)
P-value	*Definition:* probability of obtaining effect at least as large as the one observed in sample data If *p*-value is less than alpha, then hypothesis test is statistically significant.
Confidence level	*Definition:* percentage expected to get close to the same results/estimate if the research/poll/test/survey ran again Confidence level = 1 − alpha Always expressed in percentage (90%, 95%, or 99%) corresponding to percentages of the area of the normal density curve
Confidence interval	*Definition:* Upper and lower bounds (i.e., range, parameters, average) from experiment/poll/survey expected to find at a specific level of confidence Used in hypothesis testing and other methods (e.g., correlation, regression)
Sensitivity	Ability of test to correctly identify those with a disease
Specificity	Ability of test to correctly identify those without the disease
True positive	Individual has the disease, and test is positive
True negative	Individual does not have the disease, and test is negative
False positive	Person does not have the disease, and test is positive
False negative	Person has the disease, and test is negative
Prevalence	Percentage of population with the disease
Validity	*Accuracy of measure:* Do the results represent what they are supposed to measure?
	1. *Construct:* Tool measures what it is supposed to measure.
	2. *Convergent:* Tool gives similar scores as other tools on the same subject.
	3. *Discriminant:* Tool does not measure what it is not supposed to measure.
	4. *External:* Extent at which results are generalizable to the general population and/or clinical practice
	5. *Internal:* Extent at which results are true and not caused by methodological errors
Reliability	*Consistency of measure:* Can the results be reproduced under the same conditions?
	1. *Inter-rater:* consistency of measure between multiple raters (Cohen's kappa [κ])
	2. *Test–retest:* reliability of test measured over time
Evidence	1. *External:* knowledge acquired from existing literature and research
	2. *Internal:* knowledge acquired through clinical practice (e.g., data and/or observations collected from your patient) and formal education and training

Variables. Variables refer to measurable and dynamic traits or qualities. There are many subclassifications of variables used in research and statistics (Table 23.14).

Table 23.14 Variables: Types and Description

Types	Subtypes	Description
Independent *versus* dependent	Independent	▪ Affects or influences other variable(s) or outcomes
	Dependent	▪ Variable being acted on or affected ▪ Outcome
Extraneous		▪ Variables not under investigation ▪ Can adversely affect validity of results and/or study outcomes ▪ Need to identify and control them with statistical procedures and/or study design ▪ If not controlled, then referred to as *confounding* variables

(continued)

Table 23.14 Variables: Types and Description (*continued*)

Types	Subtypes	Description
Demographic		▪ *Definition:* characteristics of study subjects ▪ *Examples:* age, gender, sex, ethnicity, occupation
Continuous *versus* discrete	Continuous	▪ *Traits:* wide range of values, not only whole numbers ▪ *Examples:* age, weight, salary, temperature
	Discrete	▪ *Traits:* finite number of values, only whole numbers ▪ *Examples:* respiratory rate
Dichotomous *versus* categorical	Dichotomous	▪ *Definition:* represent traits that are either present or not present; only two categories to choose from ▪ *Example:* sex (male or female)
	Categorical	▪ *Definition:* represent traits that are either present or not present; two or more categories to choose from ▪ *Example:* race (e.g., Hispanic, Black, Asian, White)
Conceptual *versus* operational	Conceptual	▪ Broad, more abstract definition based on (theoretical) literature, experience, or both ▪ Lack of direction on how variable measured
	Operational	▪ Concrete ▪ Specific direction on how variable measured (e.g., tools)

Drug Development and Phases of Clinical Trials. Of specific interest to the clinical practice of the AGACNP is drug development. The AGACNP may have the opportunity to participate in studies or clinical trials looking at new drugs for specific illnesses or chronic conditions. The AGACNP can be an integral part of the process by obtaining informed consents, monitoring, providing patient and staff education, and assisting with data collection (Table 23.15).

Table 23.15 Phases of Clinical Trials

Phase	Procedure
Phase 1	Small study, consisting of volunteers to examine safety issues
Phase 2	Explanted study, enrolling a small number of patients who have the "disease" to see if the treatment is effective
Phase 3	Large-scale study, blinding study examining placebo versus treatment for the disease
Phase 4	Post surveillance

▶ CASE STUDY

The AGACNP is called to the bedside to evaluate a 75-year-old nursing home patient admitted for severe dehydration (blood urea nitrogen 80, creatinine 3.0, sodium 155) in the emergency department with the following vital signs: blood pressure 70/40 mmHg, heart rate 140 beats/min. The nurse has placed the patient in Trendelenburg position as this was "what they had been taught." The AGACNP wishes to change this potentially antiquated mentality to more evidence-based intervention.

The AGACNP speaks to pertinent stakeholders (e.g., nurse educator and management, higher management) and sets up an EBP committee to evaluate the current practice. The AGACNP begins by forming the research question in PICOT format: "In patients with non-hemorrhagic hypovolemic shock (P), will use of passive leg raise [PLR] (C) improve hemodynamic stability (O) within minutes (T) when compared with Trendelenburg (I)?"

The AGACNP then forms their team: staff nurses, unit nurse manager, unit nurse educator, ICU physician, and librarian. The AGACNP then proceeds with a literature search using electronic databases (i.e., CINAHL, PubMed, UpToDate). Once the search is completed, the AGACNP appraises the strength of the evidence based on design, level, and quality of evidence and finds the following articles relevant to this project (*Note:* This project is conducted in 2012, so the literature search is reflective of that time.):

1. Bridges, N., & Jarquin-Valdivia, A. A. (2005, September). Use of the Trendelenburg position as the resuscitation position: To T or not to T. *American Journal of Critical Care, 14*(5), 364–368. https://doi.org/10.4037/ajcc2005.14.5.364; http://ajcc.aacnjournals.org/content/14/5/364.full
2. Johnson, S., & Henderson, S. O. (2004). Myth: The Trendelenburg position improves circulation in cases of shock. *Canadian Journal of Emergency Medicine, 6*(1), 48–49. https://doi.org/10.1017/s1481803500008915
3. Makic, M. B., Von Rueden, K. T., Rauen, C. A., & Chadwick, J. (2011). Evidence-based practice habits: Putting more sacred cows out to pasture. *Critical Care Nurse, 31*(2), 38–62. https://doi.org/10.4037/ccn2011908

Based on this literature review, it can be concluded that although the Trendelenburg maneuver has been used for many years to evaluate fluid responsiveness, it has been associated with adverse outcomes (e.g., increasing intracranial pressure, decreased vital capacity in patients with obesity), and should not be used. Rather, PLR is a maneuver associated with fewer adverse outcomes and greater diagnostic accuracy when evaluating for fluid responsiveness.

As a result, system-wide education is implemented in using PLR for diagnosing fluid responsiveness and transiently improving hemodynamics in patients with hypovolemic shock until more definitive interventions can be implemented. Subsequently, follow-up on this education includes system-wide change in protocol.

▶ SUMMARY

AGACNPs will be called upon to improve patient care and organizational processes. Thus, the AGACNP must be able to distinguish between research and EBP as well as the difference between qualitative and quantitative research. AGACNPs are expected to be knowledgeable about the steps in implementing EBP as well as identifying and removing barriers and using facilitators to advance the process to meet the goals. AGACNPs are well positioned to advance the care of acutely and critically ill patients.

KNOWLEDGE CHECK: CHAPTER 23

1. What is the best way to describe collected data?

   A. Inferential statistics
   B. Cluster sampling
   C. Descriptive statistics
   D. Systematic sampling

2. A confidence interval for a mean is:

   A. The interval containing the unknown population mean
   B. A point in time estimate of a population mean
   C. A fixed parameter (interval)
   D. A discrete value (parameter)

3. The U.S. Food and Drug Administration approval process for drugs to get to market includes and uses multiple study phases: I, II, III IIIA, and IIIB. Phase IV studies are performed after the drug is approved for marketing and are used in market comparison. The AGACNP understands that phase II studies are:

   A. Used to determine toxicity and safety
   B. Large prospective studies to evaluate clinical efficacy
   C. The first controlled studies of the drug involving a small group of patients
   D. Performed after preliminary evidence regarding the effectiveness of the drug has been demonstrated

4. Appraisal of clinical trial includes assessment of systematic errors. Reason for systematic errors include:

   A. Multiple measurements
   B. Random chance
   C. Study design flaws
   D. Increased sample size

5. Ethnography is the study of:

   A. Nature or meaning of everyday experiences through the lived experiences of subjects
   B. Discovering theory from data systematically obtained through research
   C. Study of philosophy focusing on exploration of the inner world of individuals
   D. Study or description of a culture of groups of individuals

6. Evidence-based practice is the conscious use of current best evidence to facilitate decision-making about patient care. It is grounded in:

   A. Information found in textbooks
   B. Best evidence and clinical expertise
   C. Systematically conducted research studies
   D. Expert opinion

(*See answers next page.*)

1. C) Descriptive statistics
Descriptive statistics is the method to present data with no interpretation; it simply tells the audience what data were collected.

2. A) The interval containing the unknown population mean
The confidence level is the degree of certainty that the interval contains the unknown population parameter value. It provides the degree of assurance or confidence that the statement regarding the population parameter is correct. The more certainty desired, the wider the interval will have to be.

3. C) The first controlled studies of the drug involving a small group of patients
Phase II studies are the first controlled clinical studies of the drug involving no more than several hundred patients. The primary objective of phase II studies is to explore efficacy and, less commonly, side effects. Phase I studies determine toxicity and safety. Phase III studies are large prospective studies of clinical efficacy.

4. B) Random chance
Random errors can be introduced by chance. Variations due to chance can occur in most situations. Multiple measurements and larger sample size minimize change of systematic errors.

5. D) Study or description of a culture of groups of individuals
Ethnography is looking at the culture and meaning of individuals of the same background.

6. B) Best evidence and clinical expertise
Evidence-based practice refers to the concept that clinical decisions should be supported by the strongest evidence, one's own clinical expertise, and patient preferences and values.

7. Evidence or clinical practice guidelines:

   A. Are widely agreed upon between professional organizations
   B. Provide a strict legal protocol for AGACNPs to follow
   C. Contain best evidence, including cost-effective approaches to patient care
   D. Do not provide clinicians any protection from malpractice

8. A well-developed PICOT question helps the AGACNP:

   A. Find the largest amount of information
   B. Search for focused evidence
   C. Critically appraise the literature
   D. Cultivate a spirit of inquiry

9. Which is a well-developed PICOT question for the adult population in a critical care unit?

   A. In patients with diarrhea, will cleansing skin with soap and water reduce skin irritation immediately compared to no-rinse cleaning?
   B. In patients who are intubated, is saline lavage every 2 hours the best practice for sputum clearance?
   C. In patients who have hair on their chest, is shaving more helpful than clipping?
   D. Should patients on extracorporeal membrane oxygenation (ECMO) not be turned to prevent the dislodgment of the cannulas?

10. Which of the following databases would the AGACNP use to find the most rigorous systematic reviews?

    A. PubMed
    B. Cumulative Index to Nursing and Allied Health Literature (CINAHL)
    C. American College of Physicians (ACP) Journal Club
    D. Cochrane Library

11. What is the correct order of hierarchy of evidence, from highest to lowest, on which to base treatment decisions?

    A. Meta-analyses, randomized controlled trials, case-control/cohort studies, descriptive studies
    B. Meta-analyses, case-control/cohort studies, randomized controlled trials, descriptive studies
    C. Systematic reviews, case-control/cohort studies, randomized controlled trials, expert opinion
    D. Systematic reviews, case-control/cohort studies, randomized controlled trials, descriptive

12. The AGACNP completes a literature search and finds 30 potential articles on a particular topic of interest. To determine which of the 30 articles are appropriate, the AGACNP should first read the:

    A. Methods section of each article
    B. Discussion section of each article
    C. Abstract of each article
    D. Entire article

13. The ability to generalize findings from a study's sample to the larger population is known as:

    A. Internal validity
    B. External validity
    C. Internal evidence
    D. External evidence

(See answers next page.)

7. C) Contain best evidence, including cost-effective approaches to patient care

Practice guidelines have been developed by many professional organizations and agencies as a decision-making aid to caregivers. Most organizations attempt to incorporate the most recent available evidence and concern of cost-effectiveness into their guideline formulations. Despite an increasing level of nuance in current guidelines, they cannot be expected to account for the uniqueness of each individual and their illness. Furthermore, many discrepancies exist in guidelines from major organizations. By setting a standard of reasonable care in most cases, clinical guidelines provide protection to both clinicians (from inappropriate charges of malpractice) and patients, particularly those with inadequate healthcare resources. Even though guidelines provide the protection, they do not provide a rigid legal constraint for the conscientious physician. The physician's challenge is to incorporate the useful recommendations provided by the experts into guidelines and incorporate the guidelines into the care of each individualized patient.

8. B) Search for focused evidence

The PICOT question is used to identify the search terms for a successful and efficient focused search and begin the evidence-based research process. Focused searches will identify studies that will efficiently answer the clinical question.

9. A) In patients with diarrhea, will cleansing skin with soap and water reduce skin irritation immediately when compared to no-rinse cleaning?

The PICOT question about patients with diarrhea is well-developed because it contains comparison (cleansing with soap and water versus no-rinse cleansing), a timeline (immediately), and an outcome (reduced skin irritation). The questions concerning intubated patients and ECMO patients are not well-developed PICOT questions because there is no comparison or timeline. The question about patients with hair on the chest does not have an outcome or a timeline.

10. D) Cochrane Library

The Cochrane Library contains the most rigorous systematic reviews. While PubMed contains many systematic reviews, the quality metrics of how the systematic review is performed may vary. CINAHL provides journal articles specific to nursing but may miss key evidence from other professions. ACP Journal Club contains summaries of studies and expert clinical commentary.

11. A) Meta-analyses, randomized controlled trials, case-control/cohort studies, descriptive studies

Meta-analyses and systematic reviews of randomized controlled trials are the two highest levels of evidence, followed by randomized controlled trials, then controlled trials without randomization, case-control and cohort studies, systematic reviews of descriptive and qualitative studies, single descriptive or qualitative studies, and finally, expert committees.

12. C) Abstract of each article

Reading the abstract will provide an initial screening for potential inclusion. The initial screening will include review of level of evidence, population, intervention, and comparison groups as well as outcomes. Reading the methods sections of each article is part of the rapid critical appraisal process to determine if the study results are valid, reliable, and applicable. Reading the literature review and discussion sections can help identify further articles that may also answer the PICOT question.

13. B) External validity

External validity refers to the extent at which results are generalizable to the general population and/or clinical practice. Internal validity refers to the extent at which the results are true and not caused by methodological errors. External evidence is knowledge acquired from existing literature and research. Internal evidence is knowledge acquired through clinical practice (e.g., data and/or observations collected from the patient) as well as formal education and training.

14. Which of the following is a limitation of evidence-based practice implementation?

    A. Absence of research that explains practice

    B. Establishing linkages between academia and clinical practice

    C. Access to evidence, time, money, and clinical resources

    D. Attending conferences where research is presented outside the AGACNP's institution

15. When creating an evidence-based practice guideline, it is important to include:

    A. Systematic reviews only

    B. Traditional care model

    C. Patient values and expectations

    D. Financial data only

(See answers next page.)

14. C) Access to evidence, time, money, and clinical resources
Common limitations of evidence-based practice include needing skill in searching and appraising the literature, needing time to master these skills, needing time to implement evidence-based practice, scarce resources, and potentially limited access to evidence.

15. C) Patient values and expectations
When creating an evidence-based practice guideline, it is important to use all information available and to include the patients' values and expectations. The most well-conducted evidence-based practice guideline will not be successful if care expectations are not compatible with the patient's values.

KEY BIBLIOGRAPHY

Only key resources appear in the print edition. Access the full bibliography for this chapter on ExamPrepConnect.com.

Clarke, V., Lehane, E., Mulcahy, H., & Cotter, P. (2021). Nurse practitioners' implementation of evidence-based practice into routine care: A scoping review. *Worldviews on Evidence-Based Nursing, 18*(3), 180–189. https://doi.org/10.1111/wvn.12510

Fineout-Overholt, E., Melnyk, B. M., Stillwell, S. B., & Williamson, K. M. (2010). Evidence-based practice, step by step: Critical appraisal of the evidence: Part I. *American Journal of Nursing, 110*(7), 47–52. https://doi.org/10.1097/01.NAJ.0000383935.22721.9c

Iowa Model Collaborative. (2017). Iowa model of evidence-based practice: Revisions and validation. *Worldviews on Evidence-Based Nursing, 14*(3), 175–182. https://doi.org/10.1111/wvn.12223

Polit, D. F., & Beck, C. T. (2018). *Essentials of nursing research: Appraising evidence for nursing practice* (9th ed.). Wolters Kluwer.

Severgnini, P., Pelosi, P., Contino, E., Serafinelli, E., Novario, R., & Chiaranda, M. (2016). Accuracy of critical care pain observation tool and behavioral pain scale to assess pain in critically ill conscious and unconscious patients: Prospective, observational study. *Journal of Intensive Care, 4*, 68. https://doi.org/10.1186/s40560-016-0192-x

Part V: Practice Test

Practice Test

1. Methicillin-resistant *Staphylococcus aureus* (MRSA) is isolated from the blood of a patient who has been in the ICU of a hospital for 2 weeks. Which one of the following antibiotics is most reliable for treatment of this patient's infection?

   A. Ampicillin/sulbactam
   B. Daptomycin
   C. Doxycycline
   D. Trimethoprim–sulfamethoxazole (TMP/SMX)

2. Which of the following treatment options is *most* appropriate for a patient with acute decompensated heart failure who experiences diuretic resistance on furosemide 40 mg intravenous (IV) twice daily?

   A. Re-bolus with furosemide 40 mg IV × one dose and start furosemide IV infusion
   B. Decrease dose of furosemide to 20 mg IV twice daily
   C. Continue furosemide 40 mg IV twice daily and add bumetanide 2 mg IV twice daily
   D. Discontinue furosemide 40 mg IV twice daily and start spironolactone 25 mg PO daily

3. Which of the following intravenous (IV) treatment options is preferred in patients with hypertensive emergency due to pheochromocytoma?

   A. Labetalol
   B. Enalaprilat
   C. Phentolamine
   D. Hydralazine

4. Which of the following initial treatment options is most appropriate for a patient who experiences statin-associated muscle symptoms (SAMS) on simvastatin 10 mg PO at bedtime?

   A. Discontinue simvastatin and start atorvastatin 80 mg PO daily.
   B. Hold simvastatin and check creatine phosphokinase (CPK) level.
   C. Continue simvastatin and start gemfibrozil.
   D. Continue simvastatin and advise patient to notify provider if symptoms do not resolve in 1 week.

5. In adult patients with mild to moderate asthma, which of the following is preferred to a short-acting beta-agonist (SABA) as relief for exacerbations?

   A. Inhaled corticosteroid (ICS)/formoterol
   B. ICS alone
   C. Formoterol alone
   D. Indacaterol/mometasone

6. An AGACNP examines a patient who presented with right lower quadrant pain. The patient complains of point tenderness between the umbilicus and the anterior–superior iliac spine. This pain at this location is known as which sign?

   A. Psoas
   B. Obturator
   C. Rosving
   D. McBurney

7. A patient with cirrhosis holds up their hands flexed at the wrists. The AGACNP sees the hands start to move in a repetitive flexion manner. The AGACNP identifies this as:

   A. Dystonia
   B. Asterixis
   C. Essential tremor
   D. Parkinsonian tremor

8. Signs of dehydration include:

   A. Temperature 99.4°F, urine specific gravity 1.010
   B. Blood urea nitrogen (BUN) 20, creatinine 2.0, presence of an S_3
   C. Tachycardic with heart rate 110, blood pressure 130/74, S_4 present
   D. Dry mucous membranes, skin tenting on clavicles

9. The AGACNP appreciates a low-pitched, rough, rasping murmur at the right second intercostal space. The most likely cause is:

   A. Aortic stenosis
   B. Mitral stenosis
   C. Mitral regurgitation
   D. Aortic regurgitation

10. The AGACNP assesses a patient who is complaining of progressive shortness of breath and notes the patient has peripheral edema and crackles in bilateral bases posteriorly. What additional physical exam finding should the AGACNP be looking for?

    A. S_3
    B. S_4
    C. Split S_2
    D. Systolic click

11. A trauma patient who is hypotensive with muffled heart sounds should immediately be assessed for:

    A. Hypertension
    B. Lung sliding on extended focused assessment with sonography in trauma (eFAST)
    C. Decreased breath sounds
    D. Jugular venous distention

12. Cramping pain in the legs or buttocks that occurs while walking is called:

    A. Vasospasm
    B. Claudication
    C. Lymphedema
    D. Poikilothermia

13. A patient presents with dry, black areas on the great and fourth toes on the left foot. They have no edema or hair growth on their legs. They have faint monophasic pulses in their dorsalis pedis pulses. The most likely diagnosis is:

    A. Acute limb ischemia
    B. Deep vein thrombosis
    C. Peripheral venous disease
    D. Peripheral arterial disease

14. A patient is noted to have bilateral lower extremity edema, brownish discoloration of the distal extremities from knees to ankles. A small, shallow, weeping open wound is noted. The patient has triphasic pulses via Doppler in the dorsalis pedis pulses. What do these findings suggest?

    A. Acute limb ischemia
    B. Chronic limb ischemia
    C. Peripheral venous disease
    D. Peripheral arterial disease

15. To illicit Murphy sign, the AGACNP:

    A. Palpates deeply in the left lower quadrant (LLQ) and then quickly withdraws the hand
    B. Palpates the right upper quadrant (RUQ) deeply and asks the patient to take a deep breath
    C. Flexes the patient's right hip and bends the knee, internally rotating it
    D. Asks the supine patient to raise a knee against a hand that applies resistance

16. The AGACNP recognizes which of the following patients to be at highest risk for falls?

    A. 68 years old, post cardiac catheterization, no history of fall in past year, takes levothyroxine and atorvastatin
    B. 72 years old, presents to the ED with dysuria and fever, no history of falls in past year, takes nonsteroidal anti-inflammatory drugs for arthritis
    C. 74 years old; no history of falls in past year; takes metformin, lisinopril, and oxybutynin for urge incontinence
    D. 70 years old, reports a single fall in the past year secondary to tripping over a carpet at a friend's home, reports steady gait, assessed to have no balance or gait difficulty, takes metformin and acetaminophen

17. The AGACNP is completing a medication reconciliation for a 76-year-old patient who is admitted for exacerbation of chronic obstructive pulmonary disease. The patient has a past medication history of coronary artery disease (CAD), hypertension (HTN), and type 2 diabetes mellitus (DM). What medication would the AGACNP have concerns about for this patient who has a glomerular filtration rate (GFR) of 78 mL/min/1.73 m²?

    A. Atorvastatin 40 mg daily
    B. Alprazolam 0.5 mg BID
    C. Lisinopril 10 mg daily
    D. Metformin 850 mg daily

18. The AGACNP is completing an admission history of an 82-year-old patient status post fall at home. In addition to the chief complaint and past medical history, what additional information would be most important for the AGACNP to obtain that is known to impact hospital prognosis and is a significant indicator of mortality?

    A. Sleep–wake patterns
    B. Food intolerances
    C. Functional measures
    D. Social support network

19. A 74-year-old female patient informs the AGACNP that she is not able to reach the bathroom in time to pass urine. She states that her intravenous catheter seems to get in the way when she is trying to reach the bathroom. The patient is receiving heparin for pulmonary embolism. She expresses embarrassment because she is incontinent. What is the *best* intervention for the AGACNP at this time?

   A. Inform the patient that she should not be getting out of bed and to use a bedpan.

   B. Write an order for an indwelling Foley catheter to be placed.

   C. Tell the patient to wear incontinence pads while in the hospital.

   D. Write an order for a bedside commode.

20. The AGACNP is completing a physical assessment of an 88-year-old patient admitted for sepsis due to a urinary tract infection. What assessment finding would be of concern and require further investigation?

   A. Presence of koilonychia

   B. Altered sleep pattern

   C. Presence of skin tears

   D. Decreased tear production

21. The AGACNP admits a patient whose family reports that they have had progressive confusion for the last several years but have refused to see a provider. The AGACNP suspects that the patient has Alzheimer dementia. What pharmacologic management should be anticipated?

   A. Carbidopa–levodopa (Sinemet)

   B. Donepezil (Aricept) and memantine (Namenda)

   C. Aspirin

   D. Lorazepam (Ativan) and amitriptyline (Elavil)

22. A middle-aged female patient is being discharged from the hospital after an ischemic stroke that required intravascular reperfusion. Prior to discharge, the nurse used the Patient Health Questionnaire (PHQ) to screen for depression and notified the AGACNP that the score on the PHQ two-item screening tool is 3 and on the nine-item screening tool is 16. Based on this information, the AGACNP should:

   A. Start a selective serotonin reuptake inhibitor (SSRI) and cancel the discharge to do a psychiatric evaluation in the next 24 hours

   B. Start fluoxetine and discharge the patient with a referral for further assessment by a mental health professional

   C. Consider the PHQ screening invalid because the patient has somatic symptoms from the cerebrovascular accident that explain the high scores

   D. Give the patient a prescription for bupropion (Wellbutrin) and ask their spouse to arrange psychotherapy

23. Which of the following is a prognostic and/or risk factor for major or mild neurocognitive disorder due to Alzheimer disease?

   A. Traumatic brain injury

   B. Klinefelter syndrome

   C. Exposure to pesticides and herbicides

   D. Viral illness

598 V. PRACTICE TEST

24. Socioeconomic and cultural variations can make the diagnosis of major or minor neurocognitive changes due to Alzheimer disease difficult. Which of the following statements is true?

    A. Memory loss is considered a natural part of aging.
    B. It is easy to conduct objective cognitive assessments on those with lower education.
    C. Individuals who face fewer cognitive demands in everyday life are more challenging to assess for functional decline.
    D. Highly educated and financially well-off individuals are less likely to notice changes in cognitive function and do not access care.

25. A 50-year-old man who is relatively healthy was admitted for postoperative monitoring after a total hip replacement. He is alert and oriented and is sipping juice in a chair. He asks the AGACNP to order his home medications of alprazolam 0.5 mg PO every night at bedtime (QHS) and sertraline 100 mg PO daily that he takes for his generalized anxiety disorder. What is the appropriate action for the AGACNP?

    A. Restart the sertraline only.
    B. Restart both medications.
    C. Do not restart either medication.
    D. Offer the patient trazadone 50 mg PO QHS instead.

26. A 64-year-old man with newly diagnosed locally advanced prostate cancer, high prostate-specific antigen (PSA), and positive prostate biopsies presents with new-onset lower back pain and leg weakness with recent fall. On exam, he is noted to have decreased motor strength and deep tendon reflexes to lower extremities. The AGACNP should order:

    A. Plain films of spine
    B. Orthopedic referral outpatient
    C. Emergent MRI of the spinal cord
    D. Nonsteroidal anti-inflammatory drugs and follow-up with primary care physician

27. A 52-year-old patient recently received chemotherapy for metastatic breast cancer and presents with new-onset confusion, lethargy, and weakness. Bloodwork reveals a calcium level of 12.0. What is the *next* appropriate step?

    A. Hydration with intravenous (IV) normal saline
    B. Treatment with oral bisphosphonate
    C. Encouraging patient to drink 3 L of water daily
    D. Monitoring lab values daily

28. The number one cause of cancer death in adults in the United States is cancer of the:

    A. Colon
    B. Head and neck
    C. Lung
    D. Pancreas

29. Staging the extent or amount of cancer involvement for a person with a new diagnosis uses:

    A. Class A, class B, class C, class D
    B. Low grade, moderate grade, high grade
    C. Poor, to moderate, to well differentiated
    D. Tumor size, node involvement, metastases

30. A 40-year-old patient day 27 post allogeneic bone marrow transplant (BMT) is getting ready for discharge to home. The most important consideration for this patient on immunosuppression therapy is:

    A. Cataract monitoring
    B. *Pneumocystis* pneumonia (PCP) prophylaxis
    C. Thyroid dysfunction
    D. Transfusion therapy

31. The AGACNP is caring for an 84-year-old patient with community-acquired pneumonia. On today's lab work, the patient's creatine is 1.89 mg/dL. The two previous recordings were 1.39 mg/dL and 1.55 mg/dL. What will be ordered *next* to determine the cause of this acute kidney injury (AKI)?

    A. Renal ultrasound
    B. Urine sodium, urine creatine, serum sodium, serum creatinine
    C. Creatinine kinase
    D. Serum sodium, urine sodium, serum osmolality

32. The AGACNP is taking care of a 68-year-old patient admitted with chronic obstructive pulmonary disease exacerbation. The patient has been tachypneic in the 20s and febrile for 48 hours with poor oral intake. They were started on broad-spectrum antibiotics for presumed community-acquired pneumonia. This morning, the patient is afebrile and states they are feeling better; however, the AGACNP notes blood urea nitrogen (BUN) is now 32 mg/dL, and creatinine is 1.6 mg/dL (baseline BUN 10 mg/dL, creatinine 0.6 mg/dL); sodium is 146 mEq/L; urine creatinine is 50 mEq/L, and urine sodium 10 mEq/L. The most likely cause is:

    A. Prerenal acute kidney injury (AKI)
    B. Hydronephrosis
    C. Acute tubular necrosis
    D. Post-renal AKI

33. The AGACNP is caring for a male patient with a past medical history of hypertension, ischemic stroke, and benign prostatic hyperplasia (BPH). Home medications include metoprolol (Lopressor), lisinopril (Zestril), aspirin, simvastatin (Zocor), and tamsulosin (Flomax). The patient presents to the ED with headache and abdominal pain over bilateral lower quadrants. He reveals that he recently lost his health insurance and cannot afford his medications. Lab findings include creatinine of 3.2 mg/dL (baseline 1.1 mg/dL). The most likely cause of his renal failure is:

    A. Acute tubular necrosis
    B. Prerenal acute kidney injury (AKI)
    C. Post-renal AKI
    D. Hypertensive emergency

34. The AGACNP is caring for a 38-year-old patient who was involved in a motorcycle crash that resulted in left-sided right fracture 7 and 8 and a splenic laceration that required embolization. The patient now has acute kidney injury (AKI) with the following labs: blood urea nitrogen 65 mg/dL, creatinine 4.2 mg/dL, urine sodium 45 mEq/L. Urinalysis with microscopy shows muddy brown casts. What is the AGACNP concerned about?

    A. Acute tubular necrosis
    B. Prerenal AKI
    C. Post-renal AKI
    D. Urinary tract infection

35. A 55-year-old patient with a history of hypertension presents to the ED with shortness of breath. The history is notable for recent prolonged air travel. The AGACNP is highly suspicious of a pulmonary embolism and will obtain a CT chest with intravenous contrast. What will the AGACNP order to try to prevent contrast-induced nephropathy (CIN)?

   A. Normal saline (NS) infusion
   B. Mucomyst 600 mg PO × 1
   C. Renal consult for dialysis
   D. Sodium bicarbonate infusion

36. A new AGACNP wants to actively engage in health policy but is unfamiliar with the policy process. What *grassroots effort* could the new AGACNP use to influence and/or educate their legislator?

   A. Volunteering to help a legislator at the state level
   B. Co-drafting a bill with a legislator
   C. Calling or emailing the legislator on a stance toward a specific bill
   D. Joining a professional organization that supports legislative initiatives

37. The discharge of a patient with congestive heart failure requires that the AGACNP understand that the Medicare Severity Diagnosis Related Group (MS-DRG)–based prospective payment method penalizes the hospital for:

   A. Overspending amount of bundle payment for all services based on original admission diagnosis
   B. Any 30-day readmission on select MS-DRG–based cases even if the patient is admitted elsewhere
   C. Acceptance of a high-risk patient-case mix
   D. Not accepting the Medicare calculated cost of the related DRG

38. A multitude of factors influence health outcomes, but the *most significant factor* is:

   A. Socioeconomic status (SES)
   B. Racial and gender disparities
   C. Access to healthcare
   D. Lack of insurance

39. What should *most* influence the discharge orders an AGACNP prepares for a 68-year-old male patient with a complicated wound care treatment plan and no supplemental insurance?

   A. Part B coverage will cover 80% of wound treatment pharmaceuticals, but the patient is responsible for 20% until their deductible is met.
   B. Part B coverage will cover 80% of costs of wound care dressings, but the patient is responsible for 20% until their deductible is met.
   C. The treatment plan for wound care greatly influences the ability to discharge the patient to home care depending on frequency of care needed and level of involvement the wound requires.
   D. Home care agencies that accept a patient with requirements for wound care are responsible under their bundled payment to use dressings and wound care agents ordered by the provider.

40. The AGACNP is evaluating a 34-year-old patient who presents with a small burn on their forearm from hot coffee. The AGACNP assess the patient and notes the burn to be painful, red, and blanchable to the touch. The AGACNP recommends which *best* intervention?

   A. Topical cooling with saline
   B. Referral to a plastic surgeon for skin grafting
   C. Intravenous narcotics for pain control
   D. Evaluation for inhalation injury

41. The AGACNP is concerned that there is a delay in initiation of tube feeding in the ICU primarily due to delay in inserting small-bore feeding tubes in eligible patients. A policy exists that tube feedings cannot be given via nasogastric tubes. The practice and policy are related to the beliefs of a now-retired intensivist who proposed the policy years ago. What is the *best* potential approach for the AGACNP to change this practice?

    A. Conducting a needs assessment to see if the medical group would be interested in supporting a practice change now that the intensivist is no longer there
    B. Conducting a formal policy analysis
    C. Performing a retroactive data review of time from admission to time of small-bore feeding tube placement to evaluate the problem
    D. Bringing the issue up to the Nursing Practice Council in the ICU to gain their support in the project

42. An 87-year-old patient admitted to the ICU with four right-sided rib fractures after a mechanical fall reports occasional short-term memory loss. The family is concerned that the patient sometimes has trouble hearing, especially in telephone conversations. The patient lives independently and does not require assistance with activities of daily living. Which condition is most consistent with the stated history?

    A. Normal aging process
    B. Early signs of vascular dementia
    C. Early signs of Alzheimer dementia
    D. Benign paroxysmal positional vertigo (BPPV)

43. The AGACNP understands that falls can impact the independence of older adults. Which is the *most* modifiable risk factor associated with falls in older adults?

    A. Medication use
    B. Diet
    C. Osteoarthritis
    D. Neuropathy

44. An 82-year-old patient is admitted to the orthopedic unit after sustaining a fall resulting in hip fracture. The patient indicates that they stood up, felt dizzy, and fell. On presentation to the ED, the patient's vital signs are blood pressure 167/84, heart rate 72, and respiratory rate 15. Which medication would *most* likely have contributed to the patient's fall?

    A. Tylenol PM
    B. Diltiazem
    C. Atorvastatin
    D. Levothyroxine

45. The AGACNP is caring for a 96-year-old patient admitted to the hospital with mental status changes secondary to dehydration. The patient's adult child indicates that this is the patient's third admission in 6 months for dehydration. The AGACNP understands that older adults are at risk for dehydration secondary to:

    A. Increased perception of thirst
    B. Impaired response to serum osmolality
    C. Increased ability to concentrate urine
    D. Impaired creatinine clearance

46. An 89-year-old patient with a history of Alzheimer dementia is admitted to the hospital after a fall resulting in a fracture to the right lower extremity. The medical record indicates that the patient has severe cognitive impairment. The family is concerned that the patient may be in pain and asks how pain is assessed in patients with dementia. The AGACNP understands that patients with cognitive impairment will manifest pain by:

A. Increase in appetite

B. Decreased confusion

C. Hypotension

D. Verbal abusiveness

47. Criteria for diagnosis of irritable bowel syndrome are:

A. History of gastrointestinal intolerance to dairy products

B. Abdominal pain with distention and constipation with straining

C. Abdominal pain related to bowel movement with change in stool consistency and frequency

D. Change in bowel habit to more frequent stools persisting for more than 6 weeks

48. A 43-year female patient has been ill for 3 days and was seen in an urgent care center 48 hours before admission with abdominal cramping. A urine analysis at the urgent care center revealed +2 blood and white blood cells in the urine. The patient had been taking trimethoprim/sulfamethoxazole 160/800 mg twice per day for 3 days as prescribed. She was unable to get out of bed this morning by herself due to feeling faint, so her spouse brought her to the ED. Her admission vital signs are temperature 38.80°C, heart rate 106, blood pressure 94/56, respiratory rate 22. A complete blood count (CBC) reveals white blood cell (WBC) 13.4, hemoglobin (Hgb) 6.8, platelets within normal limits. From the patient's history and review of symptoms, the AGACNP suspects that the patient has celiac disease (CD). Along with rehydration and a gastroenterology consult, the AGACNP could order which of the following to support the diagnosis?

A. Calcium, vitamin D, vitamin K, iron, folate, vitamin B_{12} levels

B. Unit of packed red blood cells (PRBCs) to treat the patient's anemia

C. Gluten-free diet to improve the patient's symptoms

D. Immunoglobulin A (IgA) tissue transglutaminase

49. A 63-year-old female patient with a history of cirrhosis is brought to the ED with acute hematemesis and altered mental status. The patient is hypotensive and tachycardic and is vomiting blood. After intubation and fluid resuscitation, she is taken to endoscopy, where multiple large varicosities are seen. The gastroenterologist infuses octreotide and vasopressin and attempts band ligation and sclerotherapy, all of which help slow the bleeding. Laboratory studies reveal hemoglobin 6.8 g/dL, platelets 90,000/mm³, international normalized ratio 2.8. After blood product resuscitation, the patient remains borderline hypotensive at 94/55 mmHg and continues to slowly bleed. What would be the *next best temporary* treatment intervention until she stabilizes?

A. Placement of a Sengstaken–Blakemore tube

B. Transjugular intrahepatic portosystemic shunt (TIPS)

C. Hepatic transplantation

D. Continuation of fluid resuscitation and transfusion

50. A 38-year-old male patient is brought to the ED after a minor motor vehicle crash. He was found intoxicated behind the wheel with the airbag deployed. The driver states that he usually never drinks but that he was at a party and had too much. Which liver enzyme levels would lead the AGACNP to believe that this may not be an isolated episode?

A. Aspartate aminotransferase (AST) 83 unit/L, alanine transaminase (ALT) 50 unit/L, gamma-glutamyl transferase (GGT) 150 unit/L

B. AST 45 unit/L, ALT 55 unit/L, GGT 245 unit/L

C. AST 678 unit/L, ALT 828 unit/L, GGT 60 unit/L

D. AST 30 unit/L, ALT 28 unit/L, GGT 45 unit/L

51. A 68-year-old male patient is admitted from the ED with chief complaints of increased fatigue, dyspnea with mild exertion, black tarry stools, and abdominal pain. The patient rates his abdominal pain as 8 to 9 out of 10 and describes it as gnawing, with radiation to the back. The pain is constant but not always severe. The patient also notes that his abdomen is getting increasingly bigger and thinks that is why he is short of breath. He has taken Tylenol, Advil, Maalox, and Pepcid with minimal relief. This has been occurring with increased frequency over the last 48 hours, with constant pain varying from 4 to 10 out of 10. With this episode, the pain was more intense. He has not been able to sleep for two nights. Past medical-surgical history includes alcohol use disorder, esophageal varices, diabetes mellitus for 10 years, and coronary artery disease for 10 years. The patient has been abstaining from alcohol for the last 6 months. Vital signs are blood pressure 84/40, heart rate 112, respiratory rate 24, temperature 38.3°C. The AGACNP is concerned for what *priority* complication that may be occurring in this patient with liver cirrhosis?

A. Anemia with possible gastrointestinal (GI) bleed

B. Portal vein hypertension

C. Hepatorenal syndrome

D. Sepsis from spontaneous bacterial peritonitis

52. A 42-year-old male patient with a history of IV drug use and HIV, who has been only intermittently compliant with his treatment, is admitted to the hospital for emergent perforated appendicitis. A needlestick event occurs on the unit, and per hospital protocol the AGACNP orders a hepatitis panel and a CD4 count. The patient's hepatitis panel has the following positive results: immunoglobulin G (IgG), total antibody to hepatitis B core antigen (anti-HBc), Hepatitis B surface antigen (HbsAg), Immunoglobulin M antibody to hepatitis B core antigen (IgM-anti-HBc). The AGACNP interprets this test and tells the patient what the results mean. What does the AGACNP tell the patient?

A. "Your lab results are showing that you have an acute hepatitis B (HBV) infection."

B. "Your lab results are showing that you have a chronic HBV infection."

C. "Your HIV provider will most likely change your HIV medication to manage these results."

D. "Sometimes your HIV treatment can make you more susceptible to other diseases."

53. A 68-year-old patient with a past medical history of sarcoidosis on chronic steroid therapy, cirrhosis, coronary artery disease (CAD), diverticulitis, and diabetes mellitus type 2 is a patient in the ICU and develops abdominal rigidity, severe left lower quadrant abdominal pain, and acute rebound tenderness and guarding on abdominal exam. The patient becomes hypotensive and tachycardic. Laboratory data reveal rising lactic acidosis, leukocytosis, and normal serum creatinine. A STAT CT of the abdomen and pelvis reveals free intraperitoneal fluid and thickened descending colon wall with free air under the diaphragms. The most appropriate *priority* next step for the AGACNP is to:

A. Start vasopressor therapy to maintain mean arterial pressure (MAP) of 65 mmHg

B. Start broad-spectrum antimicrobial therapy

C. Give intravenous fluid boluses with normal saline

D. Consult colorectal surgery for emergency laparotomy

54. A 20-year-old female patient with a past medical history of diabetes mellitus type 1 presents with a 24-hour history of acute-onset right lower quadrant pain that started peri-umbilically and is now localized to the right lower quadrant. She has had nausea and has vomited twice, is positive for fever and anorexia, and has a low-grade temperature of 38°C. Pain intensity increases with movement. Labs are notable for a leukocytosis with bandemia. On exam, she has a positive Rovsing sign with point tenderness at McBurney point. On CT of the abdomen and pelvis, the appendix is greater than 6 mm in diameter and also demonstrates peri-appendiceal inflammatory changes that did not present on ultrasound. Based on this clinical picture, the AGACNP is concerned that the patient has:

A. Acute ruptured appendicitis

B. Acute acalculous cholecystitis

C. Gallstone pancreatitis

D. Diverticulitis

55. Hepatitis C virus (HCV) does not have a vaccine, and its incidence is underreported in the United States and across the world. However, HCV can be treated. The AGACNP is aware that the first direct-acting antiviral drug that can irradiate 90% of chronic HCV is:

   A. Ribavirin
   B. PEG-IFN-a 2a
   C. Ledipasvir-sofosbuvir
   D. Adefovir dipivoxil

56. A 64-year-old male patient is admitted with a 3-day history of initial diffuse abdominal pain. He reports anorexia, nausea, and constipation since symptom onset. Today, he awoke with fever of 38.4°C, localized left lower quadrant pain, and abdominal distention. Labs reveal hemoglobin 13.5; C-reactive protein 52 mg/L; white blood count 12,000. ED workup includes a CT of the abdomen, which shows bowel wall thickening and fat stranding. The AGACNP knows that the next step in the management plan should be:

   A. Surgical consult for exploratory laparoscopy
   B. NPO, intravenous (IV) fluid resuscitation, and IV antibiotics
   C. Gastric decompression and IV fluids
   D. Colonoscopy

57. The AGACNP has been consulted to assist with the diagnosis and management of a patient with severe hypernatremia (161 mEq/L). The AGACNP reviews the findings: 64-year-old male patient with no previous medical history recently diagnosed with craniopharyngioma is 10 days post surgical mass resection with increased urine output. Additional workup reveals serum osmolality 317 mOsm/kg, urine osmolality 100 mOsm/kg, glucose 115 mg/dL, HCO_3 24, HbA1C 6.4, serum ketone negative. Twenty-four–hour urine collection reveals polyuria (4 L/24 hours). The AGACNP orders a water deprivation test with a follow-up urine osmolality post desmopressin increasing to 850 mOsm/kg and decreasing urine output. Which is the *most* likely diagnosis?

   A. Syndrome of inappropriate antidiuretic hormone (SIADH)
   B. Central diabetes insipidus (DI)
   C. Nephrogenic DI
   D. Diabetic ketoacidosis (DKA)

58. In addition to cessation of lithium, the first-line treatment for lithium-induced nephrogenic diabetes insipidus (DI) is:

   A. Amiloride (Midamor)
   B. Nonsteroidal anti-inflammatory drugs (NSAIDs)
   C. Desmopressin (DDAVP)
   D. Clozapine (Clozaril)

59. A 40-year-old female patient with previous medical history of chronic hypokalemia and hypertension presents to the ED for headache and palpitations. Her medications include amlodipine 10 mg daily, lisinopril 20 mg daily, labetalol 200 mg 2× daily, and potassium chloride 20 mEq 2× daily. Vital signs are blood pressure (BP) 180/100 mmHg, heart rate (HR) 115 bpm. Physical exam is unrevealing with no abnormal heart tones, abdominal bruit, or peripheral edema. Initial labs are glucose 133, K^+ 2.5 mEq/L, Na^+ 136 mEq/L, HCO_3 30 mEq/L. She is given labetalol intravenously (IV) and K-Cl supplementation. Despite aggressive K-Cl supplementation (~140 mEq/day), she remains hypokalemic (K^+ 2.9). Further workup includes cortisol 15 mcg/dL, Thyroid-stimulating hormone (TSH) 3.5 milli-units/L, plasma metanephrines normal, aldosterone (plasma aldosterone concentration [PAC] 20 ng/dL), renin (plasma renin activity [PRA] 0.4 ng/mL/hr), and aldosterone-renin ratio 50 ng/dL per ng/mL/hr. Given these findings, the *most* likely diagnosis for this patient is:

   A. Pheochromocytoma
   B. Adrenal insufficiency (AI)
   C. Primary aldosteronism (PA)
   D. Hyperthyroidism

60. In DKA management, transitioning insulin infusion to a subcutaneous long-acting basal and rapid-acting insulin regimen is *most* appropriate after:

    A. Blood glucose is less than 250 mg/dL
    B. HCO_3 has normalized
    C. Anion gap (AG) has closed
    D. K^+ has normalized

61. The most common cause of hypothyroidism is:

    A. Addison disease
    B. Autoimmune thyroiditis
    C. Graves disease
    D. Exogenous glucocorticoids

62. A 58-year-old male patient with a past medical history of arthritis presents to the ED with complaints of acute-onset flank pain with radiation to the groin. He reports that the pain appears to be worse with movement. The patient also notes painful urination and blood-tinged urine. The clinical exam reveals a distressed male patient who grimaces while moving to try to find a comfortable position. He complains of severe pain in the costovertebral angle with palpitation. The abdominal exam is negative. A urinary analysis reveals the following: color = cloudy, pH = 4.5, 10 red blood cells per high-power field, 0 white blood cells (WBCs), and positive uric acid crystals. Considering examination findings and urinary analysis results, the most likely diagnosis is:

    A. Cystitis
    B. Nephrolithiasis
    C. Pyelonephritis
    D. Prostatitis

63. A 60-year-old patient with a history of type 2 diabetes mellitus (DM) and systolic heart failure presents to the ED with complaints of fatigue, painful urination and urinary frequency with urgency, and acute onset of fever and chills. The patient reports recent prostate needle biopsy. Vital signs reveal blood pressure 79/42, heart rate 133, respiration 25, temperature 102°F, and oxygen saturation 89% on room air. The patient received levofloxacin 3 months ago for similar urinary symptoms and again as a pre-procedure prophylaxis. What is the most appropriate initial course of action for the AGACNP?

    A. Obtain blood and urine cultures, initiate sepsis bundle, and admit patient to the hospital.
    B. Obtain urinalysis and culture; manage outpatient with trimethoprim–sulfamethoxazole.
    C. Consult urology.
    D. Consult infectious disease services.

64. The AGACNP is caring for a patient who was referred for chronic kidney disease with a glomerular filtration rate (GFR) of less than 10 mL/min/1.73 m² and potassium of 5 mEq/L. The patient has a history of systolic heart failure, hypertension, and type 2 diabetes mellitus. Which medication should the AGACNP immediately discontinue?

    A. Furosemide (Lasix)
    B. Hydralazine (Apresoline)
    C. Insulin determir (Levemir)
    D. Spironolactone (Aldactone)

65. An older adult patient presents with an acute change in mental status. They are found to have a white blood cell count (WBC) of 22,000 with 26% bands and lactic acid of 4.4 mmol/L. Urinalysis is positive for 3+ leukocyte esterase, 2+ nitrites, and 100 WBCs. Chest x-ray is clear. The patient has received 4 L of normal saline, and the blood pressure is 70/40. A central line is placed, and norepinephrine (Levophed) is started. The AGACNP identifies the patient's admitting diagnosis as:

   A. Urinary tract infection (UTI)
   B. Sepsis secondary to UTI
   C. Septic shock secondary to UTI
   D. Pyelonephritis

66. A possible cause of prerenal acute kidney injury is:

   A. Acute glomerulonephritis
   B. Malignant prostate hyperplasia
   C. Hypovolemia due to hemorrhage
   D. Acute tubular necrosis

67. Test–retest reliability measures:

   A. Consistency of scores over time
   B. Consistency of scores obtained from two equal halves of the same exam
   C. Consistency with which a test measures a single construct or concept
   D. Degree of agreement between two or more scores

68. An AGACNP reads a research report that indicates that the p-value was less than 0.05. The AGACNP concludes that there was:

   A. Not a significant result; it would have happened only 5/10 times through chance
   B. Not a significant result; it would have happened only 5/100 times through chance
   C. A significant result that would have happened only 5/10 times through chance
   D. A significant result that would have happened only 5/100 times through chance

69. The AGACNP's role in research includes:

   A. Principal investigator
   B. Data collector
   C. Statistician
   D. All of the above

70. Which of the following is considered a scientific method used in action-oriented learning that impacts change and a desired outcome?

   A. PDSA
   B. NQF
   C. NDNQI
   D. PICOT

71. What is the difference between quantitative and qualitative research?

   A. Quantitative research proves hypotheses.
   B. Quantitative research measures several variables.
   C. Qualitative research explores experiences.
   D. Qualitative research needs data to support the findings.

72. The AGACNP is developing a quality improvement (QI) project for decreasing falls in older adults admitted to medical-surgical floors. When preparing for the project, the AGACNP knows the highest quality of evidence will be obtained from:

    A. Randomized control trial

    B. Expert opinion

    C. Cohort study

    D. Case series

73. When developing a PICOT question, the AGACNP knows this mnemonic represents:

    A. Person, intervention, computer, occupation, and testimonial

    B. Population, intervention, comparison, outcome, and time frame

    C. Population, interaction, comparison, outcome, and time frame

    D. Person, intervention, comparison, outcome, and time frame

74. Which kind of measure captures results and is meant to improve understanding of how healthcare processes affect patient results?

    A. Process

    B. Outcome

    C. Structure

    D. Quality

75. The *first* step in the quality improvement (QI) process is to:

    A. Select a theoretical model and an implementation model

    B. Identify a care process or outcome issue

    C. Monitor data for continued improvements

    D. Implement change

76. Which of the following is an example of dissemination?

    A. Inquiring about a new quality improvement (QI) project

    B. Identifying a care process that requires improvement

    C. Publishing the results of a QI project in a peer-reviewed journal

    D. Developing a new standard operating procedure

77. An 80-year-old woman with a history of end-stage renal disease who receives hemodialysis three times a week presents to the hospital with pneumonia. She states that she would like to stop dialysis treatments. The patient is alert and oriented and able to state that she knows if she stops dialysis, she will die. Her family members are asking that dialysis be performed. What is the *best* way to proceed?

    A. Obtain a court order to perform dialysis.

    B. Perform dialysis as scheduled, as her family requested, to avoid legal liability.

    C. Have a meeting with the patient and family to discuss the decision to stop dialysis.

    D. Order an ethics consultation.

78. One of the five requirements for informed consent is:

    A. Patient must be financially compensated for research

    B. Patient must be persuaded into consenting

    C. Patient must be given 48 hours to consider the risks and benefits before they can consent

    D. Patient must receive full disclosure of risks, benefits, and alternatives

79. The AGACNP student understands they may take their certification exam through which organization?

A. American Nurses Credentialing Center (ANCC)

B. American Association of Colleges of Nursing (AACN)

C. American Geriatrics Society (AGS)

D. American Association of Nurse Practitioners (AANP)

80. The AGACNP is caring for a patient with septic shock secondary to community-acquired pneumonia. The patient requires a central venous catheter due to lack of intravenous access and increasing demand for vasopressors. After the AGACNP reviews the procedure, risks, and benefits, the patient is unable to state the reasoning for the procedure. The AGACNP knows the patient:

A. Lacks competency

B. Lacks capacity

C. Can consent for the procedure

D. Requires intubation

81. The AGACNP is caring for a patient who is deemed to lack competency. The AGACNP understands this determination comes from:

A. A judge

B. An attending physician

C. The AGACNP caring for the patient

D. The next of kin

82. The AGACNP is caring for a critically ill patient who requires a central venous catheter for administration of osmotic therapy to reduce brain swelling. The AGACNP is credentialed for this procedure and places a subclavian central venous catheter. The chest x-ray to confirm placement reveals a new pneumothorax on the side of the line placement. The AGACNP discusses this complication openly with the patient's healthcare proxy. The AGACNP is displaying:

A. Autonomy

B. Nonmaleficence

C. Accountability

D. Justice

83. Which model helps define the advanced practice role to patient population focus?

A. Synergy

B. Consensus

C. STAR

D. Collaborative practice

84. What is defined as the clinical activities within a healthcare facility that the provider has the right to perform?

A. Privileges

B. Credentialing

C. Certification

D. Licensure

85. An AGACNP student understands the ethical principle of nonmaleficence concerns:

A. Being honest

B. Keeping promises

C. Being obligated to do no harm

D. Respecting patients' right to make decisions about their own healthcare

86. The AGACNP should perform a hepatitis screening panel for which of the following patients?

    A. 55-year-old veteran who served in Vietnam

    B. 16-year-old male high school student

    C. 17-year-old female with a history of transfusion

    D. 80-year-old female with hepatic steatosis

87. The most likely victim of suicide by a firearm is a:

    A. 75-year-old man

    B. 22-year-old gang member

    C. 45-year-old hunter

    D. 30-year-old woman

88. A patient with a history of anxiety who takes lorazepam 0.5 mg TID PRN is being discharged after fracturing three ribs. Discharge medications include Tylenol, Robaxin, and oxycodone. The patient should also be prescribed:

    A. Naloxone

    B. Percocet

    C. Vicodin

    D. Ketamine

89. Healthcare disparities among Black, Hispanic, and White Americans of all age groups have been decreasing since 2014. This is largely due to:

    A. Access to health insurance

    B. Genetic modifications

    C. Better patient education

    D. Enhanced diet

90. AGACNPs discuss code status with each patient admitted to the hospital. This represents which type of prevention?

    A. Primary

    B. Secondary

    C. Tertiary

    D. Quaternary

91. A 22-year-old college student is being discharged after a motor vehicle crash. Surgical care includes splenectomy and right femur rodding. Which vaccines are needed upon discharge?

    A. Diphtheria–tetanus (DT) and human papillomavirus (HPV)

    B. Influenza and COVID-19

    C. PPSV23 and quadrivalent meningococcal vaccine

    D. Hepatitis A and B

92. Which patient requires stress ulcer prophylaxis?

    A. Female patient admitted for elective right knee replacement

    B. Male patient admitted for a ST-segment elevation myocardial infarction (STEMI)

    C. Female patient admitted for cesarean delivery

    D. Patient on mechanical ventilation for 48 hours

93. The AGACNP is caring for a patient who is on mechanical ventilation. Which strategy prevents ventilator-associated pneumonia (VAP)?

    A. Change the ventilator circuit every 24 hours.
    B. Perform spontaneous breathing trials every 24 hours.
    C. Interrupt sedation once every 48 hours.
    D. Perform spontaneous breathing trials every 48 hours.

94. An older adult male patient with stage IV lung cancer indicates that he would like to discontinue his treatment and be changed to comfort care. The patient is concerned that his family will not support his wishes and asks how to be sure his end-of-life wishes are honored. The AGACNP should *first* ask the patient if he:

    A. Has identified a durable power of attorney
    B. Has an advance directive
    C. Has discussed this with his family
    D. Would like to speak with a chaplain

95. The AGACNP is caring for a patient with a diagnosis of acute upper gastrointestinal hemorrhage. The venous thromboembolism (VTE) prophylaxis indicated at this time is:

    A. None; it is contraindicated
    B. Low-molecular-weight heparin
    C. Vitamin K antagonist
    D. Sequential compression device

96. A 29-year-old male patient had a laceration repair to his right heel 1 week ago. Although his stitches have yet to be removed, he goes swimming in a pond. A few days later, he is febrile with erythema that extends from the foot to the thigh. The right leg is edematous, the skin is tense, and his pain appears out of proportion. Labs have been sent. He is hypotensive, not responding to fluid resuscitation. Which of the following is the appropriate treatment?

    A. Obtain a STAT compartment pressure.
    B. Obtain a STAT CT scan of the right lower extremity.
    C. Obtain STAT three-view x-rays of the right lower extremity.
    D. Start a pressor, consider corticosteroids if pressure is unresponsive, consult surgery, order broad-spectrum antibiotics.

97. The AGACNP is called to the bedside of a trauma patient being admitted to the surgical ICU. The patient is on vasopressin and has persistent hypotension with a mean arterial pressure of 45. As the AGACNP prepares to place a central line, the intravenous (IV) pump alarms with "occlusion" flashing in red letters. Upon further investigation, the hand where the IV is inserted is swollen and cool to touch, and the IV does not draw or flush. Which is the *most* appropriate treatment?

    A. Stop the IV, remove the angiocatheters, elevate the extremity, and apply warm compresses.
    B. Keep the IV until the central line is placed and the position is verified, then discontinue the IV.
    C. Apply warm compresses and try to get the IV to restart to continue the infusion while placing the central line.
    D. Stop the IV and call the attending physician to alert that there was an infiltration.

98. The AGACNP is caring for a 58-year-old patient with a history of diabetes and hypertension who presents with right foot redness that has rapidly progressed over the last 24 hours. Imaging of the right lower extremity reveals gas within fluid collections tracking along fascial plans. The patient is febrile, hypotensive, and tachycardic. What is the *most likely* diagnosis?

    A. Stevens–Johnson syndrome
    B. Surgical site infection
    C. Necrotizing fasciitis
    D. Toxic epidermal necrosis

99. A 53-year-old male patient with a history of hypertension and diabetes mellitus type 2 presents with a right lower extremity wound that is not healing. On physical exam, brownish pigmentation of the skin in the lower extremities with diminished hair growth is noted. Dorsalis pedis pulses are 2+ bilaterally. A 2-cm, shallow, nonpainful, round, noninfected ulcer is noted proximal to the right medial malleolus. What is the diagnosis?

    A. Peripheral arterial disease
    B. Diabetic peripheral neuropathy
    C. Chronic venous insufficiency
    D. Acute limb ischemia

100. A 53-year-old male patient with a history of hypertension and diabetes mellitus type 2 presents with a left lower extremity wound that is not healing. On physical exam, diminished hair growth, pale atrophic skin, and nail dystrophy are noted. The patient also endorses claudication. A 2-cm painful ulcer is noted on the left lateral ankle. What type of ulcer is this?

    A. Arterial
    B. Diabetic foot
    C. Venous
    D. Stage 1 pressure

101. After using which of the following inhalers should patients be advised to rinse their mouth with water and then spit?

    A. Levalbuterol
    B. Budesonide
    C. Salmeterol
    D. Tiotropium

102. Which of the following best describes criteria for use of roflumilast in patients with chronic obstructive pulmonary disease (COPD)?

    A. Used as first-line therapy after COPD diagnosis
    B. Used only for patients with high The COPD assessment test (CAT) and Modified Medical Research Council Dyspnea Scale (mMRC Dyspnea Scale) scores
    C. Used acutely in patients with COPD as a rescue medication
    D. Used for patients with acute exacerbations of COPD

103. What is the mechanism of action of albuterol?

    A. Relaxes bronchial muscle on beta-2 receptors
    B. Inhibits acetylcholine at muscarinic receptors
    C. Inhibits IgE binding to receptor on mast cells
    D. Blocks acetylcholine in bronchial smooth muscle

104. An older adult patient with a past medical history of hypertension and alcohol use disorder presents with new-onset confusion, change in vision, headaches, nausea, and photophobia. Vital signs are temperature 101.6°F, heart rate 101, blood pressure 122/79, respiration rate 19, SaO$_2$ 93%. The AGACNP suspects the change in mental status is likely related to:

    A. Hypertensive urgency
    B. Essential hypertension
    C. Meningitis
    D. Hypertensive encephalopathy

105. A 35-year-old female patient presents with weakness, paresthesias, sensory loss, and painful eye movement with unilateral reduction in vision. The AGACNP suspects the patient has:

    A. Myasthenia gravis (MG)
    B. Amyotrophic lateral sclerosis (ALS)
    C. Multiple sclerosis (MS)
    D. Guillain-Barré syndrome (GBS)

106. The AGACNP is caring for a patient with a known brain tumor who presents with progressive weakness in the right hand. Head CT reveals the known tumor but also associated vasogenic edema. To improve the vasogenic edema, the AGACNP orders intravenous (IV):

    A. Mannitol
    B. Hypertonic saline
    C. Dexamethasone
    D. Furosemide

107. An 83-year-old male patient is admitted after a fall. Physical therapy (PT) assesses the patient to determine rehabilitation needs. The AGACNP observes that the patient ambulates slowly and has a stiff gait with minimal arm swing, and his face appears mask-like. The occupational therapy (OT) notes document hand tremors when at rest. PT and OT recommend inpatient rehabilitation for strength training and help with activities of daily living. The AGACNP is concerned the patient may have undiagnosed:

    A. Parkinson disease (PD)
    B. Myasthenia gravis (MG)
    C. Guillain-Barré syndrome (GBS)
    D. Multiple sclerosis (MS)

108. A 65-year-old male patient presents with sudden onset of right-sided weakness and numbness. Which question is *most* important to ask when obtaining a history of present illness?

    A. "What treatments have you tried?"
    B. "Where is the numbness?"
    C. "Where is the weakness?"
    D. "When did the symptoms start?"

109. A 33-year-old male patient with history of schizophrenia, alcohol use disorder, and seizure disorder is brought to the ED after experiencing a grand mal seizure. The patient is now awake. Which should the AGACNP inquire about first?

    A. Active or recent illness
    B. Environmental stressors
    C. Adherence to medication regimen
    D. Sleep habits

110. A 55-year-old female patient presents with acute-onset mental status changes with dysarthria and word-finding difficulties for the last 24 hours. Her spouse reports the patient has had a fever for a few days and is just getting over shingles. Lumbar puncture reveals clear fluid, normal glucose, protein less than 1, and 50% polymorphonuclear neutrophils (PMNs). The most likely diagnoses is:

    A. Encephalitis
    B. Seizure
    C. Primary tumor
    D. Subarachnoid hemorrhage

111. A patient with a past medical history of hypertension presents with complaints of change in vision, headaches, nausea, and one incident of vomiting. Vital signs are temperature 98.6°F, heart rate 88, blood pressure 224/118, respiratory rate 22; SaO_2 95%. While in the ED, the patient becomes progressively more confused. The AGACNP diagnoses the change in mental status as:

    A. Hypertensive urgency
    B. Essential hypertension
    C. Meningitis
    D. Hypertensive encephalopathy

112. An incarcerated patient is brought to the ED after 4 days of intermittent fever, headache, and stiffness in the neck. The patient has become progressively lethargic and confused. The AGACNP's *next* step to confirm the most likely diagnosis is to:

    A. Perform a lumbar puncture
    B. Order an MRI/magnetic resonance angiography (MRA) of the brain
    C. Order a CT scan of the cervical spine
    D. Assess for Brudzinski and Kernig signs

113. A young adult presents with a repetitive clenching of her right hand after being out with friends. She reports stress of final exams and not sleeping. With recent use of which drug should the AGACNP be *most* concerned?

    A. Marijuana
    B. Heroin
    C. Nicotine
    D. Cocaine

114. A middle-aged man presents with bilateral lower extremity weakness. He reports having had a viral illness 2 weeks prior and having recently developed neck and back pain. He says his feet were weak at first and then he noticed the weakness increasing to his knees and into his hips. He is now unable to stand. Exam reveals reduced deep tendon reflexes in the Achilles and patellar tendons. The AGACNP should order:

    A. Glucocorticoids
    B. Physical therapy
    C. Vital capacity
    D. Antiviral therapy

115. A young adult presents with complaints of facial weakness. Her eyes are mainly affected; she reports diplopia and difficulty opening her eyes. She expresses difficulty chewing and swallowing food. She reports having normal strength upon awakening and continued weakness as the day progresses. The AGACNP suspects:

    A. Bell palsy (BP)
    B. Multiple sclerosis (MS)
    C. Myasthenia gravis (MG)
    D. Guillain-Barré syndrome (GBS)

116. Which is accurate regarding symptoms and physical findings in patients with acute respiratory distress syndrome (ARDS)?

    A. Absence of bilateral crackles
    B. Bradycardia and bradypnea
    C. Hypertension more common than hypotension
    D. Absence of intravascular overload

117. A 17-year-old male patient presents to the ED after a 5-mile run. He complains of shortness of breath and chest pain radiating to the right shoulder. Vital signs are within normal limits, except for heart rate of 110 bpm. On examination, the trachea is midline, and point of maximum impulse is not displaced. Breath sounds are absent on the right side, and percussion note is hyperresonant. What is the AGACNP's *next* step?

    A. STAT chest x-ray (CXR)
    B. Arterial blood gas (ABG)
    C. Chest CT pulmonary embolism (PE) protocol
    D. Tube thoracotomy

118. A 22-year-old female patient presents with mild chest pain and shortness of breath. She has just finished a 12-hour shift in labor and delivery. She has no past medical history. The AGACNP obtains a chest x-ray that demonstrates a 20% pneumothorax (PTX) on the right side. Her vital signs are stable. What is the plan of care for this patient?

    A. Needle decompression
    B. Observation
    C. Surgical consult for video-assisted thoracoscopic surgery
    D. Discharge with follow-up studies in 48 hours

119. The AGACNP is called to evaluate a 68-year-old female patient who had a total hip replacement just over 48 hours ago. The history is significant for osteoarthritis, hypertension, and asthma. On examination, the patient is confused, hypotensive, tachypneic, and tachycardic. Lung auscultation has bronchial breath sounds on the right side. What is the *most* likely diagnosis?

    A. Community-acquired pneumonia
    B. Heart failure
    C. Hospital-associated pneumonia
    D. Acute asthma

120. A 75-year-old male patient presents with complaints of general malaise, productive cough for the last 5 days, and pleuritic chest pain. Vital signs are temperature 101.4°F, blood pressure 110/60, heart rate 115, respiratory rate 30, pulse oximetry 92%. Chest x-ray is positive for consolidation in the right upper lobe. Laboratory findings are pending. What is the *next* step?

    A. Order empiric antibiotics.
    B. Wait for laboratory results.
    C. Order an antiviral agent.
    D. Prepare for intubation.

121. A 42-year-old woman presents to the hospital with a probable diagnosis of community-acquired pneumonia. Her chest x-ray shows a large pleural effusion. The AGACNP performs a thoracentesis and obtains the following results: color: viscous, cloudy; pH: 7.11; protein: 5.8 g/dL; lactate dehydrogenase (LDH): 285 unit/L; glucose: 66 mg/dL; white blood count (WBC): 3,800/mm³; red blood cells (RBC): 24,000/mm³. Gram stain: many PMN, no organisms seen. What is the *next* step in management of this patient?

    A. Tube thoracostomy
    B. Diuresis
    C. Antiviral agent
    D. Video-assisted thoracoscopic surgery (VATS) with pleurodesis

122. A 55-year-old female patient presents with complaints of shortness of breath and productive cough of yellow sputum for the past week. Based on the patient's presentation, which ultrasound finding would the AGACNP expect to see?

    A. Absence of lung sliding
    B. Lung point
    C. A-lines
    D. B-lines

123. The AGACNP is seeing a 60-year-old female patient with emphysema. The AGACNP knows the only way to prevent continuing deterioration of the patient's lung function is for her to:

    A. Take anticholinergics as prescribed
    B. Take short-acting and long-acting beta-2 agonists as prescribed
    C. Avoid cigarette smoking
    D. Take corticosteroids as prescribed

124. The AGACNP is managing a patient with acute exacerbation of chronic obstructive pulmonary disease (COPD) in the ICU. The AGACNP is contemplating noninvasive positive pressure ventilation (NIPPV). Which finding would prohibit the AGACNP from ordering NIPPV?

    A. $PaCO_2$ of 50 mmHg
    B. Copious secretions
    C. PaO_2 of 56 mmHg
    D. Hyperinflation of lungs with flattened diaphragm

125. The AGACNP is seeing a 67-year-old male patient who is in acute respiratory failure and has a medical history of emphysema with acute exacerbations at least three times a year. The AGACNP reviews the following arterial blood gases (ABGs) on noninvasive ventilation with FIO_2 of 45%, pressure support of 12 cm H_2O, and positive end-expiratory pressure of 5 cm H_2O: pH 7.39, $PaCO_2$ 52 mmHg, PaO_2 60 mmHg, HCO_3 30 mEq/L, and SaO_2 91%. Based on this ABG, what type of acute respiratory failure is this patient experiencing?

    A. I
    B. II
    C. III
    D. IV

126. The AGACNP is called to admit a pregnant patient at 36 weeks' gestation. Vital signs are temperature 37.6°C, heart rate 100, respiratory rate 24, blood pressure (BP) 136/76, O_2 Sat 96%. Labs are basic metabolic panel (BMP) normal, complete blood count with white blood count 10.8, hemoglobin 12.0/hematocrit 36, platelet count 58,000 mm³, aspartate transaminase aspartate transaminase (AST) 200, total bilirubin 2.4, lactate dehydrogenase (LDH) 800, serum haptoglobin 20 mg/dL. The *most* likely diagnosis is:

    A. Eclampsia
    B. Preeclampsia
    C. HELLP syndrome
    D. Peripartum cardiomyopathy

127. A 36-year-old pregnant patient who has recently arrived in the United States and has had no prenatal care presents with a severe headache. Blood pressure (BP) is 170/120, basic metabolic panel shows blood urea nitrogen 24, creatinine is 1.7, urinalysis (UA) shows proteinuria. What is the most likely diagnosis?

    A. Eclampsia
    B. Preeclampsia
    C. HELLP syndrome
    D. Severe preeclampsia

128. A patient with diabetes complains of pain in the feet. They describe it as tingling, with shooting pains and intermittent burning. The AGACNP should prescribe:

    A. Lidocaine (Lidoderm) patch
    B. Ibuprofen (Motrin)
    C. Gabapentin (Neurontin)
    D. Hydromorphone (Dilaudid)

129. A patient with chronic kidney disease has bilateral rib fractures and is complaining of 10/10 pain. Incentive spirometry has dropped to 250 mL despite Lidoderm patch, Tylenol and Flexeril around the clock, and oxycodone 10 mg q4h prn. What should the AGACNP do next?

    A. Add ibuprofen 800 mg q8h.
    B. Consult anesthesia for an epidural.
    C. Consult respiratory therapy for bilevel positive airway pressure (BiPAP).
    D. Add ketorolac (Toradol) 30 mg q6h.

130. A patient who suffered a cardiac arrest and achieved return of spontaneous circulation (ROSC) is now hospital day 3. Sedation has been off for 48 hours. Vital signs: temperature 37.6°C, heart rate 90, respiratory rate 16, blood pressure 140/80, sat 96%. Vent settings are 500 × 16 40%, 5PEEP. The patient does not overbreathe the ventilator. No spontaneous movement has been noted since admission. Neurologic exam reveals absence of corneal, cough, and gag reflexes. Pupils are 4 mm and unresponsive. The next step is:

    A. Spontaneous breathing trial (SBT)
    B. CT of brain
    C. Neurosurgery consultation
    D. Formal brain death testing

131. A patient who suffered a cardiac arrest 48 hours ago remains unresponsive to pain and voice and has no spontaneous movements despite never being on sedation. They are able to breathe over the ventilator, and pupils are 3 mm and reactive. Vasopressors remain on and are difficult to wean off. MRI shows a severe anoxic brain injury. Family is adamant the patient would not want heroic measures and was made "do not resuscitate" (DNR). What should the AGACNP anticipate?

    A. Consulting palliative care
    B. Performing a spontaneous breathing trial (SBT) and extubating
    C. Referring for organ donation after cardiac death
    D. Planning a family meeting for 72 hours after return of spontaneous circulation (ROSC)

132. The AGACNP is caring for a trauma patient in the ED. The patient presented with hypotension and systolic blood pressure 88 mmHg, required bag-mask ventilation, and is stridorous on arrival. The AGACNP knows the level of trauma activation is:

    A. 3
    B. 2
    C. 1
    D. Emergency

133. The AGACNP is caring for a patient who presents after falling more than 20 feet off a cliff. The patient is conscious but is cool, clammy, and anxious. Blood pressure is 79/45, and heart rate is 134. The patient has an obvious right lower extremity deformity with a thigh that appears to be enlarging in size. The AGACNP is concerned about:

    A. Spinal shock
    B. Hemorrhagic shock
    C. Adrenal insufficiency
    D. Pulmonary embolism

134. The AGACNP is caring for a patient who presents after falling more than 20 feet off a cliff. The patient is conscious but is cool, clammy, and anxious. Blood pressure is 79/45, and heart rate is 134. The patient has an obvious right lower extremity deformity with a thigh that appears to be enlarging in size. The AGACNP will *first* order:

    A. Massive transfusion protocol
    B. Abdominal CT scan with and without contrast
    C. Dopamine infusion
    D. Lactated Ringer fluid bolus

135. A frail older adult patient who lives alone is admitted after being found on the floor. They are noted to have a body mass index (BMI) of 17. The AGACNP's *first* priority is to:

    A. Start a regular diet
    B. Monitor phosphorous levels
    C. Obtain albumin and prealbumin levels
    D. Order physical and occupational therapy and social work consults

136. A patient is brought from the scene of a car accident in which metal scaffolding fell from a bridge, impaling the patient. The patient was intubated at the scene for a Glasgow Coma Scale score of 7. The patient has obvious head and lower extremity trauma. What is the level of trauma activation?

    A. 1
    B. 2
    C. 3
    D. 4

137. The AGACNP is caring for an adult trauma patient who was involved in a heavy machinery accident in which a forklift fell onto the patient. The patient presents with heart rate 155, respiratory rate 40, blood pressure 77/45, and estimated blood loss 2.5 L. What class of hemorrhagic shock is this patient experiencing?

    A. I
    B. II
    C. III
    D. IV

138. A patient with a history of depression presents after being found at home in bed in an altered mental state after ingesting multiple substances with an unknown time of ingestion. Last known well is 24 hours ago. Vital signs are temperature 37.6°C, heart rate 105, respiratory rate 16, sat 95%. Pupils are 3 mm and reactive, and sclera have mild jaundice. The patient withdraws to pain and opens eyes briefly to voice of attending examiner for 10-second intervals. Labs reveal international normalized ratio 2.0, aspartate aminotransferase (AST) 4250, alanine aminotransferase (ALT) 3805, total bilirubin 3.6. Salicylate level is 10; acetaminophen level is 100. Comprehensive toxicology panel is pending. The most important intervention for this patient is:

    A. Naloxone
    B. Intubation
    C. Flumazenil
    D. *N*-acetylcysteine

139. A patient with a lower gastrointestinal bleed returns to the general care floor after a colonoscopy that showed a diverticular bleed. The bleeding has ceased. The patient recovered in the postanesthesia care unit. When the nurse examines the patient, they are found to be somnolent and minimally responsive to deep pain. Vital signs are temperature 37.6°C; heart rate 60, respiratory rate 8, blood pressure 110/60, sat 92% on 2 L NC. The *most* appropriate intervention(s) for the AGACNP to order is(are):

    A. Arterial blood gas (ABG) and bilevel positive airway pressure (BiPAP)
    B. Intravenous (IV) naloxone and flumazenil
    C. STAT page anesthesia for intubation
    D. Type and screen, transfuse 1 unit packed red blood cells

140. The AGACNP is caring for a patient who is 4 days post pancreas transplantation. The nurse notes that the patient has had increasing insulin requirements for 24 hours. What should the AGACNP suspect?

    A. Acute rejection
    B. Dietary habits causing increased sugar
    C. Normal postoperative course
    D. Chronic rejection

141. A 70-year-old female patient with a history of hypertension and hyperlipidemia is recovering from sepsis from a bowel perforation due to obstruction. The patient was just informed that pathology shows advanced stage IV ovarian cancer with carcinomatosis throughout the abdominal cavity. Her appetite is poor, and she refuses to eat. The oncology team is consulted, but the abdominal wound needs to completely heal (which may take 6 weeks or more) before cancer-directed therapy can be initiated. The patient asks, "What's the point?" What is the AGACNP's *next* step?

    A. Consult palliative care.
    B. Engage physical therapy.
    C. Prescribe an antidepressant.
    D. Order nutritional supplements.

142. A 60-year-old man with a history of severe chronic obstructive pulmonary disease (COPD) is admitted for rib fractures. He is adamant about his code status being do not resuscitate (DNR)/do not intubate (DNI). His ICU course has been rocky and has reached a point where he has been dependent on continuous positive airway pressure (CPAP) 20 at 100% for 5 days. This morning, he desaturated to 60% just taking his inhalers and medications and became severely anxious and short of breath. He wants to be transitioned to comfort care at home. What is the AGACNP's *next* step?

    A. Refer to inpatient hospice.

    B. Facilitate discharge home.

    C. Call anesthesia for intubation.

    D. Order 10 mg morphine and remove CPAP.

143. The AGACNP is caring for an older adult patient with end-stage renal disease and end-stage chronic obstructive pulmonary disease. The patient has a new diagnosis of pancreatic cancer on this admission. The patient tells the AGACNP they no longer want to continue with dialysis and that they want to focus on comfort. The AGACNP begins to talk with the patient about options and mentions which type of care that focuses on symptom management and does not support curative therapies?

    A. Palliative care

    B. Hospice care

    C. Home care services

    D. Rehabilitation-focused care

144. What can assist the AGACNP in identifying inappropriate medication use in older adults?

    A. American Geriatrics Society (AGS) Beers Criteria

    B. CHA_2DS_2VASc score

    C. HAS-BLED score

    D. ORBIT score

145. A 75-year-old patient with colorectal cancer is admitted postoperatively after a colon resection and ostomy creation. On postoperative day 1, the patient reports nausea but tolerates 300 mL clear liquids. The stoma is warm but unable to be fully visualized as it is covered in stool. The AGACNP should order:

    A. Total parenteral nutrition

    B. Peripheral parenteral nutrition

    C. Oral diet with dietary supplements

    D. Placement of postpyloric feeding tube

146. A young adult male patient with cystic fibrosis is being treated with meropenem for *Pseudomonas aeruginosa*pneumonia. He remains ventilated, is becoming more hypoxic, and has increased sputum production. Vital signs are temperature 39.0°C, heart rate 110, respiratory rate 26, blood pressure 100/60, sat 90% on 80% FIO_2 and 10P. What is the AGACNP most concerned about?

    A. Pulmonary embolism (PE)

    B. Carbapenem resistance

    C. Hospital-acquired pneumonia (HAP)

    D. Central line–associated bloodstream infection (CLABSI)

147. A patient has been on a ventilator for the last 3 days due to septic shock from perforated diverticulitis. Ventilator requirements increased from 40% 5P to 60% 10P overnight. The nurse reports thick white secretions and temperature 101.2°F. The morning chest x-ray shows left lower lung (LLL) infiltrate. What is the *most likely* diagnosis?

    A. Pneumonia
    B. Hospital-acquired pneumonia (HAP)
    C. Healthcare-associated pneumonia
    D. Ventilator-associated pneumonia (VAP)

148. A patient who is chronically dependent on parenteral nutrition develops a high fever of 102.8°F. The peripherally inserted central catheter (PICC line) site is reddened with purulent material. The AGACNP's *next* step is to:

    A. Start vancomycin
    B. Discontinue the PICC line
    C. Consult infectious disease
    D. Start cefazolin 2 g intravenously (IV) q8h

149. The AGACNP is caring for a 27-year-old patient admitted for preeclampsia. During morning rounds, the patient endorses dysuria and increased frequency. Urinalysis is positive for nitrates and leukoesterase. What is the diagnosis?

    A. Asymptomatic bacteriuria
    B. Uncomplicated urinary tract infection (UTI)
    C. Complicated UTI
    D. Pyelonephritis

150. The AGACNP is caring for a 27-year-old patient admitted for preeclampsia. During morning rounds, the patient reports dysuria and increased frequency. Urinalysis is positive for nitrates and leukoesterase. What should the AGACNP prescribe?

    A. Ceftriaxone
    B. Nitrofurantoin
    C. Cefazolin
    D. Meropenem

151. The AGACNP teaches a patient with methicillin-resistant *Staphyloccus aureus* (MRSA) in a wound to:

    A. Keep draining wounds uncovered
    B. Wash hands with soap and water or an alcohol-based gel only if the infected skin is draining
    C. Avoid reusing or sharing items that have direct contact with draining wound
    D. Use the chlorinated public swimming pool as it will help dry out the wound

152. The AGACNP understands the risk factors for vancomycin-resistant enterococcus (VRE) include:

    A. Previous antimicrobial therapy
    B. Residing at home with family
    C. Decolonization
    D. Streptococcal throat infection

153. A 44-year-old patient who is homeless presents to the ED with a nonproductive cough for greater than 3 weeks, night sweats, weight loss of more than 10 pounds in 2 weeks, and hemoptysis. These symptoms are most consistent with:

    A. Latent tuberculosis (TB)
    B. Active TB
    C. Bronchitis
    D. Asthma

154. The AGACNP sees a college student who reports she had unprotected sex and now presents with a urinary tract infection. She asks the AGACNP what early signs of HIV are. The AGACNP teaches the patient to monitor for:

    A. Fever, fatigue, myalgias
    B. Night sweats, weight loss, hemoptysis
    C. Fever, productive cough, pleuritic pain
    D. Fever, chills, white plaques on tonsils

155. An adult woman presents after riding a horse that reared up and fell backward onto the patient. She complains of severe pelvis pain. Vital signs are temperature 36.4°C, heart rate 120, respiratory rate 24, blood pressure 80/50, sat 95%. The figure below shows her pelvis x-ray. The AGACNP should:

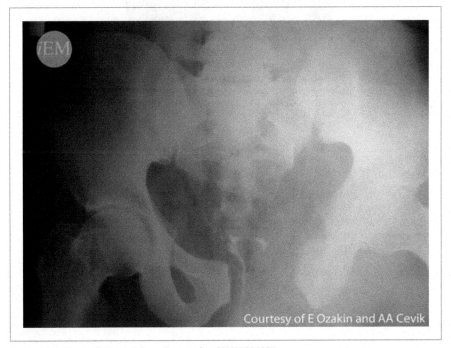

Source: https://www.flickr.com/photos/iem-student/43198254025

    A. Give 1 L normal saline bolus
    B. Apply a pelvic binder
    C. Page orthopedic surgery
    D. Transport to the operating room

156. A patient reports that, in anger, he punched a wall earlier today. The fifth metacarpal is tender to palpation and is ecchymotic and edematous. The x-ray shown below is obtained. What type of fracture is the most likely diagnosis?

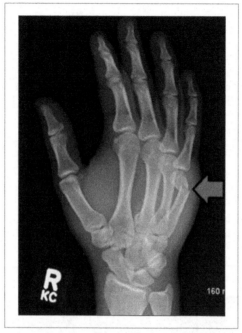

Source: James Heilman, MD, CC BY-SA 4.0 <https://cre-ativecommons.org/licenses/by-sa/4.0> , via Wikimedia Commons. https://upload.wikimedia.org/wikipedia/commons/0/0d/Fractured5thMetacarpalHead2018.jpg

A. Boxer

B. Scaphoid

C. Ulnar styloid

D. Hook of hamate

157. A 25-year-old male patient presents after falling on an outstretched right hand. Physical exam reveals tenderness in the anatomical snuffbox. There is minimal swelling but no obvious deformities. He has been icing the affected area. The best action is to:

A. Apply a spica thumb splint

B. Apply a short arm splint

C. Provide a sling and swathe

D. Refer to physical therapy

158. What test is used to diagnose de Quervain tenosynovitis?

A. Quervain

B. Finkelstein

C. Thumb

D. Lachman

159. An 18-year-old male patient presents with a swollen right hand from punching a wall after an argument. The AGACNP's exam reveals swelling over the ulnar side of the right hand. There is limited movement of the fifth metacarpophalangeal joint secondary to pain. X-rays reveal a fracture of the fifth metacarpal neck of the right hand. The AGACNP is concerned for what fracture?

    A. Colles
    B. Bennett
    C. Boxer
    D. Rolando

160. The AGACNP in the ICU is caring for a 63-year-old woman admitted with a diagnosis of intermediate/submassive pulmonary embolism. She has been resting comfortably in her bed while receiving systemic thrombolytics. Her initial presentation was notable for hypoxia, tachycardia, tachypnea, and mild hemoptysis. During evening rounds, the AGACNP notices that the patient is more somnolent. She tells the AGACNP that she has a new mild headache and is feeling nauseous. Based on this information, what is the AGACNP's most appropriate next action?

    A. Order intravenous (IV) ondansetron for the nausea, and reassess in 30 minutes
    B. Order a STAT partial thromboplastin time to ensure that the current anticoagulation is therapeutic
    C. Order a STAT head CT scan
    D. Notify the pulmonary fellow that the patient is developing signs of obstructive shock

161. A 49-year-old man recently diagnosed with unprovoked venous thromboembolism (VTE) of his right lower extremity has been receiving treatment with a direct oral anticoagulant (DOAC) and is now approaching discharge. The AGACNP in charge of his care is reviewing his discharge instructions. During the review, he asks the AGACNP how long he will need to remain on anticoagulation. How should the AGACNP respond?

    A. "You will need to continue anticoagulation for 3 months or until your deep vein thrombosis (DVT) resolves on venous duplex ultrasound."
    B. "You will need to stay on anticoagulation indefinitely because your DVT is considered unprovoked and happened in the absence of known risk factors."
    C. "You should follow up with your provider in 3 months. At that time if you have no symptoms of post-thrombotic syndrome, you may discontinue anticoagulation."
    D. "Current guidelines recommend that people with unprovoked DVT continue anticoagulation indefinitely or until an inferior vena cava (IVC) filter is placed."

162. The AGACNP is called to a rapid response. On arrival, the AGACNP finds a 49-year-old man lying on a stretcher and appearing severely ill. His nurse reports that he was awaiting a scheduled colonoscopy when he began complaining of nausea, diaphoresis, and crushing chest pressure. On exam, extremities are cool to the touch, skin is diaphoretic, and crackles are auscultated bilaterally. The patient has a history significant for hypertension and hyperlipidemia; he reports that his father died of "a heart attack" at age 42 years. Telemetry reveals sinus bradycardia with a rate of 50, blood pressure (BP) 100/58, and O_2 sat of 92%. What orders are appropriate?

    A. STAT EKG, 2 L/min oxygen via nasal cannula, sublingual nitroglycerin 1 tab, morphine 2 mg intravenously (IV), 325 mg aspirin PO
    B. STAT EKG, sublingual nitroglycerin 1 tab q5min × 3 or until chest pain resolves, morphine 2 mg IV, 325 mg aspirin PO
    C. STAT EKG, 2 L/min oxygen via nasal canula, morphine 2 mg IV, 75 mg clopidogrel PO
    D. STAT EKG, morphine 2 mg IV, normal saline bolus 250 mL over 15 minutes, aspirin 325 mg PO

163. The AGACNP is examining an 81-year-old woman who has just returned to the cardiac step-down unit after placement of a biventricular Automatic Implantable Cardioverter Defibrillator (AICD). Prior to her procedure, she was hemodynamically stable and had no abnormal exam findings. On the AGACNP's repeat assessment, however, the AGACNP is concerned that she is now hypotensive, with muffled heart sounds and an inspiratory decrease in her blood pressure of 20 mmHg. What is the most likely diagnosis?

    A. Cardiac tamponade
    B. Inferior wall myocardial infarction (MI)
    C. Sepsis
    D. Occult hemorrhage

164. The AGACNP is precepting an Advanced Practice Registered Nurse (APRN) student who is working with a male patient admitted for ST-segment elevation myocardial infarction (STEMI) related to known coronary artery disease (CAD). During the student's presentation, they describe the patient's chest discomfort as having increased in severity and frequency compared to their baseline. The discomfort occurs both at rest and with activity. The student asks how to classify these symptoms. The AGACNP responds by stating:

    A. "These symptoms are indicative of Prinzmetal angina."
    B. "The symptoms are consistent with acute aortic dissection."
    C. "This pattern of symptoms is characteristic of unstable angina."
    D. "These symptoms are best described as stable angina."

165. The AGACNP is assessing a 57-year-old man with a diagnosis of severe cardiomyopathy. He complains of terrible dyspnea, fatigue, and anorexia and tells the AGACNP that he is comfortable only at rest. On exam, the AGACNP auscultates coarse crackles throughout. His skin is warm to the touch. The AGACNP notes +3 bilateral lower extremity edema. Which of the following best describes his current New York Heart Association (NYHA) heart failure class?

    A. I
    B. II
    C. III
    D. IV

166. While caring for a patient diagnosed with hypertensive emergency and being treated with a nitroprusside infusion, the AGANCP notes that their current blood pressure reading is 150/90. One hour ago, when they were admitted, their blood pressure was 210/100. Considering this information, what is the next best action?

    A. Decrease nitroprusside infusion.
    B. Increase nitroprusside infusion.
    C. Discontinue nitroprusside and initiate labetalol infusion instead.
    D. Be satisfied with the current blood pressure and continue to monitor.

167. During patient teaching with a woman who was recently diagnosed with a stable aortic dissection, the patient asks the AGACNP why she must now take beta-blockers. How should the AGANCP respond?

    A. "Beta-blockers prevent the dissection from worsening by lowering your blood pressure."
    B. "Beta-blockers have been shown to improve outcomes by stabilizing intralumenal hematomas."
    C. "Beta-blockers work by decreasing your heart rate and reducing the contractility of your heart, which decreases the shearing forces in your aorta."
    D. "We are not entirely sure how beta-blockers contribute to improved outcomes in aortic dissection, but data show that they are beneficial."

168. The AGACNP is managing the care of a 42-year-old woman who has been admitted with new-onset dyspnea. She has a history significant for lumpectomy and radiation for breast cancer 4 months ago, and remote deep vein thrombosis (DVT) when she was in her 20s. Her current vital signs are heart rate (HR) 122, blood pressure (BP) 116/78, sat 94%. What is the clinical probability that she has a pulmonary embolism (PE)?

A. High
B. Likely
C. Intermediate
D. Probable

169. What should the AGACNP monitor when starting a patient on dupilumab (Dupixent)?

A. Cytokine concentrations
B. Blood tryptase levels
C. Liver function
D. Anaphylaxis reaction

170. The AGACNP is caring for a 62-year-old male patient who is 2 weeks status post mitral valve replacement. His nurse reports that the patient has had a persistent fever of greater than 38°C for the last 48 hours. Additionally, he has developed painful raised lesions on his hands and concerning nontender erythematous lesions on the soles of his feet. What other finding would fulfill the Modified Duke Criteria for infective endocarditis (IE)?

A. Presence of Roth spots
B. History of intravenous drug abuse (IVDA)
C. Blood culture + for a Haemophilus, Aggregatibacter, Cardiobacterium, Eikenella, Kingella (HACEK) organism
D. Janeway lesions

171. What information is important to include in discharge teaching for a patient who recently underwent mitral valve replacement with a bioprosthetic valve?

A. "You will need to take anticoagulants for at least 6 months after discharge home."
B. "You should contact your provider for prophylactic antibiotics before any invasive dental procedure."
C. "A sudden increase in discomfort is to be expected, and you can treat it at home with over-the-counter medications including acetaminophen."
D. "Anticoagulation is not indicated for bioprosthetic valves, so you will not need any new prescriptions."

172. Which therapeutics are most likely to be efficacious in treatment of symptoms associated with all types of cardiomyopathies?

A. Aspirin, statin, beta-blockers
B. Diuretics, beta-blockers, calcium channel blockers
C. Nitrates, diuretics, norepinephrine
D. Aspirin, statin, implantable defibrillator

173. The AGACNP working at the medical tent during a large concert sees a 19-year-old woman after a witnessed fainting spell. She is alert and oriented at this time, denies substance use or ingestion of alcohol, and suffered no injuries from the fall. She states she had a sudden sense of fear while standing in the large crowd and that she became light-headed and then "passed out." She is feeling better now and asks how she might prevent this from happening again. What advice should be provided based on her most likely diagnosis?

    A. "You should avoid large crowds and consider having an evaluation by a psychiatric APRN for a possible diagnosis of agoraphobia or panic disorder."

    B. "Consider limiting your intake of caffeine-containing beverages as they are known to precipitate arrythmia, which can cause fainting in some people."

    C. "Drink plenty of water to maintain your hydration, and if you feel light-headed, you can try to apply counterpressure by gripping your hands or crossing your legs."

    D. "When you stand up from your seat, be sure to do so slowly and to wait several minutes before moving to the dance floor."

174. The AGACNP is admitting a patient who has been diagnosed with acute pericarditis. They report a recent flu-like illness but are currently afebrile and without signs and symptoms of an upper respiratory infection. What medication(s) should the AGACNP anticipate ordering for this patient?

    A. Acetaminophen and broad-spectrum antibiotics

    B. Aspirin and ceftriaxone

    C. Toradol and colchicine

    D. Intravenous Immunoglobulin (IVIG)

175. The AGACNP is caring for a female patient who has presented with a 2-week history of fever. She has a history of intravenous (IV) substance use and complains of fatigue, rigors, and painful bumps on her hands and feet. Exam shows that she is ill appearing and has a fever of 39°C and a new right-sided heart murmur. What does the immediate plan for this patient include?

    A. STAT blood cultures, transthoracic echocardiogram, broad-spectrum antibiotics, infectious disease consult

    B. STAT broad-spectrum antibiotics, blood cultures, electrocardiogram, normal saline bolus of 30 mL/kg

    C. Broad-spectrum antibiotics, cardiac MRI, peripherally inserted central catheter line, addiction treatment, referral for opioid substitution therapy

    D. STAT chest x-ray (CXR), broad-spectrum antibiotics, sputum culture, O_2 at 2 L/min

Practice Test: Answers

25

1. **B) Daptomycin**
   This organism is hospital-acquired MRSA because the patient is in the hospital at the time of the infection acquisition. Daptomycin has activity against hospital-acquired MRSA. Clindamycin, doxycycline, and TMP/SMX have activity against community-acquired MRSA but not hospital-acquired MRSA. Ampicillin/sulbactam and nafcillin have activity against methicillin-susceptible *S. aureus* but not MRSA.

2. **A) Re-bolus with furosemide 40 mg IV × one dose and start furosemide IV infusion**
   An appropriate treatment for decompensated heart failure with diuretic resistance is to re-bolus and start an infusion, along with a thiazide diuretic such as metolazone. Decreasing the dose of furosemide to 20 mg IV twice daily would not be appropriate as it would provide less diuresis compared with the current dose of 20 mg IV twice daily. Continuing the furosemide 40 mg IV twice daily and adding bumetanide would not be appropriate as bumetanide is a loop diuretic like furosemide. Adding two medications from the same drug class would be a duplication of therapy. Discontinuing the furosemide 40 mg IV twice daily and starting spironolactone 25 mg PO daily would not be the best treatment option as spironolactone does not provide as much diuresis compared with a loop diuretic like furosemide.

3. **C) Phentolamine**
   Phentolamine is an IV treatment option that is preferred for patients with hypertensive emergency due to pheochromocytoma. Other treatment options that are appropriate for pheochromocytoma include nicardipine and clevidipine. Labetalol, enalaprilat, and hydralazine are not preferred for pheochromocytoma. Additionally, enalaprilat and hydralazine are not treatments of choice for hypertensive emergencies.

4. **B) Hold simvastatin and check creatinine phosphokinase (CPK) level.**
   For patients who experience SAMS, the most appropriate initial treatment option is to hold simvastatin and check CPK level to monitor for risk of rhabdomyolysis. Discontinuing the simvastatin 10 mg PO at bedtime and starting atorvastatin 80 mg PO daily would not be the best choice because simvastatin 10 mg is a low-intensity statin, and atorvastatin 80 mg is a high-intensity statin. After holding the statin and checking CPK level, it is most appropriate to start a low dose of a different statin when rechallenging a patient with SAMS. Continuing the simvastatin and starting gemfibrozil would not be appropriate because gemfibrozil interacts with statins to increase risk of SAMS and should not be used with any statin. Continuing the simvastatin and advising the patient to notify the provider if symptoms do not resolve in 1 week would not be appropriate.

5. **A) Inhaled corticosteroid (ICS)/formoterol**
   Using a combination of an ICS and formoterol is associated with better symptom control and lower risk of exacerbations than using a SABA alone.

6. **D) McBurney**
   McBurney point lies approximately 2 inches away from the anterior–superior iliac spine heading toward the umbilicus. Thus, pain at this site is McBurney sign and is highly indicative of appendicitis. Rosving, obturator, and psoas sign are other clinical signs of appendicitis.

7. **B) Asterixis**
Patients with hepatic encephalopathy who are not comatose often have a clinical finding commonly referred to as asterixis or "liver flap." It is a tremor of the hand when the wrist is extended. Dystonia causes irregular movements mimicking tremors and is often seen with abnormal postures that can be painful and limit voluntary movements. Examples of dystonia include writer's cramp and torticollis. Essential tremors are rhythmic oscillatory movements, typically of the hands, and can be divided into three subgroups: resting, postural, and intention tremors. Parkinsonian tremors are a type of resting tremor.

8. **D) Dry mucous membranes, skin tenting on clavicles**
Signs of dehydration include dry mucous membranes, skin tenting on the clavicles or the backs of the hands, and elevated BUN-to-creatinine ratio and specific gravity greater than 1.030. Patients may also complain of thirst as a symptom of dehydration. Tachycardia can be a sign of dehydration or hypovolemia but can also be caused by multiple other factors, such as fever, pain, and anxiety, and thus is not specific to dehydration. Fevers and tachypnea can cause insensible losses that can lead to dehydration.

9. **A) Aortic stenosis**
Aortic stenosis is a systolic murmur that commences shortly after the S_1, ending just prior to the aortic valve closing. It is due to the left ventricle ejecting blood over a narrowed valve and may radiate to the carotid arteries. Aortic regurgitation is a mid-systolic ejection murmur heard best at the base of the heart. Mitral stenosis is a low-pitched, rumbling, diastolic murmur heard best at the apex with the patient in the left lateral decubitus position. Mitral regurgitation is a diastolic murmur, heard best at the left fifth midclavicular line.

10. **A) S_3**
An S_3 is indicative of high ventricular filling pressures, with abrupt deceleration of flow into the ventricle such as occurs in heart failure. An S_4 is indicative of ventricular hypertrophy, causing stiffness and increased resistance; thus, assessing the patient for hypertension is important to identify the cause of the S_4. A split S_2 can be due to prolonged right ventricular systole such as in right bundle branch block, atrial septal defect, or pulmonary stenosis. A systolic click is caused by mitral valve prolapse.

11. **D) Jugular venous distention**
Hallmark signs and symptoms of cardiac tamponade include muffled heart sounds, jugular venous distention, and hypotension indicating tamponade physiology (Beck triad). Lack of lung sliding and decreased breath sounds are signs and symptoms of pneumothorax.

12. **B) Claudication**
Claudication occurs as a result of ischemia to the muscles during usage. Arterial vasospasm may cause similar symptoms, but it does not typically occur in the iliac, femoral, or leg arteries. Lymphedema refers to the edema caused by the failure of the lymph system to drain the lower extremities and does not present as cramping pain in the legs or buttocks. Poikilothermia refers to the cold temperature of an extremity that occurs with arterial compromise.

13. **D) Peripheral arterial disease**
Chronic ischemia due to lack of arterial blood flow results in skin necrosis that typically starts at the toes. Acute limb ischemia presents with severe, acute leg pain below the level of occlusion. Deep vein thromboses present with edema, commonly unilateral edema, and pulses remain palpable.

14. **C) Peripheral venous disease**
Peripheral venous disease is the result of venous congestion in the lower extremities from incompetent valves in the veins of the legs. Peripheral arterial disease results from insufficient arterial flow to extremities and results in decreased perfusion and thus decreased pulses, decreased ankle-brachial indexes, and decreased hair growth and ischemic wounds that initially appear as dry black areas on toes.

15. **B) Palpates the right upper quadrant (RUQ) deeply and asks the patient to take a deep breath**
Murphy sign is assessing for inflammation of the gallbladder. Palpating the RUQ deeply and asking the patient to take a deep breath will cause the gallbladder to descend onto the fingers of the examiner, causing irritation and compression that result in pain. Palpating deeply in the LLQ and then quickly withdrawing the hand is Rovsing sign. Flexing the patient's right hip and bending the knee, internally rotating, is obturator sign. Asking the supine patient to raise a knee against a hand that applies resistance is psoas sign.

16. **C) 74 years old; no history of falls in past year; takes metformin, lisinopril, and oxybutynin for urge incontinence**
The best initial assessment for fall risk is to ask the patient their fall history. Risk factor for fall is history of fall in the past year and medications that could potentiate falls. The 68- and 72-year-old patients do not have a fall history within the past year and are not taking medications that potentiate falls. The 70-year-old patient indicated a fall history, but it was an isolated event occurring in an unknown environment, and the patient also reports steady gait and is assessed to have no balance or gait difficulty. The 74-year-old patient is an older adult; likely has an acute infection; and takes lisinopril, which could cause orthostatic hypotension, and oxybutynin, which is an anticholinergic.

17. **B) Alprazolam 0.5 mg BID**
Alprazolam is a benzodiazepine and is on the American Geriatrics Society Beers Criteria list of potentially inappropriate medications. Atorvastatin remains appropriate for this patient who has a history of CAD. Lisinopril is also considered appropriate for treatment of CAD and HTN in the context of DM with adequate renal function. Metformin is appropriate for the treatment of diabetes because the patient has adequate GFR.

18. **C) Functional measures**
Functional measures, especially mobility, are high predictors of mortality. Sleep–wake patterns, food intolerances, and social support network are important to assess but do not have a strong association with mortality.

19. **D) Write an order for a bedside commode.**
The patient has functional incontinence related to inability to mobilize to the bathroom. Supporting mobility in older adults is important in order to prevent other complications. The patient does not require bedrest, nor would she meet the criteria for placement of indwelling catheter. Use of incontinence pads will not support the patient's mobility and would not be needed in the presence of a bedside commode.

20. **A) Presence of koilonychia**
Koilonychia is spoon-shaped nails and could represent iron-deficiency anemia. All anemias in older adults should be investigated. Aging skin is fragile and thus tears more easily, eyes are dry as a result of decreased tear production, and decreased secretion of melatonin contributes to altered sleep pattern. These are all normal findings associated with aging.

21. **B) Donepezil (Aricept) and memantine (Namenda)**
Cholinesterase inhibitors such as donepezil (Aricept) and N-methyl-D-aspartate antagonists such as memantine (Namenda) are indicated for slowing the progression of Alzheimer dementia. Carbidopa–levodopa (Sinemet) can be part of therapy for Lewy body dementia with Parkinson disease. Aspirin is indicated along with medical management for underlying vascular issues, hypertension, hyperlipidemia, and diabetes in vascular dementia. Part of Alzheimer treatment is symptom management, which can include antidepressants and anxiolytics, although benzodiazepines and antipsychotics are not first-line therapy for these patients.

22. **B) Start fluoxetine and discharge the patient with a referral for further assessment by a mental health professional**

The PHQ is a screening tool and is validated to be reliable and sensitive for depression. The scores range from 0 to 27. The first two items on the tool constitute the PHQ-2. If there is a score of zero on the first two items, there is no need to continue as a diagnosis of depression cannot be made (anhedonia and blue mood must be present, and these are the target symptoms of the two PHQ-2 questions). Once there is a score of 1 or more on the PHQ-2, the PHQ-9 (seven additional questions added to the PHQ-2) is completed. A score of 15 to 19 indicates that moderate–major depression is likely present. Stroke patients have better outcomes when started on fluoxetine. There is no need for cardiac monitoring when starting an SSRI. SSRIs are first-line therapy for depression but should be ordered only after a mental health professional has done an exam to diagnose depression. The PHQ can then be used to monitor symptoms, but no recommendation exists to base treatment on a screening tool score. The tool is valid even with somatic symptoms. Wellbutrin is not a first-line therapy, especially not without a mental health professional's assessment, and the spouse should not be asked to make a referral on their own.

23. **A) Traumatic brain injury**

Traumatic brain injury, individuals reaching midlife with Down syndrome (trisomy 21), and a genetic susceptibility polymorphism apolipoprotein E4 are all risk factors for neurocognitive disorders due to Alzheimer disease and delirium. Exposure to pesticides and herbicides is a precursor for Parkinson disease. Klinefelter syndrome may involve learning disabilities and delayed speech and language development. Viral illness, including respiratory or gastrointestinal viruses, is often a precursor to Guillain-Barré syndrome.

24. **C) Individuals who face fewer cognitive demands in everyday life are more challenging to assess for functional decline.**

Individuals who face fewer cognitive demands in everyday life are more challenging to assess for functional decline. It is more difficult to conduct cognitive assessments on people with lower educational levels. Memory loss may be considered a natural part of aging in some cultures but not always or in every culture. Highly educated and financially well-off individuals are more likely to notice changes in cognitive function and do have access to care.

25. **B) Restart both medications.**

The patient should be restarted on both medications. He is tolerating oral intake and should be allowed to take his home medications as long as there are no contraindications. Restarting benzodiazepine is important to avoid withdrawal symptoms, which could result in adverse side effects including seizures. He is alert, oriented, and at lower risk for delirium given his age and overall good health status. In older adults or patients with other risk factors for delirium, providers should be cautious with the use of benzodiazepines, and the hospitalization would offer a good opportunity to assess the tolerance of the benzodiazepine or change the treatment plan if necessary.

26. **C) Emergent MRI of the spinal cord**

The patient has prostate cancer with rising PSA and clinical findings indicating potential spinal cord compression due to prostate cancer. Emergent MRI in the spinal region where the pain is occurring is the gold standard diagnostic imaging test unless the patient cannot have MRI.

27. **A) Hydration with intravenous (IV) normal saline**

The patient is presenting with metastatic breast cancer with hyperglycemia as indicated by lab and clinical findings. Appropriate initial treatment includes hydration with normal saline.

28. **C) Lung**

The American Cancer Society states that lung cancer is the number one cause of cancer death in adults.

29. **D) Tumor size, node involvement, metastases**
The tumor, node, metastasis staging tool is used to signify the extent of the disease in cancer.

30. **B) *Pneumocystis* pneumonia (PCP) prophylaxis**
PCP prophylaxis should be initiated as prevention for PCP because post-BMT patients are at highest risk for infection on immunosuppression therapy immediately after discharge for several weeks.

31. **B) Urine sodium, urine creatine, serum sodium, serum creatinine**
The AGACNP must determine the type of AKI (prerenal, intrarenal, or post-renal). Determining the fractional excretion of sodium (FENa) will inform next steps. The patient does not have a history consistent with rhabdomyolysis, so obtaining creatine kinase not needed. Serum and urine creatinine are needed to determine the FENa, and a renal ultrasound is not appropriate at this time.

32. **A) Prerenal acute kidney injury (AKI)**
The patient presentation is consistent with a hypovolemic state, and the labs are consistent with a fractional excretion of sodium (FENa) that is less than 1%, indicating prerenal AKI. The presentation and laboratory findings are not consistent with acute tubular necrosis or post-renal AKI because the FENa would be greater than 1%. Hydronephrosis cannot be diagnosed without imaging.

33. **C) Post-renal AKI**
This presentation is most consistent with post-renal AKI. The patient has a reason for an obstructive process given the known history of BPH and the inability to take tamsulosin due to loss of insurance. Without a blood pressure reading, it is impossible to diagnosis hypertensive emergency. There is not enough information to make it possible to diagnose acute tubular necrosis or prerenal AKI.

34. **A) Acute tubular necrosis**
Muddy brown casts are highly suggestive of acute tubular necrosis. With prerenal AKI, the AGACNP would expect a lower urine sodium. There no evidence of an obstructive process, making post-renal AKI less likely.

35. **A) Normal saline (NS) infusion**
The AGACNP will order NS infusion. Hydration is the only documented preventive measure for CIN. Mucomyst, sodium bicarbonate infusion, and dialysis have not been proven to be preventive of CIN.

36. **C) Calling or emailing the legislator on a stance toward a specific bill**
Grassroots efforts are focused on action at the local level with the aim to impact change at the local, state, or national level. They are associated with bottom-up rather than top-down decision-making. Common efforts include calls or emails to legislators, gathering signatures, and attending meetings. Volunteering to help or co-drafting a bill with a legislator is active involvement and does not traditionally qualify as grassroots. Joining a professional organization is not an active strategy for engaging in policy.

37. **B) Any 30-day readmission on select MS-DRG–based cases even if the patient is admitted elsewhere**
The MS-DRG–based bundle payment considers the principal admission diagnosis, the facilities case mix and type of institution (teaching or nonteaching), and other weighting measures to calculate the prospective bundled payment. Managing the costs is then the hospital's responsibility, assuming that they are still meeting all core measures and prudent care. Therefore, overspending is an inherent risk of inefficient care. A high-risk case mix is built into the system, and Medicare does not mandate the participation of a facility in Medicare. To prevent too-early discharge of patients, a "penalty" can be placed on a hospital if there are excessive 30-day readmissions for the same medical condition, whether they are readmitted to the original facility or to another hospital.

38. **A) Socioeconomic status (SES)**
Although many factors influence health, such as racial and gender disparities and access to quality care, the single most influential factor is SES. SES is a pervasive barrier to adequate health insurance, healthcare access, ability to cover co-pays, and adequate food, housing, and environment. Statistics support the influence of SES as the predominant influence on health.

39. **C) The treatment plan for wound care greatly influences the ability to discharge the patient to home care depending on frequency of care needed and level of involvement the wound requires.**
The AGACNP must know the discharge support agencies Medicare bundled payment system to achieve a cost-effective quality discharge for the patient. Traditional Medicare does not cover any topical drugs or biologics, although they cover dressings. Nontraditional Medicare advantage plans cover wound pharmaceuticals. It is true that an 80/20 split is the percentage of payment for part B coverage; however, the key to the treatment plan is to know how to order the dressing and topical agents that are most acceptable to a home care agency. Too complicated of a plan may lead to the risk of an increased length of stay while trying to find an agency that will accept the patient. Under the Home Health Care agencies Medicare payment system called the Home Health Resource Group Prospective Payment System, agencies would be responsible for dressings and wound care but not the topical agents or biologics.

40. **A) Topical cooling with saline**
The AGACNP identifies this burn as a first-degree burn and will focus recommendations on the 4Cs: cooling, cleaning, covering, comfort; thus, cooling the area is the best intervention. Referral to a plastic surgeon for skin grafting is not indicated, over-the-counter pain management is recommended, and there is no indication of an inhalation injury.

41. **B) Conducting a formal policy analysis**
Faced with strong institutional history regarding this policy, the AGACNP needs to approach the issue carefully. The AGACNP should know that not all policies or practices in healthcare are evidence-based; therefore, a systematic approach to the problem is best. The components of a formal theoretically supported policy analysis allow the AGACNP to have a firm understanding of the issue and allow the AGACNP to set the agenda.

42. **A) Normal aging process**
Short-term memory loss and hearing loss are normal signs of aging in an octogenarian. Short-term memory loss is a part of a constellation of symptoms often described in dementia; however, it is only one of the diagnostic criteria for major or mild neurocognitive disorder, which must be present to diagnose Alzheimer or vascular dementia. BPPV is a disorder of the inner ear, often described as a sensation of spinning, and if present could explain the fall. However, given no history of dizziness coupled with hearing loss not being associated with BPPV, this diagnosis is unlikely.

43. **A) Medication use**
Medication use, especially polypharmacy with psychotropic use, is suggested to increase falls. Medication review with de-prescribing, if appropriate, is recommended as a means to prevent falls. Neuropathy and osteoarthritis are not modifiable risk factors. Diet in itself does not place the older adult at higher risk for falls unless the patient has hypovitaminosis, especially of vitamin D.

44. **A) Tylenol PM**
Tylenol PM contains diphenhydramine, which is an antihistamine and highly anticholinergic. Older adults typically have decreased clearance. Diphenhydramine is listed in the American Geriatrics Society (AGS) Beers Criteria as a potentially inappropriate medication for older adults. Diltiazem is an antihypertensive that can also contribute to falls, but in a patient who is hypotensive. Diltiazem is in the AGS Beers Criteria as a possibly inappropriate medication for patients with heart failure as it is noted to promote fluid retention; the patient does not have heart failure and is currently hypertensive with an appropriate heart rate. Atorvastatin and levothyroxine typically do not cause dizziness.

45. **B) Impaired response to serum osmolality**
    Dehydration is the most common cause of fluid and electrolyte imbalance in older adults secondary to decreased perception of thirst, impaired response to serum osmolality, and reduced ability to concentrate urine. Creatinine clearance may affect urine production but not dehydration or thirst.

46. **D) Verbal abusiveness**
    A patient with severe cognitive impairment may not be able to express pain or degree of pain appropriately. Pain occurring from a fracture is nociceptive and will likely cause constant, gnawing pain to the affected area. Understanding that this patient is likely to experience pain will guide the AGACNP to assess for pain-related behaviors such as appetite changes (likely decreased), increased confusion, and verbal abusiveness. Patients in pain typically present with hypertension, not hypotension.

47. **C) Abdominal pain related to bowel movement with change in stool consistency and frequency**
    The diagnostic Rome IV criteria clearly state that irritable bowel syndrome is defined as recurrent abdominal pain on average at least 1 day per week in the last 3 months with two or more of the following: (a) related to defecation, (b) associated with a change in the frequency of stool, (c) associated with a change in form (consistency) of stool, and (d) symptoms for more than 6 months.

48. **D) Immunoglobulin A (IgA) tissue transglutaminase**
    An overwhelming majority of people with CD will remain undiagnosed. Those who do not avoid gluten risk developing a host of debilitating complications, including anemia, peripheral neuropathies, osteopenia and bone pain, and even cancer. The single best serology testing for CD is IgA tissue transglutaminase with a sensitivity and specificity of ~98%. Although the patient should have nutrient, vitamin, and trace mineral levels checked and replaced (in this case, malabsorption is most likely the cause of her anemia), they do not diagnose CD. Diagnosis is easier while the patient is still ingesting gluten, although the popularity of gluten-free diets has made adjustments to the diagnosis process necessary. PRBCs may be required, but that is a treatment for anemia, not a diagnostic aid.

49. **A) Placement of a Sengstaken–Blakemore tube**
    The Sengstaken–Blakemore tube is a temporary measure that can tamponade the esophagus. TIPS is the best option for *definitive treatment* for this patient classified as class C cirrhotic. Fluid administration and transfusion are likely to lead to consumptive coagulopathy and progress into disseminated intravascular coagulation. The patient is not a good candidate for transplantation in an acute state.

50. **A) Aspartate aminotransferase (AST) 83 unit/L, alanine aminotransferase (ALT) 50 unit/L, gamma-glutamyl transferase (GGT) 150 unit/L**
    In patients with alcoholic liver disease, the AST/ALT ratio is usually greater than 2.0, whereas in patients with acute and chronic hepatitis, the ratio is almost always less than 1.0. The normal reference range for GGT levels varies based on the source but is generally considered abnormal for levels greater than 60 in men age 18 years or older. Modest elevations are typically seen in patients with alcoholic cirrhosis. Extreme elevations of 5 to 30× normal are typically seen in patients with intra- or posthepatic biliary obstruction.

51. **D) Sepsis from spontaneous bacterial peritonitis**
    Anemia with GI bleed, portal vein hypertension, and hepatorenal syndrome are all potential problems for this patient. However, his vital signs and pain level should lead the AGACNP to determine that sepsis is the priority complication. In patients with liver disease and increasing ascites, spontaneous bacterial peritonitis can occur without perforations and is usually a gram-negative infection that can lead to sepsis and septic shock. Although he may have anemia given his black tarry stools, his hemoglobin and kidney function are not known. Portal hypertension is the probable cause of his ascites, but it is not the priority problem.

52. **B) "Your lab results are showing that you have a chronic HBV infection."**
The lab results show the IgG antibody subclass of anti-HBc, a marker of past or current infection with HBV. Because it and the HbsAg are both positive (in the absence of IgM-anti-HBc), chronic HBV is indicated. If the IgM-anti-HBc were also positive, then that would mean that the HBV is still in an acute phase, but the immune system is responding. There are several classes of common HIV regimens that also cover HBV. The infectious disease provider will most likely review the patient's medications and compliancy. It is more likely that the patient's intermittent compliance and HIV status put him at risk, rather than his HIV treatment.

53. **D) Consult colorectal surgery for emergency laparotomy**
Based on the history, presentation, labs, and imaging findings, the patient has acute perforated colon from a probable ruptured diverticulum in the history. Perforation of intra-abdominal organs is an emergency. Clinical symptoms can range from pain to the right upper abdomen to a severe picture of acute abdomen with guarding and rebound tenderness with abdominal sepsis. The most important goal of treatment is management of abdominal sepsis with surgical control of the source infection, which is the colon contents. It is rarely diagnosed preoperatively; however, imaging can help aid in appropriate diagnosis. Final diagnosis is usually confirmed at the time of an exploratory laparotomy. Infections, trauma, medications such as steroids, malignancy, and systemic diseases like diabetes mellitus and atherosclerosis are predisposing factors. The best treatment is early surgery. Early diagnosis of perforation and immediate surgical intervention are crucial to decrease morbidity and mortality.

54. **A) Acute ruptured appendicitis**
The diagnosis is made on a characteristic history and physical examination. The classic presentation of acute appendicitis pain may start as a mild periumbilical cramping that becomes more severe and radiates to the right lower quadrant with associated nausea, emesis, abdominal swelling, and fever with positive McBurney sign. Ultrasound is the best imaging for diagnosis. The pain may radiate to the scapula or shoulder areas, especially on the right side. Other symptoms that may occur are anorexia, nausea, and emesis. Acute pancreatitis is characterized by severe, persistent, epigastric abdominal pain that may radiate to the flank and worsens while lying supine but improves when sitting up with knees flexed.

55. **C) Ledipasvir-sofosbuvir**
HCV was a chronic disease, but with U.S. Food and Drug Administration approval of ledipasvir-sofosbuvir, a new class of direct-acting antivirals, treatment is 90% successful for HCV genotypes 1, 4, 5, and 6 with a well-tolerated one-pill, once-a-day option. Ribavirin and Peginterferon Alfa-2a (PEG-IFN-a) 2a were former HCV treatments with many side effects, and adefovir dipivoxil is used in HBV treatment.

56. **B) NPO, intravenous (IV) fluid resuscitation, and IV antibiotics**
Complicated diverticulitis involves symptoms of inflammation and potential abscess, phlegmon, fistula development, or peritonitis. CT scan is the preferred mode of imaging for complicated diverticulitis, although ultrasound can be used for uncomplicated symptoms. Although it is unusual for patients to vomit, they should be made NPO and given fluid hydration and IV antibiotics until surgical need has been cleared. If conservative treatment is able to clear symptoms, colonoscopy may be considered 4 to 6 weeks after the episode to evaluate.

57. **B) Central diabetes insipidus (DI)**
The patient likely has central DI. He had a craniopharyngioma, which is associated with central DI, with increased incidence of central DI post surgical resection in up to 80% of patients for up to 2 weeks postoperatively. Additionally, the patient underwent a 24-hour urine collection confirming a true polyuria (greater than 2.5 L urine/24 hours). Additionally, he has hypernatremia with a serum greater than urine osmolality. Last, he was responsive to desmopressin during a water deprivation test; an increase in his urine osmolality and decrease in his urine output post desmopressin is highly suggestive of central DI. SIADH is unlikely as it typically presents in patients as euvolemic hyponatremia. DKA is unlikely given the normal glucose, HbA1C, and HCO_3 and the negative serum ketone. Nephrogenic DI is also unlikely; urine osmolality and urine output typically remain unchanged post desmopressin in a water deprivation test.

58. **A) Amiloride (Midamor)**

Diuretics, specifically amiloride, are considered first-line treatment for lithium-induced nephrogenic DI. NSAIDs may play a role due to blockade of prostaglandin E (2) synthesis, which is responsible for ongoing diuresis from its vasopressin antagonism. However, their use may be limited in those with nephrogenic DI given the increased risk for renal dysfunction. Clozapine is indicated in treatment of dipsogenic DI or primary polydipsia, not nephrogenic DI. Desmopressin has utility only in central or gestational DI, not in nephrogenic DI.

59. **C) Primary aldosteronism (PA)**

Given the patient's resistant hypertension that requires three medications for adequate control, chronic hypokalemia, metabolic alkalosis (also known as the clinical triad for PA), and elevated ARR and PAC with suppressed renin, the patient likely has PA. Pheochromocytoma is a consideration given the hypertension; however, the normal plasma metanephrines makes this diagnosis unlikely. AI is unlikely given the lack of (orthostatic) hypotension or hyperkalemia with a normal cortisol level. Hyperthyroidism is a consideration given her palpitations; however, the normal TSH makes this diagnosis unlikely.

60. **C) Anion gap (AG) has closed**

Transitioning an insulin infusion to a subcutaneous long-acting basal and rapid-acting insulin regimen is most appropriate once the AG has closed. Once blood glucose is less than 250 mg/dL, addition of dextrose in the parenteral fluid is warranted, and the insulin infusion continues until the AG has closed. Normal K^+ does not warrant this transition; however, hypokalemia, especially if refractory to continuous replacement, may warrant transient cessation of insulin to prevent fatal hypokalemia-induced arrhythmias. Metabolic acidosis is expected to improve post DKA treatment; however, this is not a criterion for transitioning intravenous to subcutaneous insulin in DKA.

61. **B) Autoimmune thyroiditis**

Autoimmune thyroiditis is the most common cause of hypothyroidism. Addison disease is the most common cause of primary adrenal insufficiency, whereas exogenous glucocorticoids are the most common cause of secondary adrenal insufficiency. Graves disease is the most common cause of hyperthyroidism.

62. **B) Nephrolithiasis**

The classic presentation for a patient with acute renal colic is the sudden onset of severe pain that originates in the flank and radiates inferiorly and anteriorly. The abdominal examination was negative, and unlike patients with an acute abdomen, patients with renal colic are often repositioning to try to get comfortable. The urinary analysis revealed a pH of 4.5, which suggests uric acid stones. The lack of WBCs does not support the diagnosis of a urinary tract infection. Pain involving the prostate is usually located in the perineum and radiates to the lumbosacral inguinal canals or legs.

63. **A) Obtain blood and urine cultures, initiate sepsis bundle, and admit patient to the hospital.**

The patient meets the criteria for sepsis and must be cultured, started on antibiotics, resuscitated, and admitted to the hospital for further care. Outpatient management is not possible with this patient's vital signs, and the antibiotic choice is not broad enough with the recent procedure and exposure to antibiotics. Urology consult is not warranted at this time.

64. **D) Spironolactone (Aldactone)**

Aldactone should be discontinued with a GFR this low and a potassium level of 5 mEq/L. Lasix, Apresoline, and Levemir do not require dose adjustments for this GFR level.

65. **C) Septic shock secondary to UTI**

The patient meets the criteria for septic shock because they are not responsive to fluid resuscitation, require vasopressors, and have evidence that the source is a UTI. UTI and sepsis secondary to UTI are not specific enough diagnoses. There is no confirmatory evidence to support a diagnosis of pyelonephritis.

66. **C) Hypovolemia due to hemorrhage**
    Prerenal acute kidney injury is a result of decreased flow to the kidney as potentially seen with hypovolemia. Acute glomerulonephritis and acute tubular necrosis are both intrarenal causes of acute kidney injury. Malignant prostate hyperplasia could result with post-renal acute kidney injury.

67. **A) Consistency of scores over time**
    Test–retest reliability is consistency of scores over time. Consistency of scores obtained from two equivalent halves of the same exam is split-half reliability. Consistency with which a test measures a single construct or concept is construct reliability. Degree of agreement between two or more scores is inter-rater reliability.

68. **D) A significant result that would have happened only 5/100 times through chance**
    Researchers use 0.05 as the standard level of significance. That is, researchers are willing to accept statistical significance by chance occurring 5 times out of 100.

69. **D) All of the above**
    The AGACNP's role in research can be multifaceted and includes conducting a research study, collecting data, interpreting data, and disseminating the findings.

70. **A) PDSA**
    The PDSA cycle is a widely adopted and effective model to test change on a small scale and evaluate impact on outcomes. PICOT components are the elements of a clinical question to be answered. They are used to create a search strategy for databases. NDNQI is a database that gathers data to understand factors influencing quality of nursing care and outcomes at the unit level. NQF is a set of quality indicators to develop and implement a national strategy for healthcare quality measures and reporting.

71. **C) Qualitative research explores experiences.**
    Qualitative research explores experiences, events, and meaning of phenomena, not specific data. Quantitative research looks to test hypotheses but not necessarily to "prove" them. A good quantitative research study will limit the number of variables.

72. **A) Randomized control trial**
    The highest level of evidence is derived from randomized control trails. Cohort studies would be the next highest level of evidence followed by case series and expert opinion.

73. **B) Population, intervention, comparison, outcome, and time frame**
    PICOT represents population, intervention, comparison, outcome, and time frame.

74. **B) Outcome**
    An *outcome measure* captures results and is meant to improve understanding of how healthcare processes affect patient results. Process measures allow for individuals to quantify the methods used to provide care and to determine fidelity in the use of standards of care. Structure measures capture components including manpower and use of a specific specialty unit for patient management. *Quality measure* is an overarching term and includes structure process and outcome measure.

75. **B) Identify a care process or outcome issue**
    The first step in a QI project is to identify an issue that will be addressed. Selecting theoretical and implementation models, monitoring data, and implementing change are part of the QI process but are not the initial step.

76. **C) Publishing the results of a QI project in a peer-reviewed journal**
    Dissemination is sharing what has been learned from a QI project with a broader audience. Inquiring about a new QI project and identifying a care process for improvement are done at the start of the QI process. Developing new standard operating procedure is dissemination until is it implemented/shared.

77. **C) Have a meeting with the patient and family to discuss the decision to stop dialysis.**
The patient with decision-making capacity has the right to refuse treatment under the ethical principle of autonomy. It would be inappropriate to seek a court order to perform dialysis because there is no indication that the patient lacks the legal competency to make medical decisions. Performing dialysis as requested to avoid legal liability violates the patient's autonomy. Also, the patient demonstrates capacity to make her own medical decisions as she is alert and oriented and can also state the outcome of death if she does not proceed with treatment. Facilitating a meeting with the patient and family allows the patient the opportunity to explain her choice to her family and can lead to family acceptance of patient wishes.

78. **D) Patient must receive full disclosure of risks, benefits, and alternatives**
One requirement for informed consent is that the patient must be provided with full disclosure of all risks and potential benefits of the procedure, treatment, or research before consenting. Patients should not be persuaded or coerced in any way into consenting to a procedure, treatment, or research study. Financial compensation is not necessary for research studies, although participants may be financially compensated. There is no required time period for informed consent.

79. **A) American Nurses Credentialing Center (ANCC)**
Two organizations offer a certification exam for the AGACNP student: ANCC and AACN. Note that both the Association of Critical-Care Nurses and the American Association of Colleges of Nursing both have the acronym AACN.

80. **B) Lacks capacity**
The patient's inability to state understanding of the procedure indicates the patient does not have capacity to make the decision. Competency is a legal term and thus determined by the legal system. The patient is not able to provide consent given the lack of understanding of the procedure.

81. **A) A judge**
Medical competency is a legal term that is the key to rational decision-making. Laws assume every adult is mentally competent until a court decides otherwise. Thus, only a judge can deem a person incompetent to make their own decisions.

82. **C) Accountability**
The AGACNP has an obligation to accept responsibility or to account for their actions and is doing so by disclosing this complication. Autonomy is the right to self-govern. Nonmaleficence is the obligation to do no harm, and justice is striving for fair distribution of resources.

83. **B) Consensus**
The Consensus Model for Regulation of APRN practice offers a framework and regulation for advanced nursing practice. It also defines practice in relation to patient populations, not medical specialties. The Synergy Model relates to a competency-based model matching patient needs with nurse competency. The STAR Model theory is for implementation of evidence-based practice. The Collaborative Practice Model is a framework for interdisciplinary collaboration to provide excellent patient care.

84. **A) Privileges**
Privileges are the clinical activities that a provider has the right to perform in a healthcare facility. *Credentialing* is the process by which organizations determine eligibility to provide healthcare services. *Certification* is a voluntary process by which a nongovernmental agency recognizes individuals for meeting preestablished standards, typically by taking an examination. Certification validates (based on predetermined standards) an individual's education, qualification, knowledge, and practice in a defined functional or clinical area of nursing.

85. **C) Being obligated to do no harm**
Nonmaleficence is the obligation of the provider not to do harm to the patient, including weighing risks and benefits of all testing and treatment. *Autonomy* is the right to self-govern and make decisions about one's own healthcare. *Veracity* is being honest and telling the truth. *Fidelity* is keeping one's promises.

86. **A) 55-year-old veteran who served in Vietnam**
The U.S. Preventive Services Task Force recommends screening for all adults in the United States age 18 to 79 years, including pregnant patients. Persons outside the 18- to 79-year age range should have hepatitis C testing if they have risk factors for acquiring hepatitis C.

87. **A) 75-year-old man**
Firearm suicide rates are highest in adults age 75 years and older. Since having a firearm in the home is strongly associated with suicide, strategies to mitigate firearm suicides should include depression screening and asking anyone with depression if they have a gun in the home. Homicide rates from firearms are highest among persons age 15 to 34 years.

88. **A) Naloxone**
Patients who take benzodiazepines and opioids have a higher risk for overdose. Thus, co-prescribing naloxone is recommended. Since the patient is prescribed Tylenol, Percocet and Vicodin are contraindicated as they also contain Tylenol. Ketamine is used for inpatients who have severe breakthrough pain.

89. **A) Access to health insurance**
The Affordable Care Act provided increased health insurance options for young adults, early retirees, and Americans with preexisting conditions. These were implemented in October 2013 with coverage beginning in January 2014. Expanded access to Medicaid in many states began in January 2014. This resulted in a reduction of health access disparities for Americans.

90. **D) Quaternary**
Prevention of overmedicalization is defined as *quaternary care*. *Primary prevention* aims to remove or reduce risk factors for disease (e.g., immunizations), *secondary prevention* promotes early detection of disease (e.g., Pap screening to detect carcinoma or dysplasia of the cervix), and *tertiary prevention* is aimed at limiting the impact of an established disease (e.g., mastectomy for breast cancer).

91. **C) PPSV23 and quadrivalent meningococcal vaccine**
Asplenic patients are at great risk for pneumococcal and *Neisseria meningitidis* infections. Meningitis vaccines are especially warranted in college-age patients. Flu and DT vaccines are both recommended. HPV and hepatitis vaccines are not indicated. DT is indicated at the time of admission to the hospital as prophylaxis, not at time of discharge. COVID-19 vaccine is not currently recommended.

92. **D) Patient on mechanical ventilation for 48 hours**
Two of the most important risk factors for gastrointestinal bleeding from stress ulcers are coagulopathy and respiratory failure with the need for mechanical ventilation for over 48 hours. When these two risk factors are absent, the risk of significant bleeding is only 0.1%. Other risk factors include traumatic brain injury, severe burns, sepsis, vasopressor therapy, corticosteroid therapy, and history of peptic ulcer disease and gastrointestinal bleeding. Prophylaxis should be routinely administered to critically ill patients with risk factors for significant bleeding upon admission.

93. **B) Perform spontaneous breathing trials every 24 hours.**
Daily spontaneous breathing trials are associated with earlier extubation and are a level 1 recommendation for prevention of VAP. Interruption of sedation daily is also a level 1 recommendation and should be paired with spontaneous breathing trials every 24 hours. There is no evidence to support changing ventilator circuits on a regular basis to decrease VAP rates; it is costly, so changing only when visibly soiled or when there is a malfunction is the current recommendation.

94. **B) Has an advance directive**

This is an example of quaternary care: prevention of overmedicalization. Advance directives are medical documents that identify a patient's preference for future medical care. The patient is currently competent and therefore able to explicitly determine his healthcare wishes. If the patient does not have an advance directive, then one should be developed and become part of the patient's medical record. It is also important for the patient to have a discussion with his family; however, this often evolves from completion of an advance directive or living will. The durable power of attorney should have a specific designation for healthcare and would be designated within the advance directive. Spiritual support would be beneficial to consider while the patient is developing the advance directive.

95. **D) Sequential compression device**

For acutely ill hospitalized patients with increased risk of thrombosis who are bleeding or at high risk for major bleeding, the optimal use of mechanical thromboprophylaxis with graduated compression stockings or intermittent pneumatic compression rather than no mechanical thromboprophylaxis is recommended. Chemical deep vein thrombosis prophylaxis is initially indicated; however, mechanical devices are indicated as well. When bleeding risk decreases, and if VTE risk persists, pharmacologic thromboprophylaxis may be substituted for mechanical thromboprophylaxis.

96. **D) Start a pressor, consider corticosteroids if pressure is unresponsive, consult surgery, order broad-spectrum antibiotics.**

This is a case of necrotizing fasciitis with systemic symptoms of sepsis. The patient cannot go to CT until stable. As in all cases for critical care, stabilize the patient as part of the ABCs (circulation, in this case). Septic patients need fluid resuscitation, and when the pressure does not respond to fluids, corticosteroids are often needed as well. Broad-spectrum antibiotics are needed as soon as possible as well as early aggressive surgical intervention.

97. **A) Stop the IV, remove the angiocatheters, elevate the extremity, and apply warm compresses.**

Pressors are vesicants and can cause damage to the tissues if extravasation occurs. This IV is not functional, and there are signs of extravasation. Stopping the IV and removing the angiocatheters with elevation and warm compresses help disperse the extravasation fluid. Infiltrates are harmless irritants like IV fluids. As the IV site is dysfunctional, there is no benefit to leaving it until the central line is placed.

98. **C) Necrotizing fasciitis**

Necrotizing fasciitis is a life-threatening infection of the subcutaneous tissues. It can present with signs of infection and imaging that reveals gas within fluid collection tracking along fascial plans.

99. **C) Chronic venous insufficiency**

The brownish pigmentation, strong arterial pulses, and shallow, nonpainful, nonhealing wounds on the lower extremity are indicative of chronic venous inefficiency.

100. **A) Arterial**

The finding of an ulcer on the lateral ankle combined with symptoms of claudication and exam findings of diminished hair growth, pale atrophic skin, and nail dystrophy indicate an arterial origin.

101. **B) Budesonide**

Patients should be instructed to rinse their mouth after using an inhaled corticosteroid medication such as budesonide. This will prevent oral thrush. Levalbuterol, salmeterol, and tiotropium are not inhaled corticosteroid medications.

102. **B) Used only for patients with high CAT and mMRC scores**

Roflumilast is indicated for patients with severe COPD associated with chronic bronchitis and is reserved for patients with high CAT and mMRC scores. Roflumilast is not for use as a rescue inhaler or for acute exacerbations of COPD.

103. A) Relaxes bronchial muscle on beta-2 receptors
Albuterol is a beta-2 agonist and works by relaxing bronchial smooth muscle on beta-2 receptors.

104. C) Meningitis
The patient has signs and symptoms of meningitis and risk factors that include alcohol use disorder. The patient is not hypertensive on presentation.

105. C) Multiple sclerosis (MS)
Symptoms of MS include sensory loss/impairment with weakness and optic neuritis. GBS presents with ascending paralysis, with legs being affected before arms, and subsequent loss of reflexes over a few days. In MG, the facial muscles, especially the eyelids, demonstrate ptosis, and the extraocular muscles gradually weaken with fatigue as the day progresses. ALS involves primary motor disturbances.

106. C) Dexamethasone
The treatment of choice for vasogenic edema is IV steroids, typically dexamethasone to reduce edema and improve symptoms. Mannitol and hypertonic saline are used with edema secondary to traumatic brain injury or stroke.

107. A) Parkinson disease (PD)
Classic findings of PD include bradykinesia and resting hand tremor. MG, GBS, and MS do not classically present with this constellation of symptoms.

108. D) "When did the symptoms start?"
The patient is presenting with signs of a stroke, which is time-sensitive for diagnosis and treatment. The question "When did the symptoms start?" is the most important question as the answer will dictate treatment options.

109. C) Adherence to medication regimen
Medication noncompliance is one of the most common reasons for patients with seizure disorder to have seizures. Thus, although there may be other contributing factors, the first question should determine medication adherence.

110. A) Encephalitis
The patient is presenting with neurologic dysfunction with signs and symptoms of an infection and recent viral infection, making encephalitis the most likely diagnosis.

111. D) Hypertensive encephalopathy
In hypertensive encephalopathy, the blood pressure exceeds cerebral autoregulation limits, allowing for increases in cerebral blood flow and volume. Hypertensive urgency does not have the target organ damage that is occurring here. Meningitis typically has fever, nuchal rigidity, or positive Kernig and/or Brudzinski signs.

112. A) Perform a lumbar puncture
The most likely diagnosis is meningitis. Thus, a lumbar puncture and the associated testing will confirm diagnosis of meningitis. A CT scan of the cervical spine will not confirm diagnosis of meningitis; it can rule out bony injury of the spine, but there is no indication that an injury has occurred. An MRI would confirm presence of an abscess or tumor as the cause of the symptoms, but these are not the most likely diagnoses. An MRI or MRA will not confirm diagnosis of meningitis. Eliciting Brudzinski and Kernig signs is an assessment that, when positive, leads the diagnostician toward diagnosis of meningitis but does not confirm diagnosis.

113. **D) Cocaine**

This patient is having focal seizures. Cocaine and other toxins can cause seizure due to alteration of neuronal excitability and can therefore lower the seizure threshold in a patient. Marijuana is not a cause of seizures unless it is laced with another drug. Heroin withdrawal could cause seizures, but use of heroin itself does not cause seizures. Nicotine usage has numerous long-term effects on the body, but recent usage is not a trigger for seizure activity. In general, common triggers of seizures in adults include medication noncompliance, fatigue/lack of sleep, stress, alcohol/substance use, and acute illnesses.

114. **C) Vital capacity**

This patient likely has Guillain-Barré syndrome. Classic precursors include recent viral illness and immunizations. Classic presentation is neuropathic pain in the neck and back and ascending paralysis with loss of deep tendon reflexes. Thirty percent of patients require ventilator support, including tracheostomy, thus the need for monitoring vital capacity to monitor for impending respiratory failure. Treatment is intravenous immunoglobulin. Glucocorticoids are not indicated. Physical therapy can be beneficial for the patient but is not the highest priority at this time.

115. **C) Myasthenia gravis (MG)**

MG typically affects women in their early 20s to 30s and men in their 50s to 60s. Hallmark features include weakness later in the day. Cranial and facial muscles, including eyelids; extraocular muscles with diplopia and ptosis; and chewing and swallowing muscles are commonly affected early during exacerbations. Symptoms typically improve after sleep or rest. BP affects a unilateral facial nerve, causing muscle paralysis that does not improve with rest. GBS is a polyradiculoneuropathy that causes ascending paralysis, with legs more affected than arms; it may cause complete paralysis and ventilator dependence.

116. **D) Absence of intravascular overload**

ARDS is an acute heterogeneous lung injury that is not attributed to intravascular volume overload, pulmonary edema, heart failure, or chronic lung disease. Physical findings include fever or hypothermia, tachypnea, hypoxemia with need of high FIO_2 to maintain oxygen saturation, diffuse crackles, tachycardia, hypotension, peripheral vasoconstriction, and cyanosis. Patients with ARDS have diffuse crackles and experience tachycardia and tachypnea. Patients with ARDS often experience hypotension due to higher positive end-expiratory pressure required to manage it.

117. **A) STAT chest x-ray (CXR)**

The patient is hemodynamically stable, so a CXR is indicated to accurately confirm the diagnosis. The x-ray will define extent and possible etiology for the pneumothorax. However, if the patient becomes unstable, decompression should be done immediately. An ABG is not necessary as the patient is not reported to be in acute respiratory distress. It is unlikely the patient has a PE, and a CXR would be the first diagnostic test. The patient may need a chest tube; however, a diagnosis is needed before an intervention can be performed.

118. **B) Observation**

This patient is hemodynamically stable and thus may not require intervention. Follow-up x-ray should be ordered in 6 to 8 hours and again at 24 hours to assess for expansion. Increase in symptoms warrants a chest tube or pigtail catheter. Needle decompression is needed for tension pneumothorax (PTX) when the patient develops tension physiology (becomes hemodynamically unstable). Since this is the first PTX, there is no need for a surgical consult.

119. **C) Hospital-associated pneumonia**

The patient was admitted 48 hours ago for elective surgery. Based on exam and hospitalization of more than 48 hours, hospital-associated pneumonia is the most likely diagnosis. Heart failure is not likely to have unilateral breath sounds. Asthma is a differential diagnosis, but acute asthma exacerbations do not typically have confusion or hypotension or unilateral breath sounds.

120. **A) Order empiric antibiotics.**
Antibiotics are warranted as this patient likely has community-acquired pneumonia with CURB65 score of 3 and 30-day mortality rate of 14%. Waiting for labs will only delay treatment. Antiviral agents are not indicated as he has been symptomatic for over 5 days. The patient does not need to be intubated currently.

121. **A) Tube thoracostomy**
All large pleural effusions complicated by pneumonia are most likely to be exudative. Indications for a tube thoracotomy include loculated pleural fluid, pH below 7.2, pleural glucose less than 60 mg/dL, Gm + or culture of pleural fluid and the presence of purulent material. Diuresis would not help, as this is an inflammatory process. Antiviral agents are not indicated as this is a bacterial infection. VATS is not the initial treatment for an exudative effusion.

122. **D) B-lines**
B-lines are caused by reverberations in the alveoli or interstitium. B-lines are vertical laser-like artifacts that move with respiration. They represent abnormal extravascular lung field or interstitial fibrosis. Pneumonia is expected as indicated by B-lines (focal) with possible subpleural consolidations or consolidated lung with or without shred sign, bronchograms, or effusion. Absence of lung sliding is an indication of pneumothorax. Lung point is the junction between lung sliding and absent lung sliding and is an indication of pneumothorax. A-lines are horizontal artifactual repetition of the pleural line, representing aeration of lung.

123. **C) Avoid cigarette smoking**
Smoking cessation is crucial to prevent deterioration of lung function. Anticholinergics are bronchodilators that block the bronchoconstricting effects of acetylcholine on M3 muscarinic receptors in airway smooth muscle. Beta-2 agonists are bronchodilators that relax airway smooth muscle by stimulating beta-2 adrenergic receptors. Corticosteroids decrease inflammation and swelling in the airways and are used to manage exacerbations.

124. **B) Copious secretions**
NIPPV can be used in hypercapnic respiratory failure on patients who are alert enough to protect their airway and do not have copious secretions. A patient who is in respiratory failure due to COPD exacerbation with $PaCO_2$ of 50 meets the criteria for NIPPV. A patient in acute respiratory failure with a PaO_2 of 56 mmHg meets the criteria for NIPPV. Hyperinflation of lungs with a flattened diaphragm is indicative of emphysema.

125. **B) II**
Acute respiratory failure type II is hypercapnic respiratory failure. Hypercapnic respiratory failure is caused by alveolar hypoventilation resulting in the inability to effectively eliminate carbon dioxide. Acute respiratory failure type II is characterized by a partial pressure carbon dioxide greater than 45 mmHg causing respiratory acidosis with a pH less than 7.35. Acute respiratory failure type I, the most common type of respiratory failure, is characterized by severe arterial hypoxemia that is refractory to supplemental oxygen with a PaO_2 less than 60 mmHg or SaO_2 less than 90%. Type I respiratory failure is caused by hypoxemia-damaged lung tissue. Acute respiratory failure is perioperative respiratory failure caused by a decrease in functional residual capacity due to atelectasis, ultimately causing dependent lung units to collapse. Acute respiratory failure type IV is caused by hypoperfusion of respiratory muscles in shock states. Respiratory muscles normally will consume up to 5% of cardiac output (CO). In shock conditions, respiratory muscles consume up to 40% of CO. Nothing in the patient's present medical history indicates a shock state.

126. **C) HELLP syndrome**
This patient has *h*emolysis, *e*levated *l*iver enzymes, and *l*ow *p*latelets. Eclampsia is manifested by hypertension, BP greater than 140/90 on two readings over 4 hours apart or greater than 160/110 on two readings minutes apart, and proteinuria greater than 300 mg/24 hours. *Severe* preeclampsia is preeclampsia with any of the following: platelet count less than 100,000 mcL, creatinine greater than 1.1 mg/dL or twice the patient's baseline, AST or alanine aminotransferase (ALT) greater than twice the upper limit of normal or right upper quadrant pain, pulmonary edema, and central nervous system symptoms. Eclampsia includes seizures or coma. This patient has no signs of cardiomyopathy.

127. **D) Severe preeclampsia**
Eclampsia is manifested by hypertension, BP greater than 140/90 on two readings over 4 hours apart or greater than 160/110 on two readings minutes apart, and proteinuria greater than 300 mg/24 hours. Severe preeclampsia is preeclampsia with any of the following: platelet count less than 100,000 uL, creatinine greater than 1.1 mg/dL or twice the patient's baseline, aspartate aminotransferase or alanine aminotransferase greater than twice the upper limit of normal or right upper quadrant pain, pulmonary edema, or central nervous system symptoms. HELLP syndrome is *h*emolysis, *e*levated *l*iver enzymes, and *l*ow *p*latelets.

128. **C) Gabapentin (Neurontin)**
The patient describes neuropathic pain. The best treatment for neuropathic pain is gabapentin (Neurontin). Ibuprofen, lidocaine, and hydromorphone do not work as well for neuropathic pain.

129. **B) Consult anesthesia for an epidural.**
This patient is headed toward respiratory failure due to acute pain. Aggressive pain control measures are needed to prevent intubation. BiPAP is an option to help with the impending respiratory failure but does not treat the underlying problem of pain. Treatment of pain may prevent the need for BiPAP. Ibuprofen and ketorolac are contraindicated in acute kidney injury.

130. **D) Formal brain death testing**
This patient likely suffered an anoxic brain injury. Thus far, brainstem functions are absent. Further testing is warranted to confirm brain death. While an SBT could be done, the patient is not over-breathing the ventilator and is not able to be extubated due to the current neuro exam. To demonstrate anoxia, an MRI would be more beneficial than a CT scan. There is no reason to consult neurosurgery.

131. **C) Referring for organ donation after cardiac death**
The patient may be eligible for organ donation after cardiac death and should be referred to the organ procurement organization. While an SBT is plausible, extubation is not feasible due to the patient's mental status. They can be extubated to comfort care, but donation should be explored first. Consultation with palliative care is an option, but the family seems to know what the patient would choose; thus, it is not the next best step. A family meeting may be needed, but there is no need to wait a specific time frame.

132. **C) 1**
The patient has abnormal vital signs, hypotension, and a compromised airway, making this a level 1 trauma activation.

133. **B) Hemorrhagic shock**
The patient has classic signs and symptoms of hemorrhagic shock (cool, clammy, anxious) with physiologic signs of shock. None of the patient's information is suggestive of spinal injury or involvement. There is also no information to suggest adrenal insufficiency. Given the mechanism of injury and the patient's information, pulmonary embolism is not likely.

134. **A) Massive transfusion protocol**

This patient is suffering from hemorrhagic shock and needs resuscitation with blood products. An abdominal CT will be part of the workup, but hemodynamics will prevent the patient from going to the CT scanner. Dopamine will not address the reason for the hypotension and is not the best choice of vasopressor. Lactated Ringer fluid bolus is a reasonable step, but the patient needs blood products first.

135. **B) Monitor phosphorous levels**

This patient is likely malnourished as the BMI is less than 18.5. Older adult patients who live alone may not be able to access food or cook for themselves. They are at risk for refeeding syndrome, and hypophosphatemia is the hallmark sign of refeeding syndrome. Severe hypophosphatemia can lead to respiratory insufficiency. Dental changes can make older patients require softer foods, so a regular diet may not be tolerated and can complicate the malnutrition. Guidelines do not recommend following albumin and prealbumin as markers of nutrition. While physical and occupational therapy and social work consults are needed, they are not the highest priority.

136. **A) 1**

The patient is intubated and has a penetrating trauma, making this a level 1 trauma.

137. **D) IV**

The patient has heart rate greater than 140, is hypotensive, has respiratory rate greater than 35, and has estimated blood loss over 2 L, consistent with class IV hemorrhagic shock.

138. **D) N-acetylcysteine**

The patient has an acetaminophen overdose and is in acute liver failure. N-acetylcysteine is the treatment for acetaminophen overdose. This patient, while altered, does not need to be intubated. Naloxone is for opioid overdose/overmedication, and flumazenil is used for benzodiazepine overdose/overmedication.

139. **B) Intravenous (IV) naloxone and flumazenil**

The patient has had conscious sedation for the colonoscopy and is most likely oversedated. An ABG and BiPAP can diagnose and reverse the hypoventilation but will not reverse the cause of the oversedation. Initiation of rescue BiPAP will necessitate transfer to a higher level of care, and a reversal agent may allow the patient to remain on the floor. This patient does not need to be intubated at this time. The bleeding has ceased and vital signs are stable, so transfusion is not indicated.

140. **A) Acute rejection**

There is evidence of the pancreas not functioning properly. Given the need for early identification, the AGACNP must suspect and rule out acute rejection.

141. **A) Consult palliative care.**

The patient has a terminal condition. Consult with palliative care can help her process this situation and help make decisions regarding her healthcare. While physical therapy, nutritional support, and antidepressants may be needed, they are not the highest priority, nor will they address the patient's question.

142. **A) Refer to inpatient hospice.**

Referral to inpatient hospice will allow for the patient's symptoms to be managed with intravenous (IV) medications. A discharge home is not feasible as he will experience extreme dyspnea not easily managed at home without IV medications. While medicating with morphine is appropriate for symptom management, the dose is not appropriate. The goal of comfort care medications are to treat symptoms, not to hasten death.

143. **B) Hospice care**

Hospice care focuses on comfort and symptom management and does not support curative treatments. Palliative care does support curative treatments and can be sought at any time. Home care services are not specific, and rehabilitation-focused care does not address the patient's request.

144. **A) American Geriatrics Society (AGS) Beers Criteria**

The AGS Beers Criteria for potentially inappropriate medication use in older adults provides recommendations on which medications might be inappropriate. CHA_2DS_2VASc score calculates stroke risk for patients with atrial fibrillation, HAS-BLED score estimates risk for major bleeding for patients on anticoagulation, and ORBIT assesses risk of major bleeding for patient with atrial fibrillation on anticoagulation.

145. **C) Oral diet with dietary supplements**

All patients should use the gastrointestinal tract for nutrition when able. This patient had colon surgery and can take oral nutrition early postoperatively. Thus, parenteral nutrition or a postpyloric feeding tube is not indicated.

146. **B) Carbapenem resistance**

Patients who worsen while on antibiotics should be suspected of having antibiotic resistance. Re-culture the patient to determine whether a new organism is present or whether resistance has developed. The patient has been on a ventilator; thus, ventilator-associated pneumonia is more likely than HAP. Patient information does not indicate a central line; thus, this is not a CLABSI. The patient may have a PE, but presentation with fever and hypoxia with increased sputum is not consistent with a PE.

147. **D) Ventilator-associated pneumonia (VAP)**

The patient has been on the ventilator for over 48 hours; thus, VAP is the most accurate diagnosis. Pneumonia and HAP are possible but are not the most likely diagnoses.

148. **B) Discontinue the PICC line**

This patient most likely has a central line–associated bloodstream infection. To obtain source control, the PICC line must be discontinued. Blood cultures should then be drawn to start broad-spectrum antibiotics. Vancomycin or cefazolin alone are insufficient coverage until the culture and sensitivities result. A consult with infectious disease may eventually be warranted but is not the first action.

149. **C) Complicated UTI**

Signs and symptoms of a UTI that has confirmatory urinalysis in a pregnant patient is classified as complicated UTI at a minimum. There is insufficient evidence to diagnose pyelonephritis. All pregnant patients with a positive urinalysis without symptoms require treatment for a complicated UTI.

150. **A) Ceftriaxone**

Ceftriaxone is the appropriate antibiotic coverage to treat complicated urinary tract infections (UTIs). Nitrofurantoin would treat an uncomplicated UTI. Cefazolin is insufficient coverage for a complicated UTI. Meropenem is indicated for drug-resistant organisms.

151. **C) Avoid reusing or sharing items that have direct contact with draining wound**

Patients and families should be advised to keep draining wounds covered, wash hands with soap and water or an alcohol-based gel immediately after touching infected skin, avoid reusing or sharing items that have direct contact with draining wound, and avoid sharing pools or baths to ensure a decrease in passing MRSA to another person.

152. **A) Previous antimicrobial therapy**
Previous antimicrobial therapy and residing in a long-term care facility are risk factors for VRE. Colonization, not decolonization, pressure would occur. Strep throat is not a precursor to VRE.

153. **B) Active TB**
Active TB is most consistent with a nonproductive cough 3 weeks or more in duration, fevers, chills, night sweats, and weight loss. Latent TB is often asymptomatic. Bronchitis and asthma are not congruent with the patient's symptoms.

154. **A) Fever, fatigue, myalgias**
The classic presentation of early HIV includes flu-like symptoms of fever, fatigue, and myalgias. The patient can also present with adenopathy, pharyngeal edema, recurrent vaginal or oral thrush, generalized rash, nausea, vomiting and diarrhea, or anorexia with a weight loss averaging 5 kg. Night sweats, weight loss, and hemoptysis are signs of active tuberculosis. Fever, productive cough, and pleuritic pain are classic signs of pneumonia. Fever, chills, and white plaques on tonsils are common signs of strep pharyngitis.

155. **B) Apply a pelvic binder**
This patient is likely in hemorrhagic shock from an open-book pelvic fracture. Cessation of bleeding is the highest priority. An abdominal binder will help tamponade bleeding from the pelvic bones. The patient should be given blood products, not normal saline, at this point. While orthopedic surgery needs to be consulted, a pelvic binder is more urgently needed to stabilize the patient. Additional imaging may be needed prior to transport to the operating room.

156. **A) Boxer**
Boxer fracture is the most common fractured metacarpal. Injury to the neck of the fifth metacarpal typically occurs from direct trauma (e.g., from punching an object). A scaphoid (navicular) fracture is a break in one of the small bones of the wrist that most often occurs after a fall onto an outstretched hand. Ulnar styloid fractures are usually the result of direct trauma as in sports or a fall. Fractures of the hook of the hamate are most commonly seen in athletes who use a bat or racket (e.g., baseball, tennis, hockey) and are thought to result from direct injury by the handle of the bat, racket, or club deforming or fracturing the hook of the hamate.

157. **A) Apply a spica thumb splint**
The AGACNP is concerned for scaphoid fracture based on mechanism of injury and clinical findings. Thumb spica splint is indicated with a referral to orthopedics or hand surgery. A short arm splint and sling are not appropriate. Physical therapy is not indicated during acute fracture. Occupational therapy may be needed once the fracture heals if there is weakness or contractures.

158. **B) Finkelstein**
The Finkelstein test is performed by having the patient place the thumb in the palm of the hand, then wrap the fingers around the thumb to make a fist with the thumb tucked inside. The patient tilts the wrist toward the pinky finger. Pain will occur in the radial wrist area. The Lachman test is used to assess patients who have a suspected anterior cruciate ligament injury. There is no Quervain or thumb test.

159. **C) Boxer**
Boxer fractures are the most common fractured metacarpal. Colles fracture is a fracture of the distal radius. Bennett fracture is a fracture and dislocation of the metacarpal bone at the base of the thumb. Rolando fractures are intra-articular fractures of the base of the first metacarpal, similar to Bennett fracture but more complex to treat.

160. **C) Order a STAT head CT scan**

Patients receiving systemic thrombolytics are at increased risk of severe bleeding, including intracerebral hemorrhage (ICH). Symptoms of decreased level of consciousness, new headache, nausea, and vomiting are concerning for ICH. While IV ondansetron may be an effective treatment for the patient's nausea, the priority intervention is to determine if she is suffering from ICH. Nausea is a symptom of ICH and not the primary problem. Whether the current anticoagulation is therapeutic or not is irrelevant. If the patient has developed severe bleeding, all anticoagulation and thrombolytics will be discontinued. Signs of obstructive shock include jugular venous distention; a rapid, thready pulse; and profound hypotension. These are not consistent with the patient's current clinical picture.

161. **B) "You will need to stay on anticoagulation indefinitely because your DVT is considered unprovoked and happened in the absence of known risk factors."**

Current recommendations are that patients with unprovoked DVT continue anticoagulation indefinitely. The patient will need to take a DOAC going forward to prevent recurrence. DVT resolution is not considered when determining length of therapy, and 3 months is not aligned with the current guideline recommendation for treatment of unprovoked DVT. Post-thrombotic syndrome is a complication of DVT associated with chronic pain, swelling, discomfort, and ulcer development. While one goal of appropriate anticoagulation is to reduce its occurrence, its presence does not influence duration of anticoagulation in an unprovoked DVT. IVC filters are not recommended as treatment for DVT unless an absolute contraindication to anticoagulation or chronic risk factor exists.

162. **D) STAT EKG, morphine 2 mg IV, normal saline bolus 250 mL over 15 minutes, aspirin 325 mg PO**

Based on the patient's risk factors, including hypertension, hyperlipidemia, and family history of premature cardiovascular disease (CVD), along with exam findings of acute-onset substernal crushing chest pain, nausea, diaphoresis, crackles, and cool extremities, he is most likely having a ST-segment elevation myocardial infarction (STEMI). Additionally, his bradycardia on telemetry along with low BP is concerning for an inferior wall myocardial infarction (MI). A BP of 100/58 in a patient with a history of hypertension is abnormal and likely represents hypotension. He is preload dependent and should not receive medications like nitroglycerin, which could further reduce his preload and exacerbate his symptoms. Appropriate management includes a STAT EKG to confirm likely STEMI and to localize the artery involved, morphine for pain control, a small fluid bolus to augment preload and treat hypotension, and aspirin. While an EKG, morphine, and aspirin are indicated in the treatment of unstable angina, oxygen should not be given unless the O_2 saturation is ≤90%. Nitroglycerin is also contraindicated in those having an inferior MI due to its potential to reduce preload and worsen hypotension. Clopidogrel would not be given before confirming the presence of an MI with EKG and developing a plan.

163. **A) Cardiac tamponade**

The patient is demonstrating classic exam findings of cardiac tamponade, including pulsus paradoxus (an inspiratory drop in systolic blood pressure by more than 10 mmHg), and two of the three findings of Beck triad: muffled heart sounds, hypotension, and jugular venous distention. She has likely sustained a traumatic injury during her procedure and now is bleeding into the pericardial sac and developing an effusion. While hypotension is a sign of inferior wall MI, pulsus paradoxus and muffled heart sounds are more consistent with a diagnosis of cardiac tamponade. Additionally, she has not complained of jaw or chest discomfort. Sepsis is associated with hypotension; however, there is no indication that she is infected or experiencing any other symptoms of sepsis. The priority diagnosis is cardiac tamponade, which must be immediately addressed to prevent cardiovascular collapse.

164. **C) "This pattern of symptoms is characteristic of unstable angina."**
The symptoms described by the student are most consistent with unstable angina. Unstable angina can occur with activity and at rest. It can be new onset or may represent an increase in frequency and severity from the patient's previous baseline chronic angina. Prinzmetal or variant angina is related to vasospasm of the artery and is not related to CAD. This patient has been diagnosed with STEMI and has a history of CAD. The most likely reason for his discomfort is that he has been experiencing unstable angina. Aortic dissection is associated with a tearing or ripping type of discomfort that may be felt in the back. It is not associated with changes in activity or a pattern of increasing severity and frequency. Unstable angina is characterized by a predictable pattern of chest discomfort that begins with activity or emotional stress and is relieved by rest, lasting only a few minutes.

165. **C) III**
His current NYHA classification is class III. He is experiencing moderate symptoms and is comfortable only at rest. NYHA class I includes patients with normal functional abilities. These patients can do normal activities without symptoms. NYHA class II individuals have minimal symptoms with activity and experience no symptoms at rest. New York Heart Association (NYHA) class IV includes patients with severe functional limitations. Any activity results in symptoms.

166. **A) Decrease nitroprusside infusion.**
Blood pressure of 210/100 is a hypertensive emergency. Treatment is aimed at reducing the pressure by no more than 25% in the first hour and then toward 160/100 over the next 2 to 6 hours. The patient's current blood pressure is far beyond this threshold and places them at risk for catastrophic cerebral edema. The nitroprusside should be paused or decreased to allow the blood pressure to rise toward these goals. The blood pressure is already too low, and the patient is at risk of developing cerebral edema. Further drops in blood pressure will only add to this risk. The current issue is overaggressive rate of blood pressure reduction. It is problematic regardless of the agent used. Taking no action and continuing to monitor may result in harm to the patient and is considered negligence.

167. **C) "Beta-blockers work by decreasing your heart rate and reducing the contractility of your heart, which decreases the shearing forces in your aorta."**
Beta-blockers are negative chronotropic and negative inotropic agents. They reduce shearing force in the aorta through decreasing the contractile force of the heart along with the heart rate, which prevents aortic dissections from worsening. While beta-blockers work with other antihypertensives to reduce blood pressure in these patients, it is not the primary purpose in prescribing them. Beta-blockers are prescribed for the treatment of intralumenal hematomas, but that is not the reason they are being prescribed to this patient. Beta-blockers are used to treat aortic dissection because they provide shear force reduction.

168. **C) Intermediate**
According to the Modified Wells Criteria, her clinical probability of having a PE is intermediate (malignancy within the past 6 months = 1 point, heart rate (HR) greater than 100 = 1.5 points, history of previous DVT/PE = 1.5 points) with a score of 4 points (intermediate probability = 4 to 6 points). A high probability of PE in the Modified Wells Criteria is ≥6 points. Likely and probable are not score categories in the Modified Wells Criteria.

169. **D) Anaphylaxis reaction**
Dupilumab (Dupixent) can cause hypersensitivity reactions or anaphylaxis. It is recommended when starting patients on dupilumab (Dupixent) to monitor them closely.

170. **B) History of IVDA**

Diagnosis of IE requires the presence of two major criteria from the Modified Duke Criteria, or one major and three minor criteria, or five minor criteria. Based on the patient's current exam, he is currently demonstrating three minor criteria (fever greater than 38°C, Osler nodes, and Janeway lesions); a blood culture + for a HACEK organism fulfills the required major criteria. Roth spots are considered a minor criterion that would give him a total of four minor criteria and would not fulfill the Modified Duke Criteria. A history of IVDA is minor criterion that would give him a total of four minor criteria and would not fulfill the Modified Duke Criteria. His presentation is already + for Janeway lesions (nontender erythematous lesions on the soles of the feet).

171. **B) "You should contact your provider for prophylactic antibiotics before any invasive dental procedure."**

Patients with prosthetic valves are at risk for developing IE with invasive dental procedures and are recommended to have antibiotic prophylaxis beforehand. Oral anticoagulation is currently recommended for at least 3 months after valve replacement, not 6 months. While some discomfort is expected after valve replacement surgery, any sudden increase in discomfort is not expected and should be reported to the provider.

172. **B) Diuretics, beta-blockers, calcium channel blockers**

Patients presenting with cardiomyopathy often present with heart failure (HF) symptoms and volume overload regardless of type of cardiomyopathy. These symptoms are best treated with HF-recommended medications including diuretics to decrease volume overload and beta-blockers and calcium channel blockers to decrease heart rate and increase time for ventricular filling. Aspirin and statins are not recommended to treat cardiomyopathy. While nitrates and diuretics may be useful in treatment of volume overload in patients with cardiomyopathy, norepinephrine is an afterload-increasing agent and would likely worsen symptoms of HF in these patients. An implantable defibrillator may be indicated for some patients with cardiomyopathy who are at risk of sudden cardiac death, but it is not appropriate for all patients.

173. **C) "Drink plenty of water to maintain your hydration, and if you feel light-headed, you can try to apply counterpressure by gripping your hands or crossing your legs."**

The patient's presentation is most consistent with vasovagal syncope, which is triggered by noxious stimuli, in this case the stress of standing in a large crowd. Conservative measures are recommended, including maintaining hydration and employing counterpressure exercises (hand gripping, crossing legs) if symptoms are detected. While avoiding noxious triggers may help those with recurrent vasovagal syncope, there is no indication that this patient has agoraphobia or a panic disorder. Referral to a psychiatric APRN is not indicated. While caffeine may precipitate the development of arrythmia in some sensitive individuals, there is no indication that it played a role in this patient's syncope, which is more consistent with vasovagal type and not arrythmia. Standing up slowly before ambulating may be helpful in cases of orthostatic hypotension; however, there is no indication that the syncope occurred after rising from a sitting position.

174. **C) Toradol and colchicine**

Acute pericarditis is most often viral in etiology. The symptoms are treated with nonsteroidal anti-inflammatory drugs (NSAIDs) such as toradol and colchicine. Acetaminophen is not an NSAID, and antibiotics are not indicated as the patient is afebrile and there are no signs of acute bacterial infection. While aspirin is an acceptable NSAID used to treat acute pericarditis, there is no indication for the addition of an antibiotic at this time. IVIG is used to treat certain autoimmune diseases. It is not indicated in the treatment of acute pericarditis.

175. **A) STAT blood cultures, transthoracic echocardiogram, broad-spectrum antibiotics, infectious disease consult**

Based on this patient's risk factor of IV substance use and her complaints, she most likely has infective endocarditis (IE). Initial therapy for IE includes blood cultures drawn before initiation of antibiotics, Transthoracic echocardiogram (TTE) or Transesophageal echocardiogram (TEE) to confirm endocardial involvement, and an infectious disease consult. While the patient meets some of the criteria for sepsis, patient information does not justify a bolus of IVF at this time. An EKG or cardiac MRI is not indicated. Additionally, while the patient may benefit from placement of a PICC line and will need referral for addiction treatment, these are not part of the immediate plan and are more appropriate at a later time. STAT CXR, sputum culture, and oxygen are not indicated.

Index